S0-BIM-694

SCHOOL VIOLENCE INTERVENTION

School Violence Intervention

A PRACTICAL HANDBOOK

SECOND EDITION

Edited by

Jane Close Conoley
Arnold P. Goldstein

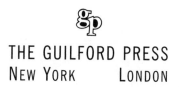

THE GUILFORD PRESS
NEW YORK   LONDON

© 2004 The Guilford Press
A Division of Guilford Publications, Inc.
72 Spring Street, New York, NY 10012
www.guilford.com

All rights reserved

No part of this book may be reproduced, translated, stored in a retrieval
system, or transmitted, in any form or by any means, electronic, mechanical,
photocopying, microfilming, recording, or otherwise, without written permission
from the Publisher.

Printed in the United States of America

This book is printed on acid-free paper.

Last digit is print number: 9 8 7 6 5 4 3 2 1

Library of Congress Cataloging-in-Publication Data

School violence intervention : a practical handbook / edited by Jane Close
Conoley, Arnold P. Goldstein.— 2nd ed.
      p. cm.
  Includes bibliographical references and index.
  ISBN 1-57230-671-8 (hardcover : alk. paper)
  1. School violence—United States—Prevention. 2. Crime prevention—Youth
participation—United States. 3. Conflict management—United States. 4. Schools—
United States—Safety measures. I. Conoley, Jane Close. II. Goldstein, Arnold P.
  LB3013.3.S379 2004
  371.7′82—dc22   2004010564

About the Editors

Jane Close Conoley, PhD, is Dean of Education and Human Development and Professor of Educational Psychology at Texas A&M University. Dr. Conoley has served as a consultant to mental health and educational agencies around the world, working to increase safety and academic achievement for children, and resilience and job satisfaction for adults, in those settings. Her research has centered on change processes that are related to increasing the acceptability of behavioral and mental health interventions in complex organizations.

Arnold P. Goldstein, PhD (1933–2002), was Professor of Special Education at Syracuse University, Director of the New York State Task Force on Juvenile Gangs, a member of the American Psychological Association Commission on Youth Violence, and a member of the Council of Representatives of the International Society for Research on Aggression. Dr. Goldstein developed three influential approaches to prosocial skills training: skillstreaming, aggression replacement training, and the Prepare Curriculum. Reflecting his role as Director of the Syracuse University Center for Research on Aggression, much of his research and teaching centered on helping youngsters replace antisocial, aggressive behaviors with constructive, alternative means of seeking life satisfaction and effectiveness.

Contributors

Amy R. Anderson, PhD, Department of Educational Psychology, University of Minnesota, Minneapolis, Minnesota

Sheldon Braaten, PhD, Department of Special Education, Ball State University, Muncie, Indiana

Gretchen Britton, MEd, School District of Philadelphia, Philadelphia, Pennsylvania

Karen T. Carey, PhD, Department of Psychology, California State University, Fresno, California

Gwendolyn Cartledge, PhD, School of Physical Activity and Special Services, Ohio State University, Columbus, Ohio

Sandra L. Christenson, PhD, Department of Educational Psychology, University of Minnesota, Minneapolis, Minnesota

Ian Cohen, MEd, Department of Psychological Studies in Education, Temple University, Philadelphia, Pennsylvania

Jane Close Conoley, PhD, College of Education and Human Development, Texas A&M University, College Station, Texas

Ellen deLara, PhD, School of Social Work, Syracuse University, Syracuse, New York

Barbara D'Incau, PhD, Counseling/Clinical/School Psychology Program, Graduate School of Education, University of California, Santa Barbara, California

Michael J. Furlong, PhD, Counseling/Clinical/School Psychology Program, Graduate School of Education, University of California, Santa Barbara, California

James Garbarino, PhD, Department of Human Development, Cornell University, Ithaca, New York

Arnold P. Goldstein, PhD (deceased), Syracuse University Center for Research on Aggression, Syracuse, New York

Marilyn L. Grady, PhD, Department of Educational Administration, University of Nebraska, Lincoln, Nebraska

Jean Haar, PhD, Department of Educational Leadership, Minnesota State University, Mankato, Minnesota

Julie A. Hirsch, PhD, Minneapolis Public Schools, Minneapolis, Minnesota

Irwin Hyman, EdD, Department of Psychological Studies in Education, Temple University, Philadelphia, Pennsylvania

Carolyn Talbert Johnson, PhD, Department of Teacher Education, University of Dayton, Dayton, Ohio

Harold R. Keller, PhD, Department of Psychological and Social Foundations, University of South Florida, Tampa, Florida

Donald W. Kodluboy, PhD, Minneapolis Public Schools, Minneapolis, Minnesota

Mary Ann Losh, PhD, Staff Development and Instructional Issues, Nebraska Department of Education, Lincoln, Nebraska

Louisa Lurkis, PhD, Department of Psychological Studies in Education, Temple University, Philadelphia, Pennsylvania

Matthew Mahon, MEd, Department of Psychological Studies in Education, Temple University, Philadelphia, Pennsylvania

Gale M. Morrison, PhD, Counseling/Clinical/School Psychology Program, Graduate School of Education, University of California, Santa Barbara, California

Richard L. Morrison, EdD, Ventura Unified School District, Ventura, California

Jerry Oestmann, PhD, Lincoln Public Schools, Lincoln, Nebraska

Scott Poland, EdD, Department of Psychological Services, Cypress–Fairbanks Independent School District, Houston, Texas

Michael E. Rozalski, PhD, Ella Cline Shear School of Education, State University of New York, Geneseo, New York

Pamela Snook, PhD, Department of Psychological Studies in Education, Temple University, Philadelphia, Pennsylvania

Susan H. Striepling-Goldstein, MS, Senior Education Specialist, Syracuse, New York

Jeremy R. Sullivan, PhD, Department of Psychological Services, Cypress–Fairbanks Independent School District, Houston, Texas

Renee C. Tapasak, PhD, private consultant, Tampa, Florida

Kenneth S. Trump, MPA, National School Safety and Security Services, Cleveland, Ohio

Mitchell L. Yell, PhD, College of Education, University of South Carolina, Columbia, South Carolina

Preface

Americans routinely identify excellent educational opportunity as a critically important national goal. Most also report that their neighborhood school is excellent and their children are safe in public school classrooms. At the same time, many citizens express concern about the overall academic achievement and safety of the U.S. public educational system.

The apparent contradiction in people's perceptions is partly explained by concentrated media and political coverage of public schooling in the United States. National reports identifying achievement gaps between U.S. students and those in other countries leave many questioning the competitiveness of a U.S. public education. Intense reporting about isolated violent episodes creates an impression of schools as armed camps that are more reminiscent of prisons than our image of places for learning. What is really happening in U.S. schools? Are children safe enough to learn?

This volume sets out to explore the complicated landscape of schooling as it relates to the safety of students and teachers. Our intent is to provide concrete, practical suggestions while not simplifying the challenge. Violence is pervasive in our country and our world. Children experience violence in their homes, neighborhoods, and churches—and in their schools. Increasing their safety in one setting absolutely requires cooperation and collaboration with many other systems. Although we strive to offer well-tested, specific strategies to increase safety, and we believe that we can have significant positive effects on children's and young people's safety, nothing we offer in this book is easy to do. Combating violence requires that adults in schools change the way they behave; organize and deliver instruction; and relate to their communities, and that they change their attitudes toward student behavior. None of these are easy adjustments, but answers do exist.

The authors in this volume are sources of tremendous information that will be immediately helpful to readers. Each of them joins me, as well, in highlighting the special contributions to this field made by Dr. Arnold P. Goldstein. Arnie died during the preparation of this work. He lives in its pages, however, because of the passion and focus he brought to improving children's lives. All who knew him were transformed by the experience of interacting with a man of such intelligence and dedication to human welfare. He was an outstanding psychologist and a treasured friend to all of us. He is sorely missed.

Special thanks go to the staff at The Guilford Press, who stood by us during difficult times. Their generosity and support made this book possible despite the loss of its special inspiration. Thank you.

JANE CLOSE CONOLEY

Contents

SCHOOL VIOLENCE INTERVENTION

PART I
Introduction

CHAPTER 1

Student Aggression

Current Status

ARNOLD P. GOLDSTEIN
JANE CLOSE CONOLEY

Pearl, Mississippi; West Paducah, Kentucky; Jonesboro, Arkansas; Edinboro, Pennsylvania; Springfield, Oregon; and Littleton, Colorado, are six, mostly rural, American towns. These are towns in whose schools, as is true for schools in the United States in general, the vast majority of students go safely to classes, do their work, learn their lessons, and do so in a school environment free from threat, harm, or danger. Yet in-school homicides occurred in each of these towns during the period from 1997 to 1999, and the topic of student violence changed from being an occasional schoolhouse concern to a broad, nationwide near-panic.

This book is about violence—its sources and solutions, its control and reduction—in the almost 90,000 schools in the United States. It is, as we shall document, a societal challenge of some magnitude, one neither to be minimized nor, as has happened, blown seriously out of proportion. The present chapter describes its recent and current status, its forms and functions, and served as a needed prelude to the rest of this book's intervention focus.

AGGRESSION TOWARD OTHER PERSONS

It is crucial to reiterate, at the beginning of this book, that for most of the 53 million schoolchildren in the United States, the school day unfolds with no threats to their safety and security—no fights, no weapons, no bullying, no theft. Much of the professional and parental public has been led to think otherwise by political hype and a media blitz. So let us begin our consideration of the school violence problem by keeping it in perspective. Yes, it is a substantial concern, which demands effective solutions. Happily for most of our children, however, it is still irrelevant to their experiences in school.

In U.S. public education, for the many decades preceding the second half of the 20th century, school-based aggression was apparently infrequent in occurrence, low in intensity, and (at least in retrospect) almost quaint in character. "Misbehavior," "poor comportment," "bad conduct," and the like, in the form of getting out of one's seat, refusing to obey a teacher, throwing a spitball, dipping a girl's pigtail in an inkwell, or even (rarely) breaking a window, seem like, and truly are, the events of another era. These events were so mild in comparison to the aggressive acts of today that it is difficult to think of the two types of behaviors as the extremes of a shared continuum. Commenting on Westin's study of urban school violence for the years 1870–1950, Bayh (1975) observes, "If, however, the system has never been totally immune from incidents of student misbehavior, such problems have historically been viewed as a relatively minor concern seldom involving more than a few sporadic and isolated incidents" (p. 3).

Rubel (1977) has correspondingly noted that the nature of fights between students has changed from words and fists to aggravated assault with lethal weapons. In a manner consistent with violence outside the schools, the years prior to the 1960s may appropriately be called the "preescalation period" in U.S. school violence. Consistent with Bayh's (1975) observations, a 1956 National Education Association survey reported that two-thirds of the 4,270 teachers sampled from across the United States reported that fewer than 1% of their students caused instance of disruption or disturbance. Ninety-five percent of the responding teachers "described the boys and girls they taught as either exceptionally well behaved, or reasonably well behaved" (National Education Association, 1956, p. 17).

1970–1990

In 1975, a U.S. Senate subcommittee headed by Birch Bayh issued a report on safety in schools. This survey of 750 school districts indicated that in U.S. schools between 1970 and 1973, homicides increased by 18.5%; rapes and attempted rapes increased by 40.1%; robberies increased by 36.7%; assaults on students increased by 85.3%; assaults on teachers increased by 77.4%; burglaries in school increased by 11.8%; drug and alcohol offenses increased by 37.5%; and the number of weapons confiscated by school personnel (pistols, knives, chukka sticks, and even sawed-off shotguns) increased by 54.4% (Bayh, 1975). The National Association of School Security Directors (1975) reported that in 1974, there were 204,000 assaults and 9,000 rapes in U.S. schools. Matters had come a very long way from spitballs and pigtails. There were 18,000 assaults on teachers in 1955, 41,000 in 1971, and 63,000 in 1975; by 1979, the number of such attacks had risen to 110,000.

The situation did not improve in the 1980s. In the 1988–1989 school year, as compared with the preceding year, school crime increased by 5% and in-school weapons possession rose by 21% in California's public schools (California Department of Education, 1989). In a similar comparison, the New York City public school system reported a 35% increase in assaults on students and school staff, a 16% increase in harassment, a 24% increase in larceny, and an overall crime rate increase of 25%. Noteworthy is the fact that the greatest increases in crime rate occurred at the elementary school level (U.S. Department of Justice, 1991).

The level of assaults on teachers in U.S. public schools was sufficiently high during this period that the vocabulary of aggression expanded to include what Block (1977) called the "battered teacher syndrome." This described a combination of stress reactions including anxiety, depression, disturbed sleep, headaches, elevated blood pressure, and eating disorders. The National Center for Education Statistics reported in 1992 that nearly one out of five U.S. school teachers reported being verbally abused by students; 8% reported being physically threatened; and 2% indicated they had been attacked by students during the previous year. A survey by the Metropolitan Life Insurance Company (1994) indicated that 11% of U.S. teachers reported being assaulted at school—in 95% of the instances, by students. (Eleven percent of the 2.56 million teachers in the United States in 1993 would be 270,000 people!)

The seriousness of these attacks notwithstanding, it must be remembered that most student aggression in U.S. schools is directed toward other students. Victimization data from 26 major U.S. cities surveyed in 1974 and 1975 indicated that 78% of the victims of personal aggression in schools (rapes, robberies, assaults, and larcenies) were students (McDermott, 1979). Ban and Ciminillo (1977) stated that in a national survey, the percentage of principals reporting "unorganized fighting" between students had increased from 2.8% in 1961 to 18% in 1974. Examining many of the data on correlates of aggression toward students, Ianni (1978) has found that 7th-graders are most likely to be attacked and 12th graders are the least likely; at about age 13, the risks of physical attack tend to be greatest. Fifty-eight percent of such attacks involve victims and offenders of the same race; the other 42% are interracial. Ianni has also found that the smaller the size of a minority group in a school, the more likely its members are to be victimized by members of other ethnic groups.

The 1989 annual school crime report from the School Safety Council noted that almost 3 million students, faculty, staff members, and visitors were crime victims in U.S. schools in 1987; 2.5 million of these crimes were thefts. Toward the end of the decade being considered here, according to the U.S. Department of Justice (1991), approximately 9% of all students ages 12–19 were crime victims in the United States; 2% were victims of violent crimes, and 7% of property crimes. In addition, 15% of these 12–19-year-olds reported that their schools had gangs, and 16% claimed that their school had experienced an actual or threatened attack on a teacher. Siegel and Senna (1991, p. 37) add that "although teenagers spend only 25% of their time in school, 40% of the robberies and 36% of the physical attacks involving this age group occur in school."

A 1990 report, aptly titled *Caught in the Crossfire* (Center to Prevent Handgun Violence, 1990), fully captures the central role of firearms in the context of school violence. From 1986 to 1990, 71 people (65 students and 6 employees) were killed by guns in U.S. schools. Another 201 were seriously wounded, and 242 were held hostage at gunpoint. Older adolescents were more frequently the perpetrators, as well as the victims. An estimated 270,000 students carry handguns to school one or more times each year. The American School Health Association (1989) estimated that 7% of boys and 2% of girls carried a knife to school every day.

1990–2002

During the 1991–1992 school year, 14.4% of New York City middle school-children reported being threatened by another student at least once each month, and 7.7% of them were in an actual fight (Youth Violence, 1991). A 1990 California survey of 5th to 12th graders revealed that in the month prior to the survey, a third of them had had personal property stolen, had been grabbed or shoved, or had seen a weapon at school. Two-thirds re-ported being insulted or cursed at by a fellow student (California Depart-ment of Education, 1990). A national crime survey (U.S. Department of Justice, 1993) reported nearly 3 million crimes per year on or near U.S. school campuses—16,000 per school day. Yet the overall trend of school vi-olence in the United States during the 1990s can perhaps best be de-scribed in capsule as "serious but not critical." Although a significant prob-lem demanding increased attention clearly existed, the condition of public education was far from the frequently claimed state of near collapse due to levels of student aggression. In fact, even given the broadly publicized six in-school shootings late in the decade, as this period progressed, the situation improved.

According to the U.S. Department of Education (2001), there has been nearly a one-third decrease in crimes against students—theft, rape, robbery, assault—from 1992 (149 crimes per 1,000 students) to 1998 (101 incidents per 1,000 students). The same source reports that during the year 2000, 90% of all U.S. schools reported "no serious violent crime" and 43% reported no crime at all.

Two broad surveys of school administrators, one reported in 1998, the other in 2000, concurred in revealing an improving situation with about ex-pressions of school violence. The National Center for Education Statistics (1998) report (see Table 1.1) indicated an improved picture in regard to stu-dent fights, vandalism, robbery, trespass, and racial tensions. The National

TABLE 1.1. Percentage of Principals Reporting Which Discipline Issues Were Moderate or Serious Issues in Their Schools, 1990–1991 and 1996–1997

Discipline issue	1990–1991	1996–1997
Student tardiness	34%	40%
Student absenteeism/class cutting	25%	25%
Physical conflicts among students	23%	21%
Student tobacco use	13%	14%
Verbal abuse of teachers	11%	12%
Student drug use	6%	9%
Vandalism of school property	12%	8%
Student alcohol use	10%	7%
Robbery or theft of items over $10	7%	5%
Gangs	[a]	5%
Trespassing	7%	4%
Racial tensions	5%	3%
Student possession of weapons	3%	2%
Physical abuse of teachers	1%	2%
Sale of drugs on school grounds	1%	2%

Note. Data from National Center for Education Statistics (1998).
[a]Item was not included in 1991 survey.

Institute of Justice (2000) survey (see Table 1.2) similarly reported decreasing levels of threats, weaponry, and violence in general.

The foregoing information reflects the views and reports of U.S. school administrators and other staff regarding the recent status of student aggression in our schools. What are the views of the students themselves? Kingery, Coggeshall, and Alford (1998) have combined the results of four 1995 surveys of very large samples of middle school students in the U.S. regarding *their* experiences of diverse indices of school violence. Because these surveys provide cross-sectional, rather than longitudinal, data, one cannot speak here to trends in student reportage. However, what can be concluded with confidence from the findings of Kingery et al. is that, in concurrence with reports from school personnel, student experiences reflect a still serious social problem affecting a substantial minority of U.S. schoolchildren adversely on an often daily basis.

The 1990s showed a declining trend in the most serious violent acts, homicide and suicide. There were an average of 42 school-based fatalities per year for the period 1992–1995, but 33 per year during 1995–1998. There has been a decline in the number of events, but, unfortunately, an increase in the number of children killed per event. Although but one such death is a terrible human tragedy, the decline in its incidence again aids us in keeping the magnitude of this serous social problem in proper perspective.

The multi-indexed declines in school violence notwithstanding, the *perception* among the schools and the general public was that it was not only increasing, but was doing so very rapidly. Whereas school-based violent deaths decreased by 40% between 1997 and 1999, poll respondents fearing an in-school

TABLE 1.2. Administrators' Perceptions of Violence as a School Problem

Perception	% of administrators responding "yes"
Violence on campus as a problem	
Very serious	4
Somewhat serious	15
Not too serious	56
Not at all serious	25
Guns on campus as a problem	
Very serious	2
Somewhat serious	0
Not too serious	27
Not at all serious	71
Other weapons on campus as a problem	
Very serious	2
Somewhat serous	6
Not too serious	50
Not at all serious	42
Likelihood that an average male junior would . . .	
Routinely carry gun on campus	
Somewhat or very likely	0
Not too likely	6
Not at all likely	94
Routinely carry gun off campus	
Somewhat or very likely	2
Not too likely	27
Not at all likely	71
Be physically threatened in school	
Somewhat or very likely	10
Not too likely	44
Not at all likely	46
Be physically threatened out of school	
Somewhat or very likely	10
Not too likely	50
Not at all likely	40

Note. Data from National Institute of Justice (2000).

shooting during this period increased by 49%. Moreover, although the actuarial probability of a school-based homicide was 1 in 2 million during 1997–1999, 71% of poll respondents thought such an event was "likely" in their community (Elliott et al., 1998). The response to this "moral panic" was (and still is) massive. Federal and local funding was significantly earmarked for control, reduction, and intervention purposes. As the United States is wont to do when faced with serious social problems, a disproportionate amount of such funding was (and still is) utilized for technological, as opposed to pedagogic, psychological, or psychoeducational means of intervention. In this era of near hysteria, a love affair with zero tolerance was born.

Zero tolerance as a violence intervention strategy actually appears to have found its initial rise to recent prominence and utilization not in school settings, but in the nation's war on drugs. The U.S. Attorney in San Diego in 1986 promoted zero tolerance as his explanation for the seizure of boats and other vehicles by anyone crossing the U.S.–Mexican border with even trace amounts of drugs (Skiba & Peterson, 1999). As noted, school systems across the United States grabbed onto this strategy in the 1990s and ran with it. In 1994, zero tolerance was codified as national policy in the Gun-Free Schools Act, requiring a 1-year out-of-school suspension for any student bringing a weapon to school. In addition, school districts were required to pass zero tolerance rules in order to remain eligible for funds under the Elementary and Secondary Schools Act of 1996. By 1997, approximately 83% of U.S. schools had in place zero tolerance policies targeted to violence and a host of related behaviors concerned with bringing alcohol, drugs, or weapons to school. Although questions remain as to whether, in actual implementation, zero tolerance punishments are too harsh, are at times meted out for infractions involving items that are only technically weapons (e.g., a nail clipper "knife") or drugs (e.g., menstrual pain reliever), are targeted disproportionately to minority students, and leave too little implementation discretion in the hands of school officials, zero tolerance remains a most popular response to perceived levels of violence in U.S. schools today.

SCHOOL CHARACTERISTICS AND AGGRESSION

The nature of leadership and governance in a school can be a major correlate of violence within its walls. A firm, fair, consistent principalship style, for example, has been shown to be associated with low levels of student aggression. High levels of arbitrary leadership and severe disciplinary actions tend to characterize schools experiencing high levels of aggression. School size is a further correlate of school violence. The larger the school, the higher its per capita violence rate is likely to be. Such a relationship, it has been proposed, may grow from the easier identification of students and by students in smaller schools, as well as from such consequences of larger schools as nonparticipation in governance, impersonality, and crowding. Crowding is a particularly salient school violence correlate, as aggressive behavior, in fact, occurs more frequently in more crowded school locations (stairways, hallways, and cafeterias) and less frequently in classrooms themselves. Other chronic "casualty zones" include lavatories, entrance and exit areas, and locker rooms. During the school day, student violence is most likely to occur during the times between classes. During the school year, for reasons that may have to do with "spring fever effects," it is more likely to occur in the spring than in the fall term (and especially in the month of March). With some exceptions, school violence is also correlated with the size of the community in which the school is located. The proportions of U.S. schools reporting serious levels of aggressive behavior are 15% in large cities, 6% in suburban areas, and 4% in rural areas. Public school students are slightly more likely to be victimized than are private school students.

CONSEQUENCES OF LOW-LEVEL AGGRESSION

Parallel to (and in many instances also underlying) the very substantial levels of student assault, weaponry, theft, intimidation, and other serious violence is lower-level aggressive behavior. Both Wilson and Petersilia (1995) and we (Goldstein, Palumbo, Striepling, & Voutsinas, 1995) have focused in depth on such low-level disorder as significant aggressive behavior in its own right, as well as a frequent precursor to and promoter of higher levels of such behavior. Wilson and Petersilia (1995) view such behavior—for example, students coming to school late, wandering the halls, writing graffiti on the walls, and throwing debris in the corridors—as the foundation upon which more serious violence rests:

> [Low-level] disorder invites youngsters to test further and further the limits of acceptable behavior. One connection between the inability of school authorities to maintain order and an increasing rate of violence is that, among students with little faith in the usefulness of the education they are supposed to be getting, challenging rules is part of the fun. When they succeed in littering or writing on walls, they feel encouraged to challenge other, more sacred rules, like the prohibition against assaulting fellow students and even teachers. (p. 149)

In the same vein, we (Goldstein et al., 1995) have written of the tendency in schools and other settings to "downsize deviance"—the tendency, as high levels of violent behavior demand the attention of teachers and administrators, to pay insufficient remedial attention to lower, less intense levels of such actions. We surveyed a national sample of U.S. teachers for *their* descriptions of in-school violent incidents and their management of them. The resultant 1,000 descriptions were classified as follows (Goldstein et al., 1995, p. 19):

Horseplay
Rule violation
Disruptiveness
Cursing

Bullying
Sexual harassment
Refusal/defiance
Threats
Vandalism
Out-of-control behavior
Student–student fights
Attacks on teachers
Use of weapons
Collective violence

The categories are arrayed roughly from least aggressive (horseplay, rule violation) to most aggressive (use of weapons, collective violence). In incident after incident, it was clear that the demands of high-level violence caused teachers to turn away from, ignore, or fail to deliver consequences for low-level transgressions.

All of us pay a heavy price for such ignoring, we believe. Aggression is primarily learned behavior. Youngsters who perpetrate low-level aggression and are rewarded for their efforts by peer approval or other means are youngsters thus primed both to continue such behaviors and to escalate their intensity. Such escalation, we have proposed elsewhere (Goldstein, 1999), may be promoted through a number of processes. These include not only the rewards of peer or self-approval, but also the high states of arousal they provide, a process of disinhibition, anticipated retaliation, and involvement in what has been termed a "character contest." In the context of group violence, rewards may come from a process termed *deindividualization*, a dynamic characterized by anonymity, modeling, contagion, diminished self-regulation, and diffusion of responsibility.

Consider the time students spend on the school bus—often a site of rowdy behavior. Our observations have revealed that serious school bus violence, such as destruction of property, pushing/tripping/attacking others, taunting or discriminatory language, attacks on the driver, use or display of weapons, and group attacks, is often preceded by very low levels of misbehavior. Examples of such low level forms include littering, eating or drinking, and being out of one's seat.

Two additional such lower-level aggressive behaviors deserve special mention. Both are very frequent in school settings, and particularly hidden or covert. One is bullying, a nasty bit of behavior that can take several possible forms (name calling, physical attack, threatening, theft, spreading of rumors, racial slurs, and shunning). The other is sexual harassment. An American Association of University Women (1993) national school survey describes the variety of ways such harassment is frequently expressed in secondary school contexts, as well as its serious negative academic and emotional consequences for the targeted youngsters (see Table 1.3). The data in

TABLE 1.3. Sexual Harassment Experiences, and Negative Consequences of These, Reported by Students in Grades 8–11

	Girls	Boys
Experiences		
Being the target of sexual jokes, gestures, or looks	76%	56%
Being touched, grabbed, or pinched	65%	42%
Being intentionally brushed up against in a sexual way	57%	36%
Being "flashed" or "mooned"	49%	41%
Having sexual rumors spread about them	42%	34%
Negative academic consequences		
Not wanting to attend school	33%	12%
Finding it harder to pay attention in class	28%	13%
Not wanting to talk in class	32%	13%
Negative emotional consequences		
Embarrassment	64%	36%
Less self-confidence	43%	14%
More self-consciousness	52%	21%
Being afraid/scared	39%	8%

Note. Data from the American Association of University Women (1993).

Table 1.4 make clear that the foundation for adolescent confusion of sex and aggression, and its consequent expression as sexual harassment, often begins in elementary school. Both bullying and sexual harassment deserve substantially greater attention than they have received to date by researchers and educational practitioners.

TABLE 1.4. Sexual Harassment Behaviors in Elementary School

Spiking (forcibly pulling down pants)
Snuggies (forcibly pulling up pants)
Flipping up skirts
Forcing kisses
Grabbing/touching another's genitals
Calling others sexually offensive names
Asking others to perform sexual acts
Threatening rape
Perpetrating sexual assault
Passing sexually explicit notes
Making gender-demeaning comments
Commenting on body parts
Using sexual profanity
Exposing genitals
Circulating pornography

Note. Data from the American Association of University Women (1993).

WEAPONS IN SCHOOLS

In contrast to the relative inattention given to sexual harassment and bullying in schools, there is considerable professional and public concern focused on more severe or intense forms of in-school aggression, particularly those involving weaponry.

The following list is a compilation, based on a variety of formal and informal sources, of the nature of such weaponry (National School Safety Center, 1993):

Guns
Knives
Screwdrivers
Mace
Pens/pencils
Baseball bats
Rocks
Bottles
Brass knuckles
Large rings
Two- and three-finger
   rings
Scissors
Stun guns
Chairs

Heavy belt buckles
Heavy false gold chains
Box cutters
Pen guns
Auto batons
Weighted gloves
Ammonia-filled spray bottles
Staples
Padlocks
Metal nail files
Steelies (ball bearings or steel
   marbles)
Nunchukus
Slap jacks
Bayonets

It is our own impression that box cutters (which often slip through metal detector scanning) are causing the most actual injury; however, guns are clearly causing the greatest concern.

Although the phenomenon of students bringing guns to schools is relatively recent, it has become sufficiently widespread that a good bit is known about the particulars of such behavior. For example, 63% of the incidents of gun violence surveyed by the National School Safety Center (1993) took place at high schools, 24% at junior high schools, 12% at elementary schools, and 1% at preschools; the types of incidents reported were intentional shootings (65%), accidents (13%), suicides (8%), hostage-taking incidents (8%), and undetermined (6%). Table 1.5 shows a breakdown of the sources from which gun-using youths obtained their weapons, as well as their stated reasons for acquiring and for using guns. Table 1.6 presents the school locations at which, and school activities during which, the guns were used. Finally, Table 1.7 describes the schools' responses to these incidents—not only the punishment of the perpetrators, but steps taken to alter the schools' environment and procedures in order to prevent the recurrence of gun violence.

TABLE 1.5. Gun Sources, Reasons for Acquiring Guns, and Reasons for Using Guns

Sources	
Friend	8%
Family member	23%
The street	14%
Gun/pawn shop	11%
Drug addict	6%
Drug dealer	2%
Someone's house or car (stolen)	2%
Other	4%

Reasons for acquiring	
Wanted for protection	53%
Enemies had guns	21%
Wanted to get someone	10%
Wanted to impress people	8%
Friends had one	5%
Wanted to sell gun	3%

Reasons for using	
Drugs/gangs	18%
Long-standing disagreements	15%
Playing with or cleaning	13%
Romantic disagreements	12%
Fights over material possessions	10%
Depression	9%
Vendetta (against "society")	6%
Racial slurs	5%
Name calling	4%
Vendetta (against school employee)	4%
Undetermined	4%

Note. N = 132. Data from National School Safety Center (1993).

Several conclusions are suggested by these data. Guns are widely available and continue to wend their way into school settings in spite of the growing use of metal detectors. Although *obtaining* a gun is an act often based on a perceived need for self-protection, *using* it is most typically a response to the perception of being disrespected (a perception that can arise from bad looks, bumps in the hall, or minor insults). Though students spend most of their school day in the classroom, guns are most often actually used during between-class transition times, in the school hallways, stairs, or similar venues. It is in these more fluid and less structured locations that the bad looks, the bumps, the perceived insults are more likely to occur. No wonder one teacher recently told us that the main accomplishment of her school's discipline committee was getting the administration to agree to 90-minute class periods, thus reducing by four the number of between-class transitions each day. The response of the schools, as noted in Table 1.7, has thus far been suspension more often than expulsion. This pattern, however, is changing rapidly, fueled by both a "get tough" political climate and pending federal legis-

TABLE 1.6. School Locations Where, and Activities during Which, Guns Were Used

Locations	
Hallways	25%
Classrooms	19%
School grounds	15%
Adjacent property	9%
Athletic facilities	8%
School buses	7%
School parking lots	5%
Cafeteria	4%
Restrooms	2%
Auditorium	1%
Undetermined	5%
Activities	
Between classes	32%
During classes	22%
After school	16%
At lunchtime	8%
During athletic events	8%
During transportation to and from school	7%
Before school	5%

Note: Data from National School Safety Center (1993).

lation. The use of expulsion is likely to increase substantially in the near future. What we hope will also grow are preventive efforts aimed at changing the ecology of the schools, so that weapons will be less likely to be present in the first place.

AGGRESSION TOWARD PROPERTY[1]

Surprising as it may seem, school vandalism data (frequency or costs) are not compiled by any of several education-relevant national-level agencies queried. A small number of states do maintain school vandalism incidence data, and most of these show moderate to substantial increases early in the 1990s with an apparent leveling off or even modest reduction later in the decade (Goldstein, 1996). Ample national statistics are readily obtainable regarding drugs, weapons, gangs, and assaults—but not regarding school vandalism.

Despite this absence of national incidence data, numerous surveys and anecdotal reports during the past 25 years suggest that school vandalism levels are high in the United States (Bradley, 1967; Casserly, Bass, & Garrett, 1980; Dukiet, 1973; Goldstein, Harootunian, & Conoley, 1994; Meaney, 1987; Rubel, 1977; Sadler, 1988; Schumacker & Leiner, 1979; Tygert, 1988). Repairs related

---

[1]See Chapter 13 for a full examination of the sources, nature, and control of school vandalism.

TABLE 1.7. Prevalent Forms of Punishment for Gun Use in Schools

Punishments

Suspension	65%
Expulsion	16%
Reprimand	19%

Environmental interventions[a]

Metal detectors
Locker removal
Locker/car search
Locker sharing (student-faculty)
Locker placement (opposite school office)
Clear or mesh bookbags
Weapon hotline
Student photo ID

Note. Data from National School Safety Center (1993).
[a]Percentages were not available for this category.

to vandalism regularly cost more than $600 million each year. Such costs reflect theft, as well as damage and destruction of school property. In 1991, for example, one of eight teachers and one of nine students in U.S. schools reported incidents of stealing within any given month (Miller & Prinz, 1991). Others reported concurring data regarding continuing high levels of in-school theft (Harris, Fray, Rees-McGee, Carroll, & Zaremba, 1987; Hutton, 1985).

Vandalism not only costs money; it typically has social costs as well. As Vestermark and Blauvelt (1978) suggest, the social cost of vandalism is the summation of three components: (1) its impact on the school's educational program, (2) its psychological impact on both students and adults, and (3) its degree of disruptiveness of group or intergroup relations. In terms of the breadth and depth of its disruptiveness on the primary educational functions of the school, the school costs of a vandalistic act may actually far exceed its monetary impact. One social cost in particular may be very high—namely, the arousal of fear among students and staff.

In terms of both their monetary and social costs, two forms of very serious aggression toward school property must be singled out for separate mention. Though both are, fortunately, rare, when they do occur the costs of both types can be immense. We refer to arson and bombings.

Karchmer (1982) estimates that 25–50% of all school fires are deliberately set. Herbert (1990) and Vernon (1979) describe two types of school-age fire setters—children under 10, whose fires are typically the results of play or experimentation, and adolescents, whose more complicated motivations may include life crises, peer or family concerns, independence and power issues, desires for revenge, or attention seeking.

School locations at which vandalistic acts are most likely to occur have been shown to have one or more of a number of specific characteristics (Goldstein, 1996). They tend to be areas of low traffic and thus reduced real or perceived surveillance. They frequently are previously vandalized sites. Already vandalized sites serve, apparently, as a trigger "for more of the same." Public places are more numerous targets. Ask youths who do not perpetrate vandalism, "Who owns the school, the museum, the bus, the library?" and they are likely to respond, "We all do." Ask the same of chronic vandals, and the response is much more likely to be "no one" (and thus, perhaps, fair game). Newer places and previously damaged (but not vandalized) areas are also more frequent targets.

The frequency, site, type, and in-school locations of school bomb incidents are described in Table 1.8 (School Security Report, 1995). Bombing is a rare but very serious aggressive vandalistic act, causing great bodily, site, and psychological damage.

A LOOK AHEAD

Violence toward persons and property in U.S. schools is substantial. Students, teachers, and staff members are its targets; physical, emotional, and fiscal injuries are its costs. Its negative impact on the basic educational mission of our schools is great—both for those who are subjected directly to such aggression and for the majority who are not. The injured student, the bat-

TABLE 1.8. School Bomb Incidents, 1993–1995

Frequency	42 incidents (with 47 bombs) in 20 states (29 explosions, 12 bombs found and removed, 6 fakes)
Schools affected	High schools (33), middle schools (7), elementary schools (2)
Types of bombs	Pipe bombs (17) Molotov cocktail bombs (7) Homemade/chemical bombs (4) Firecrackers (2) Dynamite (2) CO_2 cartridges (2) Live grenades (2) Military shell (1) Mace bomb (1) Other explosives (3) Fake bombs (6)
Typical locations	Boys' bathrooms Lockers Principal's office Parking lots Also (less frequently) hallways, windows, skylights, trophy cases, planters, stairwells, water fountains, trash cans, dumpsters

Note. Data from School Security Report (1995).

tered teacher, the violence-preoccupied principal, the fearful parent—these are its victims.

Its sources are several and probably lie as much outside the school building as within it. In all senses, schools are part of the larger communities they seek to serve. High levels of aggression in our homes, our streets, and our mass media rapidly find parallel expression in our schools. Therefore, in defining the scope of interventions to be discussed and examined in this handbook, we have made a major effort to include not only various student-oriented and school-oriented approaches, but also several targeted to the family and community forces impinging on school functioning and school violence. We hope this will make our prime message clear: School violence is complexly caused, and its optimal remediation must be of similar complexity.

We have asked the contributors to this book to keep its user-friendly, practitioner-oriented goal at center stage. Thus, although the chapters that follow are not short on addressing theory or supportive research, they are primarily devoted to diverse underlying intervention strategies and details of the operational tactics for their implementation. In the same practitioner-oriented spirit, we begin the book with a series of technique-focused presentations by a number of outstanding professional educators working at classroom, school, district, state, and national levels.

In U.S. society, in which aggression is very common, pervasively modeled, widely imitated, and richly rewarded, it is not easy to be optimistic about our collective ability to stem its tide and reverse its growth. But we also need not be pessimistic. The several dozen school violence intervention approaches whose description and examination form the substance of this book constitute a significant technology. Together, they give us the ability to have a substantial positive impact on this serious educational and social problem. Yes, we cannot be optimistic; no, we need not be pessimistic. Let us instead be realistic. "We are prepared," our chapter authors collectively assert, "to describe means for achieving a reasonable degree of violence reduction in U.S. schools." It is in this spirit this book has been written.

REFERENCES

American Association of University Women. (1993). *Report on sexual harassment in America's schools.* Washington, DC: Author.

American School Health Association. (1989). *National adolescent student health survey.* Oakland, CA: Third Party.

Ban, J. R., & Ciminillo, L. M. (1977). *Violence and vandalism in public education.* Danville, IL: Interstate.

Bayh, B. (1975, April). *Our nation's schools—a report card: "A" in school violence and vandalism* (Preliminary report of the U.S. Senate Subcommittee to Investigate Juvenile Delinquency). Washington, DC: U.S. Government Printing Office.

Block, A. (1977). The battered teacher. *Today's Education, 66*, 58–62.

Bradley, C. E. (1967). Vandalism and protective devices: Studies, conclusions, recommendations. *Proceedings of the Association of School Business Officials, 53*, 236–245.

California Department of Education. (1989). *A report of the California state legislature regarding the standard school crime reporting program for the 1987–1988 school year.* Sacramento: Author.

California Department of Education. (1990). *School crime in California for the 1988–1989 school year.* Sacramento: Author.

Casserly, M. D., Bass, S. A., & Garrett, J. R. (1980). *School vandalism: Strategies for prevention.* Lexington, MA: Lexington Books.

Center to Prevent Handgun Violence. (1990). *Caught in the crossfire: A report on gun violence in our nation's schools.* Washington, DC: Author.

Dukiet, K. (1973). Spotlight on school security. *School Management, 17*, 16–18.

Elliott, D. S., Hamburg, B., & Williams, K. R. (1998). Violence in American schools: An overview. In D. S. Elliott, B. Hamburg, & K. R. Williams (Eds.). *Violence in American schools* (pp. 120–141). Cambridge, UK: Cambridge University Press.

Goldstein, A. P. (1996). *The psychology of vandalism.* New York: Plenum Press.

Goldstein, A. P. (1999). *Low-level aggression: First steps on the ladder to violence.* Champaign, IL: Research Press.

Goldstein, A. P., Harootunian, B., & Conoley, J. C. (1994). *Student aggression: Prevention, management, and replacement training.* New York: Guilford Press.

Goldstein, A. P., Palumbo, J., Striepling, S., & Voutsinas, A. M. (1995). *Break it up.* Champaign, IL: Research Press.

Harris, J. D., Fray, B. A., Rees-McGee, S. R., Carroll, J. I., & Zaremba, E. T. (1987). Referrals to school psychologists: A national survey. *Journal of School Psychology, 25*, 343–354.

Herbert, R. L. (1990). Arson and vandalism in schools: What can the educational psychologist do? *Educational Psychology in Practice, 6*, 65–70.

Hutton, J. B. (1985). What reasons are given by teachers who refer problem behavior students? *Psychology in the Schools, 22*, 79–82.

Ianni, F. A. J. (1978). The social organization of the high school: School specific aspects of school crime. In E. Wenk & N. Harlow (Eds.), *School crime and disruption* (pp. 21–36). Davis, CA: Responsible Action.

Karchmer, C. (1982). Early intervention in arson epidemics: Developing a motive-based intervention strategy. In J. E. Chidester (Ed.), *Fire research and safety* (pp. 44–63). Washington, DC: National Bureau of Standards.

Kingery, P. M., Coggeshall, M. B., & Alford, A. A. (1998). Violence at school: Recent evidence from four national surveys. *Psychology in the Schools, 35*, 247–258.

McDermott, M. J. (1979). *Criminal victimization in urban schools.* Albany, NY: Criminal Justice Research Center.

Meaney, F. (1987). Arson, vandalism and schools. In D. Challinger (Ed.), *Crime at school* (pp. 151–159). Canberra, Australia: Seminar Proceedings.

Metropolitan Life Insurance Company. (1994). *Metropolitan Life Survey of the American Teacher: Violence in America's public schools.* New York: Author.

Miller, G., & Prinz, R. J. (1991). Designing interventions for stealing. In G. Stoner, M. R. Shinn, & H. M. Walker (Eds.), *Interventions for achievement and behavior problems* (pp. 593–616). Silver Spring, MD: National Association of School Psychologists.

National Association of School Security Directors. (1975). *Crime in schools.* Washington, DC: Author.

National Center for Education Statistics (1998). *Violence and Discipline problems in U.S. Public Schools: 1996–1997.* Washington, DC: U.S. Department of Education.

National Center for Education Statistics. (1992). *Public school principal survey on safe, disciplined, and drug-free schools.* Washington, DC: U.S. Department of Education.

National Education Association. (1956). Teacher opinion on pupil behavior, 1955–1956. *Research Bulletins of the National Education Association, 34*(2), 46–53.

National Institute of Justice (2000). *National evaluation of the youth firearms violence.* Washington, DC: Author.

National School Safety Center. (1993, May). *Weapons prevention practicum.* Practicum presented at the Conference on Disarming Our Schools, Miami, FL.

Rubel, R. J. (1977). *Unruly school: Disorders, disruptions, and crimes.* Lexington, MA: D. C. Heath.

Sadler, W. L. (1988). Vandalism in our schools: A study concerning children who destroy property and what to do about it. *Education, 108,* 556–560.

School Safety Council. (1989). *Weapons in schools.* Washington, DC: U.S. Department of Justice.

School Security Report. (1995, July). *An in-depth look at school bombing patterns.* Washington, DC: Author.

Schumacker, R. E., & Leiner, D. W. (1979). A survey of principals' perceptions towards vandalism, record keeping and prevention measures in southern Illinois. *Illinois School Research and Development, 16,* 27–37.

Siegel, L. M., & Senna, J. J. (1991). *Juvenile delinquency: Theory, practice and law.* St. Paul, MN: West.

Skiba, R., & Peterson, R. (1999). The dark side of zero tolerance: Can punishment lead to safe schools? *Phi Delta Kappan, 80,* 372–376, 381–382.

Tygert, C. (1988). Public school vandalism: Toward a synthesis of theories and transition to paradigm analysis. *Adolescence, 23,* 187–199.

U.S. Department of Education. (2001, February/March). *Community update* (No. 85). Washington, DC: U.S. Department of Education.

U.S. Department of Justice. (1991). *School crime: A national crime victimization survey report.* Washington, DC: U.S. Government Printing Office.

U.S. Department of Justice. (1993, May 19). *Bureau of Justice news release.* Washington, DC: Author.

Vernon, R. F. (1979). *Dimensions of juvenile arson and false fire alarms for the urban areas of San Diego.* Washington, DC: U.S. Department of Housing and Urban Development.

Vestermark, S. D., & Blauvelt, P. D. (1978). *Controlling crime in the school: A complete security handbook for administrators.* West Nyack, NY: Parker.

Wilson, J. Q., & Petersilia, J. (1995). *Crime.* San Francisco: Institute for Contemporary Studies Press.

Youth violence. (1991, November 25). *The New York Times,* p. 23.

PART II
Practitioners' Perspectives

CHAPTER 2

The Low-Aggression Classroom
A Teacher's View

SUSAN H. STRIEPLING-GOLDSTEIN

The days of children sitting quietly with hands folded in front of them, waiting for the lesson to begin, are long gone. In today's world many students and teachers are in an emotional and psychological, if not physical, struggle from the moment the students enter the room until they exit, either at the end of the day (elementary) or the end of the class (middle and high school). This struggle results in less instruction time for the teacher, less academic success for the student, and greater anxiety for each of them as well as for parents and administrators. Violence levels grow and the media ask, "What's happening to our schools?"

Yet some teachers' classrooms are far less frequently disrupted by violence or aggression than others'. Why do some teachers always seem to be sending students to the front office on a referral, whereas others rarely do? The teachers with calmer classrooms seem to plan and do things in such a way as to keep aggressive incidents shorter, less frequent, and less intense. This low-aggression climate enables these teachers to maintain order and provide a facilitative classroom in which learning and development occur.

This calm, facilitative environment, however, is difficult to both initiate and maintain if the rest of the "system," of which the classroom is a part, is unsupportive. This system includes all other people in the building (principal and vice principal, school psychologist, social worker, other teachers, secretaries, custodians, security, cafeteria staff, bus personnel) and those in the downtown district office as well as the significant others in the children's own families and the greater community beyond the school and family. Without the support of these parts of the system, teachers will start their careers with great energy and enthusiasm, but may either burn out and leave the profession or stay and become cynical and bitter in a few short years.

For many years people outside the teaching profession saw problems of classroom management, inadequate learning, and teacher burnout as problems of only the urban school. Urban school districts, with their broad mix of social, cultural, economic, and ethnic issues and often underfunded school budgets, struggled to find ways to deal with rising aggression and low achievement levels. Many urban schools and districts worked hard and developed effective programs that made real progress in bringing aggression levels down and academic achievement levels up. They often struggled unnoticed and unappreciated. It was often the problem schools that were noted, not the successful ones. Suburban schools were seen as immune to the problems of their urban counterparts—an oasis in the midst of chaos. However, as aggression levels continued to rise in society as a whole, it was only a matter of time before problems appeared in the suburbs. The violence at Columbine High School brought to the attention of the general public problems that had been festering for years in all our schools. We could no longer, as a nation, point our fingers and say that "they" (however we defined "they") were the problem. The problem was systemic, affecting our urban, suburban, and even rural schools. Because school violence represents a failure of several systems that surround a youngster, systemic solutions are needed.

Although there are literally hundreds of programs in existence that address both high classroom aggression levels and low student achievement, most have never been evaluated in terms of their efficacy, making it impossible for school personnel to evaluate particular programs for their unique setting characteristics. To begin the process of addressing this need for accountability, the U.S. Department of Education, in the past few years, has reviewed and evaluated hundreds of programs. The Department's Safe, Disciplined and Drug-Free Office designated 42 programs as exemplary and promising (*www.ed.gov/offices/OESE/SDFS/programs.html*). After review and evaluation, they were chosen based on their ability to actually demonstrate sustained, long-term gains on outcome criteria. This is especially valuable information for use at all levels of the educational system—teacher, classroom, school districts, family, and the larger community.

Prevention of aggression in the classroom begins long before the students step through the door on the first day of school. It begins first and foremost with teachers being sure that they are not contributing to whatever problems occur in the classroom. If student aggression is, in large measure, a result of not knowing what to do when provoked (i.e., poor social skills) plus poor ability to manage anger when it does occur, it is imperative that teachers possess a high level of social skills competence and powerful anger control resources of their own. The children we teach learn much more from what we do than from what we say. If we regularly display respect, thoughtfulness, fairness, tolerance, honesty, compassion, and concern, then we are more likely to elicit similar behaviors by our students and they are more apt to listen to what we have to say. This does not negate the necessity for solid, well thought out lessons based on a rich and varied curriculum. But we ought not expect from our students what we cannot do ourselves. Therefore, teachers' first job, before ever stepping into the classroom, is a thorough and honest inventory of their own strengths and weaknesses. Following the inventory, teachers must then seek assistance in areas in which they feel they are not as competent as they would like and need to be.

Second, prevention of aggression in the classroom begins with thinking through, as clearly and concretely as possible, the classroom demographics, organization, and procedures—all of which may influence the in-school behavior of the students. Included in this consideration are the composition of the class; the class members' probable levels of interpersonal and aggression control skills and how the teacher will deal with deficits in these skills; the physical characteristics of the classroom; teaching plans, plans for classroom community building; rules and procedures governing student behavior; available rewards and sanctions for behavior; and the nature of efforts directed at facilitating family–school collaboration. Each of these concerns is relevant to the level of classroom aggression, and thus each is considered in the rest of this chapter.

LEARNING ABOUT THE STUDENTS

There is much discussion among regular education teachers as to the advantages and disadvantages of obtaining information about students prior to having them in the classroom. For example, knowing in advance that a student received in-school suspensions eight times last term may function as an aggression-eliciting, self-fulfilling prophecy during the new term. Yet prevention begins with an understanding of the student population one will be teaching. I believe that this risk can be moderated to the extent that a teacher seeks to discern, for each student, not only how to thwart or minimize disruptiveness or aggression, but also how to facilitate classroom learning and on-task behavior. Just as teachers have reputations in a school building, so too do students. I have always thought that it is better to have "real" information (individualized education plans [IEPs], student records) than the kind of hearsay information about certain students that floats around a building.

However, IEPs and student records are confidential information, and in some schools teachers' access to them may be limited. Therefore, teachers must make do with whatever formal or informal information they can get. The things a teacher will want to know are the number of students in the class (or classes), the economic level(s) of the neighborhood(s) from which the students come, the gender and ethnic composition of the class(es), the cultural backgrounds of the students (e.g., are there any English-as-a-second-language issues for these students?), and whether the class(es) will include any special needs students.

Where does a teacher get this kind of information? The experienced teacher who has been in a building for at least a year gathers much of this information through observation. Although the specific makeup of classes changes each year, the overall population of the building usually does not. At the elementary level, class lists are usually drawn up and given to teachers in June before they leave for the summer break. After a brief scan, most put these lists away until early or mid-August. The lists are then taken out, and a serious gathering of information begins.

For secondary teachers (middle and high school), it is not unusual to receive their class lists on their first day back at school, which is often just a day or two before the appearance of students. Therefore, much of the information with which a teacher starts the year is very general. If (as in many middle schools) there is a team approach to students, the first day back is an important time for team members to meet and discuss the makeup of the group of students they will be working with. This meeting can be an opportunity to share both formal and informal information about students, as well as a chance to bring in other specialists in the building who will be dealing with the same students as the team.

For the teacher who is new to a building, this understanding takes more effort on his or her part. It is very important for this teacher to spend some time in the building talking with someone—the assistant principal, a mentoring teacher (if he or she is so lucky as to have such a person), or a building guidance counselor or social worker. If no one seems to be available, then the new teacher should specifically ask for the name and home phone number of a teacher who has been in the building for a number of years and is known by the principal to be willing to act as an informal mentor. Whether teachers are novices or veterans, it will serve them well to learn in advance about the students and situations likely to draw heavily upon their aggression management skills.

BUILDING A COMMUNITY OF LEARNERS

The creation of a community of learners is often the first task of the school year for teachers who seek classroom aggression levels that are very low and whose students achieve satisfactory academic gains. I have often heard teachers who are successful at this say, "I know I have succeeded in creating a community when exclusion from our community for inappropriate behavior is seen as the ultimate punishment by the students. When this happens, merely the threat of exclusion is enough to change behavior." With this outcome as their goal, these teachers are willing to do whatever is necessary in the first few weeks of school to create a climate of cooperation, collaboration, and respect for all learners. The time and effort spent working toward this goal differ, depending on the school level (elementary, middle, or high school).

To arm students with the diverse interpersonal skills necessary for successful community building in the classroom, during the early days and weeks of the term, particularly at the elementary and middle school levels, it is recommended that the teaching of interpersonal skills should also begin (*Skillstreaming in Early Childhood*, McGinnis & Goldstein, 2002; *Skillstreaming the Elementary School Child*, McGinnnis & Goldstein, 1997; *Skillstreaming the Adolescent*, Goldstein & McGinnis, 1997). The teaching of these skills should continue throughout the year, preferably with the whole school participating in the program. Ideally, much of this program may be done with a whole class.

During the early days and weeks of the term, curriculum is of secondary importance; community building is the teacher's pre-academic goal. Teachers and students learn and use one another's names, listen carefully to one another, and share information to discover likes, strengths, and similarities.

As much as is feasible, these activities should involve the whole class. Such community building activities can take form in preplanned games at all levels (Goldstein, 1999). These may include, for example, for younger elementary students, such things as the Jack-in-the-Name game, which helps everyone learn names quickly, or cooperative Pin the Tail on the Donkey, in which the object is for all the other players, working together, to direct the person who is blindfolded to pin the tail in the correct spot. For older elementary students and middle school students, activities may include Nonverbal Birthday Lineup, in which players are asked to line up according to month and day of birth without any talking (using paper and pencil), or Stand Up, in which group members sit in a circle with their backs to the center and arms joined as they try to stand up. A middle school, using a team approach, might include New Basketball, which is a cooperative form of basketball. In this version, there is no dribbling, everyone must pass the ball, each player must touch the ball before the shot is made, there is no shooting from beyond the foul line, other variations may be incorporated to encourage the sense of teaming and discourage the designation of "stars."

In upper elementary, middle, and high school classes (grades 4–12), classroom meetings help build a sense of "we." In a classroom meeting the chairs are set up in a circle, rules and procedures for the meeting are established, and the floor is then opened for issues of concern (e.g., use of lavatory passes, students who do not do their homework, a disruptive incident in the classroom or disorderly behavior in the lunchroom). The issues are debated and consequences decided upon by the class as a whole. Often the rules and consequences chosen by the students are harsher than those that would be applied by the teacher, and students must be guided until they become skilled in the process. Meetings can be scheduled once a week, with agenda suggestions collected throughout the week in a suggestion box. Additional meetings can be scheduled on an emergency basis. Moreover, such meetings can be a means of community building involving the whole school. If issues involving students and teachers from other rooms are raised, these individuals can be invited to the meetings involving them. Playground monitors, principals, counselors, and other staff members can also be invited to participate at specific meetings. These community-building classroom meetings not only give students an opportunity to express their needs, they provide students with the experience of a legislative process and a process of problem solving whereby the responsibility of resolution is placed squarely upon their own shoulders.

For students who meet as strangers, coming together as a "room" at the elementary level, or as a "class" at the middle school and high school levels, is difficult. All of these activities share the goal of giving students an opportunity to get to know one another. It takes time for a group identity to form. The goal of the low-aggression classroom should be to create a group identity based on cooperation rather than competition. The low-aggression classroom promotes the idea that all students can learn and help one another do well. A classroom need not be explicitly devoted to cooperative learning for students to feel that "Your learning and doing well enhances me; they don't take away from me." Research (Feshbach, 1978; Miller & Eisenberg, 1988; Reed, 1981) has shown that it is very difficult for an empathetic person to be aggressive

The chapter on empathy in *The Prepare Curriculum* (Goldstein, 1999) should be required reading for any teacher attempting to lower aggression levels, via enhanced empathy, in the classroom. If aggression levels are to be lowered it is so crucial for empathy to be enhanced, that it is worthwhile to mention a few of the several specific exercises from *Prepare* on teaching its enhancement.

Elementary teachers may use an exercise such as Tape Recordings I to teach auditory discrimination of emotions. This is done by tape recording various sentences in different tones of voice and then asking children to identify the emotion or tone. Different emotions and their relationship to different tones of the voice are thus taught. Visual discrimination can be enhanced through the exercise Taking Group Pictures. In this exercise, a Polaroid camera is used to take pictures of the children displaying an emotion in response to a story that is read. After all the children have a chance to portray an emotion and be photographed, the developed pictures are placed on a table and the class tries to match the photos with the sentences read earlier. This helps "to increase the understanding that particular facial cues communicate information about particular affective states" (Goldstein, 1999, p. 661).

Middle and high school students can use the exercise How Would You Feel? to examine cultural/racial issues and then describe the feelings related to racial issues. Each student receives an experience sheet that has a series of questions that begin with "How would you feel if . . . ?" The sheets can then be used in a whole class or, if the group is large, in small-group discussions first, followed by a whole-class discussion. The teacher uses open-ended discussion questions to elicit deeper insights from the group.

Accountability, the "back to basics" movement, expanded required curriculums, with more information and skills being added every year, more and more standardized testing, and other such pressures cause all teachers to feel that they must get to the mandated curricula as soon in the school year as possible or they will never finish. This feeling is particularly strong among middle and high school teachers. It used to be easier for elementary teachers to embrace the idea of taking time away from academics to build this sense of "we," but with the recent push toward more and more standardized testing and state and perhaps even federal norms, even they feel the crunch of "academics have to come first." It used to be that because the elementary teachers had the same students for a good portion of the day, they could more readily incorporate community-building activities into the school day without pressure. At the middle and high school levels, where teachers see a student for 40–50 minutes once a day, the pressure to begin content work immediately has always been difficult to resist. Yet beginning content work too soon often results in a substantial increase in disruptive behavior among students at *all* levels. Teachers who spend time getting to know students and having students get to know them and one another often have fewer problems in their classrooms. The better the job of laying this foundation and creating a sense of community, the better the students' academic work will be later. Time spent away from the curriculum at the beginning will indeed be made up later, when time does not have to be spent on resolving behavioral disturbances.

TEACHING PLANS AND INSTRUCTIONAL BEHAVIOR

Times of transition and change are highly stressful. The first weeks of school are among the most stressful of the school year. In anticipation of this stress, teachers who desire to create a low-aggression classroom must do as much of their planning as possible for the first weeks of school before school opens. By organizing not only materials and supplies but also the classroom itself ahead of time, a teacher can look carefully at safety and academic needs. It is important to create both a general long-range outline and a very specific 2-week teaching plan. The daily, weekly, monthly, and yearly schedules must include flexibility and activities to relieve pressure and stress; students are less likely to "go off" when they are regularly given time to unwind and regroup. Teachers also need to anticipate and take care of their own needs, as well as those of their students. Daily teaching schedules should include planning time, a real lunch (not just a sandwich on the run), and lavatory breaks. The general goal should be to humanize the environment of a classroom for both the students and the teacher as much as possible.

Teachers can and will deviate from their plans as they get to know their students and the students' abilities, but it is always better to overplan than to underplan. It is also important for teachers to have a clear understanding of their intended classroom procedures (i.e., how they want their classrooms to run) before the first day of school with students. A teacher who is well organized will be much better equipped to deal calmly with the inevitable confusion, disruption, and even chaos that can occur as everyone learns new routines.

What instructional behaviors should a teacher practice in order to keep aggression at a minimum and simultaneously deliver academic material effectively in the classroom? Kounin (1970) suggests that six particular behaviors are especially fruitful:

1. The teacher needs to stay aware of what is going on at all times. (This is the "teacher has eyes in the back of the head" effect!) Such *with-it-ness* is communicated to the class by consistent and swift recognition of (and, if necessary, application of consequences for) behaviors likely to lead to disruptiveness or more serious aggression.

2. *Overlapping*—that is, simultaneously and successfully managing two or more classroom events, be they instructional or disciplinary—is closely connected to being "with it."

3. Making smooth *transitions* without downtime from one classroom activity to another is also important. Avoiding or minimizing downtime significantly deters boredom-engendered acting-out behaviors.

4. Instructing with *momentum* is another way to minimize boredom. This means maintaining a steady sense of progress or movement throughout the particular lesson, class, or school day.

5. Maintaining a *group focus*, that is, keeping the entire class involved in a given instructional activity, diminishes the likelihood of student aggression. When the teacher attends only to a subgroup of students, the rest of the class is free for disruptiveness or mayhem.

6. Finally, an especially significant contributor to a low-aggression classroom is the teacher's communication of consistently *optimistic academic expectations*. Students live up (or down) to what is expected of them. Expecting a student to be reading at only a fourth-grade level when he or she is in seventh grade, simply because the student comes from an area of low socioeconomic status or has a sibling who is a low achiever, will probably be rewarded with continued poor performance. It is far better for teachers to let students know that they believe that the students can achieve and that the teachers will help this to happen. Teachers with high expectations are more apt to motivate their students to be more academically successful and less behaviorally disruptive. What significant others expect has a powerful influence on anyone's behavior.

RULES AND PROCEDURES

To create and maintain a low-aggression classroom, it is imperative that one teach rules, procedures, and consequences as explicitly as one teaches content. In this context, "rules" are guidelines governing appropriate and inappropriate student behaviors; "procedures" are what students need to know in order to meet their own personal needs and to perform routine instructional and "housekeeping" activities. Constant monitoring of students enables a teacher to apply consequences in a caring and consistent way. Spending time on such matters is not taking time away from the curriculum. If a teacher is spending a good portion of the day dealing with disruptions, material is not going to be covered anyway. By integrating rules, procedures, and consequences into a workable classroom routine, teachers can minimize disruptions and time spent becomes time saved.

The teaching of rules and procedures should begin on the first day of school. Ideally, a teacher meets students at the classroom door and, in a friendly but firm manner, directs students to their seats (either assigned in elementary school or random until assigned in middle and high school). This effort communicates the first procedure that the teacher expects to be followed—how to enter the classroom. It also establishes the teacher as the leader in the classroom. Often on the first day, the teacher puts his or her name and an outline of the activities for that day on the chalkboard. This sets the tone for the class and introduces another procedure: Students should always check the board for the day's assignment upon entering.

The teacher then introduces him- or herself, calls roll, and spends a large block of time involving students in the creation of rules. Rules usually come first, with procedures being taught as they come up during the course of the first week. The best rules for making rules are as follows:

- Keep the rules few in number (three to six).
- Negotiate them with the students.
- State them behaviorally and positively.
- Make a contract with the students to adhere to them.
- Send them home to parents.
- Post them in the classroom.

In an elementary classroom, where the teacher has the students for much of the day or all day, this discussion of rules and procedures will probably happen on and off throughout the first few days of school as the need arises. Elementary teachers often make the setting-up of rules their first class-building exercise. They have clear in their minds what rules they need for their class to function successfully; however, rather than just stating them, they elicit the rules from the students. This gives the students a sense of ownership and promotes adherence. Rules are always stated in a positive, behavioral way ("Listen quietly while others are speaking" rather than "Don't interrupt other people"), and time is allowed for discussion of the rules, the reason they are important, and examples.

The next step for the elementary teacher is contracting with the students to adhere to the rules. Even very young children can understand the idea of making contracts. By signing a contract, they are agreeing to follow the rules. It is also a good idea at this point to send a copy of the classroom rules home for parents to read and sign. The list of rules is sent home with a letter explaining that the whole class created the rules, their child has signed a copy of the rules, and the teacher would like the parents to review the rules with their child and sign and return the letter to indicate that they have done so. Sending rules home in this manner paves the way for home–school collaboration, discussed later in this chapter.

The last step in establishing rules in the elementary classroom is posting them. Posting rules reminds students what the rules are. In addition, when a rule is broken, the teacher can point to the posted rule for its reaffirmation.

In a secondary classroom the teacher also introduces him- or herself, calls role, and spends a large block of time presenting rules. The rules are generally the same at the secondary level as at the elementary level. However, when the teacher sees from 130 to 150 students a day, negotiating rules with them can be difficult. In middle school, some teachers list the rules (again, stated positively and behaviorally) during each class and have class discussions, during which students come up with examples of following the rules. This class-building exercise may go on for more than the first day. Other teachers divide the class into groups and have each group come up with a set of rules. In this case the teacher explains that once all the groups in all the classes have done this, the teacher will take all the ideas and integrate them into a final consensus set. A discussion of the final rules, with concrete examples, is then held with each class.

Ninth graders must also spend this amount of time on rules. In many school districts, these students are part of the high school and are in a new building with a new administration and new rules. By 10-, 11-, and 12-grades, rule-setting time may not be necessary. Instead, rules can be briefly stated and examples given.

In both middle school and high school, however, a contract to observe the rules should be made with the students. In the middle school and 9-grade, rules should be sent home in a letter to parents for signatures. In 10-, 11-, and 12-grades students should be given a copy of the rules. Rules should be posted at all levels except high school. Because at this level many teachers may use only one room, some teachers do and some do not post rules.

Classroom procedures are equally important in elementary and secondary schools. In the average classroom, between 30 and 60 procedures are necessary to keep the room running smoothly. In the elementary classroom, students usually have one or two teachers whose procedures they must learn. Middle school and high school students may have as many as eight or nine teachers, with different sets of procedures to learn. At all levels, it is well worth the time for teachers to think through, as carefully and fully as possible, how they want their classes to operate. The more thorough and complete teachers are in establishing a routine, and the more consistently that routine is followed, the smaller the chances for disruption in the classroom become. In other words, no matter what method of delivering instruction teachers are using—direct instruction, learning centers, or cooperative learning—the classroom procedures must be very structured and explicitly taught to students. It cannot be assumed that students know these things; they must be taught what their teachers expect of them. The procedures must cover everything that goes on in the room, including what to do when first entering, talking among students, obtaining help, sharpening pencils, leaving the room, returning to the room, using bathroom passes, interrupting, following fire and disaster procedures, working with classroom helpers, asking a question, disposing of trash, and any other situations that may come up in a particular classroom.

These procedures are taught as the need for them arises in the classroom. Like rules, procedures must be clearly stated, closely monitored, and consistently followed, and consequences must ensue when they are not followed. This consistency—that is, procedural expectations being clearly defined for students and enforced every time, for everyone, without exceptions—is a key factor in maintaining a low-aggression environment. Consistent application of rules and procedures provides clear expectations for students' behavior, gives students the message that the teacher is aware of their behavior, and establishes that the teacher is in charge of the classroom. Yet such consistency is difficult to maintain over time. Teachers get tired, bored, or overworked, and sometimes it seems easier to "let it go just this once." In the long run, "just this once" can become more than once, and the message students receive is that the boundary between what is acceptable and unacceptable is no longer firm. As soon as the students sense that the expectations have been lowered even slightly, they start pushing to find where the boundary is, and the foundation for the safe, low-aggression space where learning can occur begins to erode. "Every time with every child" should be the motto.

Ron Clark, one of the teachers named in 2000 as Outstanding Teacher of the Year nationwide in the Disney American Teacher Awards, knows firsthand the value of enforcing rules and procedures in his fifth- and sixth-grade classes at P.S. 83 in District 4 (a classroom in Spanish Harlem in New York City).

> He starts each new class with the same five rules, followed up with the same 50 classroom procedures that spell out acceptable behavior. "The first two weeks of school I know the kids hate me," Clark said in his native North Carolina drawl that can cajole, praise or discipline. "I don't care as long as they respect me and respect the right of the class to learn. I'm not here to be their friend. I'm here to teach them." (Sandberg, 1999, p. 12)

This set of tough behavior standards has paid off in his classroom.

> By school year's end [1999–2000], firm control and high standards translated into large achievement gains when his "low-level" class—which had not met state standards on grade 4 state tests—scored higher on grade 5 city-

wide tests in math and reading than classes labeled as "gifted." (Sandberg, 1999, p. 12)

Just as students have reputations, so too do teachers. If a teacher has been in a building for more than a couple of years and has established a reputation for being "strict" (which often means "firm but fair" in kid talk), that teacher will have an easier time creating the desired low-aggression climate. Although such teachers get new students every year, their reputations precede them, and it does not take them nearly as long as it does for a new teacher to create and maintain the desired climate.

FAMILY–SCHOOL COLLABORATION

When I wrote this chapter for the first edition of this book, I used the term *home–school collaboration* to describe the important link between the parents of the children we teach, the children themselves, and the teacher. Recently, as a result of Christenson and Sheridan's excellent book, *Schools and Families* (2001), I have changed my terminology to theirs. They make the point that

> family–school relationships are broader and, consequently, not synonymous with parent–teacher relationships. Family may refer to grandparents, older siblings, other relatives, and in some situations, surrogate parents, such as neighbors. School includes all school personnel and the emotional climate and problem solving that occur among the various professionals interfacing with families on the behalf of children and youth. Hence, family–school relationships focus on the interface of two systems for the purpose of socializing students as learners and enhancing the development of children and youth. (pg. 18)

They further state that:

> the interface between families and school must fit the specific context—or address the needs of parents, teachers, and students. Neither a "one size fits all" approach nor a focus on activities in the absence of nurturing essential attitudes among the partners will work for schools. Historically, our emphasis has been on what we do to involve families (i.e., activities) rather than how we think of the family–school relationship (i.e., attitudes) as a means for socializing and supporting students as learners. (p. 18)

This change in focus from activities to attitudes is an important one and reflects a much needed change in how we conceptualize and implement the roles of the various participants.

"The overwhelming majority of parents want to be 'good' parents, supporting their children's physical and mental development and hoping for a future better than their own. . . . A lack of knowledge about how to assist their children does not represent a lack of interest" (Rioux & Berla, 1993, p. 334). In the past most schools have sought home–school contact, but many times "contact" has meant the school (the experts) telling the parents (the nonexperts) what to do. Traditionally, it has taken the form of PTA meetings, room parenting, or parent–teacher conferences, in which the educators tell the parents about their child. There has been very little appreciation for the wisdom and knowledge many parents have. There has also not been an adequate appreciation for the desire of parents to be "good" parents, even if they do not always have the tools to accomplish their goals.

In order to maintain low-aggression classrooms, teachers must view families differently. Recognition, respect for, and appreciation of the parents and the broader family as the child's first teachers, and as their current co-teachers, together with an appreciation of both the difficulties and problems many families experience in daily life, and the strength of their commitment and contribution to the education of their children, must be the starting point of this shift in perspective. It then follows that the teacher must seek early and frequent contact and must see this contact as an opportunity to collaborate in a supportive, mutually reinforcing way.

However, teachers must remember that because of a family's own experiences with schools as students—which may have been adversarial, intimidating, or otherwise uncomfortable—they may view schools and teachers with feelings of uncertainty or insecurity. Trust is a characteristic that develops over time. A teacher's ability to create an ongoing personal relationship with family members that is friendly, warm, respectful, honest, and open will do much to build a trusting relationship.

Rights, responsibilities, roles, and resources must be clearly defined and understood by all concerned. In this way the families, the teacher, and the child have the potential to become a problem-solving team. The opportunity for the child to be successful is thus greatly enhanced. Because children who succeed in school are much less likely to be disruptive, aggression in the classroom is diminished.

How this contact happens differs with the grade level of the child. For elementary teachers, early contact often takes the form of an introductory letter to the home before school starts. The main purpose of the letter is to welcome the child and the family to the teacher's class. Some teachers write two letters, one to the parents and family (Figure 2.1) and one to the child (Figure 2.2). Teachers in the early elementary grades may use the letter to the children to invite them and their families into the classroom on a day in August to help decorate the room for the coming school year. It is an informal ice-breaking time, and the child remembers the day for the entire year. Students come to feel that the classroom is their room; parents and families have a chance to interact in a relatively stress-free way. It can be an opportunity for families to begin to understand the roles and responsibilities the

August 15, 2004

Dear Mr. and Mrs. Jones,

I am Susan Striepling-Goldstein, Elizabeth's third-grade teacher. I want to welcome you and your daughter, Elizabeth, to my class for this school year. I am really excited about the coming year and about having Elizabeth in my class. I hope that Elizabeth is looking forward to it too.

I have a full year planned for us. As well as our daily work in reading, spelling, math, science, and social studies, we will be spending time working on what I call "positive skill-building activities." I feel that it is very important that we all treat each other fairly and with consideration, so I spend lots of time reinforcing the skills that the children already have and helping them to acquire new skills. I think it is important that our class become a little community, and so we spend time doing some activities cooperatively. The social skills that we will be learning will help us to do this more successfully.

One of the things that we do is a class newspaper. This helps the children in the development of their literacy skills, and it also helps keep you, their parents, informed of what is going on in our class. Enclosed is a sample of the last edition from our class last year. Elizabeth will have the opportunity, over the course of the year, to work on all the parts of the newspaper.

We also have some special guests scheduled for the year, as well as some field trips and special projects. We'll be talking more about these things during the first weeks of school, and you will be reading about them in our class newspaper.

Mr. and Mrs. Jones, one of the most important things that will contribute to Elizabeth's having a successful year is for all three of us to stay in close contact about what is going on in school and what is going on at home. Please call me with any concerns you have. You can reach me at the school (555-2345) during the school day. Please leave a message, and I will get back to you that afternoon after the children leave, or that evening from home.

I also encourage you to visit our class and see firsthand what our day is like. To do this, please call me and arrange a time in advance. That way, we'll be sure to be in the classroom the day you would like to visit.

I love to have parent volunteers in my classroom. The school offers a brief training course for parent (or grandparent) volunteers. Any time you have to spare is appreciated—from every day to once a year, depending on your schedule. Please call the school (555-2345) if this is something that interests you, and the staff can tell you more about the training program.

Last, but certainly not least, I will be calling you sometime during the first weeks of school, just to get acquainted. Then when we meet in person the open house (this year it is scheduled for September 28th from 7 to 9 P.M.), we will already know each other a little.

I'm really excited about meeting you, and I look forward to our helping Elizabeth have a great year!

Sincerely yours,

Susan Striepling-Goldstein

FIGURE 2.1. A sample letter to parents of an elementary school child.

August 5, 2004

Dear Jamar,

My name is Ms. Striepling-Goldstein, and I am your third-grade teacher. Every August I have a special day when children and their parents or guardians can come and help me decorate our room to get ready for the new year. This year that special day will be Friday, August 25th, from 9 to 10:30 A.M. I hope you and your dad can come. Please have him call the school at 555-1234 to sign up for this event, or ask him to mail back the enclosed postcard. If you can't come on that day, we will be doing some special decorating the first two days of school, so you can help then.

Hope I'll get to meet you both on the 25th!

Sincerely,

Ms. Striepling-Goldstein

FIGURE 2.2. A sample letter to an elementary school child.

teacher expects from them in order to help their children be successful in school. It is also an opportunity for families to share with teachers their expectations for the coming school year. None of this is possible unless the individual teachers and the school they teach in appreciate and regard a child's family as a valuable resource. If this respect and appreciation can be communicated, both verbally and nonverbally by the teacher and school, much of the anxiety associated with the first days and weeks of school can be avoided.

In some schools late summer is an opportunity for teachers, along with other staff and perhaps a team of trained family members, to make home visits to the families of children in their classes. This reaching out can be valuable in any school—rural, suburban or urban—but it is especially helpful when it is a child's first year in a school or where family participation in the school has been minimal in the past. Often, a low level of participation is a reflection of a lack of awareness or opportunity, rather than a lack of desire to help one's child. Other stresses in the lives of families (e.g., lack of resources, transportation, or phone, single parenting with many younger children at home) can prevent involvement in an individual child's school life. By being positive and proactive in their approach, teachers and schools can begin the process of creating a positive, mutually supportive environment that can have a real impact on a child's school career.

Teachers in higher elementary grades use the family and child letters to introduce themselves, talk about some of the activities planned for the school year, and invite the parents and child to the first open house (which, ideally, is held early in the school year). An invitation to call the teacher at any time with questions or concerns is included (with a school telephone number). The teacher also invites the parents to visit the classroom by setting up an appointment and tells them to expect an introductory phone call within the first weeks of school, just to get acquainted. In this way the groundwork for a successful partnership with the home is laid. At this level, home visits should be a viable option for those parents whose situations make it difficult to come to school or who have no phone in their homes.

The first phone call or home visit, made before there are any problems with a child, is very important. The tone should be friendly, with the teacher saying something positive about the child and his or her academic potential. It is also very important at this initial stage to establish a collaborative atmosphere in which the family feels that they are valued members of a team whose purpose is to help the child succeed in school. Too often families are seen as "the enemy," and any contacts are made in such a way that a family gets the message that the teacher feels that the problems with the youngster are the family's fault. This immediately puts the family on the defensive and causes antagonism between the family and the child on the one hand and the teacher on the other. It is far better, through the outreach of the teacher, to make the relationship an alliance among the family, the teacher, and the child. If a problem does develop that requires contact, it is much easier to deal with a friendly, supportive family than with a hostile one. The interaction then becomes a problem-solving process in which both family and teacher try to come up with ways to modify the child's behavior. Having the support of a disruptive child's family may not solve the problem entirely, but it often helps a great deal.

At the middle and high school levels, it becomes impossible to make phone calls and/or home visits to 130–150 families. At these levels, teachers often make early initial contact with parents via a letter (Figure 2.3) introducing themselves, giving a brief course description, articulating classroom rules and homework expectations, and extending an invitation to call the teacher at school about any concerns or problems. Then, if a child is disruptive and phone contact is necessary, an initial friendly contact has been established. Teachers hope that by the time the child gets to this level, the good work of creating positive family–school relationships that has gone on in the elementary schools in the district has helped to create a positive climate in the district as a whole. Outreach by the teacher and school should continue if at all possible, especially when it is clear from former school–family interactions that such outreach is necessary to continue to create a positive climate. Again, there are ideals and realities; however, teachers and schools should strive for as many of the following conditions as possible:

- Mutually shared goals across home and school for children's learning
- Belief that parental involvement in school is paramount
- Belief that working together as partners will benefit the child's learning and development, with mutually supported roles and actions to achieve this goal
- Recognition of the value of in- and out-of-school learning opportunities for children's learning and school progress

September 14, 2004

Dear Mrs. Smith,

I am Susan Striepling-Goldstein, Jason's social studies teacher. I want to welcome you and your son, Jason, to my class for this school year. I am looking forward to a great year and I hope Jason is also.

Social studies this year, as mandated by the state of New York, will cover U.S. history from the founding to the present. We have a lot to cover and we'll be moving fairly fast, so I hope that Jason will make every effort to keep up. If at any time he is having problems, he will need to see me right away so we can be sure he doesn't fall behind. I am usually available every day after school for extra help. He should check with me in class to be sure I don't have a school meeting on the day he plans to come.

I try to keep my classroom rules as simple as possible. They are all related to helping the classroom be the best learning environment as possible for everyone. The basic ones are these:

> Speak in a positive manner about yourself and others.
> Keep your hands, arms, feet, head, and any other parts of your body in your own space.
> Speak in class only when it is your turn, and then in a manner that shows you respect yourself, your teacher, and your peers.
> Turn all your work in on time, done in a way that makes you proud of yourself.

There are also certain classroom procedures to help make the class run as smoothly as possible, such as when to use the lavatory, when to sharpen pencils, where to put completed homework, and so forth. We are in the process of learning these now in class.

I expect homework to be turned in on the day it is assigned, unless Jason has been out sick or I have spoken with you. I do not assign "busy work." What Jason has for homework will help him be successful on tests and quizzes in class. I give a short quiz each Friday at the beginning of class, which reviews the work we have done that week. Tests are given as we complete each unit. If Jason is doing his classwork and homework, he should not have difficulty on these tests and quizzes. If Jason receives a grade of less than 70 on a test or quiz, he may retake the test or quiz after school. If he gets the questions he originally missed correct this time, I will then raise his final test or quiz grade to 85. Therefore, if Jason is turning in his homework, doing his journal and special projects, and participating in class, there is no reason for him not to receive at least a passing grade of 65. My grades are figured as follows: 20% homework, 50% tests and quizzes, 20% special projects (including a class journal), and 10% class participation.

We will be doing two major research projects this year, one in the fall and one in the spring. These will involve library research (which we will be doing during class time), home interviews, a graphics component (drawings, photographs, graphs, etc.), and a final paper. I will be sending a more detailed description home to you at the time we do these projects, with suggestions on how you can help Jason be successful with his projects.

Mrs. Smith, one of the most important things that will contribute to Jason's having a successful year in social studies is for the two of us to stay in close contact about what is going on in school and what is going on at home. Please call me with any concerns you have. You can reach me at the school (555-2345) during the school day. Please leave a message, and I will get back to you that afternoon after the students leave, or that evening from home.

I'm looking forward to meeting you in the near future and having a great year with Jason.

Sincerely yours,

Susan Striepling-Goldstein

FIGURE 2.3. A sample letter to a parent of a middle school child.

- Recognition that the nature and quality of the family–school relationship influence (positively or negatively) children's school performance
- Expectation that families will be involved, and recognition that such involvement can mean different things to different families
- Expectation that teachers and school personnel will seek ways to invite parents to share in the educational process for their children, recognizing that this may "look different" to different families
- Presence of a mission statement that promotes the importance and expectation of school–family connections for children's learning (Christenson & Sheridan, 2001, p. 34)

Every phone call home should start with a positive statement about the child. Nothing puts a family on the defensive faster than to have a teacher start a conversation with a statement like this: "Your child is a real problem, and I won't stand for this behavior in my classroom." Once a teacher has put a family on the defensive in this manner, it is very difficult to gain family members' trust and help. They may argue with the teacher and deny that their child causes problems, or they may reply "Yes" to whatever the teacher says—just to get him or her off the phone. In either case, when the phone call ends, a family member may well turn to the child and agree that the teacher is a jerk and it is not worth paying attention to him or her. Either way, the chance of family help is gone. Remaining positive opens the door for families and teachers to problem solve together.

The following list summarizes positive communications strategies to be used either in direct dealings with the family or through phone calls:

- Always start with a positive message.
- Convey the desire to work together to help the child.
- Use good communication skills to promote cohesion.
- Use common language, and refrain from speaking "above" the parent.
- Use the parent's own words when possible.
- Listen quietly to what the parent says, verbalizing initially only to convey understanding (such as through "mm-hmm," "OK," or other similar, minimal encouragers).
- Express the fact that the parent's input and perspective are very important.
- Respect that the family members are experts, that they are doing the best they can, and that they want what is best for their child.
- Clearly describe expectations for school behavior and ask the parents if they agree and can support the expectations.
- Keep in mind the responsibilities of each person.
- Avoid giving advice as much as possible.
- Ask the parent for help.
- Thank the parent for listening, caring, and helping. (Christenson & Sheridan, 2001, p. 195)

Although some families will at first be surprised and a little hesitant to participate in a problem-solving session if they have not been approached this way before, most will respond positively once they realize that the teacher is sincerely asking for a collaborative relationship. Many families simply do not know how to help their children succeed in school. In low-income minority populations, the family members may not have completed many years of formal education. Research demonstrates that families on welfare, with little education, or with low-paying jobs *can* be effective in contributing to their children's success in school (Comer, 1988; Cochran, 1988). The key seems to be the teacher's being dedicated to designing ways in which parents can help their children (Epstein, 1992). Some excellent ideas for teachers to pass on to parents are suggested by Kelley (1990). Kelley recommends that teachers send the following to parents, as needed: school–home notes that rely heavily on parents' comments (see Figure 2.4), a list of daily and weekly rewards for use with children of varying ages (see Table 2.1), a parent handout explaining the use of a star chart (see Figure 2.5), and explanations and guidelines on when and how to provide sanctions for unsatisfactory behavior (see Table 2.2). In addition to behavioral guidelines, academic guidelines from the teacher on how the parents can help the child establish the "homework habit" (see Table 2.3) are useful (Olympia, Jenson, Clark, & Sheridan, 1992).

Family–school collaboration must consist of more than just phone calls, letters home, or thoughtfully designed ways of helping families to assist with homework or extending their child-rearing skills. It should include inviting the families to be a part of the learning environment of the classroom. It is often difficult for teachers to manage a classroom alone, given the variety of needs that different children have. In some schools, teachers have set up training sessions for volunteers that are run periodically throughout the school year. These sessions include such things as school rules, classroom rules, the school's expectations for volunteers and volunteers' expectations regarding their activities. In a school that has such training sessions, all volunteers who work in the building must go through this training. They can then go into classrooms and provide the additional support that teachers need. Possibilities include helping children create a classroom newsletter, forming an alliance with community resources to extend learning opportunities, volunteering for such jobs in the school that provide training and experience for outside employment for the parents, taking additional training so that they are able to make home visits on behalf of the school, teaching and working with other parents in workshop settings on curriculum and school success, and writing proposals to secure needed funds for school or parent programs (Rioux and Berla, 1993).

Ziegler (1987) presents a comprehensive review of the literature on parent involvement in schools. It has been found that students' achievement in a school where there is a high degree of parental involvement (even if the parents involved are not the children's own) is frequently greater than that of students in a school where there is virtually no such involvement. Ziegler hypothesizes that the effectiveness of family involvement "may be explained by

SCHOOL–HOME NOTE

Name Ashley   Date 4/15

CLASS _____Reading_____
    Followed instructions   Yes   So-So   No   NA
    Completed classwork satisfactorily   Yes   So-So   No   NA
    Homework test grades   A   B   C   D   F   NA
Comments:

CLASS _____Math_____
    Followed instructions   Yes   So-So   No   NA
    Completed classwork satisfactorily   Yes   So-So   No   NA
    Homework test grades   A   B   C   D   F   NA
Comments:

CLASS _____Phonics/spelling_____
    Followed instructions   Yes   So-So   No   NA
    Completed classwork satisfactorily   Yes   So-So   No   NA
    Homework test grades   A   B   C   D   F   NA
Comments:

Parent comments:
    Consequences provided last night: Ashley watched TV for an hour and had
        20 minutes of special time.

    Comments about homework: Ashley worked on her math facts.

    Other comments: Thanks for completing the note! I feel better able to help Ashley.

FIGURE 2.4. Abbreviated school–home note emphasizing parent comments. From Kelley (1990, p. 85). Copyright 1990 by The Guilford Press. Reprinted by permission.

the message children receive when they see their teachers and parents in direct, personal contact centered on the children's learning and progress" (p.3). She continues, "The more direct, first-hand, frequent and personal the parent–teacher contact, and the more visible that contact is to the child, the greater is its potential" (p. 6).

In an elementary classroom, a family member may be invited to work with an individual student on skill development or to help with a small group of children when the teacher is working with the rest of the class. Inviting a parent, grandparent, or other family member to lend a hand with a special project or to actually teach a skill, trade, or hobby to the entire class can also be effective. In some elementary schools, programs for family math and parent and child literacy have been successful.

In middle and high schools, peer pressures sometimes make families less welcomed by their own children. The challenge for middle school and high

TABLE 2.1. Daily and Weekly Rewards for Use with Children of Varying Ages

Daily	Weekly

Preschool and early elementary

Daily	Weekly
Late bedtime	Lunch at a fast-food restaurant
20 minutes with Mom or Dad	Having a friend over
Playing outside	Small toy
10–25 cents	Trip to park
Snack	Friday night late bedtime
Stories at bedtime	

Late elementary to junior high school

Daily	Weekly
Playing outside	Spending the night out or having a friend over
Computer games	Going to mall/movie with parents and friend
50 cents–$1	Wearing eyeshadow
25 cents for school snack	New T-shirt or small toy
TV	

Junior high to high school

Daily	Weekly
Use of the telephone	Going out Friday/Saturday night
$1–$3 (if money is not available in other ways)	Transportation to an activity
Not having to do the dishes	Use of car
One hour of privacy after school	Later curfew
No parental nagging after school	Going to the mall with a friend
	Money for clothes
	Double date once a month

Note. From Kelley (1990, p. 88). Copyright 1990 by The Guilford Press. Reprinted by permission.

school teachers and families is to design programs that encourage families' participation in ways that will not embarrass their children. This may involve the families' working in classes other than their own children's or working outside the classroom with students who need extra help. In both of these instances, families' connectedness to the academic enterprise in general and the school in particular is heightened; this increases the chances of families' attentiveness to their children's academic progress and their receptivity to the teacher's initiatives, should the child engage in aggressive behaviors. Although it may be harder to achieve family involvement at the secondary level, it is imperative that the attempt be made.

Aggression in the classroom always occurs within the context of the school as a whole, the neighborhood, and the larger community. Many things can be done by the individual teacher to lessen the chance of its occurring in his or her classroom. Aggression is, however, a difficult behavior to change and is remarkably consistent over time. Unless a systems-oriented approach is employed, the teacher will continually be fighting an uphill bat-

A Handout for Parents
on Star Charts

WHAT IS A STAR CHART?
A star chart is a special way of giving children positive attention. Good behavior earns stars; stars are traded in for other consequences, such as candy, TV time, play time, or a trip to McDonald's. Using star charts allows parents to provide an immediate signal that the child will earn rewards later for good behavior.

HOW TO MAKE A STAR CHART

Here is an example of a star chart parents have used to reinforce a child's good behavior.

STAR CHART FOR KATHY

Days	Make bed		Take out trash		Help wash dishes	
	Week 1	Week 2	Week 1	Week 2	Week 1	Week 2
Monday	*		*		*	
Tuesday	*		*		*	
Wednesday	*				*	
Thursday	*		*		*	
Friday			*		*	
Saturday	*		*			
Sunday	*		*		*	

Here, Kathy earned a star for each day she did the good behaviors listed on the top of the chart.

HOW TO USE A STAR CHART
1. Select target behaviors.
When parents are selecting a behavior to include in a star chart, it is best to choose a *positive* behavior. The target behavior can be the absence of a misbehavior (such as tantrums) for an interval of time. Behaviors that occur frequently (such as fighting with siblings or having tantrums) should receive stars at several intervals.

For example, Sally has tantrums about six times a day. Her mother has set up a star chart so that the day is divided into three parts—before school, after school, and after supper. Sally can earn a star for not having any tantrums during these three intervals.

2. Select consequences.
Parents and children should determine daily and weekly rewards for reaching behavior-change goals. For example, when Kathy completed her chores, she earned 25 cents and 20 minutes of special time with Dad or Mom daily. Larger rewards were provided for six of seven acceptable days.

Parents should attempt to provide truly *rewarding* consequences.

Clearly communicate to the child how many stars are needed to earn rewards.

3. Pair stars with praise.
Whenever star-earning behaviors are performed, parents should praise children.

FIGURE 2.5.   *(continued)*

FIGURE 2.5. *continued*

Do praise in a sincere manner. Do allow children to place their stars on the chart if they choose.

4. Give positive attention both right away and later.
When parents use a star chart, a child can get positive attention with a star right after a good behavior, and the child can work for special reinforcers later by trading in stars.

5. Reinforce every time the pleasing behavior occurs.
In the beginning, parents should reinforce their child each and every time the pleasing behavior occurs. Also, the child should receive a bigger reinforcer when he or she earns stars several days in a row (weekly reinforcers).

6. Reinforce small changes.
Parents should reinforce small amounts of behavior change at first, then gradually increase the amount of behavior change necessary for the bigger reinforcers.

7. Use everyday reinforcers.
Reinforcers need not be extra things, but things parents now give a child noncontingently. Examples include staying up late, watching TV, and playing outside.

8. Keep your promises.
Parents should always tell their child what he or she can earn and with how many stars. They should promise *only* something they can really give the child and should always keep their promises.

FIGURE 2.5. A handout for parents on star charts. From Kelley (1990, pp. 131–132). Copyright 1990 by The Guilford Press.

TABLE 2.2. Guidelines for Parents: Providing Sanctions for Unsatisfactory Behavior

1. Deliver only those sanctions that are planned in advance, included in a contract, and fully expected by children. Children should have full knowledge of the sanction prior to beginning the contract.
2. Always provide a rationale whenever punishment is delivered.
3. Make the sanction relatively brief, relevant to the misbehavior, and constructive. Examples: an extra chore, additional practice at writing spelling words, recopying a failed test, writing a 150-word essay about the importance of not fighting.
4. Negotiate appropriate sanctions with your child.
5. Avoid using sanctions out of anger, frustration, or embarrassment. Sanctions are intended to instruct and increase the potency of incentives.
6. Deliver sanctions in a calm manner.
7. Do not use harsh, embarrassing, cruel, or physical sanctions or reprimands.
8. If you are not fully confident of your ability to deliver sanctions calmly, avoid their use. Instead, rely solely on reward-based approaches to improving behavior.

Note. Sanctions should not be recommended to parents with anger management problems or those who tend to be excessively negative with their children. From Kelley (1990, p. 90). Copyright 1990 by The Guilford Press. Reprinted by permission.

TABLE 2.3. Developing the "Homework Habit": General Homework Guidelines for Parents

1. Establish a home environment that will encourage your child to do homework.
   a. The child should do homework in only one spot, at a desk or table.
   b. The area should be free of distractions (no noise, music, television, books, or food) and well lit.
   c. The area should be stocked with pencils, papers, erasers, and a dictionary.
   d. Make and use a "Do Not Disturb" or "Keep Out" sign for use when the child is doing homework.
2. Set up a regular time each day when homework is to be done. Establishing a routine helps to build the "homework habit."
   a. Before or after dinner is good for many students.
   b. Homework should come before television and play.
   c. Once homework is finished to your satisfaction, the child should be given free time.
   d. Even if the child does not have homework from school, you should still have the child use the mandatory homework time to do extra reading, review multiplication tables, or the like.

Note. Teachers should take time to develop specific guidelines for parents in the individual curriculum areas in which they teach. These will vary depending on the subject, the grade level, the type of homework (general classwork or special project), and the teacher's goals.

tle. In an attempt to deal with this "system," so-called full-service schools are emerging all across the United States (Dryfoos, 1994). These are schools in which school districts and community agencies are collaborating to provide services for students such as health care and social supports. The full-service schools also function as community centers, linking family support systems with child care systems. The services provided may include school-based clinics, full-day child care for 3- to 5-year-olds, before- and after-school care for 6- to 12-year-olds that includes recreation, home visitors to all parents of newborns, organized and supervised family day care for children from birth to 3 years, English as a second language for parents, general equivalency diploma (GED) classes for parents, vocational training for parents and teenagers, and recreational activities for teenagers.

I find the full-service model an exciting one, and I think it holds some keys for dealing with the aggression in our schools. First, by supporting families and involving them in the community school in real ways, we give recognition and respect to the adults who are most important in the lives of the children we teach. Second, too often a student, when asked why he or she hit, punched, shot, or killed another student, will reply, "He [she] was disrespecting me." For example, Dryfoos (1994) reported that students (at two full-service schools, I.S. 218, a middle school in Washington Heights, New York, and Hanshaw Middle School in Modesto, California), when asked why they liked their schools, said, "Everybody treats you here with respect." If respect is so important in our children's lives, then it seems to me that any environment that gives children the feeling of being respected will also lower their aggression levels.

In these challenging times, when discipline is often difficult to maintain, family–school collaboration can serve two purposes. First, when teachers create a positive relationship with families from the beginning, families and teachers can work together as a problem-solving team if behavioral problems do occur. Again, it is much easier to work with supportive families than hostile ones. Second, helping families support and encourage their children's academic achievement creates a climate in which the children have a better chance of being academically successful—and children who are more academically successful have higher self-esteem and are less disruptive in the classroom.

Teachers must break with the long tradition of isolation from families. "The process of relationship building with families must start early and continue across a child's entire academic experience" (Christenson & Sheridan, 2001, p. 203). Keeping in mind that both educators and families are concerned about the well-being of children, teachers must take the initiative of working side by side with their families in the educational process.

PHYSICAL CHARACTERISTICS OF THE CLASSROOM

Let us assume that a teacher has worked hard and has created a community of learners, the majority of whom are excited and committed to the learning process. The teacher has respect for their individual uniqueness and abilities, maintains high expectations and goals for each child, and helps each child to reach them. The teacher also regularly "catches" each child being good and praises such behavior generously, recognizing that a powerful agent of change is the rewarding of positive behavior. Finally, the teacher consistently and fairly (every child, every time) provides consequences for any behaviors that interrupt the flow in the learning process, recognizing that eliminating small problems can keep them from escalating into bigger issues.

Let us also assume that this teacher has done a good job of connecting with the students' families so that there is strong parental support, as well as an active group of volunteers who regularly help in the classroom. Furthermore, the teacher has extended the sense of community for the students to the school as a whole and even into the broader community outside school. Under these ideal circumstances, the physical characteristics of the classroom should be much like those of a comfortable workroom in someone's home. The room's features should include learning centers; desks grouped for cooperative work; books and magazines; lounging areas for reading, discussions, and downtime; displays of student work, in process as well as completed; plants and other objects that help students identify with the space and claim it as "ours."

If this teacher is in a district and in a building that facilitate this kind of environment for learning, he or she is very lucky. The reality for many teachers, particularly those working in urban and/or low-socioeconomic-status districts/schools with high neighborhood crime rates, is that the kind of support needed to create this ideal isn't there. So, just as when they are working with a child, teachers must start from where they are and build from that point.

Because the safety of staff and students is the top priority in some schools, compromises must be made. Depending on the level of disruption in a building, the physical characteristics of a classroom may include any or all of the following: The door is solidly constructed, not easily broken or broken through. It contains a window enabling someone looking in to view most of the classroom and someone inside to look out to survey the hallway. The door is attached to its frame by hydraulic dampers so that the harder one pushes, the more slowly the door closes. In addition, the door is key lockable, permitting the teacher to keep intruders out. The teacher's desk is also of solid construction and (like all the desks and tables in the room) bolted to the floor so that it cannot be used to block anyone's movement, upturned as a blockade, or picked up and thrown in the midst of a fight. Furthermore, it is placed strategically in the room to maximize the teacher's ability to see the room, move about the room, and (if necessary) escape from the room. Student desks or tables are arranged with sufficient space between them to minimize potential crowding and inadvertent bumping. Both the layout and grouping of student furniture ease movement by students as transitions take place, and promote the teacher's access to students. Any call-for-assistance devices in the room are also easily accessed by the teacher. The floor plan allows the teacher to move swiftly about the room or even to leave for reasons of personal safety.

What else might characterize this hypothetical classroom? There are no hidden corners or closets. There are no objects lying around that might serve as weapons, such as staplers or scissors. All such materials are marked for identification and kept in a locked closet under the teacher's control. The storage area is located so that the teacher is able to continue viewing the class at the same time materials are being retrieved. The room is well lit, its lights are controlled by a key (not a switch); and its windows are small and made of unbreakable material. The entire window area is covered with decorative grillwork. The interior of the room is painted (at least in part) in bright colors with a hard-surface paint. Little or no graffiti or other marks of vandalism exist in the room, because whenever such defacement takes place it is swiftly recorded, removed, and repaired. Because of hard work on the teacher's part, most of the students feel that this is their room, and vandalism is infrequent. The class's personal touch is expressed, as much as possible, with plants, a cushioned area, wall displays of student work, and similar evidence that "this is our place."

Although these accommodations will help minimize aggression, some of them plainly have a negative side. Bolting classroom furniture to the floor to prevent its being used as a weapon or blockade will also prevent its imaginative regrouping for classroom community building and other positive purposes. Grillwork over classroom windows will diminish the frequency of the single most common form of school vandalism—broken windows; it will also just as certainly increase the prison-like atmosphere that has befallen many of our schools. For these reasons, physical alterations in the classroom must be made cautiously. Changes should reflect the nature and severity of the aggression level in a particular class, school, and community. They should be considered only as interim solutions as the school and the community work toward creating a safer space for children.

A SYSTEMIC APPROACH

Although the individual classroom teacher needs to and can do much behind his or her door to build a climate of cooperation, collaboration, and respect, in order for that climate to be sustained and enhanced, it must become a systemwide goal. To that end, more and more schools are ending the isolation of the individual teacher and staff members are reaching out to each other in supportive and collaborative ways to lower aggression levels, facilitate interpersonal skills of students, and raise academic achievement levels. They are recognizing that until the issues of aggression and lack of interpersonal skills are addressed, academic achievement levels will not rise. A systems approach, as mentioned in the introduction to this chapter, is finally being seen as the only viable option for facilitating these changes.

The Delaware School

A school that has recognized the need for a proactive schoolwide approach is the Delaware School, a N–6 elementary school in Syracuse, New York. This school of 729 students is located in what was recognized in 1994 by *U.S. News and World Report* as the 12th most impoverished neighborhood of the nation's urban centers. It has a diverse student population made up of 75% minority, 40% with limited English-speaking skills, and 27% having a learning disability. The neighborhoods that the students live in have extremely high rates of poverty, drug abuse, and street violence. The majority of students come from one-parent families, and 95% receive a free or reduced-cost school lunch.

During the 1999–2000 school year only 25% of Delaware students met state academic standards, with the other 75% considered to be academically at risk and in need of specialized academic skill development. In 1998–1999 school year, this school had the highest suspension rate of all elementary schools in the Syracuse City School District (28 schools), with a total of 1,534 instructional days lost because of disciplinary action (R. DiFlorio, personal communication, 2002).

To combat these dismal statistics, the teachers and staff at Delaware banded together to address both the discipline problems and the low achievement levels. Recognizing that only a schoolwide multimodal intervention approach would facilitate lasting change in their building, they decided upon a two-pronged approach. To begin to address the academic achievement of their students, they implemented "Success for All," a research-based reading program from Johns Hopkins University (*www.successforall.net*). This is a cooperative learning model that relies heavily on social skills in order for the cooperative learning standards to be implemented effectively. To teach the social skills necessary for cooperative learning to take place, and to teach students to lower and control their anger levels, which were leading to aggressive behavior, Aggression Replacement Training (ART) was implemented. Aggression Replacement Training is a three-part program consisting of a skills component (Skillstreaming), an anger control component (Anger Control Training), and a values component (Moral Reasoning Training). It is one of the 42 exemplary and promising programs designated by the U.S. Department of Education's Safe, Disciplined and Drug-Free Office. Because the book, *Aggression Replacement Training* (Goldstein, Glick, & Gibbs, 1998), is written for the adolescent, the skills part of the program was taught from *Skillstreaming the Elementary School Child* (McGinnis & Goldstein, 1997). The other two parts of the program, Anger Control and Moral Reasoning, were modified to fit a younger population.

The program, combining Success for All and Aggression Replacement Training, was piloted in the 1999–2000 school year and implemented schoolwide in the 2000–2001 school year. The teachers found that more instruction in skillstreaming skills was related to greater reduction of aggressive behavior. The less aggressive behavior resulted in more time available for instructional activities during the school day. Out-of-school suspensions decreased dramatically, with a reduction in the suspension rate from 1,534 days lost to instruction to 936 days lost. On the New York State achievement tests given to fourth graders in the spring of 2001, math scores increased by 43% and language arts scores increased by 20%.

This school has made a commitment to its staff, students, and community to improve the opportunities and outcomes, both behaviorally and academically, of all its students. It is not an easy task to work your way up from the bottom, and it was clearly an impossible task for one teacher to accomplish alone. Not only was it necessary for individual teachers to be supported by other staff, administration, and the district as a whole, the school itself had to reach beyond the school district and into the broader community. During the summer of 2001, in a program called "Raising Readers," staff visited all first graders' homes. The purpose was to explain to parents their responsibilities in helping to facilitate their children's success in school during the upcoming year. It also gave the staff a chance to see the environments from which the children came. This has helped them to understand better the challenges that their families faced. The local American Automobile Association (AAA) provided the staff with printed directions from the school to each of the homes they visited. The school has also reached out into the community and has made connections with the Onondaga Pastoral Counseling Service. Staff from this service facilitate the small Anger Control Training groups from the school.

Dedicated administrators, teachers and staff, enthusiastic parents, a supportive central office, and supports out in the community, all working toward a common goal, are responsible for the changes going on at Delaware. In the third year of the program they continue to document gains in both academic achievement and lowered aggression levels.

Other Systemic Resources

Throughout the United States, teachers, schools, and districts are working hard, using a systemic approach to create facilitative environments for their students in which aggression levels are low, student achievement is high, and students are being adequately prepared to take their place in the 21st century. They are no longer working in isolation, but are reaching out to each other. I list here a few sources that I have found useful:

The School District of the city of Erie, Pennsylvania. This is a small urban district in the northwest corner of Pennsylvania that has reached out to Perseus House Community Youth Service Center to enhance the effectiveness of its in-school program components. The contribution of Perseus House involves parenting programs, after-school programs for youth, and the housing of an alternative education program, which are all systemic attempts to reduce incidents of in-school aggression and improve student academic achievement. Although much of the program is still in the pilot stage, initial results suggest increases in academic achievement, measured by standardized test scores, and decreases in aggression levels, measured by lower incidences of office referrals and school suspensions. *http://esd.iu5.org/district/htm.*

Chicago Public Schools. Chicago Public Schools are noted for their outreach into the surrounding community for support of their schools, from both businesses and higher education institutions (Daniels, Bizar, & Zemelman, 2001). The whole website is excellent, but explore its "Small Schools" section for some interesting ways in which it has supported a number of creative innovations. *www.cps.k12.il.us/Schools/Opportunities/Small/small.html.*

Coalition of Essential Schools (CES). This coalition is a national network of more than 1,000 schools, 19 regional centers, and a national office seeking to promote higher student achievement and to develop more nurturing and humane school communities. CES regional centers support schools in the process of change by providing opportunities for professional development and technical assistance. *www.essentialschools.org*.

U.S. Department of Education Safe, Disciplined and Drug-Free Schools Office. This website provides Internet links to its promising and exemplary programs, which many districts are using systemically to facilitate and enhance gains. *www.ed.gov/offices/OESE/SDFS/programs.html*.

Another useful website to visit is maintained by the Center for Safe Schools. *www.groups.msn.com/centerforsafeschoolsandcommunities/home.htm*.

SUMMARY

In this chapter I have considered the characteristics of a classroom setting where low levels of student aggression prevail. These characteristics include the necessity for a systemic approach to all aspects of the education process; in-depth understanding of one's students; major efforts to create a sense of community; comprehensive preplanning of classroom activities; heavy reliance on efficient, student-oriented instructional behaviors; effective development and implementation of classroom rules and procedures; a serious and continuing commitment to creatively facilitating family–school collaboration; and an array of physical alterations and accommodations in the classroom. The ideal low-aggression classroom happens only as a result of much hard work on the part of teachers, administrators, other staff members, district offices, parents, and other community members, as well as the students themselves. It happens within the context of safer schools, safer neighborhoods, and safer communities. It is not easy to achieve, but energetic efforts toward its implementation can yield substantial rewards in terms of better classroom management, higher student achievement, and higher quality of the classroom experience for everyone involved.

REFERENCES

Christenson, S. L., & Sheridan, S. M. (2001). *Schools and families: Creating essential connections for learning*. New York: Guilford Press.

Cochran, M. (1988). *Empowering families*. Ithaca, NY: Family Matter Project, Cornell University.

Comer, J. P. (1988). Educating poor minority children. *Scientific American, 259*(5), 42–48.

Daniels, H., Bizar, M., & Zemelman, S. (2001). *Rethinking high school: Best practice in teaching, learning and leadership*. Portsmouth, NH: Heinemann.

Dryfoos, J. G. (1994). *Full-service schoools: A revolution in health and social services for children, youth and families*. San Francisco: Jossey-Bass.

Epstein, J. L. (1992, March). *School and family partnerships* (Report No. 6). Boston: Center on Families, Communities, Schools and Children's Learning.

Feshbach, N. D. (1978). Studies of empathic behavior in children. In B. A. Mher (Ed.), *Progress in experimental personality research* (Vol. 8, pp. 22–28). New York: Academic Press.

Goldstein, A. P. (1999). *The Prepare curriculum: Teaching prosocial compentencies.* Champaign, IL: Research Press.

Goldstein, A. P., Glick, B., & Gibbs, J. C. (1998). *Aggression replacement training: A comprehensive intervention for aggressive youth.* Champaign, IL: Research Press.

Goldstein, A. P., & McGinnis, E. (1997). *Skillstreaming the adolescent: New strategies and perspectives for teaching prosocial skills.* Champaign, IL: Research Press.

Kelley, M. L. (1990). *School–home notes: Promoting children's classroom success.* New York: Guilford Press.

Kounin, J. (1970). *Discipline and group management in classrooms.* New York: Holt,Rinehart & Winston.

McGinnis, E., & Goldstein, A. P. (1997). *Skillstreaming the elementary school child: New strategies and perspectives for teaching prosocial skills.* Champaign, IL: Research Press.

McGinnis, E., & Goldstein, A. P. (2002). *Skillstreaming in early childhood: Teaching prosocial skills to the preschool and kindergarten child.* Champaign, IL: Research Press.

Miller, P. A., & Eisenberg, N. (1988). The relation of empathy to aggressive and externalizing/antisocial behavior. *Psychological Bulletin, 103,* 324–344.

Olympia, D., Jenson, W. R., Clark, E., & Sheridan, S. (1992). Training parents to facilitate homework completion: A model for home–school collaboration. In S. L. Christenson & J. C. Conoley (Eds.), *Home–school collaboration: Enhancing children's academic and social competence* (pp. 238–243). Silver Spring, MD: National Association of School Psychologists.

Reed, N. H. (1981). *Psychopathic delinquency, empathy, and helping behavior.* Unpublished doctoral dissertation, Loyola University of Chicago.

Rioux, J. W., & Berla, N. (1993). *Innovations in parent and family involvement.* Princeton, NJ: Eye on Education.

Sandberg, B. (1999). Respect leads to results: A top teacher's winning formula starts with high expectations. Number 9. *New York Teacher, 42*(9), 12–13.

Ziegler, S. (1987). *The effects of parent involvement on children's achievement: The significance of home/school links* (Report No. ED 304 234). Toronto: Toronto Board of Education.

CHAPTER 3

Creating Safe Schools

A Principal's Perspective

SHELDON BRAATEN

Suppose someone from the school district's central office came to you one day and said, "We are going to open a school for assaultive and violent adolescents, and we want you to accept the administrative assignment." Imagine further that the mission of this school is "zero reject, zero eject." Translated, this means that the school will accept only students who have failed to succeed in other intervention programs and who have been rejected by other schools, agencies, or youth facilities, and that the school will not "kick them out" for any reason. How would you respond? Would you say, "Sure, that sounds like an interesting and exciting challenge"? Or, as I did, "Sorry, I'm not interested. Only masochists and fools would want to do that, and I'm not either"?

At the time (1975), I was working as a special educator in an elementary program with students with emotional and behavioral disorders, and, frankly, the thought of working in a school of assaultive adolescents frightened me. After turning down the position two more times, I was finally persuaded to accept the assignment and began what was to be an 18-year lesson on creating safe schools.

The introductory lessons were dramatic. I felt fortunate in having the opportunity to work with an extraordinary staff of committed, idealistic, and energetic people; however, we quickly learned that those attributes were necessary but not sufficient to address the needs of the students in our new school. During the first 6 months we documented 305 assaults on staff members. On one day alone we dealt with 59 such assaults, and I took three of the victims to the hospital. Clearly, it was a "good news, bad news" situation. The good news was that we had the right students. The bad news was that we were paying a terrible price and had to find ways to address a host of issues quickly, beginning with safety. The facts were that despite our well-intentioned efforts and expressions of positive regard, we were taking a beating, and our mildly intrusive consequences (brief exclusionary "time outs") seemed only to increase the frequency of assaults. We quickly learned that reducing the level of violence would require much more than goodwill and our limited suppressive interventions. We would have to focus on generating prevention strategies and building a model to foster development of prosocial behavior, while concurrently taking a firm and intolerant stand against *any* display of aggression. Indeed, our very well-being, as well as that of the students, depended on it.

Unfortunately, at that time there was little in the professional literature that explained how to design such a program in a public school setting; nor were there many people we could call and ask for advice. Fortunately, we were part of a school system whose administration was willing to commit adequate resources to this undertaking, along with the support and encouragement that would be necessary to create a positive and productive environment for the students and staff. The challenging task before us was to create a comprehensive program model that would be based on the available knowledge about the "normal" development and learning processes of children and youths, as well as on effective behavior management practices. This chapter might best be described as a personal essay on lessons learned and keys to progress, with remembrance of the book title *I Never Promised You a Rose Garden*. We proceeded with a determination to succeed with students who had long histories of failure; we knew that our only real choice, and hope, was to focus much more of our energy on students' personal development and prevention measures than on strategies to suppress aggressive behaviors. We had to learn how to teach alienated and angry youths prosocial skills in ways that were developmentally appropriate and responsive to their many needs.

THE SOCIAL CONTEXT

No educator, veteran or new to the field, is unaware of the extensive attention that has been devoted to public education issues over the past two decades, and especially to the effectiveness of our schools (or the lack thereof) in meeting the needs of our nation's children and youths. Concerns related to the curriculum and academic achievement in the context of international competition have been with us since the Sputnik era. The current array of complex issues and competing agendas includes school governance, parent involvement, assessment of student achievement, cultural diversity, community support, legal mandates for a variety of compensatory and other special services, teacher competence, finance, and many others. Among all these, the most fundamental concern is the role of schools in a rapidly changing society.

During the 1990s educators and the general public became keenly aware that schools, whether urban, suburban, or rural, were no longer safe havens from the problems that many children and youths have had to face in their homes and communities. Incidents of youth violence were widely reported in the media, most notably the tragedy at Columbine High School in Littleton, Colorado. School leaders responded with steps to ensure the safety of students and staff through strict discipline policies ("zero tolerance") and an array of measures that include securing building entrances, installing metal detectors, requiring picture IDs, and hiring armed police officers.

The era also resulted in a plethora of books, articles, research reports, and countless conference presentations, community forums, and meetings on youth violence. Furthermore, new "get tough" legislation such as the Gun-Free School Zones Act of 1994 and the Safe and Drug-Free Schools and Communities Act of 1994 were enacted along with juvenile justice programs such as "boot camps."

The good news is that there have been numerous initiatives at all levels of government and by hosts of community institutions, including schools. Recent reports indicate that youth crime is at its lowest levels since the early 1970s (U.S. Department of Justice, 2003).

Clearly, some combination of the many different responses to violence has had a desirable outcome. Yet we seem unable, or more likely unwilling, to put this knowledge to work in any comprehensive or systematic manner throughout our social institutions. I fear that Dean Morris was correct in his 1977 assertion that, despite all the political rhetoric, there will be little done to seriously address the root causes of violence. In response to a reporter for U.S. News and World Report, who asked if he had any advice for the administration in Washington, Dean noted that declarations of war on crime are truisms in American politics—a popular thing to do, but one that means "we'll declare war and fulminate instead of taking the problem seriously" (cited in Commercial Union Insurance Company, 1978). I have come reluctantly to share the view of Englander, who said, "I do not get a clear message that Americans want to prevent criminal violence. They want rather to punish it" (1997, p. 152).

The recent focus in education has shifted from solving discipline and safe-school problems to the extraordinary academic accountability provisions of the No Child Left Behind Act. One emerging consequence of this shift, complicated by the tight financial restraints, is the growing number of students who are dropping out or being "elbowed out" because of misbehavior when they face certain failure on the high-stakes tests.

There are few defenders of the status quo (Lewis, 2002), and many critics have been offering reform proposals representing the spectrum of community, political, professional, and business concerns and perspectives. Although the agendas and proposed solutions vary from one proponent to the next, they all share the basic belief that something is seriously wrong (Boyd, 2003). Many observers believe that the current educational system is not working—at least not well enough—and requires a fundamental transformation (Crawford, Bodine, & Hoglund, 1993; Goodlad, 2002; Wright, 1996).

Large numbers of youths are also disillusioned, and the high rate of school dropouts indicates that they have given up the belief that continued participation in school will contribute to their personal success. It is clear that school personnel can no longer isolate themselves and their roles from the social issues of their surrounding communities. These issues include an erosion of traditional support systems, primarily family structure and functions.

This brief description of context is provided to help explain some of the factors contributing to student aggression and to underscore the complexity of the problems facing us. First, schools are part of these problems and can no longer simply remove or refer and forget troubled and troubling students. School personnel can no longer continue simply to blame students themselves, their parents, or the community for all of the serious problems they are now having to address. It has been far too easy for educators to label or otherwise identify "problem" students and assume that someone else is responsible for them.

Second, educators are very much aware that schools are being held responsible for failed practices and policies. Significant changes must be made in how schooling is delivered, and I believe the only really important measures of how well the schools succeed will be evidence of the schools' effects on the proportion of alienated, angry, and troubled youths.

Third, despite the currently popular rhetoric about getting tough with troubling students and bringing the role of schools back to basics, schools are part of an increasingly complex and diverse society and must respond to the varied needs students inevitably bring with them. That is, the schools must choose between working collaboratively with the community and being part of the solution, or continuing to be part of the problem (Lewis, 2003; Van Acker & Talbott, 1999).

Finally, there will be no simple, quick, or complete solutions. Any sincere effort to create safe or safer schools will require an unyielding long-term commitment and determination to be student focused, along with the resources necessary to ensure that schools are indeed good places to be for the students and the staff.

QUESTIONS TO BE ADDRESSED

Creating safe schools is not a simple matter of adding more security and swifter or harsher punishments. In my view, it is a process that is first based on attention to, and a continual focus on, answers to the following questions: Why do people behave the way they do? What do we know about conditions that increase or decrease the likelihood that people will behave in prosocial or antisocial ways? What do we know about the best practices and the most effective strategies for managing behavior problems? What is our vision for children and youths, and how does our specific mission help to keep us focused on that vision? What can we do to ensure that our resources are used most effectively? What can we do that diminishes our own contributions to problems and concurrently promotes the productive and prosocial development of students? What messages are sent to parents and the community, and how can we enlist them as resources in the solution? What can be done to be sure that what we offer is meaningful or relevant to the future lives of our students? How will we know that the steps we take will have the outcomes we desire?

Although the thoughts presented in the following discussion are the products of my experiences in working in a special school, the foundation for success is drawn from knowledge about normal development and effective, high-quality schools, which is applicable to all schools—whether they are regular or special settings. Furthermore, in my view, the degree to which any success is attained will not be related to the collection of specific program elements, but rather to keen attention to details.

BASIC NEEDS OF ALL STUDENTS

The very first domain of knowledge that is crucial to consider for the prevention of problem behavior, as well as intervention planning, is what we know or believe to be true about students' basic needs and development (Guetzloe, 1999). The importance of designing schools according to principles that are related to meeting the developmental needs of children and youths is generally acknowledged among educators. Clearly, these concepts have shaped the basic organization and structural differences of elementary, middle, and high schools today. That is, they were *not* created for the purpose of meeting adult needs. Yet as fundamental as these concepts are to systems that foster healthy development, we all know of examples of insensitivity to these concerns—insensitivity that often leads to schools' actually contributing to the very behavior problems they seek to eliminate.

Kauffman (2001) has discussed some ways in which schools may be responsible for some students' problem behaviors. These include insensitivity to individuals, inappropriate expectations, inconsistent management of behavior, requirements for instruction in nonfunctional or irrelevant skills, ineffective instruction in critical skills, use of destructive contingencies of reinforcement, and presentation of (or failure to provide consequences of) undesirable models of conduct. More specifically, according to Kauffman,

> the teacher's most crucial tasks as a preventative agent are to foster success and lessen the student's antisocial conduct . . . and [the teacher's] most valuable perspective . . . is to examine the student's environment to detect

factors that contribute to disordered behavior and those that encourage desired behavior. (p. 277)

The effectiveness of any school organization or specific teaching strategy is directly related to the degree to which it responds to students' varied characteristics and needs. Jones and Jones (1995) have provided an excellent summary of different psychological perspectives. This summary can help educators to understand fundamental human needs and their implications for school organization, structure, policies, and practices. In addition to the often cited work of Abraham Maslow, describing physiological, safety/security, belonging/affection, and self-respect needs, Jones and Jones (1995) describe the concepts of Stanley Coopersmith, which I have found to be especially helpful for understanding student behavior and developing responsive programs.

Coopersmith's (1967) model asserts three basic needs: significance, competence, and power. Significance is viewed as an individual's experience of being valued by someone who is important to him or her. Competence means the person's ability to perform tasks that are valued by others. Power means the person's having some sense of control over his or her environment and over decisions that affect him or her.

Trust is essential to meeting these needs. Inappropriate behavior or misbehavior may be viewed as efforts to have one or more of these needs met, even though the resulting social consequence may be negative. For example, an individual *will* find someone to provide a sense of significance. For a youth who is alienated or in trouble, that someone may be another who also feels alienated from the accepted group(s). Similarly, all students *will* be competent at something—if not reading, math, music, sports, or some other accepted skill, then at disruptions or fighting. Finally, every youth *will* express power in some way, whether as defiance or helplessness. If we understand and accept these three basic needs as true for all students, they provide explicit directions for prevention and intervention planning: Schools must ensure that each student feels valued, has the skills to make valued contributions to classes, and is offered reasonable and developmentally appropriate choices.

STUDENTS WITH PROBLEM BEHAVIORS: ARE THEY SO VERY DIFFERENT?

Before we can address the notion of serious behavior problems in our schools, we must consider a key issue rooted in how adults perceive youths in general. A Minnesota youth poll (Hedin, Hannes, & Saito, 1985) revealed that two-thirds of the students participating believed that significant adults in their lives perceived them negatively. Only 25% believed that adults held positive images of them. Furthermore, a large proportion did not believe the adults' perceptions to be accurate. According to the researchers, the results suggest that youths believe adults do not value, trust, or treat them with respect, and that this is increasingly so as the youths grow older. More recently, Csikszentmihalyi and Schmidt (1998) wrote that

> it is common for adolescents to feel that they are "second class" citizens, estranged for decision making and societal power. For teenagers, one result of being marginalized is that the seeking for respect, especially among young males, can reach pathological needs. (p. 13)

If that is what young people really think, then there should be little wonder about the source of much of their conflict with adults. Csikszentmihalyi and Schmidt further assert that their limited range of meaningful responsibilities and growing isolation from adult role models contribute to pathologies of adolescents. In contrast, they add, "those rare adolescents who have the opportunity to develop a relationship with an adult role model (parent or otherwise) are more successful at coping with everyday stresses . . . and to recover from extreme adversity" (p. 12).

Labeling students (as "emotionally disturbed," "behavior-disordered," "antisocial," "delinquent," etc.) is the typical way in which students with problems are identified for a variety of purposes, including allocating resources and determining eligibility for services. It also serves as a shorthand method to communicate information about what the labelers regard as the attributes of individual students. Although labels do serve some useful functions (particularly administrative ones), the act of labeling all too often fosters inappropriate expectations about the labeled students themselves, especially those with very challenging behavior. In particular, many educators tend to focus on the troubling behavior and to forget that these labeled students are still more like the general population than different in terms of their basic needs, wants, and developmental processes. I find that even when particular students are identified as "at risk," it remains important to cling to and build upon what they have in common with their peers, rather than to focus on differences.

A more useful approach is to acknowledge that all children and youths exhibit problem behaviors. The variance is not in kind, but in degree. The students who cause us much concern are what I would call "too kids." They engage too much or too little in particular behaviors, too often, in too many places, with too many people, over too long a period of time, and are too unresponsive to our efforts to change their behaviors. Rather than seeking some kind of new or magic treatments, we must focus on the fundamental principles that govern the learning and behavior of all individuals. Explicitly, when individuals do not know how to perform desired behaviors, we must teach them what to do. When they know how to perform desired behaviors but do not do so, we must create conditions that will elicit prosocial behavior, and provide numerous opportunities for successful practice and reinforcement.

In my view, the success or failure of prevention efforts will rest on whether we are able to diminish the belief among youths that their thoughts, their desires, their needs, and, most of all, their personal selves are not valued. The primary focus of intervention is not a matter of "taming the beast" in young people. Rather, it is a complex process orchestrated by caring adults to foster emotional and social growth, based on sensitivity to the common and variant needs of youths.

CHARACTERISTICS OF EFFECTIVE SCHOOLS

A foundation for creating safe schools, based on a prevention perspective, can begin with what we have learned about our most effective schools. Generally, an effective school is one with high student achievement and high morale among both students and staff. The pursuit of school improvement has produced many studies on effective or high-quality schools (Crawford et al., 1993). Although there are different measures of effectiveness, a review of the literature has yielded some common characteristics of these schools (Minnesota Department of Education, 1989). The following brief description of these characteristics is provided to support the assertion that the ecology of effective schools is less vulnerable to factors that contribute to student aggression and control issues.

The first characteristic is a common sense of purpose among the school staff regarding the vision, mission, or philosophy of the school, together with clearly defined goals that guide ongoing school improvement activities. This shared sense of purpose helps to ensure that the time, energy, and efforts of the staff are spent in working productively toward keeping the organization on a course that helps all students experience success in school. Second, a climate exists within these schools that supports goal setting and high expectations for both students and staff. School leaders monitor progress toward identified goals. Furthermore, the school has considerable autonomy within the school system; this enables it to determine the best means to meet its established goals and to have its own staff development program. Next, the curriculum is well organized and articulated, with time devoted to planned, purposeful, and effective models of instruction and with flexible grouping based on students' needs and learning styles. Appropriate assessment, ongoing monitoring, and instructive feedback are integral to the teaching–learning process. Behavioral issues are addressed through the consistent use of management strategies known to be effective. And, finally, effective schools have found ways to enlist parental support of school goals and to maintain parental involvement with the school.

The aforementioned first characteristic—a shared sense of the school's vision, mission, or philosophy—deserves further comment. Unfortunately, many schools have no clear and accepted philosophy and hence little sense of how to proceed when they struggle with problems. A simple but clear vision must first and foremost include a school's being a "good place to be" for all students and staff. Although the specific missions of individual schools and programs will vary to reflect the needs of their populations, a school philosophy statement must reflect the fundamental beliefs, values, and assumptions that underlie and thus guide all of the school's programs, policies, and practices. Only then can the staff determine relevant goals and objectives, work on appropriate solutions to specific problems, and set staff development agendas.

SCHOOL-BASED RESOURCES FOR DEVELOPING PROSOCIAL BEHAVIOR

Frequently, school personnel do not believe that they have the resources to respond adequately to the behavioral challenges that they face. In many instances, this may well be true. However, all schools do have resources, and they should periodically conduct an inventory and a quality analysis of these resources. An inventory is no more than a complete and accurate listing of what does exist. A quality analysis consists of a thorough examination of each item in the inventory for its strengths or assets, as well as its present weaknesses or deficits. A thoughtful and objective review of the information thus obtained can yield numerous staff-generated recommendations for school improvement, many or most of which will not require additional funding. The quality analysis process alone can help staff members focus on how to use their existing resources more effectively or improve them.

There are five types of school-based resources that can be linked to managing behavior or developing prosocial behavior: personnel, facilities, programs, specific interventions, and knowledge and skills. (Certainly, finances are also a real issue for every school.)

Personnel

The first and perhaps most important point to be made about personnel is that the staff must consist of individuals who genuinely care about students as individuals. Second, the staff–student ratio must be low enough for each student to receive a reasonable amount of attention, in order to ensure that his or her need for significance is addressed. Third, the staff should consist of individuals in different roles with varying expertise (counseling, social work, health, community liaison, etc.) to address the array of student needs. Finally, the staff must have, and productively use, the most current knowledge about effective teaching and interventions.

Facilities

The physical environment is an important consideration and can be a crucial factor in the problems that must be addressed. Aside from the obvious considerations (e.g., minimizing health and safety hazards, preventing overcrowding), school personnel must attend carefully to those environmental attributes that may either contribute to the probability of problem behavior or help to reduce risks. A thorough discussion of this topic can be found in Goldstein's (1994) *The Ecology of Aggression*, which should be read by every facility administrator.

Programs

Programs are the structured activities and services that schools offer. Included are the general curriculum, the adapted or remedial curriculum, and compensatory programs such as Title I and special education. Other programs include counseling, chemical dependence programs, recreational and vocational services, truancy prevention efforts, crisis intervention teams, parent and family support services, and social skills and behavioral incentives programs. Programs are any structured activities designed to promote the general development of all students or to provide additional support for students in need of individualized assistance. Numerous promising practices have emerged in schools, including bully prevention, conflict mediation, social skills and anger control training, and character-building programs, along with primary, secondary, and tertiary intervention models, to mention just a few. Together, these components should give the school a flexible variety of options to facilitate early identification of students who are at risk or who are already manifesting problems, as well as direct resources to ameliorate the conditions that may lead to an escalation of problems.

Interventions

Three types of interventions can be described: structural, reinforcing, and suppressive or punitive. Structural interventions are such things as clear, consistent, firm, and fair rules; appropriate assessment and feedback systems; nutrition programs; a wide variety of teaching methods and materials; conflict resolution programs; team planning and teaching; and an ongoing evaluation plan.

Reinforcing strategies include the array of tactics used to support desired behavior, ranging from thoughtful use of praise and notes home to carefully developed contract and point systems or other incentive systems. Punitive interventions must be used on some occasions to suppress unacceptable behaviors—particularly aggression, but also other behaviors that substantially disrupt an orderly and productive learning environment. Common punitive interventions include reprimands, referrals to the office, time out, suspensions, and the like. Generally, school personnel are well aware of the wide variety of intervention options available to them. A more important question has to do with how skillful staff members are in using these tools.

Too often they are applied generically, with little attention given to their appropriateness for individuals.

It is important for personnel who are distressed by students' serious problem behaviors and seek punitive solutions to be regularly reminded that although it may be essential to employ some aversive consequences, punishment by itself will not solve the problems. Punishment is a complex strategy with many possible unwanted and unintended outcomes. Furthermore, the effects of punishment vary from one individual to the next. Finally, punishment *suppresses* behaviors; it will not *eliminate* unwanted behaviors. When it is necessary to use punishment to suppress specific behaviors, it should always be part of a broader intervention plan that includes teaching or eliciting incompatible, desired behaviors and following these with high levels of reinforcement.

Knowledge and Skills

Staff development programs that encourage individual and collective growth are a vital resource for renewing commitment to a school's vision and mission, as well as enhancing the abilities of personnel to achieve the school's goals. In my view, staff development should not be limited to the occasional day devoted to a particular topic; instead, it should be a structured and ongoing school activity. Staff development is integral to a school's philosophy about learning, performance, and commitment to effective practices. It must be valued, encouraged, modeled, and reinforced by school leaders, and all personnel should be expected to participate in and contribute to the process. It can and should be an element of every staff meeting, with the agenda including information about policies, practices, and current situations.

PARENTAL, COMMUNITY, AND STUDENT INVOLVEMENT

Parental Involvement

Too often parents are viewed as part of the problem. Certainly parents and parenting practices can be factors contributing to students' problem behaviors, but they can also be resources; indeed, they can be vital in finding effective solutions. Educators must set aside notions of blaming parents and vigorously seek ways to include parents as collaborators in the effort to improve the lives of children and youths. Parents must be seen as experts on their own children, who have very valuable information about the children's needs and what will or will not be appropriate. A climate of trust can be created, based on open and honest communication and shared values. In many cases, school personnel will need to take the initiative and sustain the effort, for many parents have had unpleasant experiences with schools.

Community Involvement

There is no question that as the needs of children and youths become increasingly complex, growing numbers of demands and expectations have been placed on schools. In some ways this should not be surprising, because schools have established a history of saying, in essence, "We can do it; just give us the money." Furthermore, apart from the home, the school is where children and youths are (at least most of them). Schools alone have the mission of serving all young people. However, schools are now, more than ever, faced with the reality that they cannot achieve all their social goals alone. They must work vigorously, as one community resource, in collaboration and coordination with other such resources if they are to make a significant difference. The community has various resources, including agencies, churches, mosques, and synagogues, businesses, and caring individuals. All of these can and must be part of a collective response to meeting the needs of young people and providing an array of opportunities for healthy development. I believe that this will not happen unless and until schools take the initiative and provide the necessary leadership and coordination.

Students as Resources

Young people are not merely consumers of resources, nor do they want to be thought of as such. Indeed, the success of a prevention model will depend on providing opportunities for youths to experience significance, competence, and power through meaningful participation in and contributions to their schools and communities. Youth service programs that young people themselves help to develop can have the dual outcome of serving others in need and of building a positive and productive sense of self-worth (Emery & Richardson Turpin, 1996; Points of Light Foundation, 1995). These experiences may be crucial to any and all troubled and troubling youths.

LEADERSHIP: THE PRINCIPAL'S ROLE

It is easy to talk about what someone else should or should not do, and it is common for individuals to blame people in another role (superior or subordinate) for the problems they face. Certainly, the school principal is one of the most common targets for such blame and responsibility. The principal must respond to pressure from all sides—the central office, the building staff, parents, the community, politicians, and the students. Too frequently it is a thankless job, with endless demands and inadequate resources or encouragement. Yet there is nearly unanimous agreement that the principal provides the key to the quality of a school. Accepting the role includes accepting its responsibilities—that is, asserting leadership, advocating for all students as well as the staff, and providing a model of optimism, determination, and confidence. However, building principals cannot be blamed for the short-comings of school board members, central office staff, building staff, or members of the community. Helping troubled children and youths will take the "whole village."

CONCLUDING COMMENTS

I conclude this chapter with some personal notes. First, I strongly disagree with the current politically correct assertion that *all* students should be served in regular education classrooms regardless of the seriousness of their problems or disabilities. I do believe that there is compelling evidence against the notion of a one-size-fits-all school. There are students who, for whatever reasons, require structures and services that are best provided by an array and continuum of options, rather than added to the already chal-lenging responsibilities of regular classroom teachers and administrators. Ef-fective prevention and intervention efforts will require more options to meet individuals' needs, not fewer. Mainstream schools should and can make many changes that will increase the number of students who succeed. Such change does not imply that such schools should ignore acts of aggression or any other inappropriate social conduct. Every school must accept the challenge to teach the whole child.

Finally, I want to state that I find the often-used statement "All children can learn" offensive and degrading not only to children, but also to those who use it. Amoebas can learn! Professional educators should not even be considering such questions. The issue is not whether children can or cannot learn; rather, it is *what* they are learning—from us. I believe they should be learning about growth and development, not experiencing adults' misuse of power and control.

REFERENCES

Boyd, W. L. (2003). Public education's crisis of performance and legitimacy: Introduction and overview of the yearbook. In W. L. Boyd & D. Miretzky (Eds.), *American educa-tional governance on trial: Change and challenges: 102nd yearbook of the National Society for the Study of Education–Part I* (pp. 1–19). Chicago: National Society for the Study of Education.

Commercial Union Assurance Companies. (1978). *New clips on crime prevention.* Boston: Author.

Coopersmith, S. (1967). *The antecedents of self-esteem.* San Francisco: Freeman.

Crawford, D. K., Bodine, R. J., & Hoglund, R. G. (1993). *The school for quality learning: Managing the school and classroom the Deming way.* Champaign, IL: Research Press.

Csikszentmihalyi, M., & Schmidt, J. A. (1998). Stress and resilience in adolescence: An evolutionary perspective. In K. Borman & B. Schneider (Eds.), *The adolescent years: Social influence and educational challenges* (pp.1–17). Chicago: National Society for the Study of Education.

Emery, M., & Richardson Turpin, S. (1996). Service learning: Making the community connection. *Beyond Behavior, 7,* 15–19.

Englander, E. K. (1997). *Understanding violence.* Mahwah, NJ: Erlbaum.

Goldstein, A. (1994). *The ecology of aggression.* New York: Plenum Press.

Goodlad, J. I. (2002). Kudzu, rabbits, and school reform. *Phi Delta Kappan, 84,* 16–23.

Guetzloe, E. (1999). Violence in children and adolescents—A threat to public health and safety: A paradigm of prevention. *Preventing School Failure, 44,* 21–24.

Gun-Free Schools Act of 1994, 20 U.S.C. § 8921(b)(1).

Hedin, D., Hannes, K., & Saito, R. (1985). *Minnesota youth poll: Youth look at themselves and the world.* Minneapolis: Center for Youth Development and Research, University of Minnesota.

Jones, V. F., & Jones, L. S. (1995). *Comprehensive classroom management: Creating positive learning environments for all students* (4th ed.). Boston: Allyn & Bacon.

Kauffman, J. (2001). *Characteristics of emotional and behavioral disorders of children and youth* (7th ed.). Upper Saddle River, NJ: Prentice-Hall.

Lewis, A.C. (2002). Where is the NCLBA taking us? *Phi Delta Kappan, 84,* 4–5.

Lewis, A.C. (2003). Community counts. *Phi Delta Kappan, 85,* 179–180.

Minnesota Department of Education. (1989). *Minnesota Educational Effectiveness Program.* St. Paul: Author.

Points of Light Foundation (1995). *Everyone wins when youth serve: Building agency/school partnerships for service learning.* Washington, DC: Author.

Safe and Drug Free Schools and Communities Act of 1994, 20 U.S.C. § 7107 et seq.

U. S. Department of Justice. (2003, December). *OJJDP juvenile justice bulletin: Juvenile arrests 2001.* Washington, DC: Author.

Van Acker, R., & Talbott, E. (1999). The school context and risk for aggression: Implications for school-based prevention and intervention efforts. *Preventing School Failure, 44,* 12–20.

Wright, A. (1996). Success guaranteed: The Pathfinder Project. *Preventing School Failure, 40,* 67–72.

CHAPTER 4

The State Department
of Education's Role
in Creating Safe Schools

MARILYN L. GRADY
JEAN HAAR
MARY ANN LOSH

HISTORY

The authority for public education in the United States does not stem from
the Constitution, but rather is a "reserved" power remaining with the states.
It originates from the Tenth Amendment, which reserves to the states those
powers neither expressly given to the national government nor denied to the
state governments. However, most states have not exercised their authority
for public education directly until recent decades. Education is a state function that is largely locally administered (Alkin, Linden, Noel, & Ray, 1992).

Each state exercises its education function completely or in part through
a state department of education that has varying degrees of responsibility.
The state educational authority gains its powers and responsibilities specifically from the state's constitution and statutes (Deighton, 1971).

State departments of education emerged and became firmly established
during the period from 1812 to 1890. Although the first responsibilities of
these departments during this period were advisory, statistical, and
exhortatory, state departments of education began to come into their own
with the swift expansion of public education after the Civil War.

During the 1890–1932 period, the regulatory functions of the state departments of education were expanded with the general acceptance of compulsory education. Only a state department of education could determine
that compulsory attendance requirements were being enforced. The mainte-

nance and operational functions of the state departments of education were strengthened. The need for stronger state educational agencies that could determine whether minimum standards were being met was demonstrated.

The years from 1932 to 1953 saw the expansion of the service and support functions of the state departments of education and the emergence of their leadership role. One of the first significant leadership activities that was aimed essentially at the rural United States can be traced to statewide reorganization efforts.

From 1953 to 1970 federal influence on education increased, and state departments of education were strengthened through the concept of "federal partnership." This phase marked the beginning of the modern federal aid program for education. In many ways federal involvement was encouraged by the National Defense Education Act (NDEA) of 1958, through which the federal government dealt directly with local school districts, colleges, and universities.

The NDEA, enacted after the launching of Sputnik I, actually resulted in an upheaval in the structure of state departments of education rather than in stability. An infusion of federal funds enabled a few states to move out of their former passive roles, but the most notable effect was an imbalance within the organization of the departments. By 1950 half of the professional staff members of state departments of education were assigned to federally subsidized programs; by 1960 that percentage had risen to 56%, and in 13 states to more than 70% (Deighton, 1971). In 1963, the Advisory Council on State Departments of Education pointed out that most departments could not fully perform the duties expressly delegated to them by state legislatures because of personnel shortages (U.S. Office of Education, 1966).

Subsequent acts helped state agencies to improve and establish their leadership roles in areas such as civil rights and educational planning. In addition, state agencies have developed modern data systems and more effective personnel procedures, have found more effective ways of disseminating educational information, and have adopted modern curriculum materials. State agencies have also assumed leadership in designing and expediting research; in studying methods of financing education in the state; in providing advisory, technical, and consultative assistance; in improving working relationships with other state education departments; in identifying emerging educational problems; and in promoting teacher improvement courses (Deighton, 1971).

FUNCTIONS AND STRUCTURE OF STATE DEPARTMENTS

In general, each state department of education has four major functions or roles: regulation, operation, administration of special services, and leadership of the state program. The structure and staffing of the departments vary widely from state to state, however.

Regulation

The regulatory role consists of (1) determining that basic administrative duties have been performed by local schools in compliance with state and local laws, (2) ascertaining that proper safeguards are employed in the use of public school funds, (3) enforcing health and safety rules for construction and maintenance of buildings, (4) enforcing and determining the proper certification of teachers and educational personnel, (5) ensuring that minimum educational opportunities are provided for all children through enforcement of compulsory schooling laws and child labor laws, as well as through pupil personnel services, (6) ensuring comprehensive programs of high quality and ascertaining that required procedures are used, and (7) ensuring that schools are organized according to the law. The regulatory function of all state departments of education is based on the acceptance of the fact that education is a state function and that local school districts' operational authority flows from state statutes.

Operation

The operational role of the state education department varies greatly from state to state, with a general trend away from having the state department of education perform direct operational functions. The state department of education is the logical agency to step in and fill a need if there is no existing institution capable of doing so; as emergencies pass, however, provisions are generally made to turn the operational reins over to organizations designed to carry out specific functions, and few people would seriously propose a completely state-controlled school system operated through the state department of education. Historically, states have accepted responsibility for the operation of educational agencies and services when no other agency could provide the necessary statewide direction, especially during the developmental stages of a particular program or enterprise.

Administration of Special Services

The role of the state in the administration of special services developed because of the need for statewide uniformity and efficiency in educational services. These are services that, because of their scope, technical nature, or expense, can be offered more efficiently on a statewide basis. A state department of education can provide local school districts, the legislature, the executive office, and the general public with basic information about the status of education in the state (e.g., comparative studies and statistical information; clarification of all statutes, rules, and regulations on education).

Leadership

The leadership function of a state department of education comprises conducting long-range studies for planning the total state program of education, studying ways of improving education, providing consultant services, encouraging cooperation, promoting balance among all units of the educational system, informing the public of educational needs and progress, encouraging public support and participation, providing in-service education for all persons in the state engaged in educational work including standards, assessment and accountability systems.

Staff and Structure

Although all states have departments of education, these departments differ in structure, as well as in size and organization, and specific functions. All states have some type of state board of education, but there is great variation in the amount of control exerted by the board on the department and on the overall state educational system. Every state has a school officer responsible for the department, but, again, the responsibilities of this officer vary among the states. Some officers are political leaders and others are educational leaders, some are appointed and others are elected; some are regarded as the chief educational officers of their states and others are among many in the educational hierarchy who have state educational responsibilities.

CREATING SAFE SCHOOLS: A SURVEY OF STATE DEPARTMENTS

One area of state education departments' leadership is creating safe schools. Providing a safe school environment is imperative. For many children, schools are the safest places in their lives. The concept that schools should be safe havens has found support in law throughout the history of public schools. For teachers to teach and children to learn, there must be a safe and inviting educational environment (Curcio & First, 1993; Kaufman, 2000). In this context, we replicated our 1995 national survey (Grady, Krumm, & Losh, 1997) to determine what each state was doing to create safe havens for children.

Procedures

To obtain the information needed to answer the questions addressed in this study, we conducted interviews with individuals who work in state departments of education. Subjects were identified through a listing of persons involved with activities promoting safe and drug-free schools. In all, we were able to visit by telephone with individuals from 45 of the 50 states.

The telephone interviews were conducted during the spring of 2001. Interviewees responded to a series of school-violence–relevant questions we developed. The length of each interview was between 15 and 30 minutes. The responses to the telephone interviews follow.

Findings

Four main categories emerged from the telephone interviews: legislation, prevention, services, and collaboration.

Legislative Mandates, Initiatives, Policies

Conversations with state department of education officials often began with comments such as "Because of legislation passed we are . . . " or "Approximately a year ago, the governor mandated. . . . " Thirty-four of the interviewees mentioned legislative mandates, initiatives, or policies.

In connection to these laws, the state department of education officials are in liaison positions. They are responsible for overseeing compliance to state mandates, initiatives, and policies while providing schools with the assistance, training, and resources needed to reach compliance.

Mandates included establishing behavior standards, developing crisis and safety plans, developing policies, providing services for students in schools, and implementing specific programs such as Character Education, Codes of Conduct, Conflict Resolution, and Peer Mediation.

Mandates, initiatives, and policies were viewed as a means of reaching the ultimate goal of creating a safe school environment. As noted by one state department director, "A State Board meeting amended a state regulation that added a section on safe schools. What they said was that 'Schools will be safe for all students without exception, optimal for academic achievement and free from harassment.' "

In describing mandates, initiatives, and policies, the comments focused either on what was being addressed or on how it was being implemented. Participant comments related to "what was being addressed" follow.

"Last year legislation was passed that schools adopt behavior standards if they had not already done so. Those behavior standards were pretty loosely defined. They focused on issues of harassment, bullying, fighting and things like that."

"Current legislative session talk is about conflict mediation and peer mediation. A lot of discussion in the legislature is about anti-hate-crime legislation and how that will have an impact on schools."

"The state has legislation in place mandating that schools report certain incidents and that districts collect that information. Legislation also provides funding for program development in school climate and school safety programs."

"Basically, we were given our power under a Senate bill. It mandates that all schools create a comprehensive school safety plan. Under this bill they have to address hostage situations, incidents of weapons at school, violent incidents, bomb threats, incidents that occur in their school safety zones and during noninstructional hours."

"We are one of four states that have a regulation that mandates pupil services in our schools. So children have access to a school counselor, a school psychologist, and a school nurse."

The following participant comments are related to how legislative mandates, initiatives, and policies were being implemented:

"We go in and ensure that schools have plans in place to handle critical incidents. This is a state statute now, and schools are required to comply."

"In 1996 each school site was to have a safe school committee with a minimum of six members, made up of an equal number of parents, students, and teachers. There is current legislation to add someone from law enforcement, the fire department, and a community action agency. We also recommend that the school counselor, school nurse, custodian, and a bus driver be included in the safe school committee. They are to meet and make recommendations to their school principal regarding any school safety concerns that they feel are important."

"The General Assembly created a Center for School Safety with criminal justice services. There has been a good working relationship between the director and the Department of Education. The Center has done far more than we have been able to do in school safety. It took on the training of the school resource officers, for example."

"Legislation enacted the Safe Schools Act. It requires different sets of policies. Some of those policies were already on the books, but some statutes were moved around to create one comprehensive package. That law is to help remove disruptive students from a classroom sooner. It also allows those students to be given services much earlier on in order to intervene with disruptive behaviors. It's trying to beef up the efforts for identifying problems earlier and getting them addressed—more of an intervention strategy."

"Each school district is required to develop crisis plans and safety plans. The legislature also appropriated funds to assist the State Department of Education. We started an initiative with the State Highway Patrol here to establish a school safety hot line. The hot line gives students the opportunity to anonymously report any potential violence."

"Having these mandates and policies is just one component of the effort. It's such a complex problem that you need to address it at multiple levels and along multiple avenues. We always seem to promote the same message in many ways in order to shape social norms that will get people to either avoid the less desirable behaviors or adopt those that are desirable. Certainly, laws and policies have their place; we see that in the substance abuse prevention field a lot. If there are laws and rules, policies and mandates, they are proven to be effective in deterring certain behaviors."

Prevention

The emphasis of the state departments of education in school safety is on prevention. Twenty-two of the individuals interviewed commented extensively about prevention being key to diminishing school violence. Although the departments of education are providing services and working on documents that address three areas: prevention, intervention, and response, the strongest emphasis is on prevention.

According to the interviewees, when state departments of education are addressing prevention, they should focus on student needs and concerns. Conversations centered on the need to establish a positive school climate as well as on the need to provide student services, especially in the areas of counseling and health. Assisting with student problems and issues immediately, rather than allowing them to escalate, was noted as key to curtailing violence. Bullying, harassment, and hazing are topics that are receiving considerable attention. Twenty of the interviewees noted that either one or all three of these issues were being addressed in their states. No longer is it acceptable to look at such incidents as a norm or as "part of growing up"; rather, they are seen as crucial to whether a safe and peaceful atmosphere is being provided for students.

The following are participant comments concerning preventive measures:

"The focus is shifting. At first it was mainly weapons and drugs and things of that kind. Now it is shifting to the internal climate of the schools and what's going on there—what is causing the individuals to do what they are doing rather then how they are doing it. The aim is shifting to character building and the prevention of bullying."

"Each school system has developed a countywide action plan, which individual schools will have to incorporate into their school plans over the next year. The aim is to look at what we are doing about harassment and bullying, how we can eliminate these behaviors from our schools, how we can create safe, nurturing environments where kids feel as though they belong, where they are not harassed, and where there are consequences for harassment and bullying."

"We have developed a 'reparative program.' After any type of incident, we bring together all involved and, in a humane manner, address what happened. The idea is to establish a level of civility and order that will help kids feel safe."

"We work closely with the department of corrections, which is a progressive department and does a lot of work in reparative and restorative justice. And so we advocate that after a bomb threat, after a hazing incident, after any type of threat to the safety and security of the school or community, we bring victims and perpetrators and bystanders together and do what we can in a humane way to bring back a sense of safety and security. We believe that if you can do that right, you can make the school and community safer and more secure in the minds of people then it was before the event took place."

"We have a large grant that is placing school resource officers and probation officers in the classrooms to provide law-related education."

"Several districts employ school resource officers who are police officers with special training in conflict resolution and working toward peaceful schools. In addition, we have a school nurse in every school, and every high school has a school-based health center that provides counseling, referrals, and a wide range of services."

"We have created a Threat and Tip website in partnership with the Federal Bureau of Investigation and the net authorities. It provides a way for students to report tips anonymously via the computer. We have had a lot of tips on the website. Students can also get feedback on what they report. For instance, if a student reports that some kid has been bringing a gun to school, the student can include his e-mail address and get information back on the steps taken by the school and law enforcement.

It is also a way for parents, teachers, and students to get resources. This is an informational website for topics such as teen suicide, depression, alcoholism, and the like."

"We have anonymous hotlines. We have also endorsed some peer helping on how to recognize and reduce violence by empowering the kids to report violence."

"On the prevention side of the effort, we offer credit classes in a program called 'Get Real about Violence.' We also offer credit classes in bullying prevention, and the granddaddy of all is our 'Rough Rider Health Promotion Conference,' in which schools can team to develop an action plan that is broader in total prevention. Violence prevention can be, and is encouraged to be, a part of it. The schools do the needs assessment to decide what aspect of prevention they want to address."

"Most problems in our schools are not horrific incidents but classroom disruptions. What we find is that classroom disruptions, either physical attack on a student or fighting, are still significant problems in our schools. One of the things that we recognize is that we have kids who are coming to school with very diverse backgrounds and from very diverse communities. The behaviors that may be appropriate for their survival or their existence in those communities are inappropriate for doing well in school. So we are moving heavily in the direction of looking at schools in terms of positive behavioral interventions—teaching kids the social skills they need to be successful. One program in our department is called 'Positive Behavior Interventions.' It has schools look at schoolwide positive interventions—teaching kids what they need to know, having schoolwide policies, analyzing data. I feel very strongly that we need to look at prevention and teach kids that there are ways of getting along so that they don't have those conflicts that need to be mediated. Our focus is very much on teaching social skills."

"We are promoting violence prevention curricula. We are really going to have to concentrate on bullying. Now the governor has a bill for Character Education, and he is defining that as the Five Rs. Two of those Rs are respect and responsibility, and he wants to pass that respect and responsibility bill."

A focus of the conversations was on meeting student needs, as shown in the following comments from participants:

"A lot of what is addressed is related to school climate. We are finding that students need more counseling services as opposed to medical services—counseling services related to relationship problems and other problems that are often related to school violence. We just sent a team to do training on gay, lesbian, and bisexual students. We are providing a link for support services for kids. If we don't address the relationship issues, then the students turn to alcohol, tobacco, and violence in the school. The internal struggles and feelings of nonacceptance can be linked to school violence. I say to schools that there are certain factors—relationships, body image, and struggles with sexual orientation—that we feel are very important links to suicide. Another question, in this age of accountability and test scores, is how these pressures are affecting students. The most important question is how a student is dealing with all of these issues."

"What we are dealing with now are the other issues, the emotional and social issues. When looking at the profiles of the kids like those at Columbine, we recognize that we might be able to identify some potential candidates, but we will never be able to figure out who is actually going to commit such violence and who can't. But looking again at their profiles, we see that these kids, for the most part, were bullied, and so we recognize that bullying, teasing, and harassment are major issues in schools. We also looked at the mental health aspect and tried to put more mental health services in schools for kids."

"We want to be on top—100% in prevention of dangerous situations. We want to be ready in the event of a disaster."

Services

For the state department of education personnel charged with the responsibility of creating safe schools, the largest portion of time is spent in providing schools with services. Thirty-nine individuals described this service role. Services were categorized into two areas: the physical aspect of safety and the social and emotional aspects of safety. The physical aspect of safety included providing training, developing documents, administering funds, managing grants, and reviewing plans. The social and emotional aspects included the human side of school safety and addressing student needs. When describing social and emotional safety, discussions focused on social skills, behavior interventions, and counseling.

The following section highlights the physical or technical aspects of what state departments of education and, in a few instances, what other agencies are doing for schools. The social and emotional components are addressed in the preceding section on prevention.

Significant amounts of time and money have been spent on researching and developing information about school safety; the struggle to get that information to schools and others has been eased by technology. Thirty-two of the interview subjects mentioned websites as a method of providing information. Websites were used for posting documents, providing agency names and numbers, listing available resources, and, in increasing numbers, providing a hot line for reporting possible incidents of violence.

The physical or technical aspects of safety include three areas: training and technical assistance, workshops and conferences, and documents and resources. The following are participant comments about each of these areas. Twenty-six individuals noted their efforts to provide training and technical assistance.

"The department provided training and technical assistance in each region regarding the four components of the plan as well as other facets of school safety. A plan was written for each of the schools with assistance from advisory councils. The plans came back to the department, where each plan was reviewed and read."

"We provide information and spend a lot of time talking to districts about research-based programs surrounding conflict resolution. We also work on policy development. We are working more with groups like the National Education Association (NEA) and the Parent-Teacher Association (PTA) around this topic and are trying to reach their constituents with the best policies we can offer."

"We provide as much technical assistance as possible, everything is based on individual needs, ranging from those of large school districts to those of very small districts, as well as those of geographical areas."

"We are helping districts comply with Principles of Effectiveness. We also completed a study involving principals and lead health education teachers in middle schools and high schools. We asked questions about their backgrounds and certifications and, more important, about their staff development needs. We provide training based on this background information."

"We handle the programming aspect of the prevention programs, whether for violence, drugs, or another target. We are in the process of establishing a critical incident reporting system."

"The state legislature gave our department money to train a school safety specialist. We used the money to conduct a School Safety Specialist Academy. More than half of the participants are school administrators; some are school counselors. They are trained and sent back to the schools to pass on what they have learned. We bring in specialists for the training. The CIA, the Secret Service, and the State Police have provided programs on security, prevention of bullying, and school climate, among other subjects."

"We are providing expertise to local coordinators in how best to write measurable goals and objectives, how to identify research-based programs, and what can happen as a result of such efforts."

"We conduct classes on bomb threat management, visual weapons screening, and how to detect weapons on students. We also advise participants on how to develop their plans. We take them through the entire process. We approve the plans and provide the technical assistance training as well. We also do site surveys or site assessments, in which we go out to the school and work with the local public safety and school officials. We do a walk-through of the school and talk about policies and procedures to tighten up on their safety and security and then send them a report on our findings."

"We use funds for counseling services called Student Assistant Counselors. These are student assistant programs that help students on issues surrounding alcohol and drugs, but certainly they address issues of safety. There is a relationship between all of the behaviors involved. These programs cover a wide range of activities."

Workshops and conferences continue to be popular means of sharing information and strategies concerning school safety. Fifteen individuals noted the importance of these activities.

"We are organizing our third annual conference for preventing youth violence. This is not strictly for schools; we invite a wide spectrum of people. In most of the things we do, we try to make it a community-based presentation, because if something happens at the school, it's the community that is going to have to respond."

"We have a Safe and Healthy School Conference annually and co-sponsor a gang prevention workshop annually. These are statewide programs. We also offer monthly videoconference training in the area of health, safety, and physical education."

"We are getting ready to offer five half-day workshops around the state. They are designed especially for superintendents, assistant superintendents, and school board members, helping them to determine good local policy that supports student searches and protects students' rights."

"We had a 2-day safe school conference. We are really looking at what it takes to make our schools safe and what kinds of programs are research-based, effective programs to implement in schools."

"Right now we are planning a summer institute, to which we will invite counselors, teachers, principals, child welfare and attendance professionals, members of law enforcement, and others in the community who may be interested. We have tracks in preteen sex, bullying, and violence. We are planning a back-to-school kickoff in August. We are joining with the attorney general's office and doing a 2-day conference on health services and education and prevention."

"One of our other state agencies, the Office of Emergency Management, offers, free of charge to any school district, a 2- or 3-day in-depth training on crisis response and emergency planning. It has included new components to consider student safety, such as how to protect students if an intruder has walked into a building and evacuation plans."

Documents and other resources were described as important tools provided through the auspices of department of education personnel. Twenty participants made comments about resources that had been developed and distributed.

"The Center for Law and Civic Education, with the Attorney General's Office and the State Department of Education, has been working on a document for the last 5 years, called 'Play by the Rules.' This is a hand-out booklet for the students, given in the seventh grade, that covers every law in the state and its consequences—a means of making students aware of the new laws."

"Last summer we released our new health and education curriculum framework, which is a guideline for K–12 instructional programs on what kids need to know to be health literate. To that end, it is linked to the national assessment project, of which we are a part, that looks at what is required for safe and drug-free schools. This is a large document, but sometime soon we will have the framework part of it on our website."

"We wrote a safe school guide. A copy was mailed to every principal and superintendent. The U.S. Department of Education, the Office of Civil Rights, and the Attorney General's Office put together a manual called *Protecting Students from Harassment and Hate Crimes*, and we mass-produced it and sent it to every principal and superintendent."

"We developed a Crisis Management Resource Guide and printed more than 20,000 copies of the document. We have held 17 different workshops across the state for our school administrators, and they are still asking for them. The General Assembly approached us, wanting a model of what a crisis plan looks like. We put a document together and have reprinted it many times; we have also given several state departments of education throughout the United States permission to reproduce it."

"Four years ago schools indicated to me that they needed teaching materials in inhalant prevention. The information didn't exist, so we had to create it. We first printed 5,000 copies; these ran out and we had to do another printing. We are also trying to put as much information as possible on the website."

"We worked on two documents dealing with student searches. One was in direct response to the General Assembly, which has said, 'We want you to develop guidelines that pertain to how to conduct student searches.' Before we could finish it, the Assembly added, 'We want you to include strip searches in the guidelines.' After completing that document, we developed a School Search Resource Guide."

"A subcommittee that was co-chaired by the Department of Education and the state police expanded on the current crisis plan. We developed a flip chart with law enforcement and crisis agencies. All of our schools have these crisis plans, which include not only loss and grief issues such as suicide, accidental death, and homicide, but also physical crises in other horrific events. It covers the continuum of crises that can happen."

"We are looking at the new Culture for Lawfulness right now. This program teaches kids what will happen to their families and friends if they go to prison. It changes their attitudes. This is a 40-hour course, recommended to be taught through ninth-grade health or social studies."

"We have distributed a multilayered, multicolored crisis management guide to every parish in the state and also provided a disk so that it can be customized for every school in a parish. We joined with the Attorney General's Office and the Office of Preparedness in this effort, and it has been a huge success.

Collaboration Efforts

Nationwide, people have realized that creating safe schools is an issue of concern for all, not just for those who work in school systems. Twenty-six of the subjects shared examples of collaborative efforts among various departments, agencies, and organizations. The states' attorney generals' offices appear as frequent collaborative partners; also mentioned were law enforcement, social services, and health departments. Participant comments follow.

"We are a prevention-oriented state. We have a Prevention Institute that brings all agencies together."

"We have a subcommittee of counselors, including not just school counselors but also counselors from the Health Department, the Department of Human Services, and the private sector, working on a guide or crisis manual that will be published. They will do training as well."

"The Commissioner of Education is calling for an interagency task force on school safety to bring together people from the Commissioner level and all the state agencies and nonprofits to talk about these issues. This will include all state agencies, the president of the PTA, and the president of the NEA."

"A committee that investigates student deaths has a meeting once a month for each county. Everybody takes part—police, social workers, people from the Attorney General's Office, protective services—we all come to the table with our sides of the story and investigate case by case to see if there are any recommendations we can make to stop such things from happening."

"We join with the administrator's association, the fire marshal, and the school police and go to the Federal Emergency Management Agency (FEMA) or for training in multihazard emergency management."

"The governor and the state superintendent co-sponsored a statewide safe school summit last year. We invited national violence prevention and safety experts, including specialists in parenting. One session was for the Safe School Committee members, parents, students, and teachers, and the other session was for parents, community leaders, and other interested parties."

"We are piggybacking with the effective practice project from the governor's office and expanding on that original work. We are bringing mental health professionals into the same arena. They say 'science based'; we say 'research based,' and the reality is that every bit of it is exactly and precisely the same thing."

"We work very closely with our health education specialist, and she adds the curriculum component to all the programs I have."

"We developed a safe schools interagency steering committee that is co-chaired with our state superintendent of schools and our lieutenant governor. Several subcommittees developed as a result of that interagency committee. A subcommittee that was co-chaired by the Department of Education and the State Police expanded on the crisis plan."

"We are joining with the Attorney General's Office and holding a 2-day conference on health services and education and prevention."

"The Attorney General's Office is working with us and doing a walk-through of schools to make sure they are safe. The Attorney General's Office is also working with us to help those schools that have not completed their risk management plan or that need some more work on it."

"School safety isn't just a school problem, it is a community problem. So the community is going to have to pitch in, and that means parents, mentors, and other interested parties, have to be part of the solution and support our kids, who are trying to keep our schools safe."

SUMMARY

All interview subjects shared a focus on prevention as key to meeting the challenge of creating safe schools for all students. Those who described legislative mandates perceived the mandates as tools to strengthen and reinforce the programs, resources, and research they had identified as essential for establishing safe schools.

Research-based resources and the use of expert advice were two essentials for the training or programs provided by the state departments of education. Data collection efforts assisted in determining school needs, as well as in addressing the accountability concerns.

The state department of education personnel we interviewed are passionate and knowledgeable about creating safe schools, are confident that they are providing the type of services that schools need, and are committed to reaching the goal of providing all students with a safe learning environment. They are also busy people. Collaborative efforts, the necessity of collecting data, and the efforts to stay abreast with information and research cause these positions to be challenging and demanding. If these individuals are not organizing and providing training and resources to schools, they are attending national conferences, developing resources, or meeting with various constituents. Reaching each of the individuals we interviewed was difficult and involved many telephone calls to schedule the interviews. However, once the connections were made, the conversations were rich and detailed.

IMPLICATIONS

A state department of education provides leadership, guidance, staff development, federal program implementation, and supervision of the state school system. Although each state department's responsibilities vary by statute, the common core of duties generally includes consultative services, development and dissemination of materials that assist in the improvement of educational programs, establishment of the rules and regulations that govern standards of school operation, and accreditation of schools.

State departments also provide a conduit or connection to information not easily available at the local district level. Often this information is shared with districts via conferences/workshops, curriculum materials, on-site visits, phone assistance, websites, and networks of expertise. Local districts develop or adopt programs to serve students. These programs are, or can be, tailored to meet the unique needs of students in each school building. Assistance in learning about violence prevention programs and resources is provided through a variety of sources, depending on the structure of the state department. From our survey, it is apparent that state departments of education are important sources for connecting local school district staff with resources.

Violence often results from a complex interaction of environmental, social, and psychological factors. Among these factors are the learned behavior of responding to conflict with violence, the effects of drugs or alcohol, the presence of weapons, and the absence of positive family relationships or adult supervision. Few violence prevention programs are capable of affecting all the possible causes. The key to providing students with the skills, knowledge, and motivation they require to become healthy adults is a comprehensive program that responds to the new risks and pressures arising with each developmental stage. Addressing these risks requires a sustained effort throughout children's entire school careers (Posner, 1994, 1996).

Evaluation, or the lack of it, is a concern. Schools and school personnel may not have the expertise to evaluate and select prevention programs. Few administrators under pressure to "do something" about violence have the resources or the expertise to assess the extent of their schools' violence problems, to judge whether the programs they have chosen are appropriate for their students, or to find evidence that the programs actually work.

The key to success is knowing "which types of programs should be offered to whom, by whom, and at what age." Programs must take into account the age group being targeted, the behaviors being targeted, the selection and training of leaders, and the influence of the community. Many of the most promising strategies are family interventions that teach parenting skills and improved family relationships. The need to involve parents as well as teachers in violence prevention training programs is critical (Grady, 1995).

An emerging role for state departments of education is providing assistance in the selection and implementation of promising practices. This developing role reflects a nationwide movement among state departments of education from simply enforcing regulations to providing consultation services. The selection of promising practices includes assisting schools with the evaluation of student needs and identifying appropriate program options. Dissemination of research results, program implications, and ways to use this information locally in the development of a comprehensive plan is becoming a function for state agencies.

The ability of state departments of education to provide such assistance is dependent on their having the financial resources to do so. Historically, federal funding has provided state departments with resources that have included "flow-through" dollars to districts, as well as state agency staffers who give districts leadership assistance. Federal dollars for safe schools have been used to provide program stability. As those dollars decrease, the existence of safe school programs is threatened.

REFERENCES

Alkin, M. C., Linden, M., Noel, J., & Ray. K. (Eds.). (1992). *Encyclopedia of educational research* (6th ed., Vol. 4). New York: Macmillian.

Curcio, J. L., & First, P. F. (1993). *Violence in schools: How to proactively prevent and defuse it.* Newbury Park, CA: Corwin Press.

Deighton, L. C. (Ed.) (1971). *The encyclopedia of education* (Vol. 8). New York: Macmillian/Free Press.

Grady, M. L. (1995). *Creating safe schools.* Lincoln: Nebraska Department of Education.

Grady, M. L., Krumm, B. L., & Losh, M. A. (1997). The state department of education's role in creating safe schools. In A. P. Goldstein & J. C. Conoley (Eds.), *School violence intervention: A practical handbook* (pp. 58–71). New York: Guilford Press.

Kaufman, P. (2000). *Indicators of school crime and safety, 2000.* Washington, DC: U.S. Government Printing Office.

National Defense Education Act of 1958, Public Law No. 85–864, Title XX, Education, 20 U.S.C. § 401 (1996).

Posner, M. (1994). Research raises troubling questions about violence prevention programs. *Harvard Education Letter, 10*(3), 1–4.

Posner, M. (1996). *Youth violence: Locating and using the data.* Newton, MA: Education Development Center.

U.S. Office of Education, Advisory Council on State Departments of Education (1966). *Improving state leadership in education: First annual report, 1964–1965.* Washington, DC: U.S. Government Printing Office.

PART III
Student-Oriented Interventions

CHAPTER 5

Preschool Interventions

KAREN T. CAREY

The preschool years, generally defined as the ages from 2 to 5, constitute the most significant period for human development. "It is unquestionably the period during which the foundation is laid for the complex behavioral structures that are built in a child's lifetime" (Bijou, 1975, p. 829). Thus, the behaviors of noncompliance, aggression, and disruption that a child evidences in early life can be manifested in lifelong difficulties. However, early intervention for such problems can be effective in establishing proactive and positive interactions for young children.

The passage of federal legislation in 1986 (Preschool Education of the Handicapped Act, Public Law 99-457, amended in 1990 by the Individuals with Disabilities Act, Public Law 101-476) testifies to the importance of early intervention. This legislation mandates that educational services be provided to children between birth and 5 years of age, as well as to their families. Although educators and policy makers have given much attention to early intervention, many questions remain about the best ways to carry out interventions for young children (Barnett, Bell, & Carey, 1999).

The basic premise of any early intervention is that the least intrusive intervention that will accomplish goals for change should be used whenever possible. Interventions that can fit into, or be adapted to, existing styles of parenting or teaching should be explored first. A model for early intervention that has been found to be effective is the "naturalistic intervention" model (Barnett & Carey, 1992). Naturalistic intervention design stresses the analysis of the roles, routines, skills, and interests of the targeted child and caregivers. As a form of environmental intervention (Hart, 1985), naturalistic interventions are based on developmental studies of competent caregivers (Sigel, 1982; White, Kaban, & Attanucci, 1979). Caregivers select learning events, focus the children's attention on those that are important, and, following the children's lead, encourage curiosity and skill development. Caregivers using these skills provide some experiences intentionally and also frame serendipitous events; both types of experiences give children the opportunity to learn cognitive, behavioral, language, and affective skills.

Naturalistic interventions are guided by social-cognitive theory (Bandura, 1986), particularly the concept of "reciprocal influence." Interactions of person, behavioral, and environmental variables are analyzed and systematically assessed by means of time-series designs. Furthermore, naturalistic interventions are framed within the scientist/practitioner model. Using research to guide the development, implementation, and evaluation of interventions can provide empirical accountability and the ability to generalize from intervention research. Research-based interventions specifically designed for preschool children are limited, and thus one is often required to generalize from studies conducted with other populations. For example, interventions conducted with developmentally delayed older students can often be effective with preschool children. In this chapter, research-based naturalistic interventions for a variety of aggressive, disruptive, and noncompliant behaviors are reviewed.

TECHNIQUES FOR MANAGING PROBLEM BEHAVIORS

Problem behaviors of young children may be viewed as either excesses or deficits in desirable behaviors. However, well-designed and well-implemented interventions may increase appropriate behaviors while reducing inappropriate behaviors. Techniques used to reduce maladaptive behavior are referred to as "positive reductive procedures" (Dietz & Repp, 1983, p. 35) and are basic components of naturalistic interventions. Such techniques involve "differential reinforcement," which is used for building skills or altering patterns of behavior: Certain responses or classes of behaviors are reinforced, while others are not. Such procedures are often very effective with young children.

Differential reinforcement includes differential reinforcement of alternative behavior (DRA), in which a more acceptable behavior is substituted for the maladaptive behavior and occurrences of the acceptable behavior are reinforced. For example, if a child is unoccupied in the classroom, increasing appropriate play is an alternative behavior. Differential reinforcement of incompatible behavior (DRI) occurs when reinforcement is presented if the child performs a desirable behavior that is the opposite of the target behavior. For instance, a child cannot be both attending and off-task, or both isolated and engaged in peer play, at the same time. Differential reinforcement of functional behavior (DRF), as described by Rolider and VanHouten (1990), is based on the functional analysis of behavior: A new behavior that serves the same function as the maladaptive behavior is taught. Examples include teaching children how to receive attention appropriately, or how to escape stressful or demanding situations appropriately instead of having tantrums. Differential reinforcement of other behavior

(DRO) requires the caregiver to provide reinforcement for all responses except the target behavior. Reinforcement occurs when the child does not perform the target behavior for certain time intervals. DRO has been applied to self-injurious, aggressive, and disruptive behaviors (Poling & Ryan, 1982). Differential reinforcement of low rates of behavior (DRL) is a procedure to reduce rather than eliminate behavior, but it can be used as a first step in eliminating undesirable behaviors when behavior rates are high. For example, a child who makes numerous comments during group discussions may be allowed only a set number of comments during a specified time period.

Differential reinforcement procedures can be effective across many domains. However, appropriate alternative behaviors must be within the child's performance capabilities. DRO and DRL focus on negative and not on appropriate behavior, although DRA and modeling can be added. Self-monitoring and other feedback systems can be combined with these differential reinforcement procedures.

Modifications of the differential reinforcement procedures can be used to reduce or eliminate behavior problems. Some examples of such modifications are presented throughout the rest of the chapter.

AVERSIVE PROCEDURES AND PUNISHMENT

In many ways, punishment should be viewed as a strategy that is naturalistically used or misused by caregivers (Axelrod, 1990) and thus must be considered in many situations. For some caregivers, punishment administered to children may be reinforcing. Many commentators believe that punishment should never be used (Donnellan & LaVigna, 1990), whereas others argue that for certain behaviors involving risk, harm, or unfortunate consequences of intervention failure, interventions involving punishment may be considered at the behavioral identification stage (Axelrod, 1990). When one is considering the use of punishment or another aversive intervention, it is important to analyze the intervention with respect to the likelihood of risk or harm to the child or others, the results of a thorough problem analysis, and the likelihood of the intervention's effectiveness. Whenever punishment is used, appropriate alternative behaviors should be reinforced. Interventions that are considered aversive include time out, contingent observation, response cost, overcorrection, planned ignoring, extinction, and reprimands. These procedures are reviewed briefly.

Time Out

"Time out" is considered a punishment procedure, as it involves a child's being denied access to the opportunity to earn positive reinforcement for brief periods of time, contingent on a targeted maladaptive behavior. To be effective, the "time-in" environment must be reinforcing. Time-out durations for preschool applications should be relatively brief and are dependent on the child's history with the procedures. Isolation or seclusionary time out is not recommended for preschool children (Barnett & Carey, 1992).

Firestone (1976) evaluated the use of time out with a 4½-year-old boy in a nursery school. The child had a history of aggressive behaviors and was expelled from one nursery school at the age of 3. For every physically aggressive act, the child was placed in a chair in the corner of the classroom for 2 minutes. Physical and verbal aggressiveness decreased significantly, and cooperative play increased.

In a modified version of time out, Foxx and Shapiro (1978) used ribbons as a discriminative cue for reinforcement with older developmentally delayed students. Students were given different-colored ribbons to wear as ties and were rewarded with edibles and praise approximately every 2½ minutes for engaging in appropriate behavior. For any misbehavior, the ribbon was removed for 3 minutes, and the child was not given any edibles, praise, or access to activities during this time. The results indicated that the ribbon procedure significantly decreased disruptive behavior; however, when children were not wearing their ribbons (e.g., when they were entering the classroom), disruptive behavior reappeared. In case studies, this intervention has been found to be effective with preschool-age children as well.

Contingent Observation

"Contingent observation" involves both incidental teaching and "mild" time out from active participation in an activity (Porterfield, Herbert-Jackson, & Risley, 1976). For example, the caregiver describes the inappropriate behavior to the child (e.g., "Don't take toys from others"), as well as the appropriate behavior for the situation (e.g., "Ask for toys you want"). The child is then moved to the periphery of the activity and sits without play materials while observing other children in play. After the child watches the play of others for less than 1 minute, the child is asked whether he or she would like to rejoin the play and use appropriate behavior. Should the child respond affirmatively, he or she returns to the play. If the child does not respond or responds negatively, the child is told to sit until he or she is ready to rejoin the activity using appropriate behavior. Once the child returns to the play situation, he or she is given positive attention for appropriate behavior (Porterfield et al., 1976).

Response Cost

"Response cost" is defined as the removal or loss of a positive reinforcer held by the child if a target behavior is performed, with the result of a decrease in occurrences of the target behavior. Response cost has been applied with young children to earn points, tokens, chips, stars, checkmarks, money, or other privileges. Guidelines for the use of response cost include (1) evaluating the available natural reinforcers, (2) building in positive attention for appropriate behaviors, (3) providing the child with the reinforcer "experience", (4) defining the behaviors that determine the amounts of fines, (5) using positive reinforcement for appropriate behaviors, (6) ensuring that fines are substantial enough to change behavior, but not so large as to result in "bankruptcy", (7) administering a fine as soon as possible after each target behavior, (8) making certain there are "reserves" of reinforcement, (9) planning for collecting fines, (10) keeping records of inappropriate behavior and the response cost, and (11) evaluating the program for unplanned outcomes.

Overcorrection

"Overcorrection" involves two procedures: (1) "restitution," in which the child is required to restore the environment to an improved condition, and (2) "positive practice," in which appropriate behaviors are practiced in situations that have been associated with misbehavior, contingent on performance of the targeted maladaptive behavior. Shapiro (1979) applied overcorrection to reduce paper shredding and book tearing by a 5-year-old girl. Restitution lasted for 2 minutes and consisted of instructions to pick up all torn paper and then to clean the area (e.g., to place toys in the toy box). Physical prompting was given as necessary. Positive practice lasted for 5 minutes and consisted of looking through books with a caregiver without tearing them. Results of the intervention revealed that the behaviors were eliminated and that the improvement was sustained through 18 months after the procedures were discontinued.

Planned Ignoring

"Planned ignoring" is the withdrawal of attention in a systematic manner (Hall & Hall, 1980). "Usual attention, physical contact, and any verbal interactions are removed for a short duration contingent upon the occurrence of the unwanted behavior" (Sulzer-Azaroff & Mayer, 1991, p. 457).

When a caregiver is implementing planned ignoring, the child should first be informed of the inappropriate behavior and the plans to ignore the behavior. Specific procedures for the child, behavior, and setting should be developed. For example, when a child whines or has a tantrum, the caregiver should focus attention away from the child, show a passive expression, remain silent, and withdraw from the setting within 5 seconds.

Extinction

"Extinction," closely related to planned ignoring, refers to providing a child with no reinforcement for a behavior that was previously reinforced. Extinction has been used successfully with behaviors such as crying, whining, and tantrums. However, extinction is often extremely difficult for caregivers to implement, as the need for consistency is paramount (Barnett & Carey, 1992). Thus, unless a caregiver can commit to extinction and follow through with it consistently, it will not be effective.

Reprimands

Reprimands are perhaps the most common overt strategies for behavior control; however, when used ineffectively, they can intensify maladaptive behaviors. VanHouten (1980) provides guidelines for the use of reprimands. First, the caregiver should specify the inappropriate behavior, state why the behavior was inappropriate, and provide the child with an example of an appropriate behavior. Second, the caregiver should use a firm tone, along with appropriate nonverbal expressions of disapproval, while maintaining emotional control. The reprimand should be delivered while the caregiver is in close proximity to the child, and inappropriate behavior during the reprimand should be ignored. Finally, reprimands should be followed by other, acceptable behavioral strategies (e.g., praise). Caregivers often need training in the use of reprimands to deliver them consistently and without losing control.

In the following sections, interventions viewed by professionals and most caregivers as "acceptable" (rather than aversive) are reviewed. These include modeling and self-regulation, correspondence training, interventions for classroom management, peer interventions, compliance training, and interventions for fire setting and biting.

MODELING AND SELF-REGULATION

Modeling

According to Bandura (1986), "most human behavior is learned by observation through modeling" (p. 47). Through observing the behavior of others, children learn rules for behavior that later serve as guides for action. Modeling may have the effect of strengthening, weakening, or facilitating learned behavior. For example, many preschool children have behaviors in their repertoires that are inappropriate to the school setting (hitting, spitting, swearing). When one child behaves inappropriately and receives negative consequences, other children may become more restrained in similar behaviors.

Self-Regulation

"Self-regulation" involves self-observation or self-monitoring, judgmental processes concerning one's performance, and self-reactions. Poth and Barnett (1983) combined self-regulation with other intervention components to help with a 3-year-old boy's tic-like behavior, described as "shuddering episodes." The child's upper body and arms became tensed and rigid, and he displayed palsy-like movements in his hands for 2–3 seconds. The teacher felt that the behavior interfered with the child's classroom performance and drew negative attention from his peers. The child was taught to discriminate tense from relaxed positions and behaviors and was reinforced for completing activities where the shuddering was not exhibited. The caregiver demonstrated to the child a relaxed position, and the child was asked to show the caregiver the relaxed position. The caregiver then demonstrated the not-relaxed position, which the child was also asked to imitate. After the child practiced, he was told that he would receive a star on a special card for demonstrating the relaxed position when he was engaged in activities. The intervention was successful in eliminating the shuddering episodes.

CORRESPONDENCE TRAINING

"Correspondence training" involves training in "promise keeping" (Baer, Osnes, & Stokes, 1983). For example, a child may be asked prior to a play period, "What are you going to do in play today?" The child can be trained to reply, "I'm going to have fun and not yell at others." After the child's response, the child is directed to play; after the play period, the child is taken aside and given feedback about his or her general play behavior. If the criterion of not yelling is met, the child is praised and reinforced. If the child does engage in the target behavior (i.e., yelling), the caregiver says, "You said you were not going to yell today, but you did, so you can't have [the reinforcer]. Go back and play."

Through correspondence training, children achieve a successful history of links between verbalization and actions. It has also been found to be useful in the generalization and maintenance of responses (Stokes & Osnes, 1986).

CLASSROOM MANAGEMENT

For young children, many problem behaviors occur when they are required to interact with their peers in the classroom setting. A number of strategies have been found useful for decreasing or eliminating disruptive classroom behavior.

Classroom Rules

Classroom rules are effective for communicating expectations about classroom behavior to children. Rules can be used as a basis for determining successes and criteria for positive attention when teachers "catch" children being "good." Classroom rules are most effective when teachers follow these guidelines: (1) Develop as few rules as possible, using developmentally appropriate wording and positive statements, (2) plan and post rules prior to the first day of school, and decide what rules are appropriate to each activity, (3) provide children with brief teaching sessions to train them in the rules before activities, and (4) reduce teacher prompts and feedback gradually as the desired behavior for activities becomes habitual (Fowler, 1986; Paine, Radicchi, Rosellini, Deutchman, & Darch, 1983).

Strategies for Transitions

Transition times may be difficult for young children, and behavior problems often occur during these times. Carden-Smith and Fowler (1984) compared a teacher-monitored token system and a peer-monitored token system for reducing disruptive behavior during transition times. Three kindergarten children with disruptive behavior participated. Token systems were implemented during three transition activities: cleaning up, going to the bathroom, and waiting. The teacher explained the program, and the children received training in the procedures. The children were then assigned daily to different teams, and each team was directed to perform specifically defined transition activities. In the teacher-monitored system, children who engaged in appropriate behavior were reinforced with points by the teacher; once a certain point total was obtained, children received backup reinforcers. In the peer-monitored intervention, procedures were the same, except that a team captain was chosen for each team. Team captains monitored performance and awarded points as the teacher had done, and backup reinforcers were provided in the same manner. Although both interventions were effective in reducing disruptions during transition times, peer monitoring was superior to teacher monitoring.

Other Strategies for Disruptive Behaviors

Allen, Turner, and Everett (1970) and Pinkston, Reese, LeBlanc, and Baer (1973) described differential attention and extinction procedures to eliminate aggressive behaviors. Teachers were instructed to ignore the aggressive behavior of children and to attend only to the victims. Teachers were also instructed to attend to the children described as aggressive when they were engaged in appropriate social interaction with their peers. Results revealed decreases in aggressive behaviors and increases in positive peer social interaction.

Contingent observation has also been used to decrease disruptive behavior. Tyroler and Lahey (1980) compared the effectiveness of contingent observation and redirection procedures with a 2-year-old girl. Disruptive behaviors included aggression, crying, fussing, destroying toys, and creating dangerous situations (throwing objects, standing on counters). During the redirection phase, when the child engaged in disruptive behavior, she was told of the inappropriateness of her behavior and was redirected to a more appropriate activity ("Look at the book"). Contingent observation was then implemented, and the results demonstrated that contingent observation was more effective in decreasing disruptive behaviors than the redirection procedure was.

Kubany, Weiss, and Sloggett (1971) described the "good behavior clock" procedure for reducing disruptive classroom behavior. A 6-year-old boy who engaged in disruptive behaviors (defined as refusal to sit at his desk, refusal to engage in academic tasks, talking out, and loud outbursts) was the target of the intervention. A false face was placed over a 15-minute electric timer. The numbers 1 through 6 were placed on the face at 2-minute intervals, and a red star on the clock face indicated completion of a cycle. When the child was quiet and in his seat, he would receive a treat, which was placed in a sharing jar for distribution to himself and his classmates at the end of the school day. When the child engaged in disruptive behavior, he was given a mild prompt for appropriate behavior, and the clock was turned off. The teacher was instructed to ignore the child, and if he was quiet and in his seat after 15 seconds, he was praised and the clock was turned back on. Overall, the intervention was effective in reducing the child's disruptive behavior.

PEER INTERVENTIONS

Peers as change agents can provide powerful sources of reinforcement for learning and maintaining behaviors. Peers can model, reinforce, extinguish, and monitor behaviors even at very young ages. Furthermore, peers may have more opportunities to observe specific social behaviors than adults do.

A basic design for a peer intervention is to use a peer confederate who is close in age to the target child and who receives specific training in participating in the intervention. Peer confederates must be selected and trained carefully. Many variables may contribute to declining rates of social interaction over time, and a variety of reinforcers can be used to maintain the behavior of the peer confederates. Teacher prompts may be required, and several confederates may need to be trained to carry out the intervention. Caregivers have to monitor the intervention carefully to ensure that it is carried out as planned. Cue cards can help the confederates conduct the intervention. Specific peer initiations must be selected carefully. Such initiations may include play organizers (e.g., "Let's play"), sharing, assistance, and affection. Training of the peer confederates requires a discussion of the importance of the intervention, a description of the target social behavior, modeling and role playing of the behavior (including the behavior of the targeted child), practice, and verbal feedback (Strain & Odom, 1986, p. 546).

COMPLIANCE TRAINING

Noncompliance, or ignoring the requests of caregivers, is considered a keystone behavior that merits intervention in the home and school. Noncompliance occurs as part of a constellation of behaviors: whining, tantrums, aggressive behaviors, "talking back," aversive demands, and other behaviors related to conduct disorders.

Compliance training is based on Patterson's coercion model (Patterson, Reid, Jones, & Conger, 1975). The basis of this model is that antisocial behaviors stem from deficits in parenting skills as well as from maladaptive child behaviors. Three variables require examination: ineffective discipline, parental monitoring, and the coerciveness of child behavior. For example, a parent may respond to a child's behavior in an aversive way (an unpleasant request), the child then responds in a coercive manner (whining), and the parent then terminates the request. In such a case, the child learns that he or she can control the parent's behavior by acting in ways that are aversive to the parent.

Forehand and McMahon (1981) used a compliance training program with children ages 3–8 and their families. The program required two stages. In the first stage the parents were taught to attend effectively to appropriate child behaviors and to ignore inappropriate behavior. The parents also learned to monitor the child's appropriate behaviors effectively and to stop using ineffective methods that were linked to noncompliance (e.g., commands). Parents were trained to use rewards to increase positive parent–child exchanges and compliance. The second stage involved procedures to increase compliance with parental commands. The parents were taught to use appropriate commands and mild time out for noncompliance.

INTERVENTIONS FOR FIRE SETTING AND BITING

Fire Setting

Fires are one of the leading causes of death for preschool children (Peterson, 1988). In addition, conduct disordered children sometimes evidence firesetting behavior and, thus, early intervention is highly advisable for this reason as well.

In some cases the most important first step is to discuss with parents the seriousness of the behavior. Interviewing parents and children can reveal not only factors related to conduct-disordered child behavior, but also parental risk factors, such as family interest in fire-related activities (Kolko & Kazdin, 1989). A contract should be developed with the parents to include childproofing the home, being vigilant in monitoring child behavior, enlisting the aid of guests and others in securing lighters and matches, installing alarms and other safety equipment, and participating in a structured parent program for noncompliant children.

In other cases parents need to learn to monitor child behavior closely. Such monitoring can serve as negative reinforcement and can bring the child's behavior under control. At times parental stress or impaired functioning (e.g., parental depression) may interfere with the ability to monitor a child's behavior. Assisting parents in dealing with or eliminating the stress in their own lives can often lead to positive changes in children.

Carstens (1982) described a "work penalty threat" for treating a 4-year-old fire setter. The penalty was 1 hour of "hard labor" that did not include the child's regular chores. Examples included "scrubbing off the back porch, washing walls or cleaning the spaces between the kitchen tiles with a toothbrush" (p. 160). Most often, educational programs can be effective with children who set fires; teaching children fire-safety-related skills often satisfies their curiosity.

Biting

Biting is the leading cause of injury to children and to adults in day care centers (Solomons & Elardo, 1989). The victims of bites may suffer serious consequences, such as infections and scarring. Solomons and Elardo (1989) recommend that conflicts with and redirection of children be anticipated and that child behavior be closely monitored. They suggest that the following steps be taken when a bite occurs: (1) Use time out with the aggressor, (2) comfort the victim, and (3) examine the bite. If the skin is broken, medical attention should be sought immediately and the parents should be contacted.

When severe biting occurs at a low rate, Matson and Ollendick (1976) recommend that situations be structured to elicit the biting behavior. Mild punishment is made contingent on biting or any attempt to bite, whereas appropriate behavior is reinforced. Bites and attempted bites result in having an unpleasant mouthwash sprayed into the aggressor's mouth. Matson and Ollendick (1976) caution that ethical procedures should be followed and medical permissions should be obtained prior to engaging in such an intervention. However, intervening with low rates of behaviors often requires a prompting strategy to create occasions for the child to practice alternative behaviors.

SUMMARY

Preschools and day care centers are often the first settings in which developmental difficulties that are socially and educationally relevant surface. The role of parental behaviors and family environments is also significant. Thus, mental health professionals providing services to young children must engage in collaborative problem solving, ecobehavioral and functional assessment, and systematic evaluation of valid intervention alternatives. Analyzing problem situations, the roles of caregivers and peers, and the experiences provided to children can result in effective and successful interventions for children engaged in problem behaviors.

The use of naturalistic interventions constitutes a scientist/practitioner foundation for providing services to young children and their caregivers. Using research-based interventions by making logical generalizations to the target child in the caregiver's own setting can provide effective methods for changing behavior. In addition, naturalistic interventions constitute a fundamental approach to addressing the issues of acceptability, maintenance, and generalization (Barnett & Carey, 1992), which should be the goals of any intervention. Interventions that fit caregivers' natural styles of teaching, those that are acceptable to caregivers, and those that maintain appropriate behaviors and generalize to other situations and settings can result in the elimination of behaviors with the potential for lifelong negative consequences.

REFERENCES

Allen, K. E., Turner, K. D., & Everett, P. M. (1970). A behavior modification classroom for Head Start children with behavior problems. *Exceptional Children, 37,* 119–127.

Axelrod, S. (1990). Myths that (mis)guide our profession. In A. C. Repp & N. N. Singh (Eds.), *Perspectives on the use of nonaversive and aversive interventions for persons with developmental disabilities* (pp. 59–72). Sycamore, IL: Sycamore.

Baer, R. A., Osnes, P. G., & Stokes, T. F. (1983). Training generalized correspondence between verbal behavior at school and nonverbal behavior at home. *Education and Treatment of Children, 6,* 379–388.

Bandura, A. (1986). *The social foundations of thought and action: A social cognitive theory.* Englewood Cliffs, NJ: Prentice-Hall.

Barnett, D. W., Bell, S., & Carey, K. T. (1999). *Designing preschool interventions: A practitioner's guide.* New York: Guilford Press.

Barnett, D. W., & Carey, K. T. (1992). *Designing interventions for preschool learning and behavior problems.* San Francisco: Jossey-Bass.

Bijou, S. W. (1975). Development in the preschool years: A functional analysis. *American Psychologist, 30,* 829–837.

Carden-Smith, L. K., & Fowler, S. A. (1984). Positive peer pressure: The effects of peer monitoring on children's disruptive behavior. *Journal of Applied Behavior Analysis, 17,* 213–227.

Carstens, C. (1982). Application of a work penalty threat in the treatment of a case of juvenile firesetting. *Journal of Behavior Therapy and Experimental Psychiatry, 13,* 159–161.

Dietz, D. E. D., & Repp, A. C. (1983). Reducing behavior through reinforcement. *Exceptional Education Quarterly, 3,* 34–46.

Donnellan, A. M., & LaVigna, G. W. (1990). Myths about punishment. In A. C. Repp & N. N. Singh (Eds.), *Perspectives on the use of nonaversive and aversive interventions for persons with developmental disabilities* (pp. 35–57). Sycamore, IL: Sycamore.

Firestone, P. (1976). The effects and side effects of timeout on an aggressive nursery school child. *Journal of Behavior Therapy and Experimental Psychiatry, 6,* 79–81.

Forehand, R. L., & McMahon, R. J. (1981). *Helping the noncompliant child: A clinician's guide to parent training.* New York: Guilford Press.

Fowler, S. A. (1986). Peer-monitoring and self-monitoring: Alternatives to traditional teacher management. *Exceptional Children*, *52*, 573–581.

Foxx, R. M., & Shapiro, S. T. (1978). The timeout ribbon: A nonexclusionary timeout procedure. *Journal of Applied Behavior Analysis*, *11*, 125–143.

Hall, R. V., & Hall, M. C. (1980). *How to use planned ignoring*. Austin, TX: Pro-Ed.

Hart, B. (1985). Naturalistic language training techniques. In S. F. Warren & A. Rogers-Warren (Eds.), *Teaching functional language* (pp. 63–85). Austin, TX: Pro-Ed.

Individuals with Disabilities Act of 1990, 20 U.S.C., § 1400 (1990).

Kolko, D. J., & Kazdin, A. E. (1989). Assessment of dimensions of childhood firesetting among patients and nonpatients: The firesetting risk interview. *Journal of Abnormal Child Psychology*, *17*, 157–176.

Kubany, E. S., Weiss, L. E., & Sloggett, B. B. (1971). The good behavior clock: A reinforcement/timeout procedure for reducing disruptive classroom behavior. *Journal of Behavior Therapy and Experimental Psychiatry*, *1*, 173–179.

Matson, J. L., & Ollendick, T. H. (1976). Elimination of low frequency biting. *Behavior Therapy*, *7*, 410–412.

Paine, S. C., Radicchi, J., Rosellini, L. C., Deutchman, L., & Darch, C. B. (1983). *Structuring your classroom for academic success*. Champaign, IL: Research Press.

Patterson, G. R., Reid, J. B., Jones, R. R., & Conger, R. E. (1975). *A social learning approach to family intervention* (Vol. 1). Eugene, OR: Castalia.

Peterson, L. (1988). Preventing the leading killer of children: The role of the school psychologist in injury prevention. *School Psychology Review*, *17*, 593–600.

Pinkston, E. M., Reese, N. M., LeBlanc, J. M., & Baer, D. M. (1973). Independent control of a preschool child's aggression and peer interaction by contingent teacher attention. *Journal of Applied Behavior Analysis*, *6*, 115–124.

Poling, A., & Ryan, C. (1982). Differential reinforcement-of-other-behavior schedules: Therapeutic applications. *Behavior Modification*, *6*, 3–21.

Porterfield, J. K., Herbert-Jackson, E., & Risley, T. R. (1976). Contingent observation: An effective and acceptable procedure for reducing disruptive behavior of young children in a group setting. *Journal of Applied Behavior Analysis*, *9*, 55–64.

Poth, R. L., & Barnett, D. W. (1983). Reduction of a behavioral tic with a preschooler using relaxation and self-control techniques across settings. *School Psychology Review*, *12*, 472–475.

Preschool Education of the Handicapped Act of 1986, § 677.

Rolider, A., & VanHouten, R. (1990). The role of reinforcement in reducing inappropriate behavior: Some myths and misconceptions. In A. C. Repp & N. N. Singh (Eds.), *Perspectives on the use of nonaversive and aversive interventions for persons with developmental disabilities* (pp. 119–127). Sycamore, IL: Sycamore.

Shapiro, E. S. (1979). Restitution and positive practice overcorrection in reducing aggressive–disruptive behavior: A long term follow-up. *Journal of Behavior Therapy and Experimental Psychiatry*, *10*, 131–134.

Sigel, I. E. (1982). The relationship between parental distancing strategies and the child's cognitive behavior. In L. M. Laosa & I. E. Sigel (Eds.), *Families as learning environments for children* (pp. 47–86). New York: Plenum Press.

Solomons, H. C., & Elardo, R. (1989). Bite injuries at a day care center. *Early Childhood Research Quarterly*, *4*, 89–96.

Stokes, T. F., & Osnes, P. G. (1986). Programming the generalization of children's social behavior. In P. S. Strain, M. J. Guralnick, & H. M. Walker (Eds.), *Children's social behavior: Development, assessment, and modification* (pp. 407–443). San Diego: Academic Press.

Strain, P. S., & Odom, S. L. (1986). Peer social initiations: Effective intervention for social skills development of exceptional children. *Exceptional Children*, *52*, 543–551.

Sulzer-Azaroff, B., & Mayer, G. R. (1991). *Behavior analysis for lasting change*. Troy, MO: Holt, Rinehart & Winston.

Tyroler, M. J., & Lahey, B. B. (1980). Effects of contingent observation on the disruptive behavior of a toddler in a group setting. *Child Care Quarterly*, *9*, 265–274.

VanHouten, R. (1980). *How to use reprimands*. Austin, TX: Pro-Ed.

White, B. L., Kaban, B. T., & Attanucci, J. S. (1979). *The origins of human competence*. Lexington, MA: D.C. Heath.

CHAPTER 6

Classroom-Based Approaches

HAROLD R. KELLER
RENEE C. TAPASAK

This chapter describes a general problem-solving approach to the development and implementation of violence prevention and intervention strategies within the classroom. Other chapters in this volume address aggression and violence within the contexts of the school, home, and community.

We recognize that a teacher using proven classroom-based approaches in isolation is likely to have only minimal impact on changing student behavior without the support and commitment of those at the building and system levels. Teachers must advocate and constructively work toward the implementation of effective schoolwide approaches for violence and aggression. The school context and the degree of consistency between a classroom and the school as a whole (e.g., rules, approaches to dealing with aggression and violence, and crisis management) are important determinants in the success of any prevention and intervention strategies for addressing aggression and violence. The extent of home–school collaboration, cooperation, and consistency relative to beliefs and values concerning child development and behavior management also strongly affect the violence prevention efforts of a teacher.

There is greater impact and a higher likelihood of significant generalization effects for prevention and intervention strategies that are implemented with consistency across the ecological contexts of classroom, school, and home (as well as the broader community and cultural contexts). Indeed, recent reviews of research and national reports on youth violence (Dwyer, Osher, & Warger, 1998; McEvoy & Welker, 2000; U.S. Department of Health and Human Services, 2001) emphasize the critical importance of schoolwide approaches, school climate and school–home–community partnerships in successful intervention and prevention.

Briefly, the Surgeon General's report (U.S. Department of Health and Human Services, 2001) emphasized the following. In schools, interventions that address social context and school climate are more likely to be effective, on average, than those directed at changing individual attitudes, skills, and risky behaviors. There must be a commitment to both academic achievement and social/emotional growth within the context of interpersonal relationships that communicate adults' caring, nurturing and respect for children and youth (Dwyer et al., 1998; McEvoy & Welker, 2000). Available evidence from these sources suggests multiple characteristics of schools and school climates that are safe and responsive to all children, providing contexts for effective prevention and intervention. Such characteristics include the following:

• There is a schoolwide approach to implementing a learning climate that is consistent with research on effective schools. There is a dual emphasis on high academic achievement for all children and quality interpersonal relationships among teachers, staff and students. Appropriate social and emotional bonds are critical for a commitment to achievement and for management of behaviors. Every member of an effective school community (teachers, staff, students) must feel that he or she is a valued participant working toward meaningful goals. With high expectations for academic achievement, there must be enhanced opportunities for success and sufficient supports for progress toward success.

• There is a commitment to continuous progress monitoring and ongoing assessment that serve to identify behavioral, emotional, and academic skill needs and strengths to be addressed and enhanced. Multidisciplinary problem-solving teams are available to work with teachers to address identified skill needs. For those children with more severe problems, more comprehensive functional assessments are conducted to develop appropriate individualized interventions and support services. Resources are available that enable students to share their concerns and to feel safe expressing their feelings.

• There is an emphasis on staff development and enhanced opportunities for teachers to interact and share effective instructional and relational ideas across grade levels and buildings.

• There are attempts to actively involve families in meaningful ways with the school. Barriers to parental participation are addressed, and parents are welcomed in the school. Links to the broader community are developed so that additional supports can be provided to schools, families and students. Such approaches also are designed to increase adult–child contact time to enhance bonding, positive mentoring relationships in school, and monitoring/supervision of children.

• There is a commitment to identify problems and assess progress toward schoolwide goals.

PREVENTION

Focus on the Teacher

Effective prevention programs at the classroom level require a focus on the teacher, the skills that he or she brings to the classroom, and the kinds of schoolwide supports available to assist with challenging and aggressive behaviors in the classroom. Teachers need to understand how to derive possible meanings from observable behavior. Further, they must attempt to understand behavioral and emotional consequences of various life events or circumstances present within a child's background. At both the preservice and in-service levels, it is important that teachers acquire and continue to develop effective teaching, communication, classroom management, and problem-solving skills. These skills must be applied within a classroom environment created by a caring, nurturing, and respectful teacher who accepts and attempts to meet the needs of students within a continuum of abilities and special needs and across a range of cultural and economic backgrounds. The literature on resilient children (Doll & Lyon, 1998; Luther & Cicchetti, 2000; Masten, 2001; Wyman, Sandler, Wolchik, & Nelson, 2000) has shown that an important variable that allows at-risk children to rise above the most debilitating conditions is the presence of a caring adult in their lives. For many children, that caring adult can be and has been a teacher.

Respect, Caring, and Communication

A unidirectional demand by a teacher for respect from a student may often serve, instead, to precipitate aggressive behavior toward the teacher. Respect and caring shown *to* a student *by* a teacher are more likely to elicit respect in return and thus may serve as possible means of preventing aggressive behavior. Students, particularly at the middle school level, perceive teachers who use democratic processes and allow student involvement in decision making in the classroom as caring teachers (Wentzel, 1997). Students who perceive teachers as caring are more likely to place greater value on social responsibility and prosocial goals (Wentzel & Wigfield, 1998). Respect and caring within the classroom are typically transmitted via effective verbal and nonverbal communication skills. The application of effective communication skills in the classroom thus can serve a preventive function. In addition, the teacher who uses effective communication skills can avoid escalating a potentially violent situation and can deescalate verbally aggressive situations (Goldstein, Palumbo, Striepling, & Voutsinas, 1995). Communication skills for deescalating (and avoiding escalating) aggressive situations are discussed more fully later in this chapter.

Effective Teaching

Effective teaching (Brophy & Good, 1986; Ysseldyke & Christenson, 1993) is another crucial preventive variable. Possible precipitants of aggressive behavior for a given student may include difficulty in learning, misunderstanding or no understanding of task directions, instruction that does not match the student's current level of functioning, and instruction that is paced too rapidly for the individual. The relationship between academic underachievement and antisocial behavior, particularly aggression, is well established

(Kazdin, 1987; Patterson, 1982). Application of effective teaching skills serves a dual purpose. First, it may prevent feelings of frustration with learning, fear of failure, and other possible academically related antecedents to aggression and violence. Second, effective teaching is likely to lead to greater academic engagement. The more academically engaged a student is, the higher the student's learning outcomes are likely to be and the less likely he or she is to engage in aggressive behavior. Indeed, *academic engagement is incompatible with aggressive behavior.* This approach is in contrast to intervention strategies that target students' aggressive behaviors. Such strategies may reduce or eliminate aggressive behaviors, but will have little likelihood of enhancing learning outcomes. Effective teaching strategies can do both: academically engaged time and learning will be enhanced, reducing the probability that aggressive behavior will occur.

Classroom Management

Effective classroom management skills are a part of effective teaching, but are typically addressed separately (e.g., Alberto & Troutman, 1999; Emmer, Evertson, Sanford, Clements, & Worsham, 1984; Evertson, Emmer, Clements, Sanford, & Worsham, 1984; Kauffman, Hallahan, Mostert, Trent, & Nuttycombe, 1993; Rhode, Jenson, & Reaves, 1998; Walker, Colvin, & Ramsey, 1995). Effective classroom management motivates learning and sets the stage for productive learning.

These skills include effective individual and group student motivational strategies (e.g., the Good Behavior Game, Dolan, Turkan, Wethamer-Larsson, & Kellam, 1989), management of behavioral contingencies, timely prompting and cueing procedures, student self-control strategies (e.g., Hoff & DuPaul, 1998), room arrangement, and classroom rule structure. Since classroom management strategies are typically addressed as part of teachers' preservice education and in-service professional development, extensive coverage will not be provided here. Effective classroom management has been included as an essential component of a number of successful violence prevention programs. Examples include the Seattle Social Development Program (O'Donnell, Hawkins, Catalano, Abbott, & Day, 1995), the Bullying Prevention Program (Olweus, Limber, & Mihalic, 1998), the School Transitional Environmental Program (Felner et al., 1993), and Families and Schools Together (FAST Track, Bierman et al., 1992).

A key consideration in the implementation of successful classroom management is the integrity of the procedures (i.e., the degree to which the classroom management strategies have been implemented appropriately). Kamps et al. (2000) have demonstrated that both integrity of implementation and level of classroom structure are strongly related to reduced classroom aggression and enhanced academic engagement. In addition, access to building-level supports for classroom teachers as they develop and implement classroom management strategies is important, not only for ensuring safety and learning with individual classrooms but to the overall school environment.

Classroom Arrangement

Room arrangement can help to prevent aggressive behavior. High-traffic areas need to be free of congestion, thus reducing potential conflict. Students must be in full view of the teacher so that behavior can be easily monitored. Teaching materials and student supplies should be readily accessible in order to minimize student waiting time (when aggressive behavior is more likely). Furthermore, seats must be arranged so that students can easily see instructional presentations, to reduce the opportunity for off-task behavior (Emmer et al., 1984). Through classroom arrangement, the teacher can convey to the students, "I am here to listen, answer your questions, and help you learn."

Classroom Rules

Establishing classroom rules that are few in number, brief, concise, and clear is very important in the prevention of aggressive behavior. Positive consequences for following rules, and negative consequences for violating them, must also be clear. Involvement of the students in the establishment of rules is likely to increase rule following, since students will be more invested in what they themselves have designed. In addition to communicating classroom rules to parents, it is important to teach the classroom rules directly, not merely post them. With elementary school children, direct teaching of rules is more effective when they are stated (both orally and in writing), modeled, behaviorally rehearsed, and reinforced consistently with occasional "booster sessions" throughout the school year. Evertson et al. (1984) thoroughly describe the establishment of classroom rules and their initial implementation. Positively oriented strategies are part of most classroom management systems (Charles, 1992) and are certainly part of effective classroom management (Gettinger, 1988). These aspects of classroom rules are a major component of effective classroom structure (Kamps et al., 2000).

Cooperative Learning

Application of cooperative learning strategies within the classroom (Slavin, 1980, 1989, 1990; Slavin et al., 1985) may also aid in the prevention of aggressive behavior. Although there is little research to show the direct effects of cooperative learning on aggressive behavior, cooperative learning does enhance academic engagement and achievement. Engaging in cooperative behaviors is incompatible with aggressive behavior. Direct teaching of cooperative learning strategies is needed to counteract the competitive nature of many classrooms. Goldstein (1999) has described many cooperative games that may be used in the academic classroom and in a school's physical education classes as potential strategies for addressing violence.

Continuous Progress Monitoring

Continuous progress monitoring (Fuchs & Fuchs, 2000) is another important aspect of effective teaching. This involves frequently administered curriculum-based measurement and performance assessment that enables the classroom teacher to identify academic problems early and to develop strategies to intervene and prevent escalation of achievement difficulties. Continuous progress monitoring is effective in reducing the risk of academic failure, which is a significant risk factor for youth violence. Continuous progress-monitoring programs allow students to proceed through a hierarchy of academic skills, advancing to the next level as each skill is mastered. Since, at the preservice level, few teachers acquire a solid foundation in continuous progress monitoring and how to use results for instructional and intervention decision making, such training and assistance will need to be provided through building support teams and in-service programs.

Continuous progress monitoring for social, emotional, and aggressive behaviors allows intervention and prevention programs to be intensified or modified as indicated by the monitoring data. For those children and youth who do not respond successfully to prevention strategies, more time-intensive functional assessment approaches (Gresham & Noell, 1999) can be coordinated with classroom teachers. The availability of individualized programs is critical for successful classroom and building-wide prevention/intervention programs (Kamps et al., 2000).

Building-Level Support Teams

Teachers confronted with increasingly aggressive students need ready access to in-building supports. No matter how effective their communication, teaching, and classroom management skills, aggressive behavior presents many daily challenges to teachers. The availability of in-building, collaborative problem-solving teams (Kauffman et al., 1993; Rosenfield, 1992; Rosenfield & Gravois, 1996) is essential to successful prevention and intervention with aggressive behavior.

Such multidisciplinary problem-solving teams may include administrators, teachers, psychologists, social workers, speech/language pathologists, and other support service professionals; this allows problems to be addressed from several different professional perspectives. Supportive functions of collaborative problem-solving teams include educating about individual differences and special needs, identifying possible causes relative to behaviors or outcomes of concern, generating prevention and intervention strategies, helping to implement strategies, monitoring and ensuring the integrity of strategies, providing follow-up and troubleshooting, and evaluating the strategies' effectiveness. Such supports are critical for the development and implementation of classroom management strategies, cooperative learning, and continuous progress monitoring. Engaging in the problem-solving process not only provides teachers with needed supports, but also facilitates the ongoing development of teachers' own problem-solving skills–skills that are essential for both preventing and intervening with aggressive behavior.

Focus on the Students

Skillstreaming Approaches

Child-focused prevention programs within the school setting have been relatively general and have been derived from skills training models (Bandura, 1973) and a cognitive–behavioral tradition (Mahoney, 1974; Meichenbaum, 1977). Among the many social skills programs implemented within classrooms, the "skillstreaming" system of Goldstein and his associates is perhaps the most comprehensive and thoroughly described (Goldstein, 1999). The skillstreaming approach has been implemented in programs for adolescents (Goldstein, Sprafkin, Gershaw, & Klein, 1980), elementary school children (McGinnis & Goldstein, 1984), and preschoolers (McGinnis & Goldstein, 1990).

Many different social skills, including prosocial alternatives to aggressive behavior, are identified and may be taught directly to students via a set of four basic components: modeling, role playing, performance feedback, and transfer and maintenance of training. Training may be implemented with small groups of students or total classrooms. Evaluative research on the skillstreaming programs and on social skills training (Goldstein, 1999) generally has shown positive short-term acquisition of social skills, as well as modest transfer and maintenance effects. Direct effects on aggressive behavior of students are less clear. There is evidence that skillstreaming is more effective when it is combined with other interventions that focus more directly on aggressive behavior (e.g., anger control training) and when both teachers and parents are involved in training (Goldstein & Glick, 1987; Goldstein, Glick, Irwin, Pask, & Rubama, 1989). The efficacy of social skills training may be enhanced even further when it is applied in a prescriptive manner, based on specifically identified individual skill deficits of at-risk students (Goldstein & Keller, 1983, 1987). Social skills training is an important component in a number of successful multicomponent prevention programs. These include the Life Skills Training program (Botvin, Mihalic, & Grotpeter, 1998), Linking the Interests of Families and Teachers (LIFT; Stoolmiller, Eddy, & Reid, 2000), FAST Track (Bierman et al., 1992), and the Incredible Years Series (Webster-Stratton, 1999).

Social Problem-Solving Approaches

Social problem-solving approaches are derived from the cognitive-behavioral tradition, rely less on external input (at least in the long run), and therefore theoretically address the problems of transfer and maintenance, which are weaknesses in skills-based approaches. The training model of Spivack and Shure (1974; see Pelligrini & Urbain, 1985, for a review) has been the most successful. Training in "interpersonal cognitive problem solving" (ICPS) is done by teachers and parents. It emphasizes alternative, consequential, and means–ends thinking, as well as areas of social-cognitive competence. In addition to thinking skills, children are taught appropriate assertiveness, role taking, and awareness of social rules and conventions. Emory Cowen and his colleagues (Gesten et al., 1982; Weissberg, Gesten, Carnilce, et al., 1981; Weissberg, Gesten, Rapkin, et al., 1981) had varied success by incorporating aspects of the ICPS model into more comprehensive prevention programs.

In another variation of this approach, the program for Promoting Alternative Thinking Strategies (PATHS, Greenberg, Kusche, & Mihalic, 1998) combined ICPS with curriculum modules on emotional competence, self-control, social competence, and positive peer relations. This comprehensive program had positive effects on several risk factors associated with violence.

Second Step—A Violence Prevention Curriculum (SSVPC; Frey, Hirschstein, & Guzzo, 2000) specifically targeted violence by addressing impulsivity (via problem solving), anger management, and empathy—three variables empirically related to aggressive behavior (Camp, 1977; Coie, Dodge, & Kupersmidt, 1990; Coie & Krehbiel, 1990). The curricular packages for SSVPC, developed separately for preschool through middle school, employ modeling, role plays, homework to enhance transfer, and encouragement of parental reinforcement of newly learned skills. Positive outcomes have been sustained for up to 6 years.

The Seattle Social Development Project (O'Donnell et al., 1995) combines ICPS with prosocial skills, academic skills, avoidance of drug use, and parent training for elementary and middle school students. There are extensive long-term data and replications in other sites for the preventive effectiveness of this program for general populations as well as for children at high risk for violence (U.S. Department of Health and Human Services, 2001).

Elias and Clabby (1992) have reported an elaboration of this approach in their "improving social awareness—social problem solving" (ISA-SPS) model. Their description of 12 years of research with the ISA-SPS model is particularly important in that it describes, in detail, the implementation of the model within the complex realities of school systems. Like the research on skills-training approaches, the research on social problem-solving approaches has generally demonstrated positive short-term effects, with long-term transfer and maintenance being primarily theoretical. Improvement has been demonstrated for problem-solving thinking skills and areas of social-cognitive competence, but there has been little measurement of training effects on students' aggressive behaviors (Durlak, 1983). Prescriptive implementation of social problem solving is likely to be more efficacious, inasmuch as little is known about how individual students' developmental levels and basic cognitive processing strengths and weaknesses interact with cognitive-behavioral interventions (Goldstein, Harootunian, & Conoley, 1994).

INTERVENTION

The emphasis in this section is on addressing and intervening with aggressive behavior through a problem-solving approach. Such an approach focuses on the application of effective strategies that are specific to an individual exhibiting aggressive behavior. One strategy or set of strategies does not fit all young people. A management program for a total class is unlikely to have a significant or long-term impact on an individual student who is aggressive. The problem-solving approach is best conducted within the context of a multidisciplinary building team (Kauffman et al., 1993; Rosenfield & Gravois, 1996). A team approach potentially allows identification of a more comprehensive picture of the variables (including risk and protective factors) impacting the individual's violent and aggressive behavior.

In the development of prescriptive interventions (Goldstein, 1978), it is important to consider a number of factors: distal and proximal precipitants of the aggressive behavior, setting events, the aggressive behavior itself (quality, type, frequency, intensity, and variety), and the strengths and limitations of the aggressive individual. Application of functional assessment approaches to the individual and the contexts for his or her aggressive behavior will be helpful in the development of appropriate individualized intervention strategies (Dunlap et al., 1993). Indeed, if the aggressive and violent behavior involves a child with disabilities, a functional assessment must be used (Kern & Dunlap, 1999).

Within the problem-solving approach, the knowledge, skills, resources, and supports of the person(s) implementing the intervention must be considered. Since problems associated with violence and teaching can be highly complex, teachers must be flexible and creative problem solvers. Interventions and strategies need to be viewed as hypotheses to be tried and systematically evaluated to determine whether the desired benefits (i.e., enhanced academic engagement, increased social/emotional development, decreased violence, or decreased behaviors that have the potential of leading to violence) actually occur. The costs of implementing the intervention must be weighed in relation to the level of energy output, the extent of resources and supports needed, and the potential impact on others within the classroom.

Our own philosophy is that interventions should be implemented within the "least restrictive" educational setting, usually the general education classroom. Tobin and Sprague (2000) recommended a number of research-based alternative educational strategies for reducing violence in the school. These strategies included lower ratio of students to teachers, highly structured classroom with behavioral classroom management, positive rather than punitive emphasis in behavior management, adult mentors at school, individualized behavioral interventions based on functional assessment, social skills instruction, high-quality academic instruction, and strategies to involve parents/caregivers. We recognize that for some individuals who exhibit severe levels of aggressive behavior, the costs associated with general classroom interventions are too high in terms of energy, resources, supports, and potential impact on other students. Thus, the interventions for such students may best be implemented in more restrictive alternative educational settings.

Prevention and intervention programs that are part of a continuum of services within a building are more likely to be effective than programs with a single buildingwide (universal) approach (Kamps et al., 2000). In the former approach, students may progress to less restrictive programs within the same setting. Kazdin (1994) argues that restrictive group programs that place children in contact with deviant and aggressive peers are highly likely to produce unfavorable results with children whose initial problems were not severe. Thus, in considering interventions involving placement of children into more restrictive settings, it is important to avoid iatrogenic effects (i.e., outcomes in which negative effects of an intervention outweigh potential positive benefits).

Precipitants of Aggressive Behavior

Understanding within School Precipitants

A functional assessment process is a particularly fruitful approach to identifying antecedent conditions and setting events for aggressive behavior. Understanding the potential precipitants of a student's aggressive behavior is important to the problem-solving process for at least two reasons.

First, examining precipitants to the aggressive behavior will help the teacher and support personnel to identify those factors that are under their control within the classroom. They can hypothesize about many possible factors that may have triggered or caused a particular set of aggressive behaviors. Only those precipitating factors that are under the control of classroom professionals are fruitful ones to pursue within the problem-solving process. Even if some hypothesized factors are accurate (e.g., there is a genetic component in a student's aggressive behavior; the student is a victim of abuse; the student spends inordinate amounts of time watching violent TV and videos and playing violent video games), entertaining those hypotheses within a problem-solving process has little likelihood of resulting in potentially helpful classroom interventions for the aggressive behaviors. For the greatest chance of successful intervention, an individual teacher or school-based team engaging in a problem-solving process must constantly focus un those precipitants that are operating within the classroom context.

Second, to the extent that collaborative involvement of families and community agencies is fostered, the targets of a functional assessment and the potential range of precipitating events can be increased. Indeed, the most successful prevention and intervention programs for violence are those that actively involve the home, school, and community (U.S. Department of Health and Human Services, 2001).

Understanding beyond School Precipitants

It is important to recognize that many precipitants of aggressive behavior are beyond the control of the teacher or school. Recognition of such distal precipitants (e.g., the student's having been abused at home, having been teased on the bus, needing to "save face" with peers, being hungry) is necessary for creating the kind of caring and nurturing classroom climate needed for prevention/intervention programs to be effective (McEvoy & Welker, 2000).

Responding to agitation resulting from such "out-of-classroom" events with active listening and empathy communicates a sense of caring and helps to establish a setting where effective interventions can be implemented. For example, a child who has experienced teasing and or a fight on the bus or playground before entering the classroom may be "on a very short fuse" that could precipitate aggression in the classroom later that morning. An awareness of that event (e.g., through a good communication system with bus drivers or playground supervisors, or through an understanding of body language communicating agitation) may result in a teachers merely taking a couple of "private" minutes to express sympathy and actively listen to the student, thereby defusing a potentially aggressive situation.

Skills in understanding child development, distal precipitants of aggression, nonverbal cues, and those of active listening and empathy are best acquired through experience paired with in-service staff development. Few novice teachers enter the classroom with these kinds of skills. The point here is not to create teachers as school counselors or mental health professionals. Counseling as an intervention strategy, in general, has *not* been found to be an effective intervention for violence and aggression (U.S. Department of Health and Human Services, 2001). Rather, it is important that classroom teachers develop and use skills that are essential to the establishment of caring and nurturing classroom climates that enable successful interventions and preventions.

Recognition of distal precipitants also can be important to the problem-solving process and to the immediate reactions of school personnel to an aggressive situation. Recognition of factors that are beyond the control of the school does not absolve the individual student from accepting responsibility for his or her aggressive actions. However, such recognition may help the teacher maintain a personal distance from the aggressive action, engage in effective problem solving, and/or respond immediately to an action in a way that deescalates a situation. A teacher who learns that a student is behaving aggressively toward the teacher because of some unrelated event can realize that the aggression is not truly directed at him or her. By not personalizing the attack, the teacher can more easily engage in problem solving about how to prevent the aggressive behavior in the future and will have a greater likelihood of developing an effective individual intervention. The teacher will be less likely to engage in a power struggle with the student which could escalate the situation. A teacher's reaction that includes a calm voice, empathic comments, and or redirection helps to deescalate the situation.

Defusing Strategies

To illustrate this point and some effective strategies for defusing a potentially violent situation, consider a frequent pattern with many agitated individuals. A student who is agitated often manifests this agitation initially through some form of anxiety. An increase or change in level or amount of behavior (e.g., pacing, difficulty in sitting still, tapping fingers or a pencil, changed pitch or volume of voice, rapid talking) is a typical cue of anxiety. Verbally, the student may ask questions. It is important at this point in the sequence to listen to the questions. If they are information-seeking questions, the teacher should try to respond directly to a question by providing the information sought, even if the teacher "knows" that there is anger underlying the question. Sometimes the agitation and anxiety may be related to a fear of the unknown or to misunderstanding a given task. When the teacher provides the requested information, the student's anxiety is reduced and the agitation is deescalated.

Sometimes the questions a student asks may be more challenging in nature. In this case it is important to ignore the challenge in the questions and simply redirect the student to the task at hand. In addition, the teacher must be aware of the nonverbal aspects of the situation, especially those relating to personal space. Invading the personal space of an agitated individual, particularly by physically confronting the individual in a face-to-face mode, may be perceived as threatening and may therefore escalate a situation. A particularly effective nonverbal approach is to stand near an agitated student, just outside his or her personal space and at a 45- or 90-degree angle, while communicating with the student. Such a supportive stance communicates respect for the student and his or her personal space. It allows the student an opportunity to choose between communication (and deescalation) and escape (a choice that may not be optimal, but is more desirable than direct physical confrontation with the teacher). It also serves to maintain personal safety for the adult (outside the reach of a fist or foot).

A still higher level of agitation may take the form of defensiveness, in which the student becomes more overtly angry, with louder and more confrontational comments. Here, an appropriate verbal response is to set limits, using a calm voice. Effective limit setting involves stating clear, concise, reasonable, and enforceable directions. Offering choices, along with consequences for each choice, is desirable. For example, "Return to your math work, finish it, and you can use the computer; if you continue your (present) behavior, you will need to go to Ms. Jones's room to cool off." When choices are offered, it is better to offer a positive choice and its consequence first, then a negative choice (persisting in the agitated behavior) and its consequence next. Reversing the order of the choices (i.e., stating the negative choice first) is likely to result in the student's not even hearing the positive choice and its consequence, and thus escalating the situation. Stating choices allows the student the opportunity to assume control over his or her own behavior, which is ultimately where control belongs.

Communicating with the student at each level of agitation in a calm, low voice is helpful as well. It is not merely the content of the communication that is important, but also how the content is stated. Remaining calm is more easily managed when the adult has depersonalized the interaction and not allowed him- or herself to enter into a power struggle with the student. If the student's agitation is still at a verbal level, it is best to respond only verbally. This is not a time to attempt to intervene physically. Moreover, if the student is defensive and confrontational, this is not a time for engaging in reasoning with the student. The student will not hear any reasons for alternative behaviors at this point. Limit setting that is brief and concise is most likely to be fruitful.

If the level of agitation escalates to physical threats against the adult, it is usually not easily predicted whether the student will follow through with the threats. The wisest course at this point is to seek help and ensure the safety of the other students. This may be done by trying to isolate the individual (offering the student an opportunity to go somewhere else and cool down) or by directing other students to leave the area.

The sensitive teacher can interpret the behavior of his or her students. At the earliest point possible in the preceding sequence (i.e., when a student appears unhappy or anxious), the teacher needs to invite the student to go to a quiet setting away from the other students. The student should be provided with the opportunity to express his or her feelings (verbally, in writing, or through drawings) either to the classroom teacher, school counselor, or another school professional of his or her choice. This approach can be highly effective in preventing mild upset from escalating into anger, agitation, and violent behavior.

After verbal deescalation strategies have been effective, it is important to reestablish effective communication with the student and engage in reasoning about alternative courses of action in the future. This is now a teachable moment for that student, and perhaps for others in the class, about how to handle similar situations in the future in a more effective manner. At earlier stages in the sequence of agitation, such reasoning approaches are unlikely to be effective.

It is important to recognize that deescalation strategies may not always be effective with each individual on each occasion. The creative problem-solving process also involves thinking through situations in advance and developing a plan for the possibility that a given strategy may not be effective. Having alternative plans available (including, for example, a request for help from the office or a team member) facilitates a teacher's ability to remain calm, which reduces the emotional component of the situation for everyone involved.

In summary, it is important for teachers to learn to recognize the precipitants of aggressive behavior so that they can focus on those precipitants that are under their control within the classroom setting. In addition, learning to recognize that some aggressive behavior is precipitated by events outside the classroom context can help a teacher demonstrate caring and create a supportive classroom climate. Such recognition also can help a teacher depersonalize the situation and engage in effective problem solving and verbal deescalation strategies before an incident escalates to a physically aggressive level. Goldstein et al. (1995) provide detailed descriptions of these and other verbal deescalation strategies for managing student aggression.

Setting Events for Aggressive Behavior

It is important within a problem-solving approach to examine potential setting events (locations, activities) that seem to set the occasion for aggressive behavior. Recording those occasions when some form of disciplinary action is needed for aggressive behavior, as well as the circumstances surrounding the behavior, may help teachers and other personnel identify consistent times or places in which the behaviors occur. For example, a given student's aggressive behavior may be more likely to occur at transitions between activities or locations, in certain areas of the room or building, or during certain academic activities. Determining consistent patterns may allow teachers to develop effective prevention or intervention strategies. A functional assessment approach will be helpful in identifying setting events.

Aggressive Behavior: Quality, Type, Frequency, Intensity, and Variety

When a teacher is engaging in problem solving, it is important to consider the aggressive behavior itself. The quality and type of aggressive behavior, whether verbal or physical, will help determine the kind of staff response needed to reduce or limit the aggressive behavior. The teacher's response has to match the aggressive behavior being exhibited; over- or underreaction to aggressive behavior is likely to raise the level of aggressiveness. For example, responding physically to verbal aggression is likely to result in the student's engaging in physical aggression. Responding to the anxiety reactions of an agitated student with limit-setting directives, rather than supportive verbal reactions, is likely to escalate the situation. Responding to physical aggression with verbal reasoning at the time of the physical aggression is also unlikely to be successful. Zero tolerance and out-of-school suspension policies have not been found to be effective interventions for reducing the incidence of minor infractions. Developing and implementing strategies to prevent even minor aggressive behavior is of primary importance.

Solo Physical Aggression

Addressing physical aggression in the classroom requires in-service training in school safety procedures and extensive practice. Merely reading a book or attending a workshop is not a sufficient means for learning how to apply the needed skills in a timely, appropriate, effective, and safety-conscious manner. There is considerable variation across schools and districts in whether and how teachers should handle potentially aggressive or aggressive students. Physical aggression directed toward a teacher generally takes one of two forms: a strike (in which an object such as a fist or foot comes in contact with a target) or a grab (e.g., choke, wrist grab, bite, bear hug, hair pull). A teacher needs to have basic knowledge and skills for responding to both forms of physical aggression in a manner that maintains the safety and security of both the teacher and all students. Safely responding to strikes requires blocking and moving skills (Goldstein et al., 1995), whereas reactions to grabs call for an understanding and application of basic principles of leverage and momentum (Goldstein et al., 1995).

Physical Aggression Involving Two or More Students

When physical aggression involves two or more students, it is important for the teacher not to engage in heroics and attempt to intervene in solo fashion. A team approach is the best strategy, with team members well trained in verbal deescalation strategies as well as physical intervention strategies.

The advantages of a team approach over a solo intervention include safety in numbers (without overwhelming the students), the opportunity for feedback during debriefing (relative to the situation and the team's response), and the presence of witnesses (for accountability). Team members assume a variety of roles in situations of such physical aggression. First, an attempt must be made to remove the audience or isolate the combatants. Second, the situation must be assessed accurately and quickly as to who is involved, what has occurred, and what is now happening. Third, an array of well-practiced intervention strategies must be available to the team members. Finally, once the situation has been brought under control, an attempt must be made to interview those involved (as well as witnesses) and to begin getting the student participants to think about and engage in alternative and more constructive approaches to solving problems (i.e., approaches that do not involve physical aggression).

Goldstein et al. (1995) describe a number of physical interventions and restraint techniques for dealing with such situations. Again, training and practice are required for safe and effective use of the strategies. We believe that nonviolent physical crisis interventions that maintain the dignity, safety, and security of all involved are most helpful. Such interventions are designed to be used for brief durations, with the goal being to assist the students to regain self-control as quickly as possible. Only those levels of force required to get a situation under control are to be used. If the level of violence is so severe that more intense forms of restraint (e.g., placing an individual on the ground in order to restrain him or her) are required, it is best to involve appropriately trained school security staff rather than teaching staff.

Alternative Educational Settings

The frequency, intensity, and variety of aggressive behaviors may also determine the restrictiveness of the educational setting in which aggression-related interventions are most effectively applied. Research has demonstrated that aggression is a highly stable form of behavior (Olweus, 1979). Two general onset trajectories for youth violence have been identified (Loeber, Farrington, and Waschbusch, 1998). One, an early-onset trajectory, in which children become seriously violent before age 13, results in youth who generally commit more crimes, and more serious crimes. The late-onset trajectory is one in which violence begins in adolescence and usually ends with transition into adulthood. Less is known about late-onset violence prevention, particularly for those serious violent offenders who emerge without apparent warning signs in their childhood (U.S. Department of Health and Human Services, 2001).

The frequency, intensity, and variety of aggressive behaviors are strong indices of how far along the developmental continuum of aggression a given individual has moved. The more frequently a child or youth engages in aggressive behavior, the more intense the aggressive behaviors, and the wider the variety of aggressive behaviors, the farther along the child or youth is on the aggression continuum. The farther along the aggression continuum the child has moved, the more intense the interventions to bring about changes in aggression must be. Therefore, interventions with a student who engages in aggressive behavior with high frequency, at very intense levels of aggression, and/or in a wide variety of aggressive behaviors may be best implemented within more restrictive alternative educational settings.

Characteristics of the Aggressive Individual

Another consideration in a problem-solving approach to interventions for aggressive behavior is the set of characteristics (both strengths and limitations) that the aggressive individual brings to the situation. The primary focus should be on the prevention of aggression and on strengthening individual assets and protective factors surrounding the individual. For those individuals for whom preventive strategies have not been effective, interventions unique to the specific characteristics of the aggressive individual are more likely to be effective.

Goldstein and Keller (1987) have conceptualized aggressive acts as involving a number of covert and observable events or skills. Identification of one or more of these as playing a part in a student's aggression may help a teacher or other school support staff member to develop classroom interventions to address the student's unique needs. These covert and observable events/skills include (1) cognitive and academic skill deficits, (2) arousal-heightening interpretation of external stimuli, (3) heightened affective arousal, (4) ineffective communication, (5) mismanagement of contingencies, (6) prosocial skill deficits, and (7) prosocial value deficits. A description of each event/skill and possible interventions for each follows.

Cognitive and Academic Skill Deficits

Before any of the individual-specific interventions described here are applied, it is important to determine whether the student has the capability to use the training. Many of the interventions require considerable cognitive skills on the part of the participants. More extensive modeling, role playing, and guided practice may be needed by some students. Within an academic setting applying effective instruction, one must constantly ask whether the instruction is at the appropriate level for the individual student. Instead of implementing complex interventions to address aggressive behavior, teachers may find that modifying instructional levels, approaches, and/or programs may reduce academic frustration and thus decrease aggression. Flexibility and creativity in instructional programming is critical. Use of peer and volunteer tutoring, as well as cooperative learning strategies, are important approaches, particularly for aggressive students who have missed instructional/learning time. Coordinated planning with parents/caregivers and with before- and after-school care programs can increase instructional/learning time. A focus on enhancing academic engagement and increasing academic achievement through effective teaching is a major component of many of the successful comprehensive violence prevention programs (U.S. Department of Health and Human Services, 2001).

Arousal-Heightening Interpretation of External Stimuli

A particular external event may trigger aggression, not because of anything inherent in the event, but because the event is accompanied or followed by kinesthetic and other physiological cues that signal anger to the individual. The individual presumably engages in anger-arousing self-statements (e.g., "That kid is cutting me off in the lunch line, and I'm going to get him"). An intervention that can be used to address this problem is anger control training (Feindler & Fremouw, 1983; Lochman, 1992). Anger control training focuses on triggers, cues, reminders, reducers, and self-evaluation. "Triggers" are the external events and internal interpretations or self-statements that serve to provoke anger arousal. "Cues" are the internal physiological experiences that uniquely signal anger arousal for the individual student. "Reminders" and "reducers" are self-control strategies for reducing anger arousal in any situation; these strategies include self-instruction and effective coping self-statements. Finally, "self-evaluation" enables participants in anger control training to determine how well they apply the self-control strategies. Anger control techniques are most effective when delivered by staff well trained in their application. Training in these techniques can be conducted by support services staff (e.g., school counselors, school psychologists, school social workers) and or teachers. Ideally, conducting anger control training in the classroom with teachers involved is likely to be most effective in terms of students' generalizing the self-control strategies.

Another approach to intervening in anger-arousing interpretations of events is to focus on the accuracy of the interpretations. Some students misread common teasing by peers and interpret the peers' statements or body language as hostile. Thus, they respond with anger and aggression. Interventions that address such misinterpretations and help students understand the meanings of words or body language are likely to be effective.

Heightened Affective Arousal

Teaching self-relaxation techniques (Jacobson, 1929, 1964) may be helpful for the individual who has the skills to recognize the internal bodily cues of anger arousal. In addition, it must be noted that most aggression involves more than a single individual. As indicated earlier in the discussion of verbal deescalation techniques, a number of intervention strategies can serve to reduce anger arousal. Modeling calmness through the use of body language (relaxed posture) and a soft, calm voice can be helpful. Encouraging talking (allowing venting, in an appropriate context without an audience) can be helpful in reducing anger. Open-ended questions and requests for descriptions of what happened, rather than judgmental statements and questions, are effective tactics for eliciting talking as an alternative to physical aggression. Active listening (through attention to the speaker, verbal reflection, and genuine interest) to the content of what is said, as well as its underlying meanings and feelings, is helpful in reducing anger arousal. Providing support both nonverbally and verbally can be helpful as well. Indicating that nonaggressive alternatives exist, and that the adult is willing to help the angry student attempt such alternative problem solutions, communicates active support and provides the individual with choices (doing the latter is necessary for the student to attain self-control).

Anger is often maintained or escalated because of a fear of "losing face" (a reputation/identity issue), because a student feels that not backing down is valued by other students. Thus, yet another effective tactic is to help the individual "save face." This can be done by removing any spectators from the confrontation and by helping the individual retreat or back down in a manner that does not involve the perceived loss of power. Again, effective professional development for teachers in the use of these strategies is crucial. These approaches are particularly helpful in establishing a positive climate for effective instruction and effective intervention.

Ineffective Communication

Some students engage in aggressive behavior because ineffective communication skills have served to escalate the aggression between two individuals. Sanger and her colleagues presented qualitative data on delinquent girls and described relationships between pragmatic language and violence (Sanger, Moore-Brown, Magnuson, & Svoboda, 2001; Sanger, Moore-Brown, Montgomery, Rezac, & Keller, 2003). Speech/language pathologists can work in the classroom and with teachers to facilitate the pragmatic language skills of children as a possible means of preventing aggression. They may assist in training to address ineffective communication skills, which can affect skills in problem solving (Elias & Clabby, 1992), and negotiation (Goldstein & Rosenbaum, 1982), as well as conflict mediation (Goldstein & Keller, 1987). Negotiated and agreed-upon settlements of aggressive conflicts are often tenuous at best. Since solutions are hard to reach and frequently easy to dissolve, the establishment of written contracts can be another effective intervention for communication problems. The behavioral literature has extensive coverage of behavioral contracting (e.g., Walker, 1990).

Mismanagement of Contingencies

In addition to strengthening communication, negotiation, and problem-solving skills as means of reducing or avoiding aggressive behavior, teachers and support personnel can train students, or others in the students' environment, to rearrange contingencies in order to strengthen desirable behaviors incompatible with aggressive behavior. There is an extensive behavioral literature on the systematic arranging of contingencies to increase and decrease particular behaviors in an individual's repertoire (e.g., Alberto & Troutman, 1999; O'Leary & O'Leary, 1977; Patterson, 1982). A critical assumption behind this approach is that desirable, prosocial alternative behaviors already exist in the individual's behavioral repertoire, but are rarely exhibited. Functional assessment is an important step in planning the rearrangement of contingencies. Staff development in behavioral strategies and staff support for the implementation and monitoring of behavioral programs are important. A positive support, rather than punitive, emphasis is critical for effective behavioral programs (Tobin & Sprague, 2000).

Consideration of the contingencies that influence the aggressive behavior of an individual must to some extent address the potential motivations for the behavior. This is particularly pertinent when teachers and schools use suspension or sending students to the office as a consequence for aggressive behavior. If the behavior is escape motivated, because of something aversive in the classroom setting, then removal from the classroom following the aggressive behavior serves as a reinforcer for aggression. For example, if a student does not do well in a particular academic subject, then the classroom may be aversive to the individual at the time the subject is taught. If aggressive behavior has resulted in removal from the classroom and its accompanying failure experience, then it is likely that aggressive behavior will be strengthened as a means of escaping the aversive situation. The student is likely to engage in aggressive behavior in order to avoid an unpleasant academic subject and classroom.

Prosocial Skill Deficits

An aggressive individual may not display alternative prosocial behaviors because he or she simply does not know how to do so. When such behaviors are weak or lacking altogether, they must be directly taught. There are a variety of curricula for directly teaching social skills to address the prosocial skill deficiencies of aggressive individuals (e.g., Cartledge & Kleefeld, 1991, 1994; Cartledge & Milburn, 1995; Goldstein et al., 1980; McGinnis & Goldstein, 1984, 1990; Sheridan, 1995). These curricular packages may be used in the classroom and taught by teachers, support professionals, and paraprofessionals who have had appropriate training or in-service staff development.

Prosocial Value Deficits

An individual may learn to control his or her anger, communicate effectively with others, and engage in alternative prosocial behaviors, but may still choose to behave in an aggressive manner. An intervention strategy designed to change underlying values—particularly values pertaining to regard for the needs and perspectives of others—may be needed. Goldstein (1999) has described one such prosocial values training strategy, based on the cognitive-developmental theory of Kohlberg (1976). The approach makes use of dilemma discussion groups, in which a group leader first assesses participants' level of moral reasoning, then presents each individual with cognitive conflicts at progressively higher stages of moral reasoning. As this description suggests, the demands on the group leader are extensive; there is also minimal documented evidence for the efficacy of this approach as a separate intervention.

In another approach, Goldstein and Glick (1987) have incorporated prosocial values training as one component within a comprehensive aggression replacement training package that includes anger control training, prosocial skills training, and parent training. Although they demonstrated direct training effects for anger control and prosocial skill acquisition, as well as a reduction in aggressive behaviors, there were limited direct training effects on prosocial values. We believe that focusing on such internal processes as prosocial values, however desirable, presents change agents with a formidable long-term task. An alternative approach to addressing an individual's choice of aggressive behaviors over alternative prosocial behaviors is to focus on problem-solving skills. The efficacy of problem-solving interventions is greater (Elias & Clabby, 1992), and there is demonstrated long-term maintenance (U.S. Department of Health and Human Services, 2001).

Teacher/Staff Member Considerations

An important concern with the implementation of interventions developed within a problem-solving approach is the person (or persons) responsible for carrying out the intervention. Does the teacher or staff member have the knowledge and skills needed to implement the interventions? Does this person have the necessary resources to implement the interventions effectively? Are there supports available to help this person design, implement, monitor, troubleshoot, and evaluate the efficacy of the interventions? Without such knowledge, skills, resources, and supports, the best-designed interventions for aggressive behavior are likely to fail. As stated earlier, professional development and opportunities for teachers to interact and share effective instructional and intervention ideas are critical for a building implementing effective prevention and intervention programs. Throughout this chapter, we have noted areas where staff development is crucial for successful implementation of classroom-based strategies. Further, in-building collaborative and multidisciplinary problem-solving teams (Kauffman et al., 1993; Rosenfield, 1992; Rosenfield & Gravois, 1996) can play a valuable role in the process. In addition to providing the necessary support functions indicated previously, such teams are additional human resources in the intervention process; team members can be particularly helpful in the initial implementation phases. Through the collaborative consultation process within a problem-solving approach (Conoley & Conoley, 1982; Rosenfield, 1992; Rosenfield & Gravois, 1996), they can serve to enhance the teachers' knowledge and skills as well. Involvement of parents and community agency representatives in the problem-solving process also increases the likelihood of success, as multiple contexts in the child's life become mobilized to attain common goals.

Implementation Costs

When determining which interventions to employ to address the aggressive behaviors manifested in the classroom setting, one must consider the relative costs of implementing the interventions. The extent of resources and supports, both within the classroom and in the broader school and community, must be considered. How much energy must the staff expend in order to carry out the intervention effectively? Can the intervention be conducted within the context of the particular classroom's instructional and management demands? It is also important to consider the potential impact of the intervention on other students in the classroom context. As noted earlier, in cases where the costs are too high in terms of energy, resources, supports, and potential impact on other students, the interventions may be implemented most appropriately in more restrictive alternative educational settings. It is important to note that prevention approaches targeting all students are cost-effective, in the long run, in comparison to individually focused intensive intervention programs initiated after more severe levels of aggression and violence are established.

MONITORING TREATMENT INTEGRITY AND OUTCOMES

The costs of aggressive behavior to society are so high, and the complexities of aggression so great, that it is critical for the effectiveness of prevention and intervention programs to be evaluated. The problem-solving approach advocated within this chapter consists of problem identification, problem analysis, plan implementation, and plan evaluation. Because it is not always possible to determine the optimal intervention for a given individual engaging in aggressive behavior, the problem-solving process of systematically generating and testing hypotheses is essential. Application of continuous progress monitoring is essential, so that strategies can be changed if unsuccessful for a given student.

Treatment integrity is a critical concern in the determination of an intervention's efficacy. It must be documented that the intervention was conducted in the manner in which it was designed. This is particularly important when an intervention is carried out by staff members other than the intervention's designer(s), following staff training or collaborative team problem solving. If the intervention was not implemented properly, then failure to bring about change in the aggressive behavior cannot be attributed to the inefficacy of the intervention. Too often prevention and intervention programs have been deemed unsuccessful, with no attention paid to the integrity with which the program was implemented. It may be that a given program was ineffective, but it could have been ineffective because it was not implemented properly. Kamps et al. (2000) demonstrated that the stronger the implementation of a prevention program, the greater the success of the program in terms of breadth and duration of effects. Staff training and monitoring of implementation are critical for successful prevention and intervention.

Evaluation of an intervention's efficacy must also involve multiple measures at multiple levels (Goldstein & Keller, 1983, 1987). Measures must include not only aggression and problem behaviors, but also changes in associated risk and protective factors. Such multimethod, multilevel evaluation allows the generalization of effects, as well as any unanticipated effects of an intervention, to be assessed. The question of generalization of effects relates to the importance of using both proximal and distal measures. "Proximal" measures are those measures that assess the direct and immediate effects of an intervention. For example, the proximal effects of prosocial skill training can be determined with role-play measures of the specific social skills that were taught during the intervention. Without such proximal evaluation for acquisition, there is little need to examine more important generalization ("distal") effects. That is, has the intervention had effects on the daily life of an individual student (e.g., school success, school truancy, discipline notices, suspensions, contact with police and/or the judicial system)? Has the specific skill training led to judgments of greater competence by significant others in the student's environment?

Another concern of treatment evaluation is with social validity (Kazdin, 1977). That is, there must be concern not only with whether significant change in target measures has taken place, but with whether the attained changes are meaningful and important to the individual student and to the student's significant others (e.g., teachers, parents, caregivers, siblings). Application of both quantitative and qualitative methodologies are needed to evaluate programs and their effectiveness.

The individualized intervention approach recommended here does not lend itself to large-sample inferential research designs for evaluating an intervention's efficacy. Furthermore, the reality constraints of school practitioners do not make such evaluation designs feasible. Time-series research methodology is more appropriately applied to the demands of the school setting and individualized interventions. Although time-series methodology has been developed within the context of behavioral approaches, its application is not limited to such interventions (Barlow, Hayes, & Nelson, 1984; Hersen & Barlow, 1976; Kazdin, 1980; Kratochwill & Levin, 1992). With thorough record keeping and documentation of intervention processes, data from individual students can be aggregated over time for application of inferential statistics. Such aggregation of individual data will permit consideration of the generality and specificity of intervention effects with respect to student and problem characteristics and will enhance the development of effective individualized interventions. Data can be aggregated not only across students, but also across staff members within a school setting. Finally, collaboration with researchers at nearby colleges and universities may allow the use of more elaborate control group and large-sample inferential designs within the context of educating students. Monitoring treatment integrity and program outcomes should not have to be done by the classroom teacher. Support from building teams and district evaluation specialists is essential to the program evaluation process. In addition, the development of collaborative research partnerships between public and private schools and colleges and universities would be of mutual benefit.

In summary, we believe that a proactive, multilevel problem-solving approach to preventing and reducing aggression in the classroom is optimal. Prevention must be the primary focus, as much greater costs are involved when we intervene after aggressive behavior has escalated and moved farther along the developmental trajectories. These greater costs are evident both fiscally and in terms of effects on all those involved. Individualized problem solving is likely to be more effective than the frequently used reactive approach of suspension and expulsion. Although reactive strategies may solve immediate problems, they do not solve long-term problems within individuals, the classroom, or broader ecological contexts.

REFERENCES

Alberto, P., & Troutman, A. (1999). *Applied behavioral analysis for teachers* (5th ed.). Englewood Cliffs, NJ: Prentice-Hall.

Bandura, A. (1973). *Aggression: A social learning analysis*. Englewood Cliffs, NJ: Prentice-Hall.

Barlow, D. H., Hayes, S. C., & Nelson, R. (1984). *The scientist practitioner: Research and accountability in clinical and educational settings*. Elmsford, NY: Pergamon Press.

Bierman, K., Coie, J., Dodge, K., Greenberg, M., Lochman, J., & McMahon, R. (1992). A developmental and clinical model for the prevention of conduct disorder: The FAST Track Program. *Development and Psychopathology, 4*, 509–527.

Botvin, G. J., Mihalic, S. F., & Grotpeter, J. K. (1998). *Life skills training*. Boulder, CO: Center for the Study and Prevention of Violence.

Brophy, J. E., & Good, T. L. (1986). Teacher behavior and student achievement. In M. L. Wittrock (Ed.), *Handbook of research on teaching* (3rd ed., pp. 328–375). New York: Macmillan.

Camp, B. W. (1977). Verbal mediation in young aggressive boys. *Journal of Abnormal Psychology, 86*, 145–153.

Cartledge, G., & Kleefeld, J. (1991). *Taking part: Introducing social skills to children*. Circle Pines, MN: American Guidance Service.

Cartledge, G., & Kleefeld, J. (1994). *Working together: Building children's social skills through folk literature*. Circle Pines, MN: American Guidance Service.

Cartledge, G., & Milburn, J. F. (1995). *Teaching social skills to children and youth: Innovative approaches* (3rd ed.). Boston: Allyn & Bacon.

Charles, C. M. (1992). *Building classroom discipline* (4th ed.). White Plains, NY: Longman.

Coie, J. D., Dodge, K. A., & Kupersmidt, J. (1990). Peer group behavior and social status. In S. R. Asher & J. D. Coie (Eds.), *Peer rejection in childhood* (pp. 67–99). New York: Cambridge University Press.

Coie, J. D., & Krehbiel, G. (1990). Adapting intervention to the problems of aggressive and disruptive rejected children. In S. R. Asher & J. D. Coie (Eds.), *Peer rejection in childhood* (pp. 178–201). New York: Cambridge University Press.

Conoley, J. C., & Conoley, C. W. (1982). *School consultation: A guide to practice and training*. Elmsford, NY: Pergamon Press.

Dolan, L., Turkan, J., Wethamer-Larsson, L., & Kellam, S. (1989). *The good behavior game manual*. Baltimore, MD: The Prevention Program. (Also available on the Internet at *www.bpp.jhu.edu*)

Doll, B., & Lyon, M. A. (1998). Risk and resilience: Implications for the delivery of educational and mental health services in schools. *School Psychology Review, 27*, 348–363.

Dunlap, G., Kern, L., dePerczel, M., Clarke, S., Wilson, D., Childs, K., White, R., & Falk, G. (1993). Functional analysis of classroom variables for students with emotional and behavioral disorders. *Behavioral Disorders, 18*, 275–291.

Durlak, J. A. (1983). Social problem-solving as a primary prevention strategy. In R. D. Felner, L. A. Jason, J. N. Moritsugu, & S. S. Farber (Eds.), *Preventive psychology: Theory, research, and practice* (pp. 31–48). Elmsford, NY: Pergamon Press.

Dwyer, K., Osher, D., & Warger, C. (1998). *Early warning, timely response: A guide to safe schools*. Washington, DC: U. S. Department of Education.

Elias, M. J., & Clabby, J. F. (1992). *Building social problem-solving skills: Guidelines from a school-based program*. San Francisco: Jossey-Bass.

Emmer, E. T., Evertson, C. M., Sanford, J. P., Clements, B. S., & Worsham, M. E. (1984). *Classroom management for secondary teachers*. Englewood Cliffs, NJ: Prentice-Hall.

Evertson, C. M., Emmer, E. T., Clements, B. S., Sanford, J. P., & Worsham, M. E. (1984). *Classroom management for elementary teachers*. Englewood Cliffs, NJ: Prentice-Hall.

Feindler, E. L., & Fremouw, W. J. (1983). Stress inoculation training for adolescent anger problems. In D. Meichenbaum & M. E. Jaremko (Eds.), *Stress reduction and prevention* (pp. 451–485). New York: Plenum Press.

Felner, R. D., Brand, S., Adan, A. M., Mulhall, P. F., Flowers, N., Sartain, B., & BuBois, D. L. (1993). Restructuring the ecology of the school as an approach to prevention during school transitions: Longitudinal follow-ups and extensions of the School Transitional Environment Project (STEP). In L. A. Jason, K. E. Danner, & K. S. Kuraski (Eds.), *Prevention and school transitions* (pp. 103–136). New York: Haworth Press.

Frey, K. S., Hirschstein, M. K., & Guzzo, B. A. (2000). Second Step: Preventing aggression by promoting social competence. *Journal of Emotional and Behavioral Disorders, 8,* 102–112.

Fuchs, L. S., & Fuchs, D. (2000). Analogue assessment of academic skills: Curriculum-based measurement and performance assessment. In E. S. Shapiro & T. R. Kratochwill (Eds.), *Behavioral assessment in schools: Theory, research, and clinical foundations* (2nd ed., pp. 168–201). New York: Guilford Press.

Gesten, E. L., Rains, M. H., Rapkin, B. D., Weissberg, R. P., Flores de Apodaca, R., Cowen, E. L., & Bowen, R. (1982). Training children in social problem-solving competencies: A first and second look. *American Journal of Community Psychology, 10,* 95–115.

Gettinger, M. (1988). Methods of proactive classroom management. *School Psychology Review, 17,* 227–242.

Goldstein, A. P. (Ed.). (1978). *Prescriptions for child mental health and education*. Elmsford, NY: Pergamon Press.

Goldstein, A. P. (1999). *The prepare curriculum* (2nd ed.). Champaign, IL: Research Press.

Goldstein, A. P., & Glick, B. (1987). *Aggression replacement training: A comprehensive intervention for aggressive youth*. Champaign, IL: Research Press.

Goldstein, A. P., Glick, B., Irwin, M. J., Pask, C., & Rubama, I. (1989). *Reducing delinquency: Intervention in the community*. Elmsford, NY: Pergamon Press.

Goldstein, A. P., Harootunian, B., & Conoley, J. C. (1994). *Student aggression: Prevention, management, and replacement training*. New York: Guilford Press.

Goldstein, A. P., & Keller, H. R. (1983). Aggression prevention and control: Multi-targeted, multi-channel, multi-disciplinary. In Center for Research on Aggression (Ed.), *Prevention and control of aggression* (pp. 338–350). Elmsford, NY: Pergamon Press.

Goldstein, A. P., & Keller, H. R. (1987). *Aggressive behavior: Assessment and intervention*. Elmsford, NY: Pergamon Press.

Goldstein, A. P., Palumbo, J., Striepling, S., & Voutsinas, A. M. (1995). *Break it up: A teacher's guide to managing student aggression*. Champaign, IL: Research Press.

Goldstein, A. P., & Rosenbaum, A. (1982). *Aggress-less*. Englewood Cliffs, NJ: Prentice-Hall.

Goldstein, A. P., Sprafkin, R. P., Gershaw, J. J., & Klein, P. (1980). *Skillstreaming the adolescent*. Champaign, IL: Research Press.

Greenberg, M. T., Kusche, C., & Mihalic, S. (1998). Promoting alternative thinking strategies (PATHS). In D. S. Elliott (Series Ed.), *Blueprints for violence prevention*. Boulder, CO: Center for the Study and Prevention of Violence, Institute of Behavioral Science, University of Colorado at Boulder.

Gresham, F. M., & Noell, G. H. (1999). Functional analysis assessment as a cornerstone for noncategorical special education. In D. J. Reschley, W. D. Tilly, & J. P. Grimes (Eds.), *Special education in transition: Functional assessment and noncategorical programming* (pp. 49–79). Longmont, CO: Sopris West.

Hersen, M., & Barlow, D. H. (1976). *Single case experimental designs: Strategies for studying behavior change*. Elmsford, NY: Pergamon Press.

Hoff, K., & DuPaul, G. (1998). Reducing disruptive behavior in general education classrooms: The use of slf-management strategies. *School Psychology Review, 27*, 290–303.

Jacobson, E. (1929). *Progressive relaxation*. Chicago: University of Chicago Press.

Jacobson, E. (1964). *Anxiety and tension control*. Philadelphia: J. B. Lippincott.

Kamps, D., Kravits, T., Rauch, J., Kamps, J. L., & Chung, N. (2000). A prevention program for students with or at risk for ED: Moderating effects of variation in treatment and classroom structure. *Journal of Emotional and Behavioral Disorders, 8*, 141–154.

Kauffman, J. M., Hallahan, D. P., Mostert, M. P., Trent, S. C., & Nuttycombe, D. G. (1993). *Managing classroom behavior: A reflective case-based approach*. Boston: Allyn & Bacon.

Kazdin, A. E. (1977). Assessing the clinical or applied significance of behavior change through social validation. *Behavior Modification, 1*, 427–452.

Kazdin, A. E. (1980). *Research design in clinical psychology*. New York: Harper & Row.

Kazdin, A. E. (1987). *Conduct disorders in childhood and adolescence*. Beverly Hills, CA: Sage.

Kazdin, A. E. (1994). Interventions for aggressive and antisocial children. In L. D. Eron, J. H. Gentry, & P. Schlegel (Eds.), *Reason to hope: A psychosocial perspective on violence and youth* (pp. 341–382). Washington, DC: American Psychological Association.

Kern, L, & Dunlap, G. (1999). Developing effective program plans for students with disabilities. In D. J. Reschley, W. D. Tilly, & J. P. Grimes (Eds.), *Special education in transition: Functional assessment and noncategorical programming* (pp. 213–232). Longmont, CO: Sopris West.

Kohlberg, L. (1976). Moral stages and moralization: The cognitive-development approach. In T. Lickona (Ed.), *Moral development and behavior: Theory, research and social issues* (pp. 31–53). New York: Holt, Rinehart & Winston.

Kratochwill, T. R., & Levin, J. R. (Eds.). (1992). *Single-case research design and analysis: New directions for psychology and education*. Hillsdale, NJ: Erlbaum.

Lochman, J. E. (1992). Cognitive-behavioral intervention with aggressive boys: Three-year follow-up and preventive effects. *Journal of Consulting and Clinical Psychology, 60*, 426–432.

Loeber, R., Farrington, D. P., & Waschbusch, D. A. (1998). Serious and violent juvenile offenders. In R. Loeber & D. P. Farrington (Eds.), *Serious and violent juvenile offenders: Risk factors and successful interventions* (pp. 13–29). Thousand Oaks, CA: Sage.

Luthar, S. S., & Cicchetti, D. (2000). The construct of resilience: Implications for interventions and social policies. *Development and Psychopathology, 12*, 857–885.

Mahoney, M. J. (1974). *Cognition and behavior modification*. Cambridge, MA: Ballinger.

Masten, A. S. (2001). Ordinary magic: Resilience processes in development. *American Psychologist, 56*, 227–238.

McEvoy, A., & Welker, R. (2000). Antisocial behavior, academic failure, and school climate: A critical review. *Journal of Emotional and Behavioral Disorders, 8*, 130–140.

McGinnis, E., & Goldstein, A. P. (1984). *Skillstreaming the elementary school child: A guide for teaching prosocial skills*. Champaign, IL: Research Press.

McGinnis, E., & Goldstein, A. P. (1990). *Skillstreaming in early childhood*. Champaign, IL: Research Press.

Meichenbaum, D. H. (1977). *Cognitive-behavior modification: An integrative approach*. New York: Plenum Press.

O'Donnell, J., Hawkins, J. D., Catalano, R. F., Abbott, R. D., & Day, E. (1995). Preventing school failure, drug use, and delinquency among low-income children: Long-term intervention in elementary schools. *American Journal of Orthopsychiatry, 65*, 87–100.

O'Leary, K. D., & O'Leary, S. G. (1977). *Classroom management*. Elmsford, NY: Pergamon Press.

Olweus, D. (1979). Stability of aggressive reaction patterns in males: A review. *Psychological Bulletin, 86*, 852–875.

Olweus, D., Limber, S., & Mihalic, S. (1998). Bullying prevention program. In D. S. Elliott (Series Ed.), *Blueprints for violence prevention*. Boulder, CO: Center for the Study and Prevention of Violence, Institute of Behavioral Science, University of Colorado at Boulder.

Patterson, G. R. (1982). *Coercive family process*. Eugene, OR: Castalia.

Pelligrini, D. S., & Urbain, E. S. (1985). An evaluation of interpersonal cognitive problem solving training with children. *Journal of Child Psychology and Psychiatry, 26*, 17–41.

Rhode, G., Jenson, W., & Reavis, H. (1998). *The tough kid book: Practical classroom management strategies*. Longmont, CO: Sopris West.

Rosenfield, S. (1992). Developing school-based consultation teams: A design for organizational change. *School Psychology Quarterly, 7*, 27–46.

Rosenfield, S. A., & Gravois, T. A. (1996). *Instructional consultation teams: Collaborating for change*. New York: Guilford Press.

Sanger, D. D., Moore-Brown, B., Magnuson, G., & Svoboda, N. (2001). Prevalence of language problems among adolescent delinquents: A closer look. *Communication Disorders Quarterly, 23*(1), 17–25.

Sanger, D., Moore-Brown, B. J., Montgomery, J., Rezac, C., & Keller, H. (2003). Female incarcerated adolescents with language problems talk about their own communication behaviors and learning. *Journal of Communication Disorders, 36*, 465–486.

Sheridan, S. M. (1995). *The tough kid social skills book*. Longmont, CO: Sopris West.

Slavin, R. E. (1980). *Using student team learning* (rev. ed.). Baltimore: Center for Social Organization of Schools, Johns Hopkins University.

Slavin, R. E. (1989). When does cooperative learning increase student achievement? *Psychological Bulletin, 94*, 429–445.

Slavin, R. E. (1990). Achievement effects of ability grouping in secondary schools: A best-evidence synthesis. *Review of Educational Research, 60*, 471–499.

Slavin, R. E., Sharan, S., Kagan, S., Hertz-Lazarowitz, R., Webb, C., & Schmuck, R. (1985). *Learning to cooperate, cooperating to learn*. New York: Plenum Press.

Spivack, G., & Shure, M. B. (1974). *Social adjustment in young children*. San Francisco: Jossey-Bass.

Stoolmiller, M., Eddy, J. M., & Reid, J. B. (2000). Detecting and describing preventative intervention effects in a universal school-based randomized trial targeting delinquent and violent behavior. *Journal of Consulting and Clinical Psychology, 68*, 296–306.

Tobin, T., & Sprague, J. (2000). Alternative education strategies: Reducing violence in school and the community. *Journal of Emotional and Behavioral Disorders, 8*, 177–186.

U.S. Department of Health and Human Services. (2001). *Youth violence: A report of the Surgeon General*. Rockville, MD: U. S. Department of Health and Human Services, Centers for Disease Control and Prevention, National Center for Injury Prevention and Control; Substance Abuse and Mental Health Services Administration, Center for

Mental Health Services; and National Institutes of Health, National Institute of Mental Health.

Walker, H., Colvin, G., & Ramsey, E. (1995). *Antisocial behavior in school: Strategies and best practices*. Boston: Brookes/Cole.

Walker, J. E. (1990). *Behavior management: Practical approach for educators* (5th ed.). Columbus, OH: Merrill.

Webster-Stratton, C. (1999). *How to promote social and emotional competence in young children*. Thousand Oaks, CA: Sage.

Weissberg, R. P., Gesten, E. L., Carnilce, C. L., Toro, P. A., Rapkin, B. D., Davidson, E., & Cowen, E. L. (1981). Social problem-solving skills training: A competence building intervention with 2nd–4th grade children. *American Journal of Community Psychology, 9*, 411–424.

Weissberg, R. P., Gesten, E. L., Rapkin, B. D., Cowen, E. L., Davidson, E., Flores de Apodaca, R., & McKim, B. J. (1981). The evaluation of a social problem-solving training program for suburban and inner city third grade children. *Journal of Consulting and Clinical Psychology, 49*, 251–261.

Wentzel, K. R. (1997). Student motivation in middle school: The role of perceived pedagogical caring. *Journal of Educational Psychology, 89*, 411–419.

Wentzel, K. R., & Wigfield, A. (1998). Academic and social motivational influences on students' academic performance. *Educational Psychology Review, 10*, 155–175.

Wyman, P. A., Sandler, I., Wolchik, S., & Nelson, K. (2000). Resilience as cumulative competence promotion and stress protection: Theory and intervention. In D. Cicchetti, J. Rappaport, I. Sandler, & R. Weissberg (Eds.), *The promotion of wellness in children and adolescents* (pp. 133–184). Washington, DC: CWLA.

Ysseldyke, J., & Christenson, S. (1993). *The instructional environment system-II: A system to identify a student's instructional needs*. Longmont, CO: Sopris West.

CHAPTER 7

School Crisis Teams

SCOTT POLAND

Ronald D. Stephens, the executive director of the National School Safety Center (NSSC), has said that there are two types of schools in this country—those that just had a crisis and those that are about to have one (Stephens, 1994). Stephens has also pointed out that many schools have been "caught with their plans down" (Stephens, 1989). My colleagues and I (Poland, Pitcher, & Lazarus, 1995) cite surveys showing that only about 25% of schools have a crisis plan, and note that only one state, South Carolina, has formally legislated crisis planning for schools.

It is very difficult to gather actual incidence figures for school violence and other tragedies that affect schools. Furlong and Morrison (1994) have pointed out that there *has* been a real increase in school violence; however, media coverage has made the problem seem worse than it really is. Schools have been proven to be safer than their communities.

It is difficult to get exact figures on the number of homicides or suicides that occur at school each year. Federal government researchers reported 105 such deaths in the years 1992–1994 ("Data Released," 1995). These researchers also found the following when they surveyed high school students:

- 11% had brought a weapon to school in the last month.
- 25% had been offered, sold, or given an illegal drug.
- 4.4% had missed a day of school in the last month because of safety concerns.

The number of young people who are fearful at school seems to be growing, unfortunately. A 1993 study of 24,000 secondary students found that 50% of them follow conscious strategies to avoid harm at school (Porter, 1996). Porter (1995b) has also noted that juvenile arrests for murder and other violent crime have soared over the last decade, largely because of the increasing availability of drugs and guns.

The role of school personnel in organizing crisis teams and affecting the entire area of school crisis and violence can and must be an active one. Pitcher and Poland (1992) have pointed out that most crisis planning is done in the aftermath of traumatic events. Unfortunately, school personnel lack training, preparation, and planning in this important area, and many have a tendency to believe that a crisis will not occur at their school. However, one only has to read the newspaper to be struck by the volume, intensity, and severity of school crisis situations. I have come to the conclusion that any event that might be imagined as too horrific to ever occur has already happened and a school has dealt with it. Schools not only are increasingly recognizing their responsibility in regard to school crises, but are increasingly being held liable for such crises. The trend to hold schools more accountable has been emphasized repeatedly (Pitcher & Poland, 1992; Poland et al., 1995; Stephens, 1994, 1995). Schools have not been required to report figures on crime and violence up to this point; however, recent national legislation requires such reporting by universities and colleges. One can predict that more accountability will be required of schools and administrators in the very near future.

SCHOOL CRISIS HISTORY: WHAT HAVE WE LEARNED?

One of the first school crisis incidents to gain national attention was the kidnapping of a busload of schoolchildren in Chowchilla, California, in the early 1970s. This incident and the school response was reviewed in detail by Terr (1983), who pointed out that once the children escaped their kidnappers after being buried underground for 3 days, nothing was provided for them in the way of counseling support by either the school or the local mental health authorities. Pitcher and Poland (1992) have noted that the prevailing view in the mental health field at that time was that children who experience a crisis are resilient and will bounce back. Terr (1983) examined this very point and found that 5 years later, 100% of the Chowchilla children had clinical symptoms of depression, fear, or anxiety.

Elsewhere (Poland, 1994), I have cited several examples of schools that were much more responsive following a crisis; they took steps to return students to school as quickly as possible and provided counseling and group processing activities at school. Sandall (1986) described a very active school response in Cokeville, Wyoming, following a bomb explosion and fire in an elementary school. The school administrator took a number of steps to manage the crisis and provide leadership to the entire community. The following specific steps were taken in Cokeville:

- A town meeting was held to give everyone the facts.
- Children were encouraged to return to school as soon as possible.

- Faculty meetings were held not only to help the faculty members cope, but to outline how they could help their students.
- Children were given an opportunity to express their emotions, as well as permission to express a range of emotions.

Sandall emphasized that those children who verbalized their feelings about the incident the most openly recovered the most quickly. A key point was made by the principal, who quoted the old Western saying that once you fall off a horse, you need to get right back on again to minimize your fears.

A tragic shooting occurred at an elementary school in Winnetka, Illinois, near the end of the school year in 1988. This incident was described in detail by Dillard (1989), who was the school psychologist. Dillard was at the central office when the incident occurred and made immediate plans to go to the school, only to be told by superiors to stay away. Dillard had no idea about what might be appropriate duties to perform, but felt a need to go to the scene. Dillard became the advocate for the students' being provided processing opportunities at school; in fact, meetings were held with students and parents throughout the summer.

Prior to the shootings at Columbine High School, Littleton, Colorado, in April 1999, the most violent event to occur on school grounds in the United States took place in Stockton, California, in January 1989. A gunman opened fire on students and teachers on the playground at Cleveland Elementary School. Armstrong (1990) and Busher (1990) discussed this tragedy, in which 5 children were killed and 29 wounded. They emphasized that previous crisis drills conducted on that very playground resulted in lives' being saved. The school took numerous steps to give everyone concerned the facts and to deal with the problems resulting from many parents' and some students' not being proficient in English. However, Armstrong (1990) pointed out that although many mental health workers were quickly brought to the school, a number of teachers chose not to allow them into their classrooms. The teachers, as a group, were reluctant to discuss the incident and wanted to receive extra pay to stay after school to share their feelings. The administration did not authorize extra pay, nor was long-term counseling assistance provided to students until parents marched on the central office and got the attention of the local news media. Pitcher and Poland (1992) have discussed the reluctance of school personnel, in this case and many others, to process crisis incidents. A recommended strategy is to call a faculty meeting for the purpose of assisting the faculty to help students, but first to help the faculty cope.

These are only a few of the many crisis events with which schools have dealt. There is an emerging trend for schools to be more active following a crisis. It is known today that although children are resilient, it is necessary for schools to take a number of steps following a crisis. Pitcher and Poland (1992) have cited key principles outlined by the National Institute of Mental Health:

- School mental health workers are encouraged to seek out children who need their help.
- Children need to be provided with opportunities to express their emotions and to be given permission to express a range of emotions. The most common reactions of children to a crisis are fear of future bad events, regression in behavior, and difficulty in sleeping.
- Parents need to be provided with information about childhood reactions to crisis and need to be given specific suggestions about how to assist their child. This can often be accomplished by conducting a meeting with parents as quickly as possible.

A review of the school crisis literature indicates that some important lessons can be learned from those who have experienced a crisis. The NSSC gathered together administrators who had experienced a severe crisis and developed an excellent training film entitled *School Crisis under Control* (NSSC, 1991). The administrators themselves provided the following advice about school crisis for other administrators:

- Recognize that it could happen to you. Crisis situations occur even in the best schools.
- What you learn in one crisis situation will help you in the next situation, although no two crisis situations are alike.
- Crisis team members must understand their duties, and crisis plans must be updated annually.
- Everyone must be alert for crises, and crisis intervention is an "inside job" that involves a prepared staff, student body, and community.

GAINING ADMINISTRATIVE SUPPORT FOR CRISIS PLANNING

It may seem that all administrators recognize the need for crisis planning. There have been many moving first-person accounts of how administrators dealt with a tragedy. The simple fact, however, is that most school administrators have had no training in this area and have very high levels of denial. A statement by Carden, an administrator whose school a gunman held hostage, summarizes the attitude of many administrators: "School officials are reluctant to face this. It's like a will—people are afraid to write one because they think they will die if they do!" (quoted in Jennings, 1989, p. 27). General obstacles to crisis planning in the schools, pointed out by McIntyre and Reid (1989), include the following:

- There is a myth that taking action will make the crisis worse.
- There are territorial issues exist about whose job crisis planning is, and it is often not listed on anyone's job description.

- Schools often lack the needed resources for planning, and administrators often lack the time.
- Few curriculum units are devoted to safety topics, conflict resolution, or problem solving.

Peterson and Straub (1992) emphasize that school administrators have a clear legal obligation to make crisis plans. They cite the growing legal trend to hold a third party (i.e., the school) responsible for failing to take reasonable steps to prevent a crisis or manage a crisis situation. Several states have begun to enact legislation to address the area of school crisis planning (Brock, Sandoval, & Lewis, 1995). As noted at the beginning of this chapter, the most significant legislation was passed recently in South Carolina, where schools are now required to have a crisis plan. However, several surveys (cited in Pitcher & Poland, 1992) indicate that few schools have a crisis plan, and a concern for those that do have plans is that the plans are often gathering dust on a shelf and are not a part of conducting school on an everyday basis.

School crisis planning must be viewed as a constantly evolving task, and, according to Stephens (1994), it must be listed as a priority in the job descriptions of administrators and other school personnel. What advice is there for educators who are unable to persuade principals and superintendents to devote time to crisis planning? Burneman (1995) has pointed out that those who cannot get administrative support for crisis planning may want to focus their energy on other topics; however, it is very important to be persistent in writing crisis plans and providing reluctant administrators with books, journal articles, and newspaper clippings about crisis situations. The sad reality is that most school crisis planning takes place only after a tragedy occurs. I have fielded numerous calls from school personnel around the country who were in the midst of a crisis, and the common theme of these calls is that everyone wished more planning time had been devoted to clarifying the responsibilities of crisis team members and developing plans. The following biblical quotation summarizes the need for crisis planning today: "I must work the works of him that sent me, while it is day: the night cometh, when no man can work" (John 9:4, King James Version).

THE ORGANIZATION OF SCHOOL CRISIS TEAMS

There is a growing literature to guide schools in developing crisis teams (Brock et al., 1995; Johnson, 1993; Poland & Pitcher, 1990; Peterson & Straub, 1992; Ruof & Harris, 1988; Slaikeu, 1984; Watson, Poda, Miller, Rice, & West, 1990). Elsewhere (Poland, 1993), I have emphasized three key points for schools to follow:

1. Staff members must review the crisis situations that have already occurred, with an emphasis on how the event could have been either prevented or managed better.
2. Each school or district must examine its own resources and circumstances and make a plan that fits its situation and needs.
3. School crisis planning must be based on a theoretical model.

Theoretical Model for Crisis Planning

School crisis planning is a very broad area, and it is difficult for schools to decide exactly where to begin with what seems to be an overwhelming task. It is essential that schools begin with a theoretical model to guide all of their efforts. Caplan (1964) developed a famous model, which emphasizes that there are three levels of crisis intervention. This framework has been elaborated on in regard to the schools and has been found to encompass all areas of crisis planning, including such diverse areas as law enforcement, transportation, school safety, and curriculum issues (Pitcher & Poland, 1992; Slaikeu, 1984). Schools must develop crisis plans at all three of the following levels:

1. "Primary prevention," which consists of activities devoted to preventing a crisis from occurring. Examples include conflict resolution, gun safety, safe driving, and suicide prevention programs.
2. "Secondary intervention," which includes steps taken in the immediate aftermath of a crisis to minimize the effects of the crisis and keep it from escalating. Examples include evacuating students to a safe place away from danger and leading classroom discussions on death and loss immediately after a death in the school family.
3. "Tertiary intervention," which involves providing long-term follow-up assistance to those who have experienced a severe crisis. An example is monitoring and supporting the friends of a suicide victim a year after the suicide and being alert to a possible anniversary effect.

Schools have a tendency to view crisis intervention as having only one level, secondary intervention. Poland et al. (1995) pointed out that those present at one high school described in great detail what they thought and did in the immediate aftermath of the shooting of the assistant principal, but it was difficult to convince school officials of the ongoing needs for assistance for the faculty and students, or of the need for prevention activities to reduce the bringing of weapons to school. The crisis provided an opportunity to create prevention programs and develop crisis teams that could improve the school's ability to respond to such events, but it was hard to convince the school staff of this. Indeed, the most common school reaction to a crisis is to ignore it, because of lack of training or fear that a response will worsen the situation or result in an administrator being criticized (Oates, 1988). Schools that do respond to a crisis are only rarely implementing previously thought-out intervention plans. It is imperative that schools make their plans today and organize them on the basis of Caplan's (1964) model. Every school has already experienced some type of crisis event and needs to review the handling of the event with a critical eye as to what worked and what did not. Schools need to anticipate what additional types of crisis events might occur and make plans to deal with them.

Developing Crisis Teams

There is not a great deal of literature available on how to organize crisis teams in schools. What qualities or characteristics should crisis team members have? Burneman (1995) addressed this question and cited these important qualities for potential crisis team members:

- A broad perspective on life
- Ability to project multiple consequences
- Willingness to challenge ideas and work cooperatively toward a solution
- Ability to think clearly under stress
- Flexibility
- Familiarity with the school system and community
- Availability

I have also stressed the importance of choosing crisis team members who are known to stay calm and who are motivated to make a difference (Poland, 1995). Each school or district must look at its own resources and then choose one of the following three options as teams are organized:

1. A building team, in which every member works in the same building. The obvious advantages are that team members know one another and the student body and that they can easily meet on a routine basis to review crisis plans. This approach works well when a school is large enough to have campus personnel in important positions (e.g., nurse, counselor, psychologist, and security liaison).

2. A district team, in which every member is employed by the school district. This arrangement makes communication and crisis planning more difficult than when a building approach is utilized. A counselor or nurse may have to cover several locations, and the psychologist may have to be called from the central office. It is important that a representative from each high school be included on the team, because the literature and experience clearly indicate that high school students are more at risk for violent and accidental deaths.

3. A combination district and community team, in which some team members are employed by the district and others (e.g., medical personnel, mental health workers, or police officers) are employed by community agen-

cies. This arrangement is more difficult to organize, but it is what many small and rural school districts need in order to develop comprehensive plans. A district should never be in the position of establishing relations with outside agencies after a crisis has occurred.

Planning meetings should be held with representatives of all the agencies that are going to be involved. Some schools have been frustrated by a lack of response from community agencies. It is important that schools and districts make initial plans and get crisis planning started while continuing to try to involve agency personnel. It is particularly important to be cautious about outside professionals who call a school on the day of a crisis and volunteer to help; their credentials and expertise must to be examined to ensure that they have the needed skills. The ideal arrangement is to locate and interview these professionals before a crisis occurs. This process is especially important if local ministers are to be called on for assistance, because of probable differences of opinion among denominations about the handling of crises.

Schools that have building crisis teams may still need to call for extra assistance from the district or central office. Johnson (1993) has discussed the difference between a centralized and an on-site team. Elsewhere (Poland, 1994), I have cited incidents in which a centralized team was not called by a building administrator after a student death, and I have stressed the need for centralized teams to solve entry issues. A campus administrator may either fail to call the centralized crisis team or fail to implement its suggestions. The team members must publicize their services and establish credibility and may need to add a member from a resistant campus to their team. Site or building teams are in the best position to work on prevention, and centralized or district teams can assist with intervention after a crisis has occurred. A practice that works well is to call in counselors from feeder schools, as these counselors may already have relationships established with the students who have experienced a crisis. A sample organizational chart that may be used for any of the three types of crisis teams is provided in Figure 7.1.

How many members should a crisis team have? The purpose of a team is to delegate duties, because it is simply not possible for one administrator to do everything that is needed in the aftermath of a crisis. There are school districts that have 20-member teams and 200-page crisis plans. However, I have cautioned against writing plans that are so lengthy that school personnel will not review them on a regular basis (Poland, 1993); the plans should be made part of everyday school planning. The question of team size is an administrative and commonsense one. Schoenfeld (1993) has recommended 1–2 members for every 100 students, but this would not be very practical for a high school of 3,000, as it would necessitate a crisis team of 30–60. If the team is very large, then it is hard to schedule meetings and communicate with all members. Conversely, a team that is composed of only 2 or 3 people

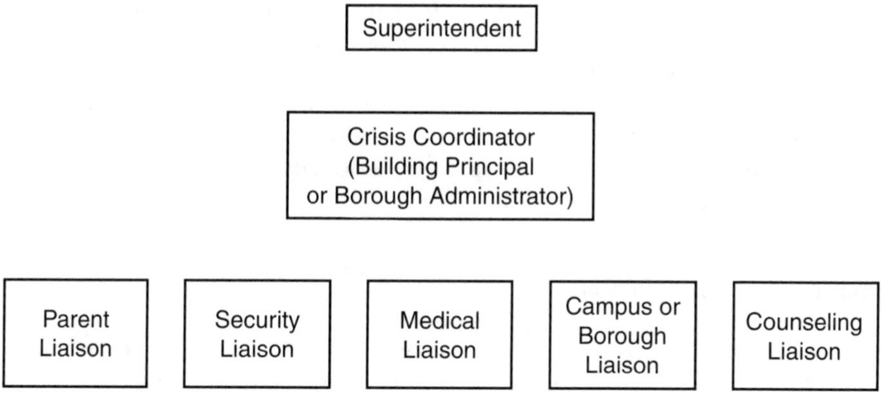

FIGURE 7.1. Sample organizational chart.

will be too small, especially when one member might be away for some reason. Poland and Pitcher (1990) recommended a team size of 4–8. At a minimum, the team should include the following members to assist the responsible administrator: (1) a medical liaison, (2) a security liaison, (3) a parent liaison, and (4) a counseling liaison. This would result in a team of 5. All of these liaisons could have other school staff members appointed to assist them. Two additional team members who may be useful are a media liaison and a campus liaison. The building principal may want to fill those roles rather than delegating them.

Peterson and Straub (1992) have developed school crisis plans that outline the roles of three key school professionals: teacher, counselor, and principal. Pitcher and Poland (1992) described a six-member crisis team in great detail stressing that team members should be chosen for their ability to do the job and that all duties should be arranged according to Caplan's (1964) model. All team members should be asked what they are doing to prevent a crisis from occurring, not just what they are going to do in the immediate aftermath of a crisis. The following is an example of relevant duties for an emotional or counseling liaison:

1. *Primary prevention.* Implement curriculum programs in areas such as suicide prevention, drug education, gun safety, safe driving, bicycle safety, and conflict resolution. Locate counseling assistance in both the school district and the community, and become familiar with the most common reactions of children and adolescents to a disaster. Determine where in the school counseling services can be provided, given existing space limitations.

2. *Secondary intervention.* Provide small-group and individual counseling after a crisis. Advocate for opportunities for students to express their emo-

tions through classroom activities such as discussion, writing, and artwork. Provide assistance to school faculty members. Talk to surviving classmates of deceased or injured students.

3. *Tertiary intervention*. Provide follow-up counseling to the most affected students. Be alert to birthdays or anniversary dates, which may be especially difficult for survivors. Guide the school community toward creating appropriate projects or memorials.

Training Crisis Team Members

It is not possible to specify all the areas of training for team members, and it is obvious that each member will need some specialized training. Crisis team members must view their training as a constantly evolving process as more and more is learned about school crisis. The following list provides an initial foundation for training and suggestions for all team members:

1. Crisis definition and theory should form the basis of planning (see the preceding section "Theoretical Model for Crisis Planning").
2. Planning for many different types of school crises must occur.
3. Childhood reactions to crisis vary by ages; however, the most common reactions are worry about the future, decline in school performance, regression in behavior, and problems with sleeping.
4. Children's understanding of death varies by developmental stages.
5. Everyone must be given the facts about a crisis in order to dispel rumors.
6. Permission must be given to express a wide range of emotions, and everyone must be given an opportunity to tell his or her story.
7. Each individual has his or her own unique history of loss, and unresolved issues may resurface.
8. The severity of a person's crisis response is affected by the event's intensity and duration, as well as the person's own stability.
9. Emotional support must be provided as soon as possible, and staff members and students who have experienced a crisis should be kept together.
10. The school should be kept open and viewed as a source of support.
11. Children are more resilient than adults, but they still need help.
12. Mental health workers must seek out those who need their help after a crisis.
13. Parent meetings are very effective means of assisting children, in that they help parents to understand the typical childhood reactions to a crisis and help parents respond with patience, love, tolerance, and support.
14. Crisis team members should meet frequently to evaluate the progress of crisis management.

15. A checklist of crisis steps should be developed to guide the team's actions.

16. A calling tree should be developed to enable the administrator to alert school personnel to a crisis so that they can begin planning.

17. Policies and procedures must be created that will ensure a close working relationship with the local police and judicial authorities.

18. Communication issues (e.g., who calls the superintendent and other school personnel who need to know about a crisis) should be clarified.

19. Crisis team meetings must be conducted to process and review crisis team activities, with emphasis on how to prevent or better manage crisis events.

ISSUES SCHOOL CRISIS TEAMS SHOULD ADDRESS

Communication Issues

Stephens (1994) has pointed out that schools need better communication systems than they currently have. The NSSC (1991) has recommended that schools have the latest communication devices and has suggested the following:

- Intercoms should be modernized, and portable buildings and playgrounds should be connected via intercoms or outside speakers.
- An emergency kit should be developed; this may include such items as fax machines, portable phones, a copy of the emergency contact card for each student, a copy of the school's floor plan, and bullhorns.
- Schools need a clear emergency signal.

Pitcher and Poland (1992) discussed a three-part approach to communication: Schools and school districts have a need to communicate within buildings, between buildings, and with community resources and agencies. We describe how our school district began using school computers for communication at first, because of the inadequacy of the telephone system. In a second phase, private phones were installed in the office of each principal. Following the phone installation, all administrators were issued two-way radios. The current radio system has a general communication channel and an emergency channel. The emergency channel is monitored all day and is reserved for police and medical emergency situations. Communication codes have also been developed to alert building crisis team members as to the nature of a crisis. One school utilizes the following phrase over the intercom to indicate that someone has a gun in the office area: "There is a phone call for Dr. Gun in the office." Previously rehearsed steps are then taken.

A school that does not have any of the modern equipment just described may consider having all teachers write their names on both red and blue tags and place these on their key chains. Red means a medical emergency; blue means an administrative emergency. A responsible student should be chosen who will take the message to the office in case of an emergency when the teacher cannot leave the rest of the students.

Media Policies and Procedures

A number of articles have been written concerning the relations of schools with the media (Bark, 1989; Elliot, 1989; Jay, 1989). The authors of all of these have stressed the need to develop positive relations with the media before a crisis occurs. It must be acknowledged that the media have a job to do and that each school needs to have a trained spokesperson to conduct interviews. These authors also suggest that media representatives should be provided with the materials necessary to do their jobs; "stonewalling" the media and forbidding representatives to step onto school grounds are not recommended strategies.

Pitcher and Poland (1992) have discussed the development of a media policy that emphasizes cooperation and containment. Media representatives are not allowed to roam the halls and film grieving students, but they are allowed to interview the principal or his or her designee. Peterson and Straub (1992) make similar recommendations and give examples of setting limits and utilizing written statements to avoid confusion. In addition, the school can use the media to publicize the support that is available at the school and in the community for those affected by a crisis (Poland, 1993). Elliot (1989), who addresses public relations issues, gives examples of how important it is for the top administrator to go to the scene of the crisis to show care and concern, as well as to clarify positive actions that are being taken. Many school districts are starting to provide training to district-level administrators and principals about how to interact with the media. Poland and Pitcher (1990) have pointed out that perhaps what did most to broaden the support base for psychological services in their district was not only the response to a major crisis, but the ability to represent the district well in a series of media interviews.

Transportation Issues

Poland and McCormick (1999) have described the role of the transportation department in crisis intervention and have emphasized the need for district planning. We describe in detail a 4-hour in-service training session provided to all bus drivers, which covered behavior management, crisis intervention, suicide intervention, and coordination between bus drivers and the building crisis teams. The transportation department had in place emergency procedures to cover accidents and mechanical failures; however, there was little coordination with the rest of the district. The bus drivers were very receptive to the in-service session and asked many important questions about how, as the single adult on a bus, a driver is supposed to manage accidents and situations involving violent or out-of-control students. It is very important to screen bus drivers carefully and provide them with training about how to interact with students. Safety devices being used on buses include two-way radios and surveillance cameras. Manufacturing standards for school buses in regard to such matters as gas tank location, seat belts, and pop-out windows have been discussed by Rota (1989), but no national standards have been established to date.

School Design and Safety

Most schools today were designed before security became an issue. There are many recommendations for increasing school safety through structural design (Pitcher & Poland, 1992). The NSSC has published numerous materials on this issue and has staff members available to tour schools and make recommendations. School safety officers have made the following recommendations ("Is Your School Built for Safety," 1995):

- School staff members must take responsibility for school safety and increase their supervision.
- A combination of approaches is needed.
- Nooks and crannies in the school should be eliminated.
- Restroom supervision should be increased by eliminating restroom doors or separate faculty restrooms.
- Trees and shrubs should be trimmed to increase visibility.
- All doors except one clearly identified entrance that is monitored by the school staff should be locked.
- All school staff should be trained to question visitors, and students should be taught to alert staff when visitors are in the building.
- The community needs to be involved in helping keep the school safe.
- Security alarms should be installed.

A dramatic example of designing a school with safety in mind is the Townview Magnet Center in the inner city of Dallas, Texas. The construction cost was $41 million, with $3.5 million of this sum devoted to security technology—including 37 surveillance cameras, six metal detectors, five full-time police officers, and intruder-resistant gates (Porter, 1995a).

One of the best-known school safety officers in the United States is Alex Rascon, chief of security for the San Diego, California, schools. Rascon (personal interview, 1996) recommends a combination approach to making schools safer; he does not support having federal funds go only to gadgetry (e.g., metal detectors). Rascon also recommends the removal of student lockers, as they are places to hide weapons and contraband.

Crisis Drills and Readiness Activities

The importance of conducting crisis drills was emphasized by Patricia Busher, the principal of Cleveland Elementary School, Stockton, California, which was the scene of one of the worst incidents of school violence in U.S. history. She emphasized in an NSSC (1991) training film that she is convinced that having practiced the evacuation of her playground saved lives. Historically, schools have conducted fire drills as often as once a month. It is clear, however, that a fire is not the only or even the most likely crisis that might occur at school. Poland and Pitcher (1990) have described how conducting crisis drills made the crisis intervention program in their district come alive, especially because the drills themselves were conducted initially by the top administrators in the district. Elsewhere (Poland, 1993), I have described planning steps for school crisis drills:

1. Planning begins with a paper-and-pencil activity in which the crisis team is presented with five possible crisis situations and each team member records his or her hypothetical response.
2. Team members discuss their anticipated responses and select one scenario to simulate each semester, with precautions taken not to alarm staff and students unduly.
3. It is important to inform the public of the need for crisis planning and the conduction of drills.
4. The use of dramatic props, such as starter pistols and simulated blood, should be avoided.
5. A sign should be placed in the area where a drill is to be conducted, clearly stating that a drill is taking place. In addition, all relevant agencies should be notified in advance that this is a drill.
6. At least some drills should involve moving staff members and students to a safer location.
7. An objective staff member from another building or the central office should observe the drill and give feedback to the crisis team.
8. The crisis team members should meet regularly and review their activities, with the emphasis placed on continual improvement.

Pitcher and Poland (1992) have described the evolution of their district's crisis drills from a few surprise drills' being conducted by central office personnel to each building either conducting its own drill or summarizing how it handled an actual crisis. These summaries are sent to the director of psychological services for feedback and accountability.

An example of what *not* to do in conducting a school crisis drill occurred in Dallas, Texas, where a newspaper headline read, "Lincoln Officials Stage Fake Shooting" (Marcias, 1992). There was much criticism of the drill because local authorities thought a real shooting had taken place, as did a number of teachers and students, who had extreme emotional reactions.

It is essential, however, for some type of crisis drill activity to be conducted at school. School officials should plan those drills carefully, with the emphasis always placed on improvement. The school crisis literature includes many testimonials to the fact that students are not going to do what they need to do in a moment of crisis unless school staff members have practiced it with them and have clearly emphasized the need for students to follow the directives of an adult with no questions asked. A sample crisis drill is described in Table 7.1.

PRACTICAL EXAMPLES OF HANDLING SCHOOL CRISIS SITUATIONS

Coping with a Death

Stevenson (1986) estimates that 1 of every 750 students dies or is killed each year. This means that all schools must cope with the deaths of students, and sometimes with the deaths of faculty members and parents as well. Pitcher and Poland (1992) have emphasized that school personnel, especially counselors, need to be aware of the developmental stages that children go through in their understanding of death. They recommend that the principal verify a death and then notify the faculty through a calling tree or in a faculty meeting. It is important to give school personnel an opportunity to work through their own issues about death and loss before having to assist their students.

If it is not possible to utilize either of these notification methods, then the teachers should be given a hand-delivered memorandum providing them with specific information and ideas about how to assist their students. Poland and Pitcher (1990) have developed a tip sheet for teachers in dealing with death and recommend an in-service training session whose purpose is

---

TABLE 7.1. Sample Crisis Drill: One District's Approach

Secondary school: A female student has been shot in the foot (a pistol she was carrying in her purse has discharged). The incident has occurred in the front of the school by the flagpole, with other students nearby. You are first notified of the incident when several hysterical students rush into the office. The student has a younger brother who attends the same school. The superintendent's secretary will role-play the victim's mother; please call her.

Elementary school: A group of unsupervised boys have been playing near a high-voltage tower on the playground. One boy has received a severe electrical shock. You are first notified of the incident when several hysterical students rush into the office. It is reported that several students became so frightened that they left the school grounds. The injured boy has younger siblings at the school and an older brother in junior high school. The superintendent's secretary will role-play the victim's mother; please notify her.

The secondary and elementary schools in this district were given these respective scenarios, with the following identified task: "Please respond to this incident according to the district crisis intervention procedures. District personnel are on the scene to role-play and ask questions. This is a practice drill, and the appropriate district personnel should be alerted; however, it is not necessary to notify agencies outside the district."
A crisis visitation team composed of central office administrators was present to role-play the crisis. The involvement of top administrators in this indicated to the

principals that it was important. Crisis visitation team members were assigned these specific roles to play:

- Victim
- Bereaved classmate
- Mother of the victim
- Father of the victim
- Law enforcement officer
- Media representative
- Angry citizen

The crisis visitation team members were told that the purpose of the drill was to assess the ability of the individual school to respond to a simulated crisis, and to give each school's staff members feedback so that they would be better prepared for a real crisis. A list of questions was provided for each role played by crisis visitation team members. The questions for the media representative and the bereaved classmate are listed here:

Media representative
- Who meets you?
- To whom are you allowed to talk?
- Who is the building spokesperson?
- Are you allowed access to the entire campus?
- Are you allowed to photograph or interview students?

Bereaved classmate
- Who is available to comfort you?
- Are you unsure whether to remain at school or to go home?
- Will the school be safe and normal tomorrow?
- You have other friends who are upset. Who could talk to your friends or to your class?
- Is your friend going to be all right?
- How can you help your friend?
- How could this have happened?

The deputy superintendent accompanied the crisis visitation team. He delivered the notification of the crisis and documented the overall response through the following questions:

- Who was identified to go to the scene? Was this a reasonable choice of personnel?
- Was the building crisis team called in?
- Were the superintendent and the public information director notified? If so, by whom?
- What plans were stated to restore order and direct students? By whom?
- What plans were stated to contact the parents of the injured student? By whom?
- What plans were stated to call the local police? By whom?
- What plans were stated to call the director of security? By whom?
- What plans were stated to notify the victim's sibling(s)? By whom?
- What plans were stated to communicate to the faculty what happened? By whom?
- What plans were made to follow up on the medical condition of the injured student? By whom?
- What plans were made to follow up at school with those most affected? By whom?
- Was the entire crisis team involved in handling the incident?
- Was teamwork emphasized?
- Was it evident that the crisis team members had given prior thought to their respective duties?

to empower teachers so that they can help many students by supporting the expression of a range of emotions. Teachers can provide various beneficial classroom activities for expressing emotions: talking, writing, artwork, music, or activities to assist the family of the deceased. Teachers have had students make a list of all the good things and positive memories of the deceased and have prepared students for funeral attendance. Schools have often underestimated the impact a death may have. Oates (1988) stresses that schools should ask three questions in trying to estimate the reaction to a death and to help decide how many mental health professionals will be needed to assist upset staff members and students:

1. Who was the deceased? Was he or she a long-time or popular member of the community? If so, then many people will be upset.
2. What happened to the deceased? Violent and unexpected deaths, such as murders and suicides, are more difficult to deal with.
3. Where did the death occur? A death that occurs at school will be much more traumatic.

Poland and McCormack (2000) have recommended that two additional questions be asked:

4. What other recent tragedies have occurred, and how did they affect this particular school community?
5. Was another member of the school community responsible for this death?

It is better to send too many mental health professionals to the school to deal with emotionality than not enough. Lazarus (1993) discusses the model of debriefing recommended by the National Association for Victims' Assistance. This debriefing process involves allowing all those who have experienced a crisis or a loss to tell their stories. Schoenfeld (1993) has stressed the need for risk screening, based on both exposure and other risk factors. Exposure has to do with physical proximity to the tragedy in terms of what was observed. Other important risk factors are the following:

- Familiarity with the victim
- Previous trauma or loss
- Individual psychopathology
- Family psychopathology
- Concern about family members' safety

Finally, Poland et al. (1995) have described the need to locate counseling space. We recommend that the room in which student discussion groups are held be no larger than a normal classroom.

Planning for Evacuation

Most schools have a plan to evacuate students from the building, but schools need to consider what to do if the students cannot return immediately to the building. All schools need an emergency communication kit, as previously recommended (see the earlier section "Communication Issues") to provide for basic needs. Poland, Pitcher, and Lazarus (2002) have stressed the need to locate a place where staff members and students can go to wait comfortably, such as a neighboring school, church, or business. Teachers may even want to put together activities that can keep students occupied, and young students may even need some personal items to reduce their anxiety, such as stuffed animals or pictures of parents. One principal emphasized that keeping her entire elementary school outside for an entire afternoon because of a gas leak was difficult. She commented that the next time they would have such basic items as water, bug spray, and activities to amuse the students (N. Samson, personal communication, September 1996).

It is also important to locate places within the building for staff members and students to take cover. In case of natural disasters such as tornadoes or earthquakes, refuge should be sought in the areas of the building recommended as the safest by the architectural firm that designed the building. Many schools have also faced the situation of an intruder in a building with a weapon. In such situations, several key points will help ensure student safety (Poland, 1993):

1. Students should be taught a signal that means "Take cover underneath furniture."
2. Each teacher should lock all classroom doors, turn off lights, and silently await the "All clear" signal from the building administrator.
3. Procedures to evacuate students quickly from the playground and cafeteria should be practiced; students should also be taught where to take cover in these locations.

Dealing with Bomb Threats

No one can tell a school administrator whether to evacuate each time a bomb threat is received: however, evacuation is the safest course of action. Most school plans call for someone to stay behind and look for the bomb. It is important that these school personnel receive training about the various types of bombs they might encounter, as well as where to look for them. The NSSC (1989) makes recommendations about what information to try to obtain from a caller who notifies the school that there is a bomb. The receptionist needs to stay calm and ask questions like the following:

- "Where is the bomb, and what type is it?"
- "When will it go off?"

- "Why was it placed, and who are you?"

The receptionist should also try to identify voice characteristics of the caller and any background sounds. Pitcher and Poland (1992) have described what *not* to do, using the example of the principal who panicked, grabbed the intercom, and yelled for everyone to evacuate 5 minutes before the bell for Christmas vacation. The principal even forgot to identify himself, and many students thought that it was a joke and refused to follow evacuation procedures.

Intervening in Fights

Schools often struggle with how to respond to fights. How much can a teacher reasonably be expected to do to break up a fight? Many teachers believe that they are liable if they do not physically take action to stop students from fighting.

Stephens (1994) has emphasized that school personnel should not try to be heroes, but should document all incidents of fighting and call police when fights occur. Pitcher and Poland (1992) suggested that one of the most effective strategies schools can employ is to remove the audience from the vicinity where the students are fighting. This involves a number of crowd control techniques. Violent students should also be given choices and not threatened with consequences while they are agitated. It is also very important to give violent individuals personal space and to talk with them in a calm manner and to maintain eye contact. Administrative policies must clearly specify the expectations for school personnel in this area. School personnel need training in how to stop violence from escalating and how to prevent fights from starting. School principals in Houston, Texas, have commented that recently adopted policies (which make all students charged with fighting appear in court and pay fines of $200) have greatly reduced the number of fights.

Coping with Natural Disasters

Peterson and Straub (1992) describe the broad impact of natural disasters, which frequently result in fear, helplessness, and hopelessness. They point out that because of the often widespread destruction and the fact that (unlike many crisis situations) natural disasters cannot be prevented, but only prepared for, the emotional reactions are severe. Signs of posttraumatic stress disorder found in the aftermath can include the following: (1) depression in adults, (2) increased illnesses in both adults and children, (3) truancy in teens, (4) increased substance abuse, and (5) general anxiety. Poland et al. (1995) have emphasized that school-age victims of disasters should resume their daily routine as soon as possible and should be allowed to help with cleanup activities. The Red Cross has outlined four phases in disaster recovery: (1) heroic, (2) honeymoon, (3) disillusionment, and (4) construction.

Lazarus (1993) discussed a number of recommendations in the aftermath of Hurricane Andrew. During a disaster, some children may be separated from their families or parents and will need extra assistance, and most children will exhibit signs of posttraumatic stress disorder. The school can provide a bridge to the community, and can serve as a familiar place where victims can come to get not only emotional assistance but shelter as well. Gostelow (personal communication, March 1996) has emphasized the importance of victims' discussing their reactions and has suggested that counselors forget the word "feelings" because many people are more comfortable with the term "reactions." Gostelow also points out that victims should be helped to gain a sense of control over small issues, and that school personnel should be told to come to a meeting to learn how to assist the children who have experienced a disaster, when in reality the meeting will focus on ventilating the reactions of the school personnel.

Lazarus (1993) describes a number of very important activities that took place in Florida to prepare children who were victims of Hurricane Andrew prior to the next hurricane season. Lazarus stressed that children must be active participants in the prediction and preparation process, that the prized possessions of children should be safeguarded, and that they need to be taught where to locate shelter. A natural disaster is difficult for all victims, but a prepared school crisis team can provide invaluable assistance to the school and the community.

The Oklahoma City Bombing: Coping with a Large-Scale Disaster

The bombing of the federal building in Oklahoma City on April 19, 1995, which killed 169 people and injured hundreds, had a tremendous impact on the area's schools and raised many questions about how schools can respond to such a staggering tragedy. How can the schools coordinate their crisis teams' efforts with those at the city, state, and national levels? The major focus of attention in Oklahoma City was on the recovery efforts and the rescue workers themselves. Many questions had to be raised about how to assist school personnel and children who were greatly affected by the tragedy. Walker (1995) stressed the importance of listening to the children of Oklahoma City who were affected by the bombing. Walker's recommended interview protocol included the following:

- Understanding the bombing in terms of what, how, and why
- Expressing thoughts and feelings, both initial and ongoing
- Making choices, both initially after the bombing and in the following days
- Discussing what others such as adults did to help initially, and what else they can still do to provide help

A similar format is provided in a publication by Shaw (1995) entitled *The Terrible Scary Explosion Book*. This publication is intended to be read to a child by an adult, and many opportunities are provided for the child to express feelings and ask questions.

The Oklahoma City school superintendent asked for help from other parts of the country, as more than 300 of the district's students said that a family member or someone else close to them had been killed or injured. I was privileged to be part of an assistance team put together by the U.S. Department of Education. The team, consisting of psychiatrists, psychologists, and social workers with crisis expertise, was assembled and sent to Oklahoma City for several days. We met with administrators, counselors, teachers, students, and business leaders and developed a response and recovery plan for the school district. The single greatest accomplishment was getting the local school system included in the federal grant that provided disaster relief funds to work on mental health issues. The Oklahoma City schools received $1.4 million to hire counselors to work with those affected by the tragedy for a 1-year period ("Oklahoma City Schools," 1995). It is important to note that the counselors were in the school every day and were completely accessible to teachers and students.

Other accomplishments of the team included the following:

- Targeting those students most affected
- Making plans to deal with the emotional impact of the bombing of the federal building
- Developing training programs for teachers and administrators
- Addressing the numerous school safety concerns voiced by students

School administrators must think about how their crisis teams can integrate and work with all levels of government. The tragedies of September 11, 2001, illustrate that massive crises, demanding multilevel coordination, must receive planning attention. There are resources to assist the schools, and it is the wise administrator who asks for assistance.

Intervening in Youth Suicide

The Centers for Disease Control and Prevention (CDC), indicating that youth suicide rates are at or near an all-time high, has published a resource guide for preventing youth suicide (CDC, 1992). This guide makes a number of recommendations for the schools:

1. School programs need to link up more closely with community resources.
2. More programs need to focus on reducing access to lethal weapons, especially guns.

3. Suicide prevention programs need to link up with other programs for high-risk youths, such as alcohol use, dropout, and pregnancy prevention programs.
4. The lack of evaluative data on prevention programs is a great obstacle to improving prevention efforts. School systems and local and state agencies need to improve data collection and implement proven intervention programs.
5. Programs need to be developed to focus on the 20- to 24-year-old population, which has a suicide rate twice that of teens.

The problem of youth suicide is sometimes overlooked because of the many other problems of young people today. Homicide has now become the second leading cause of death for teenagers, with suicide now the third leading cause of death. A recent CDC (1992) survey found that 8% of high school students had already attempted suicide, 27% had seriously contemplated it, and 16% had made a plan to commit suicide. Recent research has emphasized that the suicide rate for 10- to 14-year-olds has more than doubled in the last decade, whereas the suicide rate for 15- to 19-year-olds rose only 28% (Lawton, 1995).

Schools have been reluctant to face the problem of youth suicide. Harris and Crawford (1987) have documented that few schools have any training in suicide prevention or a plan in place. Slenkovich (1986) cited one of a growing number of cases in which schools have been sued after the suicide of a student. Schools have been ordered to pay monetary damages to the parents of deceased students (McKee, Jones, & Barbe, 1993). The key issue is not whether the school somehow caused the suicide, but whether the school failed to take reasonable steps to prevent it. Schools have a responsibility to have prevention programs in place, to foresee that a student who is threatening suicide is at risk, and to take steps to supervise that student and obtain psychological help for him or her. School personnel must also notify parents whenever they have reason to believe that a student is suicidal. I recently testified in federal court against a school district that failed to take appropriate action when aware of a junior high student's suicidal intent. The student did commit suicide, and the jury found the school district partially liable ("School District Partially Liable," 1995).

Elsewhere (Poland, 1989), I have applied Caplan's model to the problem of youth suicide and outlined the roles of the schools as the following: (1) detection, (2) assessment, (3) parent notification, and (4) referral and follow-up. All school personnel who interact with students (including such personnel as secretaries, bus drivers, and cafeteria workers) must be taught the warning signs of suicide and must be empowered to follow procedures to alert the appropriate personnel and get assistance for a suicidal student. When school personnel are provided with correct information about the problem, many commonly held misperceptions can be addressed. It must be emphasized that no one should keep a secret about suicidal behavior. School psychologists and counselors are the logical personnel to assess the severity level. It is very important that these personnel receive training on how to interact with suicidal students and what questions to ask. The key recommendations are these:

1. Try to remain calm, and seek collaboration from a colleague.
2. Gather case history information from the student and approach the student as if he or she were planning a trip.
3. Ask specific questions about the suicidal plan and the frequency of suicidal thoughts.
4. Emphasize that there are alternatives to suicide and that the student is not the first person to feel this way.
5. Do not make any deals with the student to keep the suicidal thoughts or actions a secret, and explain the ethical responsibility to notify the student's parents.
6. Have the student sign a no-suicide contract, and provide the student with the phone number of the local crisis hot line.
7. Supervise the student until parents have assumed responsibility.

Poland et al. (1995) have clarified that a key question is not whether the parents should be called (because that is a given), but, rather, what to say to the parents and how to elicit a supportive reaction from them. Parents have sometimes been uncooperative and have minimized the suicidal ideation or actions of their child; school personnel must be firm in their recommendation that counseling assistance is needed. Parents have become angry at school personnel in this notification process and have tried to forbid them from interacting with their child again. This situation is covered in the state of Texas by legislation stating that under the circumstance of suicide, personnel such as physicians, psychologists, and counselors need not obtain parental permission to work with a minor. When parents refuse to get emotional assistance for a suicidal child, a referral must be made to the local child protective services agency. It is absolutely essential that the appropriate school personnel follow up and provide emotional support, regardless of what the parents do.

Berman and Jobes (1995) have pointed out that the most common factors in youth suicide are depression, substance abuse, conduct problems, recklessness, impulsivity, and gun availability. More than a decade of work on this problem has revealed a prevalent pattern: Young people almost always tell their friends about their suicidal plans, and, unfortunately, their friends do not always look to adults for help. Many professionals believe that the single action that would reduce youth suicide most is to reduce gun access to troubled youths. Sixty percent of male youth suicides and 47% of female youth suicides involve guns (American Psychological Association, 1993). School personnel must also be familiar with the concept of the "precipitating event"—that is, the event that a suicidal adolescent views as the "last straw" and that causes the adolescent to take suicidal action.

Schools also need to make "postvention" plans for what to do after a suicide occurs. "Few events in a school are more painful or potentially more disruptive than the suicide of a student" (Lamb & Dunne-Maxim, 1987, p. 245). The American Association of Suicidology (AAS) has published school postvention guidelines that include the following (AAS, 1991):

- Don't dismiss school or encourage funeral attendance during school hours.
- Don't hold a large-scale school assembly or dedicate a memorial to the deceased.
- Do provide individual and group counseling.
- Verify the facts, and do treat the death as a suicide.
- Do contact the family of the deceased.
- Do emphasize that no one is to blame for the suicide.
- Do emphasize that help is available, that suicide is preventable, and that everyone has a role to play in prevention.

The AAS postvention guidelines also include the following recommendations, which encourage the media not to dramaticize the suicide:

- Don't make the suicide front-page news.
- Don't print a picture of the deceased.
- Avoid details about the method.
- Do not report the suicide as the result of simplistic, romantic, or mystic factors.
- Do emphasize that there are alternatives to suicide, and publicize where to get assistance.

I have emphasized the importance of following carefully made postvention plans and stressed that there is much that is not known about suicide clusters and contagion (Poland, 1989) (although the CDC is now in the midst of a multiyear study). School psychologists also need to know that not everyone agrees with the guidelines developed by the AAS. In particular, the recommendations made by Phi Delta Kappa International (1988) are in conflict with those of the AAS on key points. Phi Delta Kappa recommends that the death not be treated as suicide and suggests that all concerned be forbidden to use the word "suicide" in order to protect the privacy of the family. A school administrator who has not thoroughly researched this area might also, following these guidelines, call for having all students who want more information about the death to gather in a large assembly. This would be a mistake. Experience has shown that, when large numbers of students gather, emotionality is difficult to manage. It is essential to tell the truth, but a classroom setting is much more manageable than an assembly.

There is also disagreement on the question of what information should be made available to students through curriculum presentations. I have discussed this issue in great detail and recommended carefully planned units that teach the warning signs of suicide and ways to get assistance (Poland, 1989). This unit should be carefully integrated with the discussion of other mental health problems in U.S. society. Several states (e.g., California, New Jersey, Florida, and Wisconsin) have passed legislation requiring schools to provide curriculum presentations on suicide prevention.

Dealing with Guns in the Schools

Almost all national media sources, including television, newspapers, and magazines, have recently publicized the severe problem of young people and guns. President Clinton commented on this problem in his televised address to the nation on health care in September 1993, in which he stated, "We have the only country in the world where teenagers can roam the streets with semiautomatic weapons and be better armed than the police. We must do something about that!"

"How many guns come to school on a daily basis?" is a question that many educators have asked, along with, "How can we keep guns out of our schools?" Guns may well constitute the single greatest threat to student and educator safety today, as indicated by statistics in Houston, Texas, showing a 600% increase in accidental gun deaths among children from 1988 to 1992, and more than a 100% increase in juveniles charged with murder from 1988 to 1992 (Poland, 1993). O'Donnell (1995) has discussed the need for numerous strategies to be implemented to reduce firearm deaths among children. One such strategy is a national trend to hold adults accountable through prosecution when a child is injured or killed with a gun (Sharp, 1995).

Colorado is the latest state to address the problem of young people and guns, with 1993 legislation making it illegal for a minor to possess a handgun unless involved in adult-supervised training. Poland et al. (2002) discussed the U. S. Secret Service study of school violence that found most perpetrators of school violence obtained the guns from their own homes. Many questions have been raised about parental responsibility. The parents of the Columbine perpetrators are currently being sued by the families of many victims. To date, no national changes or initiatives have kept guns away from children despite passionate U. S. Congressional testimony from the parents of several victims of school violence.

Many schools have focused exclusively on the strategy of keeping guns off campus through the use of metal detectors. Hanson (1993b) discussed the effectiveness of walk-through metal detectors, noted that numerous schools have found metal detectors to reduce the number of guns brought to school, and cited surveys of students reporting that metal detectors were a deterrent. I have stressed that the schools must try not only to make it difficult to bring a gun to school, but also to create a climate in which students immediately report the presence of a gun on campus to administrators (Poland, 1993). A few schools are starting to address the questions of gun ownership and gun safety in the curriculum. One such program is in place in the Dade County (Florida) schools (Pitcher & Poland, 1992). The program has as its goal to reduce handgun deaths and injuries to children and consists of the following strategies:

1. Students in grades K–12 are informed of the dangers of guns through three presentations a year.
2. Students hear from the victims of gunshots themselves, and the legal implications of a minor's being injured with a gun owned by an adult are emphasized in community awareness presentations.
3. "Say no to guns" posters are utilized, which contain famous last words such as "I was only angry for a moment," "I thought it was a toy," and "I didn't know that it was loaded."

There are several similar curricula designed to reduce the current epidemic of gun deaths of children. Roth (1993), in reviewing the recommendations of the 3-year Task Force on Youth Violence released by the American Psychological Association, stressed the availability of guns as a major reason for the high levels of youth violence. The phrase "The trigger pulls the finger" sums up the dilemma we face with young people. Guns are more accessible to young people than ever before, and they are using them. We can only hope that through education and information in the schools, the next generation of Americans will choose not to have a gun in every other home. A valuable source of information about children and gun deaths is the Children's Defense Fund (25 E. Street N.W., Washington, DC 20001). This group cites the following figures about gun violence:

- More than 5,000 children are killed by guns each year.
- The total number of children killed by firearms rose 144% from 1986 to 1992.
- A gun in the home is 43 times more likely to be used to commit homicide, suicide, or an accidental killing than it is to be used to kill in self-defense.

The Children's Defense Fund (1996) is very active politically and publishes various materials, including posters on gun safety and violence issues that affect children.

The Gun Safety Institute (320 Leader Boulevard, Cleveland, OH 41114) publishes a curriculum on gun safety. This group also outlines the reasons that young people are attracted to guns: power, excitement, safety, and comfort with aggression (Gun Safety Institute, 1995).

PREVENTION

Every crisis that is dealt with needs to be examined carefully, not only for how it could have been managed better, but for how it could have been prevented. Elsewhere (Poland, 1994), I have described how building principals in one district asked for a checklist to follow when a crisis occurs. The checklist that was eventually developed included questions not only about intervention but also about prevention; it appears in Table 7.2.

Pitcher and Poland (1992) have recommended beginning prevention efforts with programs to address the leading causes of death for children, which are accident, homicide, and suicide. Personal safety units need to be added to the curriculum to address not only guns, but also cars and bicycles. A number of Texas schools have implemented programs to encourage

TABLE 7.2. Crisis Intervention and Prevention Checklist

❑ The crisis coordinator (principal) becomes aware of the crisis and notifies the crisis liaisons.

❑ The crisis coordinator clarifies the duties of the various liaisons and supervises the crisis intervention activities.

❑ The crisis coordinator or a designee notifies the superintendent of the crisis.

❑ The crisis coordinator interacts with media representatives as needed.

❑ The crisis coordinator or a designee notifies the district public information director of the crisis.

❑ The law enforcement liaison notifies the district security director and appropriate local law enforcement personnel and coordinates their activities as needed.

❑ The medical liaison contacts emergency medical personnel and provides medical assistance as needed.

❑ The student liaison directs activities to ensure the safety and emotional well-being of the student body.

❑ The campus liaison communicates specifics of the crisis to the faculty and gives the faculty guidance on how they can assist in crisis management.

❑ The counseling/psychological liaison provides needed emotional support to affected students, family, friends, faculty, etc.

❑ The parent liaison communicates to concerned parents orally and/or in writing.

❑ The crisis coordinator conducts a faculty meeting, after the students have gone home, to discuss the crisis.

❑ The crisis coordinator conducts a debriefing meeting with the crisis team. This meeting processes the crisis event and clarifies follow-up activities for the team.

❑ The crisis coordinator updates the superintendent and the public information director on the resolution of the crisis.

❑ The crisis coordinator discusses with the crisis team ways to prevent further crisis situations of this type.

Note. Adapted from Pitcher and Poland (1992, p. 149). Copyright 1994 by The Guilford Press. Adapted by permission.

the use of bicycle helmets and have established "safe ride" programs to reduce the number of teenagers who drive while under the influence of alcohol or other drugs. Among the most difficult concepts to get across to young people are the finality of death and the fact that death can happen to them. It is also apparent that schools must provide programs to teach students to solve conflicts without violence. Curriculum units for this purpose have been developed by several companies, and a national mediation organization trains school personnel to teach students to mediate disputes without violence. Students are presented with figures on incidents of violence and are provided with information about the role of drugs and alcohol. Anger is examined as a natural emotion, and role-play scenarios and discussions focus on alternatives to aggression. The need for collaboration between schools and communities through education and modeling of conflict resolution, and the need for a national campaign to reduce youth violence, have been stressed by Curry (1993), Johnson and Johnson (1995), and Osofsky (1995).

In addressing the areas of prevention, it is important to examine the predictive factors of violence as outlined by the American Psychological Association Task Force on Youth Violence (Roth, 1993): child abuse, ineffective parenting, violence at home, media violence, poverty, prejudice, substance abuse, and gun access. These factors all have many implications for schools, and it is clear that many societal factors are involved. Texas state representative Mike Martin made the following comment concerning youth violence: "In five years we have seen a transformation of young people that has been unprecedented in our history and we at the legislative level have got to respond" (quoted in Hanson, 1993a, p. 22a). The schools must focus more on prevention, as must all of U.S. society; answers to the increased level of youth violence in our schools and our communities will not come easily. A number of preventive programs have been reviewed by Prothrow-Stith and Quaday (1995), and one program in Pittsburgh, Pennsylvania, includes the following comprehensive steps:

- Working to provide a safe environment for all schoolchildren and school staff members
- Hiring a full-time violence prevention coordinator
- Establishing a culturally sensitive K–12 curriculum
- Establishing a forum for students to have input in program design
- Developing programs specific to sexual assault
- Targeting antigang activities to schools where multiple gangs are present
- Evaluating programs and using the information gleaned to adapt them
- Providing support for transitions from school to work, and providing economic opportunities for high-risk youths

One of the most helpful tools that a crisis team can develop is a plan to guide the actions of everyone if a crisis should occur. For example, a flip chart is used by the schools in my school district (Cypress–Fairbanks Independent School District, Houston, Texas). All school personnel (including substitutes) are given this flip chart, which outlines what to do in a variety of crisis situations. The flip chart is printed in the colors of the school and is updated each year. The specific types of procedures covered are as follows:

1. Emergency plan
2. Serious injury
3. Media procedure
4. Evacuation procedure
5. Teacher checklist
6. General procedures and information
7. Take-cover procedures
8. Gas leaks
9. Hazardous material spills
10. Bomb threats
11. Earthquakes
12. Severe windstorm
13. Flooding
14. Weapon on campus
15. Explosions
16. Children left at school
17. Kidnapped or missing students
18. Suicide danger
19. Severe storm/weather policy
20. Loss of power/utilities
21. Fallen aircraft
22. Intruder in building with a weapon
23. Threatening person(s) outside building

CONCLUSIONS

Stephens (1995) has emphasized that crisis planning in the schools is an "inside job" that involves a committed staff, students, and community; he has also cautioned that schools must not get "caught with their plans down." The general strategies recommended by Stephens and in this chapter to make schools safer are the following:

1. Reducing the presence of guns, weapons, gangs, drugs, and nonstudents on campus
2. Establishing a positive school climate with outstanding leadership and extensive community involvement
3. Designing schools with safety as an objective, and maximizing surveillance and supervision of students
4. Developing cooperative and collaborative relations between schools and all agencies that serve young people

There is much that schools can do to improve their management of crisis situations through advance planning and constantly evolving crisis plans. It is imperative that school crisis teams be formed to provide leadership in this important area, and that plans at all three levels of crisis intervention be developed. One former school security chief compared a school crisis to a military battle and asked, "Would a general ever send his troops into a battle without a plan?" (K. Trump, personal communication, December 2003). He further stressed that schools must be involved in homeland security planning and that a terrorist attack could occur at a U. S. school. Unfortunately, we must probably conclude that there will be more school crisis situations next year than we are presently experiencing and that the next decade will bring increased accountability for school administrators in the area of crisis planning. It is important for school staffs to make crisis plans today, *before* a crisis strikes.

Our schools and our society as a whole must place more emphasis on prevention. According to Howell (1993), a recent report from the United Nations found that the United States has the highest level of youth violence and the most young people living in poverty of any industrialized nation in the world. This has occurred because U.S. society has not put enough emphasis on children and programs to serve them.

Many educators have commented that our schools are safer than our communities. This is probably true, but we can continue to improve our efforts at school while working on the much bigger problem in our society. Our schools today must have well-organized crisis teams whose members all know their roles in a crisis and are all committed to making school a safer place. Schools must not only take steps to protect themselves from the world around them, but must also protect themselves from within. Almost every student who commits a violent act has discussed it with his or her friends. We must have in place curriculum programs that teach young people alternatives to violence and the importance of getting adult assistance when someone is homicidal or suicidal. It is my belief that preventive curriculum programs will not be implemented widely in our schools without legislative mandates.

REFERENCES

American Association of Suicidology (AAS). (1991). *Postvention guidelines for the schools.* Denver, CO: Author.

American Psychological Association. (1993). *Violence and youth: Psychology's response.* Washington, DC: Author.

Armstrong, M. (1990). Stockton school shooting. In S. Poland (Chair), *Crisis intervention in the schools.* Symposium presented at the meeting of the National Association of School Psychologists, San Francisco.

Bark, E. (1989, April 23). Imagemakers tell clients to be honest with the media. *Houston Chronicle,* p. 4e.

Berman, L., & Jobes, D. (1995). Suicide prevention in adolescents. *Suicide and Life-Threatening Behavior, 25*(1), 143–154.

Brock, S., Sandoval, J., & Lewis, S. (1995). *Preparing for crisis in the schools: A manual for building school crisis response teams.* Brandon, VT: Clinical Psychology.

Burneman, B. (1995). *On-site crisis response plan for school systems*. Ardmore, OK: Clasara Foundation.

Busher, F. (Chair). (1990). *Tragedy in Stockton school yard*. Symposium presented at the meeting of the National Association of School Psychologists, San Francisco.

Caplan, G. (1964). *Principles of preventive psychiatry*. New York: Basic Books.

Centers for Disease Control and Prevention (CDC). (1992). *Youth suicide prevention and resource guide*. Atlanta, GA: Author.

Children's Defense Fund. (1996, June/July). *CDF report* (Vol. 17, Nos. 7, 8). Washington, DC: Author.

Curry, J. (1993). *Violence in our schools: How to proactively prevent and defuse*. Thousand Oaks, CA: Corvin.

Data released on school associated deaths. (1998). *School Violence Alert, 8*(10), p. 2–4.

Dillard, H. (1989). Winnetka: One year later. *Communique, 17*(8), 17–20.

Elliot, J. (1989, April 21). Public angry at slow action on oil spill. *USA Today*, p. 1b.

Furlong, M., & Morrison, G. (1994). Introduction to mini-series: School violence and safety in perspective. *School Psychology Review, 23*, 139–151.

Gun Safety Institute. (1995). *Solutions without guns: A curriculum guide*. Cleveland: Author.

Hanson, E. (1993a, October 14). Public hearings set on youth violence. *Houston Chronicle*, p. 22a.

Hanson, E. (1993b, October 16). Dramatic arms deterrent cited in metal detector use in schools. *Houston Chronicle*, p. 36a.

Harris, M., & Crawford, R. (1987). *Youth suicide: The identification of effective concepts and practices in policies and procedure for Texas schools* (Monograph No. 3). Commerce: Center for Policy Studies and Research, East Texas State University.

Howell, R. (1993, September 26). U.S. has worst rate for youth violence. *Houston Chronicle*, p. 8a.

Is your school built for safety or designed for disaster? (1995, May). *School Violence Alert*, p. 1.

Jay, B. (1989, January). Managing a crisis in the schools. *National Association of Secondary School Principals Bulletin*, pp. 14–17.

Jennings, L. (1989, October 4). Crisis consultants share lessons they learned from school violence. *Education Week*, pp. 1, 27.

Johnson, D., & Johnson, R. (1995). *Reducing school violence through conflict resolution*. Alexandria, VA: Association for Supervision and Curriculum Development.

Johnson, K. (1993). *School crisis management*. Alameda, CA: Hunter House.

Lamb, F., & Dunne-Maxim, K. (1987). Postvention in the schools: Policy and process. In E. Dunne, J. McIntosh, & K. Dunne-Maxim (Eds.), *Suicide and its aftermath* (pp. 245–263). New York: Norton.

Lawton, M. (1995, May 31). Suicide rate among youths soaring. *Education Week*, p. 5.

Lazarus, P. (1993). Preparing our children for the hurricane season: A psychological perspective. *Florida Association of School Psychologists, 20*(3), 4–6.

Marcias, A. (1992, October 7). Lincoln officials stage fake shooting. *Dallas Morning News*, p. 7a.

McIntyre, M., & Reid, B. (1989). *Obstacles to implementation of crisis intervention programs*. Unpublished manuscript, Chesterfield County Schools, Chesterfield, VA.

McKee, P., Jones, W., & Barbe, H. (1993). *Suicide and the school*. Horsham, PA: LRP.

National School Safety Center (NSSC). (1989). *School safety checklist*. Malibu, CA: Author.

National School Safety Center (NSSC) (Producer). (1991). *School crisis under control* [Film]. Malibu, CA: Author.

Oates, M. (1988, fall). Responding to death in the schools. *Texas Association for Counselor Development Journal*, pp. 83–96.

O'Donnell, C. (1995, September). Firearm deaths among children and youth. *American Psychologist, 50*(9), 771–775.

Oklahoma City schools get federal aid for counseling. (1995, November 29). *Education Week*, p. 2.

Osofsky, J. (1995). The effects of exposure to violence of young children. *American Psychologist, 50*(9), 782–788.

Petersen, S., & Straub, R. (1992). *School crisis survival guide*. West Nyack, NY: Center for Applied Research in Education.

Phi Delta Kappa International. (1988, September). *Responding to student suicide: First 48 hours* (Current Issues Memo). Bloomington, IN: Author.

Pitcher, G. D., & Poland, S. (1992). *Crisis intervention in the schools*. New York: Guilford Press.

Poland, S. (1989). *Suicide intervention in the schools*. New York: Guilford Press.

Poland, S. (1993). *Crisis manual for the Alaska schools*. Juneau: Alaska Department of Education.

Poland, S. (1994). The role of school crisis intervention teams to prevent and reduce trauma. *School Psychology Review, 23*, 175–190.

Poland, S. (1995). Suicide intervention. In A. Thomas & J. Grimes (Eds.), *Best practices in school psychology* (Vol. 3, pp. 459–470). Silver Spring, MD: National Association of School Psychologists.

Poland, S., & Lieberman, R. (2002). Best practices in suicide prevention. In A. Thomas & J. Grimes (Eds.), *Best practices in school psychology* (Vol. 4, pp. 1151–1161). Bethesda, MD: National Association of School Psychologists.

Poland, S., & McCormick, J. (1999). *Coping with crisis: Lessons learned*. Longmont, CO: Sopris West.

Poland, S., & McCormick, J. (2000). *Coping with crisis: A quick reference guide*. Longmont, CO: Sopris West.

Poland, S., & Pitcher, G. (1990). Best practices in crisis intervention. In A. Thomas & J. Grimes (Eds.), *Best practices in school psychology* (Vol. 2., pp. 259–275). Silver Spring, MD: National Association of School Psychologists.

Poland, S., Pitcher, G., & Lazarus, P. (1995). Best practices in crisis intervention. In A. Thomas & J. Grimes (Eds.), *Best practices in school psychology* (Vol. 3, pp. 445–459). Silver Spring, MD: National Association of School Psychologists.

Poland, S., Pitcher, G., & Lazarus, P. (2002). Best practices in prevention and management. In A. Thomas & J. Grimes (Eds.), *Best practices in school psychology* (Vol. 4, pp. 1057–1080). Bethesda, MD: National Association of School Psychologists.

Porter, J. (1995a, September 6). State of the art school seeks to take a bite out of crime. *Education Week*, p. 6.

Porter, J. (1995b, September 26). Report on juvenile crime brings calls for new policies. *Education Week*, p. 6.

Porter, J. (1996, January 17). Poll finds fear of crime alters student routines. *Education Week*, p. 5.

Prothrow-Stith, D., & Quaday, S. (1995). *Hidden casualties: The relationship between violence and learning*. Pittsburgh: National Health and Education Consortium.

Rota, K. (1989, December 12). Safety changes are still evolving. *USA Today*, p. 1a.

Roth, B. (1993, August 11). Psychologists take up youth violence fight. *Houston Chronicle*, p. 4a.

Ruof, S., & Harris, J. (1988). Suicide contagion: Guilt and modeling. *Communique, 16*(17), 8.

Sandall, N. (1986). Early intervention in a disaster: The Cokeville hostage/bombing crisis. *Communique, 15*(2), 1–2.

Schoenfeld, M. (1993). *Crisis response team: Lessening the aftermath*. Foresthill, CA: Author.

School district partially liable for student suicide, pays $165,000. (1995, November). *Your School and the Law*, p. 1.

Sharp, D. (1995, August 29). Gun laws target parents. *USAToday*, p. 2a.

Shaw, T. (1995). *The terrible scary explosion book*. Norman: Oklahoma School Counselor Association.

Slaikeu, K. (1984). *Crisis intervention: A handbook for practice and research*. Boston: Allyn & Bacon.

Slenkovich, J. (1986, June). School districts can be sued for inadequate suicide prevention programs. *The Schools' Advocate*, pp. 1–3.

Stephens, R. D. (1994). Planning for safer and better schools: School violence prevention and intervention strategies. *School Psychology Review, 23*, 204–216.

Stephens, R. (1995). *Safe schools: Handbook for violence prevention*. Bloomington, IN: National Education Service.

Stevenson, R. (1986, December). How to handle death in the schools. *National Association of Secondary School Principals Bulletin*, pp. 1–2.

Terr, L. C. (1983). Chowchilla revisited: The effects of a psychic trauma four years after a school bus kidnapping. *American Journal of Psychiatry, 12*, 140–146.

Walker, J. (1995). *Listening to the children: Interview guide*. Unpublished manuscript, Georgia Counseling Associates, Atlanta, GA.

Watson, R., Poda, J., Miller, C., Rice, E., & West, G. (1990). *Containing crisis: A guide to managing school emergencies*. Bloomington, IN: National Education Service.

CHAPTER 8

Interventions for Aggressive Students in a Public School-Based Day Treatment Program

JERRY OESTMANN

For more than 15 years the Behavioral Skills Program (BSP) has provided day treatment services to students who have severe behavioral, emotional, and mental health problems, and over that time there have been changes. The staff of BSP would agree with Sprague and Walker (2000) that today's students with emotional and behavioral disorders (EBDs) are increasingly violent, have more severe pathology, and have experienced more risk factors and community problems as compared with students even a few years ago. Sugai (1996) found that every classroom has students who need special help for behavioral issues, but up to 10% of these students may need highly intensive and specialized educational and therapeutic services. Our staff has commented that the BSP serves the upper 10% of this 10%. Not only do students have more problems, but the demand for BSP services has increased because of the more severe problems. From 1995 to 2000 the number of students identified as emotionally and behaviorally disordered (EBD) in our school district has increased by about 12%, but the number of students served each year at BSP has increased more than 60%.

This chapter first provides a general description of day treatment for children and youth based on a psychoeducational approach. Then key ingredients needed for a successful public-school-based day treatment program to remediate and prevent aggressive behavior in students with severe EBD are presented. Methods of operation used at BSP are presented as practical examples of how to put in operation a treatment philosophy focused on creating a safe and trusting environment and preventing aggressive behavior at BSP, in referring/home schools, at home, and in the community. Specifically, methods to provide individualized, intensive, comprehensive, and sustained services are presented. In addition, two more essential ingredients for a successful program, a cohesive team and humor, are presented.

DEFINING DAY TREATMENT

Most day treatment programs employ psychological treatment and education in an integrated psychoeducational approach. Day treatment settings are usually designed to have a "school-like" environment. Students spend most of their day in a classroom with a small staff–student ratio, the daily routine is consistent and structured, and curriculums are modified to motivate and aid students with learning disabilities or other cognitive deficits. Academic programming in day treatment is often limited to remedial instruction of basic academic skills. A few programs are fully accredited and teach advanced academics, art, music, computer skills, and vocational skills (Baenen, Stephens, & Glenwick, 1986; Sayegh & Grizenko, 1991; Zimet & Farley, 1985).

Psychological interventions usually incorporate elements of many theoretical approaches. Behavioral, ecological, cognitive, developmental, family systems, and client-centered approaches, along with psychiatric care, all play a significant role in treatment. Treatment often includes intensive individual, group, or family therapy focused on personal issues such as oppositional and aggressive behavior, depression, anxiety, trauma recovery, family issues, or other psycho-emotional problems. Social skills training is usually provided with a focus on development of behavior self-management, building positive social relationships, emotional coping skills, and communication abilities. Day treatment programs often use systematic behavior management plans involving level systems, token economies, verbal deescalation and redirection, time-out rooms, and other behavioral interventions and crisis intervention techniques. A few programs provide case management and other support services, including therapy to students' families (Baenen et al., 1986; Gabel & Finn, 1986; Topp, 1991; Zimet & Farley, 1985).

As a special education and mental health service, school-based day treatment provides advantages over both more restrictive placements and less restrictive options. First, highly restrictive out-of-community or out-of-home placements have not demonstrated success either in long-term change in children's functioning and mental health or in improvements in parents' or schools' abilities to manage their children (Koyanagi & Gaines, 1993). Highly restrictive placements are often inappropriate at best and may instill long-term behavioral and emotional problems at worst (Behar, 1980; Stroul & Friedman, 1986). In contrast, day treatment, regardless of theoretical orientation, appears to produce positive results in behavior change and returning the child to a less restrictive setting (Baenen et al., 1986; Kutash & Rivera, 1995; Sayegh & Grizenko, 1991; Zimet & Farley, 1985). Second, day treatment may prevent more restrictive placements by providing a level of treatment that is more intensive than less restrictive alternatives or an intermediate placement for children leaving more restrictive settings but who are not ready to be mainstreamed (Gabel & Finn, 1986). Third, community-based day treatment programs can facilitate a gradual transition of the child to less restrictive settings and provide access to professionals who can work directly with parents and teachers (Gabel & Finn, 1986; Koyanagi & Gaines, 1993; Sayegh & Grizenko, 1991; Zimet & Farley, 1985). This prevents disruption in family, peer, and community relationships, avoids stigmatizing the child and family, and decreases family dependence on restrictive placements (Gabel & Finn, 1986; Sayegh & Grizenko, 1991; Zimet & Farley, 1985). Fourth, day treatment services may be more cost-effective than residential treatment. Grizenko and Papineau (1992) found that the annual cost of day treatment was almost one-sixth the cost of residential care. Hambleton (2001) reported that more than 50% of the 22,000 juveniles incarcerated in Nebraska in 1998 could have been served in a treatment program. The cost to the state for one day of incarceration was $165, whereas the cost of a community treatment program was less than $50 per day. Cost-effectiveness can also be inferred from the history of results of community services provided to other disability groups, which indicates that less restrictive placements can provide services at a lower cost than institutional settings (Knitzer, 1982).

Day treatment also has advantages over less restrictive services such as outpatient psychotherapy, special education, or consultation. First, many schools are reluctant to integrate psychological treatment in the classroom beyond basic behavior management techniques (Koyanagi & Gaines, 1993). In fact, special education has come under severe criticism for emphasis on behavior control over teaching academic and social skills and failure to use counseling and mental health services (Epstein, Cullinan, Quinn, & Cumblad, 1994). In contrast to special education alone, day treatment has the advantage of combining special education with an intensive mental health treatment program and behavior intervention milieu. This multidisciplinary approach is more appropriate for students in need of continuous therapeutic intervention. Second, outpatient programs may not provide the level of safety required to serve many children with severe EBDs. Concerns about security and liability in the event a child with EBD harms him- or herself or others has led schools, social service agencies, and juvenile courts to use more restrictive programs than might be necessary (Behar, 1980; Stroul & Friedman, 1986). Children with moderate or severe EBD may be so disruptive at home, in the community, or at school that outpatient and family support services are not adequate to meet their needs (Duchnowski, 1994; Gabel & Finn, 1986; Koyanagi & Gaines, 1993; Satterfield, Satterfield, & Schell, 1987; Sayegh & Grizenko, 1991; Topp, 1991; Zimet & Farley, 1985). Traditional outpatient services may reduce disruptive behavior but may not lead to generalized improved behavior across settings or normalize and repair relationships with teachers and peers who are not involved in the treatment (Grizenko, Papineau, & Sayegh, 1993). Day treatment can provide a self-contained and secured environment that allows the child to participate in school, home, and community life. In addition, day treatment can provide continuous collaboration with all involved to increase the effectiveness of the services supporting the child (Gabel & Finn, 1986; Koyanagi & Gaines, 1993; Sayegh & Grizenko, 1991; Stroul & Friedman, 1986; Topp, 1991; Tuma, 1991; Zimet & Farley, 1985).

KEY INGREDIENTS IN DEVELOPING A PROGRAM: THE PHILOSOPHICAL FOUNDATION

The philosophy of a school-based day treatment program serves as the foundation on which the attitudes and beliefs of staff members are based, establishes a benchmark by which success can be measured, and states specifically what the program will do. The primary philosophy of BSP is to create a safe and trusting relationship with each student as a way to prevent aggression and manage violent crises effectively. Students with EBDs need to develop trusting relationships with adults who are positive role models. Without first developing trust, students will not respond to intervention techniques in crisis situations. Students need to be certain that the adults can respond rapidly and competently to violent and aggressive behavior. Such a philosophy leads to the development of interventions and treatments that go beyond analyzing antecedents and consequences. The day treatment staff need to be experts in helping students change deeply ingrained negative identities and beliefs, restore rational thinking and behavior, and resolve trauma, internal turmoil, and conflict in their relationships with parents, teachers, and peers.

Creating a safe and trusting relationship with our students is our philosophical foundation, but a philosophy must also provide a structure that states specifically what the program will do. The key operational philosophy of a school-based day treatment program should be to remediate and prevent further deterioration of educational, emotional, and behavioral problems. To be effective, a day treatment program must have a clear philosophy based on prevention. As a means to that end, the program must provide individualized, intensive, comprehensive, and sustained services as essential ingredients (Kauffman, 1999). There are two additional essential ingredients for a successful program; a cohesive team and (last but not least) humor. Day treatment has a mission to address the interaction of children with their home and school environments based on assumptions that (1) children benefit most from treatment that involves the family, (2) interventions should be implemented in the most natural setting possible, and (3) structured and consistent interdisciplinary programs are critical (Zimet & Farley, 1985).

AN OPERATIONAL PHILOSOPHY

In talking with colleagues, BSP staff have found that when programs are being planned, a great deal of time is spent designing a level system, deciding what reinforcement schedules to use, or deciding how many therapy groups to conduct. When BSP started, plans were laid out on paper in great detail, but when our students started coming we found that they did not fit the paper plans. So we went back to work and started developing the program around the needs of the students who were actually coming to us. This meant (and still means) that the program could easily look very different from year to year, month to month, or even day to day.

Individualized Programming

Special education for children with EBDs has been criticized for being only a placement focused on control, rather than a well-planned, individually tailored, and empirically based method of intervention (Simpson, 1999; Knitzer, Steinberg, & Fleisch, 1990). Our staff members use dozens of intervention techniques and structured programs found in the literature. We have learned that there are no cookbook answers or one-size-fits-all approaches. There are, however, guideline questions that can be used to develop systematic, individualized, and empirically based interventions (Simpson, 1999). First, the team must ask which behavior is the right one to target. For example, impulsivity and hyperactivity should be targeted before working on developing empathy for others. Second, the team must ask whether the intervention will do more harm than good. Choosing to use self-monitoring of off-task behavior might increase the student's anxiety, which in turn may increase aggression or work refusal. Third, the team must determine how the intervention will be evaluated, particularly as to how it will affect the student. A student with obsessive negative thoughts about himself may become enraged if he has a progress chart posted in the class next to those of students who are doing better than he. Fourth, the method of evaluation should match the desired goal. If the goal is to improve a student's ability to make inferences from a story she just read, she should not be evaluated on her decoding skills. Fifth, the intervention should be based on methods that have acceptance at large in the field. For example, Pelham and Waschbusch (1999) report there are only three, out of more than a dozen, treatments for attention-deficit/hyperactivity disorder based on sound empirical evidence (i.e., behavior modification, stimulant medication, and a combination of both). Finally, the team must consider whether the intervention will prevent the use of other options. For example will punitive measures prevent the use of positive problem solving? Using these questions in the team process can help target efforts to the right problem, at the right time, and in the right way.

A school-based day treatment program should be an intervention model and not just a placement in which to house a troubling student. Part of developing an individualized intervention is to provide a service approach that implements new strategies. We have tried to develop a program in which there are differences between what happens at BSP and what happens in regular classes or special education resource rooms. An important difference is in the fundamental approach to education. Students in regular school settings are expected to acquire a specific quantity of academic knowledge and skills for their given grade level. For example, students in the fifth grade are expected to achieve district-established academic objectives for fifth grade by the end of the school year. In our program, by contrast, the focus is not on a quantity of academic material covered each year; instead, the focus is on acquiring new skills at a student's own rate. Skill quality and skill mastery are as important as the quantity of material each student covers each year. This progressive approach has reduced student frustration and resulted in significant academic success. In several cases we have determined that students were acting out in regular classes because of their academic skill deficits. We have had successful results with these students by focusing on helping them gain academic skills, rather than working on behavior management or mental health issues.

A second difference is that the role of teachers in our program is drastically altered from that of teachers in regular classrooms. In regular classes, teachers may challenge and test the limits of the students' knowledge, thus focusing on what the students do not know rather than on what has been mastered. Most children strive harder to achieve in such circumstances, but in our experience, children with EBDs lose interest and stop trying. If they are set up for possible failure in this way, then, in their minds, the teacher is the enemy. So no matter what procedure the teacher uses to manage behavior, it will not work. Instead, children with EBDs must be constantly set up for success. The teachers in our program expend great effort in helping each child to be successful and reinforcing even small degrees of progress.

A third distinct difference between day treatment and regular school classes lies in teachers' reactions to behavioral problems. What happens in a regular class when a student makes a mistake in performing a math exercise? Maag (1995) noted the answer is that the teacher usually does not get mad but may review the concept with the student, provide extra assistance, and have the student correct the paper. But if the student makes a mistake in behavior, what happens? Usually the teacher gets angry, assumes the student knew what to do but chose not to use the appropriate behavior, and reprimands the student publicly. If this approach is used with students with EBDs, they will withdraw and refuse to work, engage in behavior to avoid the work, or act out their frustration, boredom, or anger. A BSP student told his mother the reason he did better at BSP was that teachers put up with a lot from him but did not change their attitude toward him. When he got mad, they let him cool down; next they would say, "It was a bad moment, let's make the rest of the day better," and then they would make a plan. In contrast, the mother reflected that at his other school, when he apologized, the teachers rehashed the incident, brought up the past, and threatened negative consequences. In a school-based day treatment classroom, the occurrence of a behavior problem is seen as an instructional opportunity. Such occurrences give the teacher or therapist a chance to teach a behavioral skill a student does not know, or to retrain skills and motivate the student to perform correctly. The mindset should be that the student is still developing the skill, rather than that the student has mastered the skill and should always perform it flawlessly (Maag, 1995). What must happen in day treatment is for students to learn behavioral strategies that will help them to eventually accept more traditional educational approaches. The day treatment staff must also work with the students' referring/home schools to create conditions in the regular classes that will accommodate the students with EBDs without generating continual power struggles and conflict.

Creating an individualized intervention for each BSP student entails more than writing an individualized education plan (IEP). Individualizing services means using different approaches to academic learning, behavior management, and mental health treatment for each student. It means planning interventions as a team with a clear focus on the outcome for the student. Finally, individualizing intervention means creating an environment that is positive and accommodating to each student's needs and seeing problems as opportunities for change.

Intensive Services

Intensive treatment and educational services is usually understood to mean that the program has a small student-to-staff ratio. But how small should this ratio be, and what types of staff are needed to provide intensive services? In a world of budget constraints, the answers to these questions cannot be guesswork. The best way to answer them is to focus on the needs of students. BSP has a ratio of students to direct services staff (e.g. teachers, paraprofessional educators, psychotherapists, and behavior intervention specialists) of approximately 4:1. This ratio was developed from experience in working with our students. We know that there is a high probability that at any time a student will get frustrated with work, have trouble understanding new concepts and skills, be embarrassed by a public mistake, or become distracted, hyperactive, or disruptive to others. These situations can become violent. It is also important to keep the teacher and the paraprofessional educator in the classroom as much as possible so that the learning experience can continue to flow smoothly. If it is at all possible, it is best to provide extra support in the classroom to help the student get back in control and on a positive track.

There are, however, many times in the day where at least one student is not able to remain in the classroom and needs one-on-one help. Such one-on-one interventions are primarily used in two situations. First, help outside the class may be the best learning environment and a way to avoid aggressive behavior when a student is not dangerous but refusing to work, needs a quieter, less distracting place to work, is having an emotionally tough day, or needs help in a certain subject or task one-on-one. The use of out-of-class intervention can keep a student on task, teach positive behavior choices, or help the student cope with emotions so he or she can return to class as soon as possible.

The second circumstance in which one-on-one intervention outside the classroom is necessary is one in which a student is threatening to become or is dangerous and it is possible to safely remove the student from the classroom. In such situations the student must be engaged in positive problem-solving interventions away from the threatening situation with a neutral staff person. If the student cannot be removed safely or has reached the point of needing to be physically restrained, the other students should be evacuated and engaged in a positive activity. The deescalation process should then occur with the student in the classroom. For safety purposes, it is important never to leave a staff member alone with an agitated student.

Students in day treatment programs are there because they do not have the appropriate behavioral skills or it is extremely difficult for them to regulate their emotions. They routinely use aggression when angry, anxious, frustrated, or otherwise stressed. These students often need a secluded area to vent their aggression and work with staff to deescalate and engage in positive decision making. They need a safely designed time-out room with continuous staff monitoring.

The cycle of tantrums, rage, and threatening behavior can last a few minutes to several hours. These crisis situations can be long and taxing events for the student in crisis, for the students who are trying to stay in control, and for staff. The day treatment program needs sufficient staff so that teachers and paraprofessional educators can stay in the classroom and therapists can continue their therapy schedule. The behavior intervention specialist is the person we depend on to assist the student in crisis. In a crisis situation there must be enough staff to rotate so that everyone can cover his or her other duties, and yet have an adult immediately available to the student in crisis to help deescalate aggressive behavior. Rotating staff also ensures that the staff involved in monitoring and deescalating the crisis have a positive attitude and neutral emotions.

The average amounts of time students at BSP required out-of-class, one-on-one attention in the year 2000–2001 are displayed in Table 8.1. Some stu-

TABLE 8.1. Average and Total Hours in Out-of-Class Interventions for BSP Students in 2000–2001

Elementary students	1st quarter (n = 32)	2nd quarter (n = 34)	3rd quarter (n = 35)	4th quarter (n = 43)
Average 1:1 hours/student	10.6	5.7	7.6	8.2
Total 1:1 hours/quarter	339.2	200	267.7	334

Secondary students	1st quarter (n = 38)	2nd quarter (n = 30)	3rd quarter (n = 36)	4th quarter (n = 37)
Average 1:1 hours/student	4.9	5.6	4.2	2.6
Total 1:1 hours/quarter	185.8	169.6	151.6	99.8

dents required very little of this time, and classroom interventions were sufficient to help them with their behavior problems. Students with the most severe pathology required the lion's share of one-on-one intervention. In the first quarter of 2000–2001 two elementary students accounted for more than 30% of the elementary time out-of-class. Fortunately, these students responded to interventions, and their out-of-class time was reduced by more than 50% for one and 70% for the other student. The total number of hours devoted to one-on-one intervention out-of-class can provide a guide as to how much staff time is needed in a day treatment program. In the year 2000–2001, the elementary students needed more than 1,140 hours of one-on-one assistance and the secondary students needed more than 604 hours, for a total of over 1,744 hours of intervention.

It is interesting to note the differences in the amount of time between the elementary and secondary students in one-on-one interventions. I can speculate as to the reasons for the differences, based on my experience working in the program. I suspect there are both student- and staff-related reasons for the difference in out-of-classroom time. Goani, Black, and Baldwin (1998) cited several studies that documented patterns in maladaptive behavior often found with children with EBDs, and we have witnessed these at BSP. First, the younger the children, the more they need adults to help them learn to cooperate, think of others, and control emotions and impulses. Elementary students with EBDs seem to be developmentally stagnated at the "terrible twos." They often rely on tantrums and fighting to make their wants and needs known or to express hurt, frustration, or anger. Previous learning has trained many of our students to continue a tantrum for a long period of time. Their experience is that eventually adults will break down and they will get what they want, or get out of doing what they were trying to avoid. Our younger students are extremely persistent in these attempts and sometimes have episodes lasting hours.

We often see our younger "criers" start to use aggression directed at hurting others, stealing, and school failure between second and sixth grades. At this age they rely on adults to stop them from hurting others and are not very concerned about the consequences of their behavior. They tend to be hypersensitive, fearful, and "horriblize" minor events (e.g., not getting a turn, not being first in line, or a teasing comment from a peer). Elementary students need adults' help to deal with problems because they lack problem-solving skills. These and other factors require that adults spend a great deal of time in one-on-one interaction to help the elementary age student. By the time our students are middle schoolers they are trying to act like older role models. They do not seek adult assistance. They make their own decisions even when they know the consequences are not in their best interest. When secondary school students become threatening, we have found that monitoring them and then initiating problem solving with a neutral adult in the hall or the therapist's office usually leads to a quicker and more positive resolution than classroom-based intervention.

These general comments do not apply to all our students. Some of the younger students display very mature coping skills, and some of the secondary school students act out for hours at a time on an almost daily basis. What is clear is that effective day treatment programs absolutely require adequate numbers of staff trained to handle violent or potentially violent situations.

Comprehensive Service

Providing comprehensive wraparound services is extremely difficult. It is not possible for any one program or agency to provide a full array of services to students with EBDs. It is also difficult to maintain close contact and consistency between agencies that are providing various services to children and their families. This section describes the attempts BSP staff make to ensure as much cooperation as possible with the family, the referring/home school, social services and other agencies, and the community.

We have found that providing a school-based day treatment program has created a unique opportunity for the school system. Usually teachers in special education settings have little opportunity to work with those outside the school system on behalf of their students. An important objective for school-based day treatment is to prevent violence outside the program. BSP staff members have intimate knowledge of their students that can be communicated to parents and other family members, referring/home-school teachers, and other professionals involved in each case. In a recent instance, the therapist was aware of a student's anger at his father in regard to abuse of his mother. The student had not told anyone else. This information was helpful in treatment of the family; it helped the teacher understand why the student was so aggressive in her class, and it helped the student's probation officer, who was not getting much cooperation from the student. There are many other cases in which staff members have played a vital role in explaining students' behaviors to others.

Consultation with Referring/Home Schools

The focus of BSP is to help students to be as successful as possible at their referring/home schools. In our program, most students spend at least part of the day at their referring/home schools. The time a student spends there depends on his or her progress toward achieving behavior goals and emotional stability. We have found that in most day treatment settings, the student is at the program building the entire day until released from the program. Few programs provide transportation and other supports to involve the student in the referring/home school while still receiving day treatment services. The referring/home school staff is included as part of the BSP team. This inclusion of the referring/home school staff on the team provides a focus for the consultation process and makes consultation a two-way street. The referring/home school staff must be treated with respect and offered options and support; second-guessing and criticism are counterproductive. A mindset that we always try to maintain is that the referring/home school staff members are assumed to be doing the best they can with the resources they have.

The close relationship with the referring/home school allows the respective staffs to communicate directly and daily if necessary. If a student is having a bad day, the student can be kept at the day treatment program and the referring/home school can be informed as to why the student will be absent. This procedure often prevents an incident that would be unsafe or would harm the student's inclusion at the referring/home school. If a student has problems at his or her referring/home school, consequences can be provided in both settings. This lets the student know that the staffs of the two buildings are working together. If the student is treated consistently across settings, the motivation to perform well at the referring/home school is enhanced. These efforts maintain the student's positive relationship with the referring/home school, thus adding to the attraction of increasing time there.

For example, Jason is a seventh grader who became belligerent and assaulted a peer at his referring/home school. The team decided that the referring/home school and the student needed a short break from each other before positive problem resolution could occur. A plan was developed so that Jason could be at BSP full-time for 2 days instead of being suspended. The BSP staff worked with Jason and the situation at the referring/home school. After 2 days the problem was resolved, and Jason resumed his previous schedule at his referring/home school.

Case Management in the Community

We have found that case management is essential for building collaboration among all the agencies involved with a student. If services are not coordinated across agencies and among professionals, the efforts of all involved are jeopardized (Nelson & Pearson, 1991). Students with EBDs and their families frequently have multiple personal, family, and community problems that necessitate involvement with several agencies and systems (Koyanagi & Gaines, 1993; Nelson & Pearson, 1991; Stroul & Friedman, 1986). Our staff members serve in a case management role that is a resource to parents and community agencies involved with the student.

"Case management" means that our staff members perform several functions that help prevent students' aggressive behavior, both in and out of the program. A case manager acts as a liaison between the client and the community. Case management creates positive communication and understanding among all involved. In addition, it reduces duplication of effort, prevents agencies from contradicting one another's efforts and authority, and ensures that responsibilities fall to those who can most appropriately provide a particular service in a given circumstance (Stroul & Friedman, 1986).

The day treatment staff members should work to coordinate their efforts with those of probation officers, police, case workers, and residential services in providing consistency and structure across settings. A particular concern is coordinating treatment with outside psychotherapists who may be treating the family or providing specialized treatment to the student (e.g., treatment of sexual abuse). By coordinating and communicating, the day treatment staff can support other treatment efforts and make modifications in interventions, based on the input of the outside therapists or other professionals. In the day treatment setting, we have found that a psychotherapist is the most logical person to act as a case manager.

Finally, case management provides a unified effort that the student is aware of; the student knows that the use of violence will have consequences involving others in his or her life. A dramatic example of outside agencies' spontaneously collaborating with our program happened a couple of years ago. A student and his mother went to the doctor. They began to fight in the doctor's office, and the police were called. The police department had worked closely with us and knew the family. They put the student and his mother in separate police cars and brought them to us. When they arrived, the student's therapist worked with the officers, the student, and his mother to resolve the situation.

Case Management with Outside Placements

Case management ensures continuity of care when a student is placed outside the program for a period of time and may return. Students may be hospitalized by the family or social services, or incarcerated by the courts, because of problems at home or in the community. Our psychotherapists make every effort to communicate with outside placements. If this communication does not occur, nothing may be heard about a student for several weeks. Often no one will contact the program for information about the student's behavior or achievement at school. When the student does return to the family, there may be no information provided regarding the evaluations done, interventions recommended, or medications prescribed. The program may never get information about the problems that led to the placement. Without this information, the student may be returning to an environment that is not equipped to accommodate him or her. More important, the cycle of emotional and behavioral problems may continue or even worsen, and may thus lead to more restrictive placement, if information is not shared. As case manager, the psychotherapist can make sure that someone in the new placement knows what has happened in the past treatment. In addition, if it is likely that the student will return, keeping a connection will facilitate this process. Finally, maintaining a connection with students builds rapport because the students know the program staff has not abandoned them and wants them back.

Working with Parents

A teacher new to our program remarked that some of our success with parents resulted from the fact that the parents are supported and asked to participate in the decisions made about their child's program. From the very first time parents come in contact with our program, they must be assured that they can trust the staff and that their children will be safe. Some families are reluctant to let outsiders become involved in their family issues. This guardedness may be an attempt to deny or cover up family dysfunction or to avoid therapeutic change. We have found that it is important not to jump to this conclusion and that there are many reasons for families to be less than enthusiastic about their child becoming a day treatment student. For many families, handling a problem within the family may be a normal cultural expectation. Parents may be wary because in the past they were made to feel blamed and see themselves as unsuccessful parents. They are sometimes in danger of losing their jobs because of the frequent need to rush to school in response to demands to remove their child. They are afraid that we too will call them to get their child. Some parents have been to many therapists, attended parenting classes, put stickers on charts on refrigerator doors, used time out, and so on. By the time they get to day treatment, they may be less than willing to try one more idea. Often the parents we work with are suspicious of the motives of the school personnel, dread hearing from school, and cringe at the idea that school officials expect parents to be able to change their children's behavior. Many parents are concerned that their children will be in a setting that exclusively serves students with EBDs. They are fearful that other students may influence their child to have bad behavior. A number of parents have been in treatment programs or have had negative experiences as students in school; these previous experiences may be a source of distrust. These parents need some support in order to trust the staff enough to try to make changes. When parents do not trust the staff, they will not be supportive of the interventions used.

We consider anyone acting in the parental role—parents, guardians, surrogate parents, foster parents, residential staff members, or others—as essential team members. There must be ongoing communication and cooperation, as well as a reciprocal positive relationship, between parents and staff. Parents may be involved in traditional ways, such as by attending school events and serving on individualized education plan (IEP) teams. Parents should also have considerable daily input in the intervention plans, plans for reintegration to home schools, and other issues related to their children's education and treatment. Ideally, parents will also agree to be involved in family therapy; however, in our program the parents cannot be required to participate because of special education laws.

On each of our teams, we designate a member (or members) as being responsible for parent contact. Having one primary contact person prevents parents from being contacted redundantly on the same issue and avoids inconsistent communication. Usually, the psychotherapist maintains the closest contact with parents. Whatever the case, psychotherapists and teachers should offer frequent support through phone calls and home visits to discuss the student's progress.

There are several techniques for building trust with parents. One is for staff members to try to make frequent contacts to talk about the positive things their children have done. Many parents have told us that our program is the first in which anyone has said anything positive about their children or them. A staff member should contact a parent not only when a major behavioral incident occurs, but when a student exhibits success. When a parent is contacted, rapport can be built and the parent's defensiveness can be reduced by taking a few simple measures. If a problem has arisen, the staff member should identify the problem and options for its resolution, rather than merely discussing the student in negative terms. The parent should be involved by the staff in routinely scheduled sessions to address family and community issues affecting the student's progress. If a family is seeing an outside therapist, the program should cooperate with and support any special behavioral programs occurring in the home or residential setting.

Psychotherapists must be willing to work after school hours and go to students' homes to accommodate the families' needs. Psychotherapists are often asked to go to homes in crisis situations. In a recent incident, a student ran away from home. The parent was very upset. The therapist went to the child's home to support the parent and helped the parent communicate with police. As the crisis was resolved and the child was found, the therapist worked with the family to make sure the child would not run away again.

BSP staff have found many opportunities to help parents with problems they are having. The staff members should do all they can to use these situations to build rapport and help parents find solutions to the problems. Such efforts can reduce family stress and the risk of violence in the home. For example, many parents of our students say that their children are not allowed to participate in community activities (e.g., soccer or midget football) or that they cannot get any day care providers or even relatives to provide after-school care for their child. BSP staff have taken an active role in helping parents find care. This care may be furnished by private providers or a therapeutic program. We are very fortunate that a collaborative partner of BSP, the Child Guidance Center, has an after-school day treatment service that uses our building. This service not only provides skilled care after school hours, but actively works to get students with EBDs involved in positive activities in the community and provides additional support and therapy services to the students and parents. Our staff has also worked with parents to find clothes, food, and medical care and to meet other family needs.

We have learned that parents who are able to be effective case managers can reduce conflict at home. It is important that parents learn how to be their families' case managers in order to get services they need. The psychotherapist or other staff members can teach parents how to perform many case management functions, support their efforts, and answer questions. As noted earlier, case management functions include planning services, communicating with others involved and informing various agencies as to what other agencies are doing, and working positively with police, the judicial system, social services, residential or family support agencies, and medical services on behalf of a child. Parents can become powerful advocates if they are taught to monitor progress and intervention success, broker and acquire services, and act as liaisons between various service/resource providers (Stroul & Friedman, 1986).

Therapeutic Crisis Intervention and Use of Police

It would be great to say that with the right behavior management plan, a well-designed education curriculum, and an excellent psychotherapy regimen, all violent behavior can be prevented. But this is not the case. Most students referred to our program exhibit physical aggression at one time or another. Day treatment staff members must be given the training and facilities to respond quickly and therapeutically to frequent incidents of aggression.

Our methods of crisis intervention are guided by two premises. First, the safety of everyone is the top priority. If a physical intervention procedure cannot be carried out safely, it should not be tried. Second, physical intervention is not the solution to a crisis. The end of a crisis comes about when the parties involved have been able to bring about a safe, positive, and equitable solution. Solutions do not happen through intimidation, but through discussion and agreement.

In our program, we have taken the stand that if a student assaults another student or staff member, there should be definite consequences. Students need to know that we will do all we can to keep the program a safe place to be. This may mean the involvement of police. Our program has developed a close relationship with the local police department. Officers routinely stop by and visit informally. This gives the officers a better understanding of our program and of the students. In addition, police officers often have experience with some of our families. It is very helpful if we know an officer who is familiar with the family and can call on him or her if we have a concern. In a recent incident a mother called the therapist with a family problem, but she was afraid to call the police herself. The therapist called an officer who knew the family. They worked together to resolve the issue without serious incident.

Officers are sometimes called in crisis situations. If a younger student runs away from the program, the police are notified to help locate and return the student. In the event of an assault, the standard procedure is that parents are notified and the police are called to investigate. Most officers consult with staff members and take a low-key approach in interviewing students. The officer answering a call determines whether a criminal assault has occurred and cites the offending student if this is the case. Usually the student is released to the program, but he or she may be taken to the juvenile justice facility or to a hospital if the officer determines that either is appropriate. The student is usually referred to the department's youth aid section. Parents and the student meet with youth aid officers and plan consequences for each case. If the student's situation dictates it, he or she may be referred to juvenile court.

This procedure has never been a threat to the program's relationship with students. The appropriate use of the police does not burden officers with needless calls. Students who are victims of assault recognize that an additional step has been taken to ensure safety. Students who commit assaults understand that there are consequences and that staff members will work with them and their victims to resolve conflict and maintain safety.

There are several crisis intervention programs. All of our staffers have been trained in "therapeutic crisis intervention" (TCI; Budlong, Holden, & Mooney, 1993). TCI provides clear guidelines on when and how to perform a physical intervention. If a physical intervention is used, staffers should expect an initial reaction of a dramatic escalation in aggression. Carrying out an intervention safely may require two to five staff members, and the intervention may last an hour or longer. The physical intervention process must include a gradual and sequential release process as a student calms and is willing to comply with expectations. This process should never be rushed. The intervention should never be considered over until the student and all those involved have participated in a positive resolution of the incident. This should happen as soon as possible after the physical intervention is complete (Budlong et al., 1993).

According to TCI, staff members should be aware of three major concerns in using physical intervention techniques. First, physical interventions require that staff be aware of their own emotions. It is essential to be emotionally neutral when physical intervention is used. Day treatment staff endure verbal and physical abuse of every description, including profanity, as well as racial and personal attacks. Staff members can expect to be spit on or bit. Staff should not take these attacks personally, but should work to resolve situations in a positive process. If a staff person cannot remain calm and rational, he or she needs to be able to ask for help from other team members to intervene with the student.

Second, staff members need to be aware of the student's feelings and know the meaning behind the behavior in order to intervene safely. The use of physical intervention should be based on a known history of the student. Physical intervention may not be appropriate for students who are sexual abuse survivors. Students who have significant cognitive deficits may not be able to benefit from the verbal deescalation and conflict resolution components of the intervention. Some students are simply too big or strong to be physically restrained safely. Still other students are inadvertently reinforced by the restraint process. Alternative or modified procedures should be designed for students for whom physical restraint is inappropriate.

Third, staff members must be aware of the physical environment in a crisis situation. The physical environment may provide resources or barriers to verbal or physical interventions. The staff members need to be aware of and use resources to calm the student. They must also assess the safety of the environment before initiating a physical intervention. For example, a physical intervention is not appropriate in a stairwell or in a store or other public area.

Physical intervention is a tool to maintain safety and prevent future violence. Use of physical intervention should not be the primary management technique in a day treatment setting. For physical intervention to be used therapeutically, staff members must be well trained and must continually practice the techniques.

Working with parents, physicians, human service agencies, juvenile justice and police agencies, and others involved in the life of a child with EBDs is a challenge. Kauffman (1999) stated that effective prevention requires that programs be designed to address chronic and severe problems at all levels and to bring the problems into control, with the goal of long-term management and problem resolution. This phase of the mission is perhaps the most difficult to accomplish, and BSP staff members are continuously trying to improve in this area.

Sustained Intervention

The Behavioral Skills Program (BSP) is the most restrictive placement provided to Lincoln public school students with EBDs. A student is placed in the program only after all less restrictive interventions have failed. Placement is usually long-term, with an average length of stay of 19.27 months. The program was designed to supplement special education and mainstream services provided in the student's regular school or referring/home school. The ultimate goal of the program is to help a student regain full-time placement in a regular classroom setting with appropriate accommodations. But some students spend most of their school careers involved with BSP. Some students who have left the program successfully have had to return once or twice before finally finding their places in their regular schools. We also have a number of students with episodic mental health problems that must return in times of crisis and are then able to return to their regular schools when their mental health is stabilized.

Understanding Student Behavior

As part of a sustained program the BSP staff members focus on developing a very detailed and intimate understanding of each student. To maintain a safe atmosphere, it is important to understand why a student is in day treatment. Most students referred to us have already experienced a wide variety of behavior management approaches, applied by both parents and professionals. The students may have had years of placement in special education classrooms with experienced and skilled teachers. They may have seen numerous psychotherapists, been placed in one or more hospital settings, or perhaps been adjudicated. If any of the previous attempts to correct problems had worked, the students would not have been referred to day treatment. The day treatment staff must provide the means and motivation for students to change their behavior and beliefs and resolve their emotional turmoil and trauma.

We have found that the students referred to us exhibit severe and pervasive aggression for a variety of reasons. Like all children, our students have feelings of anxiety, get scared, and worry. However, unlike other children, those with EBDs usually have multiple life experiences that put them at risk for severe emotional and behavioral maladjustment (Koyanagi & Gaines, 1993; Nelson & Pearson, 1991). These problems can be some of the reasons that children with EBDs have long-term, frequent, and intensively aggressive behaviors. Students served in day treatments experience many risk/stress factors (Koyanagi & Gaines, 1993; Nelson & Pearson, 1991). These risk factors include experiencing physical or psychological trauma, living in dysfunctional families and dangerous communities and neighborhoods, and/or having multiple psychological, cognitive, or physical developmental disabilities (Singh, Landrum, Donatelli, Hampton, & Ellis, 1994; Epstein et al., 1994; Koyanagi & Gaines, 1993; Nelson & Pearson, 1991; Grizenko & Sayegh, 1990).

Although the students we have worked with do experience a number of risk/stress factors, most students also have a variety of other reasons or purposes underlying their behavior. For a small number of students, their aggressive behavior may stem from their natural temperaments. Often, however, aggressive behavior is motivated by the students' emotional states, attitudes, or beliefs. Our experience is that students with EBDs often have an overriding fear of getting hurt, both physically and emotionally. They are easily frustrated or feel trapped and threatened. Often our students recognize that their behavior is dysfunctional and know the appropriate skills, but do not know what to do to stop themselves from acting out inappropriately. Their worldview is often fatalistic; they feel that nothing will make their lives better. Some students do not recognize that they are rejected by most peers, but accept rejection as a fact of their existence.

The students we have served often have trouble thinking and acting coherently. Some students are genuinely surprised when the outcome of their aggressive behavior does not achieve their desired results. These students may misinterpret routine circumstances as threatening, or they may not realize the inappropriateness of their responses. Other students have difficulty controlling their impulses. Their moods can change rapidly and escalate predictably to aggression. Sometimes students are simply tired or do not feel well because they are not cared for at home and are therefore easily irritated and noncompliant.

Aggression, of course, is also motivated by antecedents and consequences. Some students use aggression to avoid academic work or to reduce the expectations of parents or teachers. We have found that if students feel unsafe, they may use aggression to make sure they are not victimized and may build a tough image by victimizing others. Children who distrust others use aggression to maintain emotional distance and avoid rejection from others. Many students are tougher than others and find that the abuse of others can be intrinsically and tangibly very rewarding. Aggression is stimulating and exciting because it enhances self-importance and makes others look less powerful.

These are but a few of the individual causes of our students' aggression. Students with EBDs are not only perpetrators of violence; they are often victims of aggression. In our program we try to recognize this dichotomy as it operates in a student's behavior. The in-depth understanding of a student's unique situation and the underlying causes of his or her behavior will lead to the creation of interventions to meet the individual's needs.

A COHESIVE TEAM

The use of a team approach is one of the most important ingredients of success in helping staff members work together to achieve the goals of the program. The success of a program is dependent on how much the staff members trust one another, how well they collaborate in making decisions, and how well they support each other's efforts. All team members play a critical role in making sure that decisions are made with the primary criterion of what is best for the students.

Teams serve an organizational and program management purpose that helps create a safe, stable, and positive environment for students. Teams should have a high degree of autonomy, responsibility, and power to make the ongoing decisions in the operation of the program. Intervention and treatment methods, curriculum and teaching activities, students' schedules at referring/home schools, and many other decisions should be made by the team, and not by school administrators.

The team process should provide support in several forms. The team process builds a "can do" attitude among staff members. Day treatment programs are often pressed to stretch resources and serve more and more students with increasingly severe problems. The team structure prevents staff members from feeling isolated and unsupported under this stress. Team support creates an atmosphere that frees the staff to be creative in finding ways to serve more students while still maintaining quality.

Teams also provide support for handling students safely. In working with violent students, there are times when a one-on-one situation can be very threatening. If a student is in crisis, it is essential that more than one staff person is involved and the situation is handled in a way that does not intimidate the student. When two or three adults are supportively involved, physical aggression can be avoided and a positive conflict resolution obtained.

Even the most patient staff member can get frustrated with a student. In our program, team members spend a great deal of time learning how to "read" one another, and they practice working cooperatively. Because of these efforts, one team member can ask another to take over a situation when the first member feels unable to deal with a student. There are also times when certain staff members must handle a situation and leave their regular duties. For example, a teacher may need to leave his or her class to work out a problem with a student. The teacher must be confident that the paraeducator will be able to continue the class and that other staff members will be willing to go into the class and help out without being asked.

Finally, the team creates a professional identity for the staff. Team building is an ongoing process of staff collaboration. Teams facilitate the melding of various philosophies, create staff cohesion, and promote positive communication styles and problem-solving techniques. Team members must work constantly to overcome personal and professional differences and develop cohesion. Inevitably, there will be times when staff members do not get along well; the team structure enables them to resolve these conflicts and regain the ability to provide a "best-practice" level of intervention. The team process helps staff members to develop and use skills to teach students how to manage their behavior and facilitates the best quality of education and treatment.

The team structure makes it easier for members to communicate and modify interventions throughout the day and allow for quick decision making. In our program it is often said, "If you miss a day, when you come back the program has completely changed." This adaptability reduces the chance of violence, because interventions for a student can be changed according to his or her present needs and circumstances.

Currently at BSP there is an elementary team for grades 1–6 and a secondary team for grades 7 and up. Each team is structured and operates differently to meet the unique needs of each grade group. We have tried, as much as possible, to structure the schedules and classes for each team to resemble a regular school setting. The elementary team currently has six teachers, six paraeducators, three full-time psychotherapists, two part-time psychotherapists, and one behavior intervention specialist. Each elementary teacher teaches multiple grade levels, and students are matched on the basis of their academic and treatment needs. Most elementary teachers teach all subjects, and the students have the same teacher all day. Most of the 5th- and 6th-grade students are with two teachers who team their curriculum. Thus, one teacher teaches all the language arts and the other covers mathematics, social studies, and science. This is done because in our district some sixth-grade students go to middle schools and some go to elementary schools. This structure helps our students transition to schools where students change classrooms for some periods. The psychotherapists are assigned caseloads, and most of their time is spent with the students assigned to them. The elementary staff meet and consult informally several times a week to make team decisions and have at least one formal staffing a week.

The six secondary teachers teach their subject specialties, and students move from class to class each period just as they would in a middle school or high school. The entire secondary team meets twice a day. This is done for two reasons. First, all the teachers and psychotherapists have contact with each student on a daily basis and need to know what is going on with each student at all times. Second, the team uses a "level" system for students, and they meet each day to determine the level each student will start on the next day. The secondary team has two full-time psychotherapists, two psychotherapists who split time between BSP and duties outside the program, two behavior intervention specialists, and one recreation therapist who also assists the elementary team. To facilitate decision making, the secondary team has smaller treatment teams made up of teachers, psychotherapists, and behavior intervention specialists. The treatment teams develop individual plans for students assigned to them and then present the plans to the entire secondary team for input and implementation.

Staff Members and Their Roles

Each BSP team member plays a variety of complementary roles. The roles of staff members are so varied that at times it is difficult to tell who is the teacher, the administrator, the psychotherapist, the paraeducator, or the behavior intervention specialist. A visitor to the program may see a psychotherapist helping a student with academic work, a teacher serving lunches, or a paraeducator talking quietly with a distraught student. In fact, it is important that all staff members, including the bus drivers, secretaries, and custodians, receive training in how to work with aggressive students. The roles and expertise of teachers, psychotherapists, paraeducators, behavior intervention specialists, intern therapists and student teachers, administrators, bus drivers, secretaries, and all other staff members are expanded and interwoven in a successful team. Although all team members are important, staff members who are most directly involved in the education and treatment of students with EBDs have some unique qualifications and special roles to play in a day treatment setting.

Teachers

Ideally, all our teachers have impeccable professional skills. Teachers are expected to be knowledgeable about their subject matter and able to organize and communicate academic information and skills meaningfully and effectively. To meet each student's needs, teachers must go beyond remedial instruction and be able to develop a more enriched curriculum, experiential or functional learning programs, or vocational training. Teachers must also motivate students to achieve academically and evaluate their achievement fairly and objectively. We believe these professional skills are defining characteristics of good teachers; however, these skills, though necessary, are insufficient for work with students with EBDs. Webber, Anderson, and Otey (1991) have stated that personal characteristics such as responsiveness, warmth and affection, supportiveness, flexibility, confidence, and honesty are required to bring about success. We have also found that a sense of humor and the ability to develop positive, trusting relationships with students are also critically important attributes. We have found that our best teachers have "megalevels" of these personal characteristics.

To teach students with severe EBDs, even more than professional skills and the aforementioned personal characteristics are needed. These teachers must be highly skilled in behavior management and able to teach academic and behavioral skills simultaneously. Teachers are responsible for creating an environment in the classroom that builds students' self-confidence, teaches behavioral skills, and reinforces the students' use of appropriate behavior choices. Teachers spend a great portion of their time helping students learn to be happy and positive and to enjoy the activities in the classroom.

Teachers in our program must also have the unique skill of incorporating psychological treatment, not just behavior management, into the educational process. Day treatment teachers must be knowledgeable about how to deal with mental health and family dysfunction that manifest in behavior problems in the classroom. They need to know community and cultural issues that may affect the students' behaviors, emotions, and attitudes. Teachers must communicate and work cooperatively with social services and juvenile justice agencies regarding the students' treatment and educational progress. In short, a day treatment teacher provides an integrated treatment and educational setting to meet each child's needs.

Paraeducators and Behavior Intervention Specialists

A common denominator of all direct care services to children or adults with disabilities is a heavy reliance on staff members who are not certified as professionals. BSP uses paraeducators (paras) in each class to assist the teacher, and behavior intervention specialists (BISs) to assist all staff and students. The roles of these staff members are critical. They are chosen for their ability to develop positive relationships with students yet maintain appropriate relationship boundaries. BSP paras have responsibilities for helping students with academic work, charting progress on behavior goals, and intervening with students who are aggressive or distraught. A para must understand the teacher's plans and know each student so that he or she can take over the class if a teacher must leave the room or in order to help a substitute teacher get through the day. Behavior intervention specialists deescalate aggressive students by using nonaversive techniques, help students with social behavior, monitor time-out areas, keep data on students' time out of class, and complete documentation of behavior incidents. The BIS staff members must know how to do safe interventions, resolve conflict situations positively on a one-on-one basis, and know the specific academic and treatment needs of each student. Neither type of staff member should be cast in the role of "bouncer" "go-for" or "substitute parent." There should be opportunities for paras and the BISs to interact with students in positive situations. At BSP all staff participate in physical education (PE) and recess activities, eat lunch with the students, and take active roles in special activities, such as school craft sales or basketball games between students and staff and the local Sertoma club. All professional staff members need to reinforce that paras and BIS staff have the same status as any other staff members. This can be done by giving them leadership tasks, listening to their opinions, and making sure that they are aware of any decisions that affect their roles. Both BSP paras and BISs often develop activities for the class, provide information a student has confided in them, and participate in developing intervention plans.

Psychotherapists and Recreation Therapist

The role of psychotherapists in our program is quite different from the usual role of therapists in clinics, private practice offices, hospitals, or other traditional treatment settings. The psychotherapists act as mental health assessment and treatment professionals, consultants to staff and parents, case managers, and liaisons to outside therapists, physicians, and community agencies. The psychotherapists are also responsible for doing all they can to create change in the referring/home school and family environments that will help students. The psychotherapists in our program are critical in preventing aggression, because of their knowledge and skills in developing interventions that go beyond behavior management. The multiple problems, the wide variety of pathology and psychological issues, and the various cognitive abilities of day treatment students require therapists to have a broad range of treatment skills. Therapists incorporate psychoeducational, cognitive-behavioral, ecological, and systems methods, as well as family therapy and other models in treatment. The school-based day treatment setting allows psychotherapists to intervene at the time and place a problem occurs and to work with everyone involved in developing a solution. BSP therapists must have the necessary skills to work with parents of all types. Many of the parents of our students have (or have had) severe mental health or other disabilities, have abused (or been abused by) their children or spouses, and/or are living under a great deal of ongoing stress. Many of these parents have had negative experiences with schools and psychotherapists in the past. The therapists must be able to deal with these issues while also serving the students.

Clearly, psychotherapists working in day treatment settings have an interesting and challenging position that requires a high level of experience, knowledge, and energy. BSP provides the therapists with a unique opportunity to be very accessible to students. The therapists must be able to maintain a therapeutic relationship with students, yet be authority figures who set limits and administer consequences, and be involved in physical interventions. In addition, the therapists must understand classroom culture and be able to provide practical interventions for teachers. They must be ready, willing, and able to participate in the classroom, as well as in the lunchroom, in the gym, on the playground, and on field trips. The therapists have to be willing to accept other team members' points of view and incorporate those views in treatment. In short, the psychotherapists must have an attitude of willingness to do whatever is needed, whenever needed, to create a partnership between education and treatment.

In addition to the psychotherapists, the recreation therapist plays a critical therapeutic role. Students with EBDs frequently exhibit aggression on the playground, in PE, or while playing in the neighborhood. Parents often tell us that their children have been kicked out of every organized recreation program and day care they have tried. These children have difficulty following the rules of games and sports, handling competition, and cooperating with peers in games and sports. The recreation therapist helps students learn how to compete and cooperate, develop social and physical skills, understand sports rules, and enjoy physical education, sports activities, and common, ordinary play throughout the day.

Bus Drivers

The school bus drivers are a critical part of providing services to our students and in supporting the referring/home schools. Our buses run on the students' schedules. We may have two or three students from the same school, but if student A can handle only an hour at the regular school and student B can handle a half-day, we make two runs to that school. Likewise, if student C does better in the morning in a regular school and student D does better in the afternoon, we run two routes if possible. These routes and schedules can change on an almost daily basis. The drivers also change routes at a moment's notice in case of a crisis. For example, they try to get a student early if he or she is in crisis at the referring/home school, pick the student up at home if he or she is suspended from the referring/home school, or drive BSP staff to the referring/home school in crisis situations so we can safely transport the agitated student to BSP. The drivers are incredibly patient with families and referring/home schools that may not get students out to the bus on time and do not complain when we ask them to return for a student who missed the bus. Our drivers are a valuable source of information, as they overhear student conversations and observe behaviors. Their reports have helped us stop aggressive behavior before it happens and have alerted us to conflicts and issues students are having at home that they witness.

Ironically, in the BSP building there is intensive support and rapid intervention, there are immediate consequences for dangerous behavior, and highly aggressive and older students are generally separated from younger or less aggressive students. But on the bus all types of students ride together (with the exception that elementary and secondary students are not transported together), and the only adult is the driver. Typically, the behavior problems that occur on the bus are the result of challenges, trash talk, or teasing. When fighting and aggressive provocation occur, we have implemented several solutions. One is simply having the bus driver return to the program without confronting the students. The driver can radio ahead to have staff members meet the bus and intervene. In the event that a severe assault is occurring, the bus driver calls police and evacuates the nonaggressive students from the bus.

No matter how many safety measures have been instituted, the most important preventive intervention is to employ bus drivers with calm personalities who will not create power struggles with students. In addition, teachers and psychotherapists must communicate closely with the drivers. Drivers should be given the information needed to understand the students' behavior and the motivation for their behavior. The staff should also provide support to the drivers by discussing the interventions that they can use if incidents occur on a bus. This can be as simple as reminding the drivers of a common strategy—a power struggle can often be avoided if you remember to lower your voice as a student raises his or hers—or setting up a reward program for good bus rides. A recent incident illustrates the point. On the way to the home/referring school, a sixth grader started to pick on another student. The driver prompted the student to stop, and when he did not, the driver turned back to BSP without further comment. The driver had been told that the student would try to bargain to avoid the consequences. When the student offered to be good if they went on, the driver calmly told the student that he had already made his choice. The driver returned the student to the program, where a therapist took over the problem solving while the student waited for the late bus.

School Nurse Paraprofessional

The nurse paraprofessional has been invaluable in straightening out communication with referring/home school nurses, parents, and physicians concerning medications for students. Many conflicts over whether a student is to have mediation, or whether there have been medication changes, happen each day. It is important that the nurse para have knowledge of each student's medications to ensure they are given appropriately. Many aggressive behaviors can occur because medications were not given properly and the student was not able to control his or her emotions and behavior on his or her own. The nurse para is also responsible for administering medications and treating students who are ill, think they are ill, or are injured. The interpersonal relationship skills of the nurse para have prevented a great deal of student resistance to taking medications and helped to comfort students when they were angry or upset about an illness or injury.

IT'S GOTTA BE FUN

A final ingredient in developing a day treatment that is necessary for success is one that cannot be taught. To have a successful program, staff have to know how to have fun. This can take several forms. One of our teams is reserved, yet knows how to make the students happy and feel cared for. Its members are quiet, but they can laugh at themselves and give each other a good-natured hard time. The other team is boisterous and extroverted. The students learn that teachers and therapists are people too and that having fun does not mean putting others down or exploiting others to get a laugh. Creating an atmosphere where positive humor and a positive focus are maintained serves many purposes. Fun builds safety and trust by reducing tension and threat. Fun also allows staff members to be creative and flexible and to help students without "controlling" them. Fun and positive attitudes can disarm the power of students' verbal and physical abuse, as well as their negative emotions and attitudes. We cannot pretend that working in a day treatment program is not highly stressful. Fun combats burnout. Team members must remember to laugh at themselves. This ingredient helps everyone to face the next day.

SUMMARY AND CONCLUSIONS

Day treatment programs have become more common in schools as the number of children identified with severe EBDs has increased. Such programs vary in the types of treatments offered and in educational philosophies and procedures. They also vary in the types of students accepted, the amount of help given to reintegrate students into less restrictive settings, and the scope of services provided to families.

Because of the aggressive behavior of students with EBDs, the staff members of day treatment programs must be able to prevent aggression and intervene safely in violent situations. The philosophy of the program is the foundation to building a secure environment. The program philosophy must prioritize the establishment of safety and trust in a positive, supportive relationship between staff and students.

To design an effective program, staff members must develop a complete understanding of the antecedents, consequences, and meanings of the students' behavior. In addition, there must be an understanding of the motivations, attitudes, beliefs, and emotions underlying the behavior. Each student's level of risk factors, and history of abuse and other psychological trauma, must also be considered in the treatment process.

Day treatment programs must provide a very different approach to serving students than is available in either more restrictive or less restrictive settings. The success of the program depends as much on the interpersonal skills of staff members as on their professional skills. A team approach provides the structure to support staff members and allows them to work cooperatively.

Day treatment programs must develop procedures to prevent violence at the program, in the referring/home school, at home, and in the community. Consultation and support for referring/home schools and families can prevent violence and maintain consistency in behavior management across settings. Day treatment can provide case management services to ensure that the program's goals and interventions dovetail with the efforts of other agencies involved. The involvement of parents requires a concerted effort by the day treatment staff. Parents of children with EBDs may need a great deal of support. Staff members must build trust with parents through frequent contact, by providing practical help with family problems, and by seeking parental input for program interventions.

Although the prevention of violence is possible to achieve, crises involving aggression cannot be totally eliminated. Day treatment staff must be well trained and practiced in a structured plan of crisis intervention and deescalation. To ensure safety, staff members must be capable of using interventions in a therapeutic manner. Physical control does not terminate a crisis. Only when the student and staff are involved in nonaggressive resolution of the conflict is the crisis over.

In serving aggressive students, day treatment programs face many problems that must be addressed in the future. One problem is how to serve students who may not have the cognitive reasoning abilities to benefit from verbal therapeutic intervention. A second problem, a concern is expressed by teachers of our students, is how to serve students with learning disabilities and other handicapping conditions. Teachers may not have the particular skills, resources, or experience to serve these students, and it is often difficult to create the experiential or functional educational program these students need. Third, students' families often have severe problems. It is sometimes difficult to undo 12–16 hours of time at home or on the street with 6 hours of time in treatment each day. Fourth, it is often difficult to determine when it is time to refer a student elsewhere or when to terminate treatment because of lack of progress or truancy. When resources are scarce, it is hard to justify keeping a spot for a student who is seldom present. Then there is the problem of where else the student can be referred to. Often, there is nowhere else for the student to go, or the student will not be accepted anywhere else because of aggressive behavior or poor prognosis.

These are just a few of the problems for programs that serve extremely aggressive or violent students. The methods outlined in this chapter are not a blueprint that can be replicated in every community or neighborhood. Day treatment programs will vary in design and programming, depending on the needs of the students and on the nature of the community or school district. In this chapter, just a few methods to prevent aggression and intervene in crises have been presented. New experiences and situations are encountered every day at BSP. We hope that the ideas offered here will be a foundation for readers to be innovative in dealing with their unique situations.

The payoff for developing programs of this type is that highly aggressive students can be served in school- or community-based settings. In addition, in the research our program has conducted in the last few years to determine program outcomes, the findings thus far have been positive. Students have improved not only behaviorally but academically, and more restrictive placements have been prevented. These outcomes provide evidence that day treatment programs can be a worthwhile investment for public schools.

REFERENCES

Baenen, R. S., Stephens, M. A., & Glenwick, D. S. (1986). Outcome in psychoeducational day school programs: A review. *American Journal of Orthopsychiatry, 56,* 263–270.

Behar, L. (1980). Financing mental health services for children and adolescents. *Bulletin of the Menninger Clinic, 54,* 127–139.

Budlong, M. J., Holden, M. J., & Mooney, A. J. (1993). *Therapeutic crisis intervention.* Ithaca, NY: Family Life Development Center, Cornell University.

Duchnowski, A. J. (1994). Innovative service models: Education. *Journal of Clinical Child Psychology, 23*, 13–18.

Epstein, M. H., Cullinan, D., Quinn, K. P., & Cumblad, C. (1994). Characteristics of children with emotional and behavioral disorders in community-based programs designed to prevent placement in residential facilities. *Journal of Emotional and Behavioral Disorders, 2*, 51–57.

Gabel, S., & Finn, M. (1986). Outcome in children's day treatment programs: Review of the literature and recommendations for future research. *International Journal of Partial Hospitalization, 3*, 261–271.

Gaoni, L., Black, Q. C., & Baldwin, S. (1998). Defining adolescent behaviour disorder: An overview. *Journal of Adolescence, 21*, 1–13.

Grizenko, N., & Papineau, D. (1992). A comparison of cost effectiveness of day treatment and residential treatment for children with severe behaviour problems. *Canadian Journal of Psychiatry, 37*, 393–400.

Grizenko, N., Papineau, D., & Sayegh, L. (1993). Effectiveness of a multimodal day treatment program for children with disruptive behavior problems. *Journal of the American Academy of Child and Adolescent Psychiatry, 32*, 127–134.

Grizenko, N., & Sayegh, L. (1990). Evaluation of the effectiveness of a psychodynamically oriented day treatment program for children with behaviour problems: A pilot study. *Canadian Journal of Psychiatry, 35*, 519–525.

Hambleton, K. (2001, June 10). *State takes giant steps in juvenile justice. Lincoln Journal-Star*, pp. C1–C2.

Kauffman, J.M. (1999). How we prevent the prevention of emotional and behavioral disorders. *Exceptional Children, 65*, 448–468.

Knitzer, J. (1982). *Unclaimed children: The failure of public responsibility to children and adolescents in need of mental health services.* Washington DC: Children's Defense Fund.

Knitzer, J., Steinberg, Z., & Fleisch, B. (1990). *At the schoolhouse door: An examination of programs and policies for children with behavioral and emotional problems.* New York: Bank Street College of Education.

Koyanagi, C., & Gaines, S. (1993). *All systems failure: An examination of the results of neglecting the needs of children with serious emotional disturbance.* Alexandria, VA: National Mental Health Association.

Kutash, K., & Rivera, V. R. (1995). Effectiveness of children's mental health services: A review of the literature. *Education and Treatment of Children, 18*, 443–477.

Maag, J. W. (1995). *Behavior management: Theoretical implications and practical applications.* Unpublished manuscript, University of Nebraska.

Nelson, C. M., & Pearson, C. A. (1991). *Integrating services for children and youth with emotional and behavioral disorders.* Reston, VA: Council for Exceptional Children.

Pelham, W. E., & Waschbusch, D. (1999). Behavior therapy with ADHD children. In H. Quay & A. Hogan (Eds.), *Handbook of disruptive behavior disorders* (pp. 255–278). New York: Plenum Press.

Satterfield, J. H., Satterfield, B. T., & Schell, A. M. (1987). Therapeutic interventions to prevent delinquency in hyperactive boys. *Journal of American Academy of Child and Adolescent Psychiatry, 26*, 56–64.

Sayegh, L., & Grizenko, N. (1991). Studies of the effectiveness of day treatment programs for children. *Canadian Journal of Psychiatry, 36*, 246–253.

Simpson, R. (1999). Children and youth with emotional and behavioral disorders: A concerned look at the present and a hopeful eye for the future. *Behavioral Disorders, 24*, 284–292.

Singh, N. N., Landrum, T. J., Donatelli, L. S., Hampton, C., & Ellis, C. R. (1994). Characteristics of children and adolescents with serious emotional disturbance in systems of care: Part I. Partial hospitalization and inpatient psychiatric services. *Journal of Emotional and Behavioral Disorders, 2,* 13–20.

Sprague, J., & Walker, H. (2000). Early identification and intervention for youth with antisocial and violent behavior. *Exceptional Children, 66,* 367–378.

Stroul, B. A., & Friedman, R. M. (1986). *A system of care for severely emotionally disturbed children and youth.* Washington, DC: Child Development Center, Georgetown University.

Sugai, G. (1996). Providing effective behavior support to all students: Procedures and processes. *SAIL, 11*(1), 1–4.

Topp, D. B., (1991). Beyond the continuum of care: Conceptualizing day treatment for children and youth. *Community Mental Health Journal, 27,* 105–113.

Tuma, J. M. (1991). Mental health services for children: The state of the art. *American Psychologist, 44,* 188–199.

Webber, J., Anderson, T., & Otey, L. (1991). Teachers' mindsets for surviving in BD classrooms. *Intervention in Schools and Clinics, 26,* 288–292.

Zimet, S. G., & Farley, M. D. (1985). Day treatment for children in the United States. *Journal of the American Academy of Child Psychiatry, 24*(6) 732–738.

CHAPTER 9

Gang-Oriented Interventions

DONALD W. KODLUBOY

The increase in gang activity on school campuses across the nation has produced a heightened level of awareness (Miller, 2001; Howell & Lynch, 2000; Esbensen, 2000; Goldstein & Kodluboy, 1998). Miller reports that gangs are present in a record-breaking 3,700 localities, including cities, towns, and counties. Yet analyses of gang-related activity in a school or school system are often avoided until the number of gang members reaches a significant portion of the student population.

Communitywide concern may swiftly rise to broad-based, public demands for action when the community is shocked by the occurrence of a major event involving students in or near a school building. The precipitant most likely to generate such demands for action is the shooting of a student on or near a school building (Prophet, 1990; Huff, 1990; Stephens, 1989). This chapter emphasizes practical methods of responding to the gang problem in and near schools.

SCHOOL-AGE STREET GANGS: BASIC ISSUES

Definitions

In any discussion of gang education, prevention, and intervention, the first task is to frame questions carefully and to define the essential terms of the issue. What is a gang? What is the prevalence of gang members and gang-related activity in or near school? What is the threat of this presence and activity to students' receiving and benefiting from an education? Finally, what is the threat of gang activity to the future of students currently in school? Educators first must determine who is at risk for or currently involved in gang activity and who are the potential victims of such activity. Basically, what is a gang, who is involved, what difference does it make to the school, and what can educators do about it?

Definitions of a "gang" range from broad to extremely narrow, as do definitions of "gang-related activity" (Esbensen, 2000; Spergel, 1990; Huff, 1990; Goldstein & Huff, 1993; Maxson & Klein, 1990; Klein & Maxson, 1989). The broadest definition is that a gang is a continuing group of two or more persons who identify themselves a gang by name and/or symbolism and who engage in antisocial behavior. Some more restrictive definitions also require recognition by community individuals or agencies, negative perception by the community, history of delinquent or criminal acts, and perhaps some hierarchy or vertical structure (Winfree, Fuller, Vigil, & Mays, 1992; Spergel, 1990; Huff, 1990). Youth gangs tend to evolve over time in response to community pressures, so their impact is also likely to change over time.

For school officials, a simple definition best serves the needs of students, parents, and educators. A street gang is a group of two or more youth who have a visible presence over time in a community, who have public unifying verbal and or visible symbols, who engage in a broad range of delinquent or criminal activity, and *who recognize and respond to intergroup rivalry* (Miller, 2001; Esbensen, 2000; Goldstein & Kodluboy, 1998). For example, a gang may display visible hand signs, wear specific colors, display specific tattoos, engage in multiple, differing criminal acts, respond aggressively to a like-minded but rival group, and who been present in the community for several months or longer.

A gang may be small and local, perhaps loosely affiliated with several similarly named groups across town. It may be part of a broad gang family across several cities or states and may be locally led or, far less often, subordinate to a hierarchical leader in another city or state. All forms of street gangs are possible in the public schools of both small and large cities across the nation. Single-issue gangs, such as white supremacists gangs who engage in a restricted range of delinquent or criminal activity, related to their ideology, although not street gangs, nonetheless present a significant threat to the school and community in which they appear (Goldstein & Kodluboy, 1998).

Plausible Deniability and Community Inertia

School systems, like city governments (Trump, 1998; Huff, 1990; Jankowski, 1991), are prone to ambivalence about or outright denial of gang presence or the significance of gang presence in the schools (Kodluboy & Evenrud, 1993; Gaustad, 1991). The problems presented by gang members are generally dealt with through application of individual disciplines according to district discipline policies, application of general dress codes, or private parent meetings. Were it not for the specific problems posed for school systems by gang presence, such an approach might be sustainable. However, the increasing gang presence in cities across the United States, the increasing width of the age range of gang affiliation, the increasing frequency and severity of violence among gang members, and the increasing public fear generated by gang-related activity all suggest that a more specific approach is advisable.

Miller (April 2001), writing for the Office of Juvenile Justice and Delinquency Prevention (OJJDP), reports that by "the late 1990s, 3,700 identified localities in the United States, about 2,550 cities towns and villages and 1,150 counties . . . reported the presence of gang problems" (p. ix). Overall, 60% of all cities reported gang presence. "A Gallup poll showed American parents are most worried about two problems in the schools: violence and gangs, and lack of discipline" (Koklaranis, 1994, p. A1).

Marian Wright Edelman of the Children's Defense Fund notes, "Never has America permitted children to rely on guns and gangs, rather than parents and neighbors, for protection and love" (quoted in Holstrom, 1994, p. 6).

John B. Reid, of the Oregon Social Learning Center, asserted, "Gangs are taking the place of parents" (quoted in Graves, 1994, p. A1). Graves (1994) further remarked that four major influences increase the probability that a student will commit an act of violence: drug and alcohol use, access to guns, association with a gang, and exposure to violence in the mass media.

Burnett and Walz (1994) state that gangs play a significant role in the steady increase in school violence. Gaustad (1991) noted that the presence of gangs in a school increases the likelihood of violence. Gang or drug disputes are the leading cause of gun violence in schools (Lane, 1991). Zagar, Arbit, Sylvies, and Busch (1990) and Busch, Zagar, Hughes, Arbit, and Bussell (1990) have demonstrated that the four strongest predictors of whether a youth will kill someone are intrafamilial violence, learning disability, drug or alcohol use, and gang membership.

Howell and Lynch (2000) identify a strong correlation "between the presence of gangs and both guns and drugs in school" (p.1). Students are more likely to report a gun in school, drugs in school, and victimization in schools with gangs than in schools without a gang presence.

A survey of 700 U.S. city school districts by the National League of Cities (1994) revealed a significant increase in school violence in nearly 40% of these districts. In addition, "Nearly forty percent said student or neighborhood gangs were a significant factor in school violence" (National League of Cities, 1994, p. 1). "Fifty-two percent of the midsize cities view gangs as a serious influence, and 72% of the largest cities say they are part of the problem" (National League of Cities, 1994, p. 7). Thirty-nine percent of 700 city school districts reported gang activity as a factor of concern. Increasingly, districts across the nation have developed or work closely with school police units of five or more officers, who engage in intervention and prevention activities or who primarily conduct investigations of gangs in the school system.

Gang activity is common in most large urban school districts. Howell and Lynch (2000) report, "The incidence of gangs in schools nearly doubled from 1989 to 1995" (p. 1). Spergel et al. (1994, p. 1) stated that currently "the

United States has some 1,439 gangs and 120,636 gang members." Klein (1995) reported that the gang situation is worsening and gangs have become more violent across the United States.

Gang-Related, Gang-Involved, Gang-Independent

"Gang-related activity" is sometimes broadly defined as any antisocial behavior committed by or among gang members, and sometimes more restrictively defined as antisocial behavior occurring as a discernible function of gang membership or for a discernible benefit to the gang itself. The former, broad definition is sometimes referred to as the "Los Angeles definition," whereas the latter, narrow definition is referred to as the "Chicago definition" (Maxson & Klein, 1990).

School officials should use both definitions, as appropriate to the event being described, for careful recording of data over time about incidents involving gang members. The rationale for this dual tactic is that:

1. All instances of delinquent behavior involving gang members can be captured, and
2. Careful and prescriptive allocation of resources to benefit individual students and the school as a whole can be made.

Example one: If for instance, multiple incidents of violence involve a single gang member, but do not involve other or rival gang members, then individual school and community-based individual or family intervention may be necessary, with perhaps some intervention by the school police liaison or school resource officer. This example is one of gang-involved but probably not gang-related activity.

Example two: If incidents of school violence involve several gang members or occur between rival gang members, continue in the community before or after school, appear to have damaging effects on other members of the school community, and appear to have a specific gang function or benefit to one or both gangs, then greater and gang-specific intervention will likely be necessary. This example is one of probable gang-related motivation, rather than simple gang member involvement. Careful monitoring of confirmed or suspected gang-involved students over time, to identify further similar or related incidents, will determine whether a "look-back" review over time is necessary and whether reclassifying an incident is advised.

How Big Must This Problem Be before I Worry?

Gangs in school may be small, that is, 2–12 members, or large, that is, greater than 12 members. A gang may exist in only one school or across schools in a city. Some gangs are indeed nationwide, across many cities and states, maintaining close or loose affiliations with "branch" members. For example, some gangs may exist primarily in a given neighborhood, extend across an entire metropolitan region, or, in the case of the "supergangs" of the Midwest and West Coast, extend across state lines, with membership numbering in the thousands.

Large gangs, such as the Crips and Bloods of the West Coast or the Gangster Disciples of the Midwest, have both a relatively well-defined hierarchical structure of adult leadership and a number of less cohesive, adult-dominated and/or primarily youth-composed subsets across many states and regions of the nation. Both extremes may exist within a single gang and within a given city.

Street Gangs

Youth gangs are primarily ethnic gangs, are relatively homogeneous, and are made up mostly of marginal youths within a population already defined by the greater society as marginal (Fagan, 1989). The reader is cautioned not to assume a necessary relationship between ethnicity and gang membership. Ethnic gangs form as a response to multiple marginality variables of racism, economic stresses, community disorganization, and others; "social conditions, not genes create gangs" (Goldstein & Kodluboy, 1998, p. 73). Nation-wide, 48% of gang members are African American, 43% are Hispanic–Latino, 5% are Caucasian, 4% are Asian. These figures represent averages from various surveys and include multiethnic gangs (Goldstein & Kodluboy, 1998). The ethnic makeup of gangs in a community generally reflects the overall ethnic composition of the community. Increasingly, gangs are expanding their membership across ethnic groups. Persons from other ethnic groups are included as social, economic, or other stresses may dictate. Indeed, in some Midwestern locales, formerly all-African-American gangs now have all-European-American subsets or "sound alike" white gangs with the same name as African American gangs.

Many marginal youths who have no discernible association with adult gang members, or even with other gang-involved youths, may nonetheless profess a strong and pervasive personal affiliation with an established gang. Others may demonstrate little visible or professed gang affiliation in school, whereas their life outside school is occupied with significant gang-related criminal activity. Gang-affiliated youths may "gang bang" (i.e., engage in gang-related criminal activities) in or near school or only away from their school or neighborhood.

It is important to note that although gang affiliation or identification is always a risk factor, gang membership is not necessarily a permanent affiliation or lifetime condition for most school-age youths. Most gang members leave the gang after their first year of affiliation (Howell & Lynch, 2000). There is no rigid, archetypal pattern of gang affiliation or leaving the gang that can describe each individual student. Few studies of leaving the gang have been published (Decker & Van Winkle, 1996), but enough information is available to caution school staff to avoid inadvertently reinforcing the commonly held belief that the only way out of a gang is to die or go to prison.

Which of My Students Is a Gang Member or Affiliate?

When it is known that gangs are present in the community, how is an educator to know who is involved? Self-reporting is an important indicator of either actual gang affiliation or a student's self-perception. That is, students may indicate gang membership either because they are actually affiliated with a gang or because gang membership is perceived to give them status or protection in the community.

Students generally join gangs for the same reasons any adolescents affiliate with any group. The most common reasons for joining a gang are to have friends, access to girlfriends, social opportunities, economic opportunities, and protection (Fagan, 1989). Students sometimes simply walk away from the gang, sometimes are "beaten out" of the gang, and sometimes simply "age out" or mature and spend less and less time with the gang. Many do indeed die or go to prison before they decide to, or are able to, leave the gang alive and intact.

Determining who is a gang member requires some care, as well as some basic gang education, for administrators. Students generally join a gang between the ages of 10 and 13. This may occur through simple affiliation or hanging out with other gang members; through casual encounters with gang members (e.g., at a party or at school); or, less often, through being actively recruited or even being "walked in " or "blessed in" (i. e., publicly accepted into the gang) by older gang members (Fagan, 1989).

Students who are alleged or who declare themselves to be gang members may be members in name only; loosely associated fringe or marginal members, also referred to colloquially as "wannabes"; core or hard-core members; or former members who retain some limited social affiliation with active gang members. Students may form a brief but intense gang identification (accompanied by frequent or serious delinquent acts) before maturing, leaving the gang behind, and moving on to more socially appropriate endeavors. Others may move in and out of gang life, always remaining at the fringe and rarely engaging in the more serious violent or other criminal acts of the gang. Still others may move in and out of gang affiliation, switching gang affiliation as frequently as more conventional youths change their conventional peer associations. Some youths join a gang at an early age, commit increasingly serious offenses, and remain in a continuing criminal association with the gang well into their adult years. The age of leaving a gang is increasing, as gangs are becoming a permanent (albeit nonlegitimate) subculture within urban and, with growing frequency, suburban areas. Gang members are increasingly choosing to remain active in both social and criminal gang activities later in life (Spergel, 1990).

Risk Assessment by Degree

In the school setting the degree of gang involvement may be assessed by determining the amount of time a student is interacting with gang members, both in school and in the community, and the severity and/or risk of *both* the gang-related and gang-involved activities in which the student engages in school and in the community. Such a risk assessment is best performed by trusted and knowledgeable staff who have access to both school and community information.

A school social worker, counselor or psychologist may be best trained to conduct such an assessment. In some districts, such as those with close relationships with local law enforcement, a school liaison or school resource officer is also able to conduct or support such an assessment. The function of this assessment is to provide prevention and intervention resources to the student, school staff, and family, to prevent further gang activity by the student, and to reduce harm to the student and to the student body at large. It is not the function of such an assessment to support justification for moving the student to another school unless there is an extreme risk of injury to the student.

Initial Response

Recently, communities have become concerned about overidentification of youth as gang members. For this reason, several states have prepared restrictive definitions of gang membership. For example, in Minnesota, a 10-point criterion list has been developed. For individuals to be identified as gang members, they must display at least 3 of the 10 listed criteria:

- Being arrested with other gang members
- Displaying gang tattoos
- Admitting gang membership
- Wearing gang-specific symbols
- Being in photos with gang members displaying gang symbols
- Frequently associating with known gang members
- Having name on a gang document such as a roster
- Being identified by a reliable source
- Corresponding with gang members and writing or receiving correspondence about gang activity
- Writing gang graffiti on walls, paper

For school officials, such a criterion list is helpful and advisory, but not compelling. A more flexible standard of identification is acceptable, provided that the purpose is to provide or prescribe support to the student and family. In either instance, keeping identifications private and not accessible to the other students is critical to prevent further marginalization of the student, if not violence directed toward the student.

In addition, lists of danger signs or indicators of gang affiliation, useful for determining the status of a given student, are available in the literature (Stephens, 1991; National School Safety Center [NSSC], 1988, 1991). It is important to note, however, that students who exhibit such warning signs may or may not actually be gang-involved. Some students affect gang attire and behavior simply for status, others do so for the vicarious excitement of identifying with the "thug life," and yet others do so for the assumed protective factor of belonging to a powerful or intimidating group. With the increasing significance of media images in the lives of students, "gangster chic" dress, language, music, and aspirations are increasingly common among U.S. adolescents in general (Kodluboy, 1994, 1996).

Students who are not gang members but who affect gang affiliation, must nonetheless be cautioned that to display gang affiliation, (1) marginalizes the student, (2) increases the risk of violence against the student by real gang members, (3) increases the risk of violence toward the school resulting from the student's ersatz display of gang affiliation, and (4) decreases the likelihood of supportive responses from adults and youth who encounter the student in the community and in school.

Self-Identifying Gang Membership

Although the general lists of indicators are important and useful for school staffs, Winfree et al. (1992) note that self-definition by reputed gang affiliates approximates the probability of antisocial behavior more closely than does a more restrictive definition. The authors propose that self-defined gang members may be more motivated to prove their status through antisocial activity than gang members defined as such by others. Fagan (1989) also notes that self-reports by gang members most closely reflect the reality of gang membership and activity.

For school officials, the path to accurate determination of gang membership varies with their locales. For cities with long-standing and well-established gangs, the determination problem is simple. For cities with an emerging gang problem, it is more perplexing. The risk of defining students as members of gangs that do not exist or are relatively insignificant is real, as is the risk of a premature and disproportionate community response. Conversely, denying gang membership is no guarantee of lack of affiliation. Careful observation over time and developing a trusting relationship with the student will be necessary to determine the reasons for the original suspicion of gang affiliation. For example, it is common for a youth to be peer identified, however inaccurately, as a gang member only because the youth has a sibling or cousin who is a known and admitted gang member.

TYPOLOGY OF GANGS

No single, archetypal gang can be described with any reliability. School personnel may be required to contend with gangs that are primarily protective, social, fighting, or entrepreneurial in nature. In a large enough school or district, each type of gang may be encountered. As noted earlier, a gang usually draws its members from a single ethnic group (i.e., it is primarily Asian, African American, Hispanic, or white); somewhat less commonly, a gang may be multiethnic. As also noted earlier, in cities where gangs are well established, older students who are gang-involved may have certain ties to adult gang members or leaders. However, in cities where gangs are a relatively new phenomenon, there may be little adult connection. In communities where gangs have been historically absent (e.g., communities of recent immigrants from Southeast Asia), gangs have only recently evolved, and connections with adult gang leaders are less common. Such gangs are only now maturing into their own unique structures. In planning gang prevention, and especially gang violence prevention strategies, school officials must take into account the range of identities encountered when the specter of youth gang violence is present. Failing to distinguish among different types of gangs, their current status in the community, their stage of evolution, and their function for the students who are involved may result in either a significant over- or underreaction to the problems gangs present.

Although most communities generally deny the existence of a gang problem until gangs are well established (Spergel, 1990; Jankowski, 1991; Huff, 1990), other communities inadvertently assign an identity to emerging gangs that is disproportionate to their actual impact. This may occur when the local media, social activists, politicians, and private or public agencies inadvertently inflate and romanticize the gangs' significance to marginal youths. Such youths are frequently vulnerable to the perceptions of an emerging gang's strength and influence in a community (Jankowski, 1991).

Proportional Response

School officials must take great care neither to overreact nor to underreact to the very real threat of gang-related activity in school; one approach may exacerbate and the other may neglect the problem (Kodluboy & Evenrud, 1993; Goldstein, Glick, Carthan, & Blancero, 1994). Although there is no research to suggest that gangs can be defined into or out of existence, it appears quite possible to push marginally affiliated youths closer to the gang core than might occur if a proportionate response is developed to a gang presence in a community. Administrators must focus on gathering and carefully reviewing information from multiple sources to determine the existence of new or known gangs, as well as their presumed numbers, leaders (if any), criminal history or intent, motivation for moving into the community, impact in other communities (if relevant), and probability of impact in the school.

The rise of crack cocaine use and its spread across the United States which overran the late 1980s and 1990s, brought entrepreneurial gangs, also called "business" or "instrumental" gangs, to the forefront of our knowledge about gangs. Such gangs spread across the nation from coast to coast, even infiltrating small Midwestern towns that had never before encountered the phenomenon of gang activity. The supergangs of the West and Midwest found a niche in smaller and more distant cities, especially those with large airports or on interstate highways. Some of these gangs were engaged in direct recruitment of school-age youths to serve as drug runners, lookouts, or full-fledged members. Although the growth in this activity has leveled off and perhaps declined somewhat, some students continue to engage in drug selling as a function of or as a side activity to their primary gang involvement. Students who join business gangs do so primarily for protection, illicit recreation, and monetary gain.

It is important for school personnel to bear in mind that although most gang affiliation begins through normal social contacts outside school, active gang recruitment also occurs in and near schools (Spergel, 1990). It is common for gang members present in a school to challenge new students with the question "Who do you claim?" or "Where are you from?" meaning "With which gang are you affiliated?" Such interactions are "red flag" indicators, calling for further investigation by trained staff members.

INTERVIEWING PRESUMED GANG MEMBERS AND THEIR FAMILIES

Individual students who are reported to be gang members, or who give visible indications of gang affiliation through associating with known gang members or through displaying gang attire, language, or behavior, should be approached individually—preferably in private—for an interview to determine the degree of affiliation, if any. The purpose of the interview is to (1) determine the significance of the student's gang affiliation for the school setting, (2) assess the need for referral for further assessment or intervention, as appropriate, and (3) begin an immediate and ongoing threat assessment for the student, any potential rivals, and the school as a whole.

Limits of Confidentiality

Before beginning the interview, the staff member should secure a private location, or in an emergent situation, at least one out of sight and sound of other staff members, students, or parents. The interviewer should give the reason for the interview and state the limits of confidentiality that can be kept by the staff member. It is important never to say, "This is off the record," "This is just between you and me," or anything similar unless this is truly the case. Generally, it is necessary to inform the student being interviewed that the interviewer must break confidentiality if (1) the student threatens some other person in a specific and credible manner, (2) the student indicates impending harm to self or others, (3) the student reveals physical or sexual abuse, or (4) the student identifies a credible, emergent, and urgent threat to his or her own safety, other students, or the school environment. If there is any uncertainty or controversy between staff members regarding confidentiality, consult with the school district attorney or data privacy specialist to discuss mandatory reporting issues applicable to the situation.

During some interviews, before the student is given the "limits of confidentiality" warning, the student may blurt out some threat or past action that the staff member is legally bound to report or otherwise respond to. When this is necessary, it is sometimes possible to convince the student that it is necessary to break the confidence and to achieve the student's consent to do so. It is always preferable to obtain a student agreement to break a confidence, even though such consent is not legally necessary when mandatory reporting is compelled. Vigorous, competent, and sensitive attempts to gain the student's consent are strongly encouraged. These attempts maintain credibility with the student and the student's peers. If a staff member becomes known as one who routinely, without warning or without apparent reason, seeks and then disclose what students perceive as confidential, effective gang intervention and prevention will become difficult if not impossible. Nonetheless, when mandatory reporting is required, staff must sacrifice relationships with students to respect the law and prevent harm.

Whom Do They Trust?

If a staff member becomes known as one who is knowledgeable about gangs, knowledgeable about the student's culture, otherwise trustworthy, fair across the board to all sides of a dispute, consistent, tough but always available to encourage and reward prosocial behavior, students will beat a path to the door of that staff member. It is not uncommon for students to seek out such a staff member before an incident occurs, so that the staff member can intervene early and prevent problems. When students see staff members who are always appropriately encouraging, willing to help whenever needed, never take sides in a dispute, and apply the rules consistently to all parties, trust will follow, and information will flow allowing timely prevention and intervention.

The Interview

The interviewer may wish to begin the interview by not saying anything specific about gangs, but rather by simply asking the student about observed behavior and academic problems, the significance of the student's changes in clothing, jewelry, graffiti-marked assignments or folders, or the like. The response of students is generally determined by their presumption of the interviewer's knowledge of local gangs. The rule of thumb is that the more an interviewer is presumed to know about gangs, the more students will tell him or her. If the student accurately discloses some gang affiliation, the interviewer can move on to gathering specific details of involvement. If the student minimizes or denies gang affiliation, the interviewer should describe his or her concerns (revealing some knowledge of gang representing practices in the process) and then again ask the questions about gang affiliation. Most gang-involved students freely discuss their involvement if they know that the interviewer has at least a basic knowledge about gangs.

In questioning a student, the interviewer must always remember to say, "I am not accusing you of being a gang member, but can you tell me the significance of . . . ?" Only after the basic facts of the presumed gang affiliation have been discussed, and the student has been informed of the interviewer's concerns, should the interviewer ask whether the student is actually involved with a gang. If the student professes some gang involvement, the interviewer should next determine the amount of time the student spends with other gang affiliates and the activities in which they engage. The gang-involved student should be informed that it may be necessary to contact his or her parents to ensure everyone's safety. Ideally, the decision to do so should involve the student. For suspected, but not confirmed, gang involvement, parent contact may be delayed only if the risk is perceived to be very low or absent. When gang involvement or gang-related behavior is of greater concern or impact, informing the parents in a timely manner is necessary. The best way to approach parents is with open-ended questions, described in a following section on home visits. The student should also be informed of school policy (which is generally zero tolerance for gang activity), offered any assistance needed for academic or social success in school, and assured of support for any and all appropriate behavior in school. Students generally are relatively truthful about gang affiliation, sometimes reeling out the "full story" over time, withholding facts as their personal self-interest requires.

Identifying Gang Members

It is necessary for school staff members to encourage, praise, and otherwise recognize any and all appropriate academic and social behavior of gang-involved students. The effort should focus on developing the non-gang-related aspects of a student's social repertoire and facilitating expression of those conventional values that are held by all but the most extreme gang members (Fagan, 1989). Whatever the level of students' gang involvement may be, most retain some conventional values, commonly including respect for school, work, and family. It is at this interface of shared values that school-based gang intervention with individual students must occur (Kodluboy & Evenrud, 1993; Kodluboy, 1994; Goldstein & Kodluboy, 1998).

With the rare exception of gang members coming to school purely for criminal purposes or purely to recruit new gang members, gang-involved students who come to school probably remain amenable to some form of intervention, as evidenced by the fact that they still come to school.

Educators in cities with an emerging gang problem often assume that gang membership is largely tangential to school concerns. Educators in cities with well-defined gang problems—especially those who have experienced significant gang impact on student attendance, safety, and mobility, as well as makeup of the student body—tend to take a far more decisive approach to gang prevention, intervention, and response.

The Home Visit

It is sometimes necessary and advisable to make a visit to speak with a gang-involved student's parent or guardian in the home setting. Each school district should have a policy regarding (1) who should and can make home visits, (2) under what circumstances home visits should be made—that is, when a parent or guardian cannot be contacted during the day and yet interaction is critical, or when it is desirable to speak with a parent in a comfortable, nonthreatening setting, (3) basic safety protocols for staff to follow, and (4) reasons and anticipated outcomes for a home visit. In many jurisdictions, teachers routinely and safely make home visits on a regular basis. In other jurisdictions, because of the physical risk present in some neighborhoods, making home visits is limited to daylight hours, requires the presence of two persons, and allows for an individual staff member's judgment as to whether to leave his or her vehicle to enter a dwelling if any threat is perceived. In some jurisdictions, home visits may be prohibited because of local dangers or limited during some specific time period because of community upset and a temporary increased risk of violence. In many jurisdictions, community crime prevention officers or community liaison officers accompany school staff members. Visiting staff members may be provided with cell phones, school district two-way radios, and, sometimes, school security staff to accompany them. Whatever the case in a given district, district policy should be closely followed.

Practical Matters Often Not Taught in College Education Courses

If school district policy encourages home visits and if staff members determine a need to make such a visit, some practical advice is appropriate. If a potential threat is perceived before the visit but staff members persist in making such a visit, consider asking the school resource officer or police liaison to accompany them on the visit or to conduct the visit themselves. In some jurisdictions, community crime prevention officers or community liaison officers accompany school staff members.

Travel Considerations

Before driving to a student's home, you may wish to speak with your school resource officer or school liaison officer, or you may wish to call the local police precinct or district office to ascertain any community unrest or risk at the address being visited. They will be happy to assist you.

While driving to the dwelling, observe unusual or suspicious "street scenes," such as aggregations of persons who look at you with sustained stares or who make intimidating gestures or movements. If a neighborhood is known to be a center of street-level drug dealing, be cautious to not drive down a blocked street unless an escape route is apparent. In heavy traffic, always remain at a distance behind the car in front of you so that you can clearly see the vehicle's rear tires where they touch the ground. This allows you to easily drive around the vehicle if necessary and if you cannot back your car to safety. Always keep doors locked. Avoid alleys unless you are certain they are safe. You may wish to park directly in front of the dwelling if you feel unsafe walking any distance. Conversely, if you have a greater fear of later vandalism to your car by the student being visited, and if it is safe to do so, you may wish to park down the block and walk.

The Dwelling

Gated yards should always be visually scanned for (1) signs of ill-tempered dogs, (2) areas where persons of ill-intent might secret themselves to the surprise of a visitor, (3) conspicuous gatherings of apparent gang members or other wayward persons, (4) any hostile words or gestures of persons in the immediate vicinity. If a threat is perceived, it is strongly encouraged that staff calmly, but with authority, leave the area immediately. When driving to a dwelling, drive around the block to assess potential threat. Avoid driving in an alley unless absolutely necessary. In many situations, driving in an alley only increases risk to the visiting staff and presents difficult or limited opportunities to quickly depart the setting if a threat becomes apparent. Open the car window and listen for sounds that may indicate threat. When in doubt, do not leave your car, rather, leave the area, return to the school, and meet with your school police officer to reconsider the home visit.

Upon exiting your vehicle and then approaching a dwelling on foot, display a school-issued photo identification badge in a conspicuous manner. If you do not have such a photo identification badge, get one before making home visits. Carry a legal pad holder or similar device to demonstrate that you are there for official business. When you encounter persons outside the dwelling or in the hallways of an apartment building, cordially greet them and ascertain the degree of threat if any. Appear confident, walk with ease and authority, and exude whatever presence you can muster. Feel free to identify yourself when asking for information, for example, say, "Good morning . . . I'm Dr. Don from the school. Is Ms. Watkins's apartment on this floor?" or, if looking for a truant student and encountering several agemates of the student, "Hi, guys, I'm Dr. Don from the school . . . is Jason around to-day? He is not in trouble . . . I'm worried about him and I just want to make sure he is OK."

Although staff members are rarely at any real threat when making home visits for gang-related reasons, it is always necessary to take these simple precautions to increase safety, decrease risk, and increase the likelihood of a successful visit. Before knocking on the door of a house or apartment, or entering the dwelling itself, look for any signs of gang activity, such as gang graffiti, bullet holes, or similar indications of gang presence. Identify yourself verbally and keep your ID badge clearly visible. Students and sometimes parents will not open the door if they think you are somebody other than a school official, such as a probation officer or a police investigator. If you are greatly concerned, but persist in entering a hallway or dwelling, step to one side as you knock on the door and have your ID badge clearly visible for persons within to see the badge through a peephole or a crack in the door as it is opened. If you become fearful at any time, leave the area immediately.

Experienced home visitors will have a briefcase, notebook, or umbrella in hand in case an unfriendly dog should greet them. The function of the object is to offer a chewable alternative to one's arm or leg, allowing time for the dog owner to restrain the animal. If a dangerous dog is known to be on the scene, many wise visitors will call the family ahead and ask to have the dog restrained before the visit. For an unannounced visit, calling out to family members to restrain their dog before opening the door is strongly advised. For visitors wisely fearful of dogs, rescheduling the visit for another time or at a dog-free location is advisable

House Rules

Upon entry, honor any apparent house rules—the family is not in your "house"; rather, you are in theirs. For example, if the persons present in the home are wearing shoes, you may enter wearing shoes. If you notice that all persons in the home are shoeless, as is common in the homes of most Southeast Asian families, remove your shoes upon entering. If offered refreshments, accept them; take time to speak casually before getting to the point of the visit; allay any apparent fears of the family before speaking about gang issues, and let the parent(s) know that you are there to seek their advice and support in collaborating on solving a problem evidenced by their child. Greet all persons in the dwelling respectfully and with deference, especially elders. This is their home and you are a guest. Do not sit until invited to do so.

Begin by saying, "Thank you for letting me come visit today. We have some concerns about Tyrone's behavior at school . . . are you noticing anything similar at home or in the community?" "I have no reason to believe that Tou is a gang member, but we have noticed that he is doing some things that gang members do . . . do you have any concerns about such behavior?" "Josh is a great kid, but he has been hanging out with some troubling students as school . . . have you noticed any change in his behavior?" Such inquiries generally open the door to a discussion.

If the parents agree that there is some gang activity, be prepared to collaborate on a school–home plan for enhancing and monitoring academic and social behavior. In addition, have a ready list of phone numbers for community agencies that may assist the family, and bring along a release-of-information form so that the school can interact with those community agencies. Always ask whether there is any current involvement with the courts or a mental health or other community agency to expedite communication and program planning. Always ask, "How can I help you?" and "What advice do you have for us?" Listen respectfully.

I have visited homes to encounter deeply concerned and helpful parents, hardworking but overwhelmed families, and both single- and two-parent families who teach by example and uphold high social values that have somehow escaped their children. Conversely, I have also visited homes occupied by numerous pit bull dogs, battered gang members fresh from their latest confrontations, and intoxicated students and parents. At times parents have insisted on going to their son's room to rouse him because he was sleeping on a mattress under which their guns were stashed. I have met with distraught parents who expect, and sometimes ask, school staff to take their children to jail. Expect the best of the visit, but be prepared for significant functional and sometimes safety challenges.

Upon entry into the home, remain in the living room, dining room, or kitchen of the house. Do not enter a student's room unless with the parent. Avoid the basement, attic, and garage unless accompanied by law enforcement personnel. Remember how you got into a room, house, or apartment, and be mentally prepared to leave the same way as expeditiously as necessary. Generally a staff member should not enter a home if there is no responsible adult present, even if the staff member knows the minor children who are present. Male staff members should avoid entering a home if only a female adult is present. Female staff members should ascertain the risk of entering a home with only adult males present and should politely reschedule the visit for a time when a two-person team can perform it. These issues are rarely spoken of, but are almost always on the minds of staff members who make home visits. Follow district policy. If policy does not address such issues, ask supervisors for advice and guidance before making a home visit. If you have a reasonable fear of violence, do not make the visit. Reschedule the meeting at school or ask a police liaison officer to make the visit.

Going to Court

On occasion, a staff member may receive a subpoena or a request from a parent to attend a court proceeding involving his or her gang-involved child. Each district should have a policy regarding timely and appropriate response to a subpoena or court order, and the policy must be available to members of the staff who request such information. When attending court as directed by a subpoena, court order, or parental request, all aspects of data privacy laws and confidentiality rules must be followed. Staff members should request advice from the district counsel as to what can or must be said and what information requires a direct order from the court before they can respond.

Having considered these issues and requirements, upon reporting either verbally or in writing to the court or to officers of the court, the staff member must be careful to (1) describe the behavior of the student objectively and with specific examples, (2) avoid psychologizing and generalizing, (3) stay within direct observations, (4) avoid unwarranted assumptions, and (5) be cautious of predicting future behavior beyond reasonable extrapolations from existing data. The courtroom is not the place to make points that are not supported by instances of fact. When opinions are requested, such opinions should reflect best practice and common practice of one's profession. School psychologists, for example, are expected to give somewhat different comments and opinions than are teachers; the converse is true as well.

If asked for an opinion regarding disposition of a case for gang-involved students, especially when the behavior resulting in the court referral is related to gang membership, relationships, and activities, it may be appropriate to ask the court for increased court supervision of the student, preferably for the entire school year. It is also often wise to ask for court support for the parent in encouraging, if not mandating, the student to participate in some after-school, supervised prosocial activity, social skills instruction, or mental health treatment, as appropriate.

SIGNIFICANCE OF GANG MEMBERSHIP FOR SCHOOLS

The primary significance of gang membership for schools is that gang members represent a significant subgroup of students who are more likely to be at risk and to present risk to other students than the general adolescent population (Cromwell, Taylor, & Palacios, 1992; Esbensen, 2000; Felgar, 1992; Goldstein & Kodluboy, 1998; Howell & Lynch, 2000; Huff, 1990; Resnick & Blum, 1994; Spergel, 1990). Spergel et al. (1994, p. 1) report that "75% of youth gang members had prior police records" and that youth gang membership is "associated with significantly higher levels of delinquency and index crimes. The rate of violent offenses for gang members is three times as high as for non gang delinquents."

Gang members are likely to be poor students; are more likely to engage in more high-risk behaviors affecting health and safety than non-gang-involved adolescents; tend to be more like institutionalized adolescents than like typical adolescents; are likely to have poorer academic performance, poorer attendance, and a greater history of delinquency than their peers in general; are more likely to be in alternative educational placements than peers; are more likely to remain gang-affiliated later in life than gang members of the past were; are likely to have an early onset of delinquency with serious criminal involvement; and are likely to affiliate with other like-minded youths who are engaged in gang pursuits (Spergel, 1990; Huff, 1990; Cromwell et al., 1992; Resnick & Blum, 1994; Hagedorn, 1988; Fagan, 1990; Klein, 1995).

Gang members, as marginal members of already marginalized populations (Fagan, 1989), have been well conceptualized as "defiant individualists" who receive support for deviant behavior from the gang structure, but who accept only limited control from that structure (Jankowski, 1991). Indeed, the view of many gang members as risk takers appears to have some legitimacy. Resnick and Blum (1994) studied adolescent health risk and behavioral correlates. The index group of the study consisted of adolescents who had engaged in nonabusive sexual intercourse at or before age 10 years, as contrasted with those who abstained until after 16 years of age. The index youths (primarily males) were more likely than controls to indicate gang involvement, including both personally participating in gangs and having friends in gangs. Such youths, accounting for 3.4% of a school population, were also more likely to have lower academic performance, to engage in unprotected sex at adolescence, to be involved in unplanned pregnancies, and to display suicidal intent or action.

The core concern within the risk portrait of gang membership is a fear of gang-related violence in or near a school. The scope of violence affecting the nation's schools is indeed daunting, with gang violence contributing to the problem. According to the National School Boards Association, gang-related violence is among the "top five types of violent incidents reported in schools during 1993" (Sautter, 1993, p. 156). A 1993 Harris Poll of students in grades 6–12 found "widespread fear of violence at school" (Lantieri, 1995). Lantieri states that more than 400,000 violent crimes are reported at or near a school each year. Sautter (1993) reports that more than 3,000,000 crimes are committed each year in the 85,000 schools of the United States. Extrapolating from a 1991 U.S. Department of Justice study, Sautter projects that violent crimes in school settings affect 430,000 student victims in a school year. The 1991 study used by Sautter also found that 13% of public high school seniors had been threatened with a weapon.

The degree of violence experienced by many of the nation's youths is numbing. During a 4-year period, a single high school in New York City recorded 70 students "killed, shot, stabbed or permanently injured on the school grounds" (Morrow, 1992, p. 23). Half of the 1,900 students in Thomas Jefferson High have "some kind of puncture wound on their body at any given time" (Morrow, 1992, p. 23).

Neighborhood gang disputes over some real or imagined slight, drug sales, or territory often move to or near the schoolyard. On a sunny, warm March day in 1994, I personally witnessed and participated in the emergency management of such an event. Forty children attending an urban school were pinned to the ground as a gang dispute erupted into gunfire adjacent to the playground. Two teenage gang members mistook several approaching youths for gang rivals only because of the color of the clothing they were wearing. One teen fired six .44 magnum rounds at the purported rivals while frightened students lay in the sand.

In 1993 a gang dispute took place across the street from Sullivan High School in Chicago. Shots were fired, killing a 15-year-old freshman (Sautter, 1993). In 1987, another gang dispute resulted in the murder of a student on a Portland, Oregon, high school campus (Prophet, 1990). Felgar (1992) reports several gang shootings on or near campuses, including a 1983 shooting in Compton, California, where gang members opened fire and killed five students. Such incidents are tragic and deeply disturbing for staff, students, and community residents; unfortunately, they are occurring more often as the prevalence of gangs in schools and communities and the degree of social disorganization in U.S. neighborhoods increase.

Gang violence is more commonly seen near the school campus than in the school itself. Spergel (1990; Spergel et al., 1994) notes that gang activity involving students increases as the distance from the school door becomes greater. In gang-infested neighborhoods, merely getting to or from school can be a challenge to both gang-involved and non-gang-involved students. As a result, students sometimes carry weapons for protection from gang violence, among other reasons, even if they are not gang members (Gaustad, 1991; Felgar, 1992).

The role of the school as a locus of interaction where gang members meet and where new relationships are formed is significant. Curry and Spergel (1992, p. 288) note that for African American students, gang involvement and delinquency are "found to be associated with the presence of gang members in classroom and home." The authors also note the failure or inability of schools to comprehensively meet the needs of Hispanic students and cite this as one factor contributing to the "growth of delinquent youth gangs as social alternatives to traditionally legitimized forms of social organization" (p. 289). Spergel (1990) notes that gang members are found in disproportionate numbers in alternative educational sites and programs for students with special needs; they account for 20% of such students.

Gang members commonly state that in some neighborhoods, "if you didn't go to school with your hat cocked a certain way . . . you didn't get in and out of the building without being robbed or jumped" (Robson, 1990, p. 69). Spergel et al. (1994) note that although extremes of gang violence do not generally occur in schools, "gang recruitment and especially planning of gang activities may occur on school grounds and may be carried out after school is dismissed" (p. 4). Goldstein (1994) notes that school gun violence arises from gang or drug disputes 18% of the time.

Bastian and Taylor (1995) report a supplement to the National Crime Victimization Survey that reveals some of the unique problems presented to schools by gang activity. Schools where gangs are reported by students as present or possibly present are more likely than schools with no reported gang presence to have:

- Students who come from homes with incomes of less than $30,000
- More students of color to serve
- More students reporting victimization
- An urban rather than nonurban location
- Students reporting being afraid of attack both at school and on the way to or from school
- Students reporting that they avoid private areas of the school and campus (e.g., restrooms) more than public areas
- Students reporting greater ease in obtaining drugs

Thornberry, Krohn, Lizotte, and Chard-Wierschem (1993) note that the onset of delinquency committed by individual gang members is concurrent with the onset of gang membership. Subsequently leaving the gang shows a corresponding decrease in individual acts of delinquency. Lyon, Henggler, and Hall (1992), in an examination of institutionalized male offenders, found greater delinquency, greater aggression, and less social maturity among gang members than among nonmembers.

It is apparent that gang-related violence has multiple implications for school staff members and students. When threatening behavior or violent action has occurred on or near campus or along student travel routes to and from school, the district should, in documenting the disruption, determine whether the event was gang-related. Specifically, the school administration should document the activity itself, the names of participants, apparent gang contribution to the event, and the impact on staff, students, families, and the community. This will enable the administrators to determine access points for intervention and to anticipate any further violent disruption as a function of the index event.

PREVENTION AND INTERVENTION

Basic Issues

A basic premise for school systems in responding to gang-related issues is that no amount of intervention (i.e., practices put into effect after gang-related behavior has been observed) can substitute for prevention. Unfortunately, both prevention and intervention activities are often poorly researched and rarely evaluated. Klein (1995), reviewing the prevention and suppression literature, notes that few programs have been shown to be effective and that some may even be harmful. Esbensen (2000) and Miller (2001) review current explanations for the growth in gangs, citing risk factors such as (1) the presumed lucrative drug trade, (2) immigration pressures, (3) public awareness of common gang names and activities through the media, (4) internal migration of gang members, (5) government policies that inadvertently maintained and increased the legitimacy of social practices that engender gang activity, (6) increase in the number of female-headed households, which allowed gangs to assume the role of the missing male in a household, and (7) the overwhelming presence of gang subculture and images presented in a positive light in the media.

This last variable, that is, the role of the media in youth violence in general, is well validated despite the repeated denials of the industry. Bushman and Anderson (2001) clearly demonstrate that there is a strong positive causal, not merely correlational, relationship between media violence and aggression in youth.

Staff members are cautioned to pay careful attention to the music that is commonly allowed at school parties and dances, the video games that youth commonly use on school computers, and the dress of students. Staff may be adventitiously reinforcing gang- and other violence-related student behaviors by allowing the display and enjoyment of these items under the schoolhouse roof.

Esbensen (2000) divides prevention efforts into primary, focusing on the entire at-risk population; secondary, focusing on greatest at-risk individuals; and tertiary, focusing on individual gang members. Gottfredson and Gottfredson (1999) note that gang and violence prevention efforts in schools are generally implemented with marginal, if not inadequate, training in the prevention/intervention model, too few implementation staff members, too little supervision, inadequate data collection, and low fidelity of treatment.

Mihalic, Irwin, Elliott, Fagan, and Hansen (2001) describe promising and model programs for violence prevention that are instructive to schools wishing to implement prevention programs and wanting to select community-based programs with which to collaborate. The approach is research based and data driven in that only programs that follow best practices in the field are described as promising. Especially instructive for schools are bullying prevention programs such as that described by Olweus (1993), Big Brothers and Big Sisters, a long-term, well-supervised mentoring program, and Life Skills Training, a direct instruction social skills and refusal skills training program. The Midwestern Prevention Project, also known as Project STAR, which is a school–community collaboration project, and Functional Family Therapy and Multisystemic Therapy projects for community referral choices, which are programs focus on functional parent and student client social skills development. The essence of these programs that is direct instruction in specific social skills and their implementation in the context of the school, the family, and the community.

Gottfredson (2001) recommends supporting programs that are research based, have a competent evaluation component, and are part of a broader school environment. Programs likely to be effective are characterized by (1) clear rule setting, (2) communicating clear expectations for behavior, (3) consistent enforcement of rules and expectations, (4) providing rewards for compliance, and (5) punishment for noncompliance. These observations are consistent with all available research, which supports a strong behavioral component, including a cognitive-behavioral component, for social skills instruction. Simply stated, effective programs include (1) specific target behaviors to be learned, (2) consistent feedback for both appropriate and inappropriate behavior, (3) actual direct instruction in the skills to be displayed, and (4) opportunities for repeated practice of the desired behavior. Such programs will likely result in social gains and reductions in problem behavior in the school. Conversely, programs that are theory driven, deficient in data, ambiguous in terms, and inconsistent in instruction and feedback, are less likely to show a positive effect.

In discussing prevention and intervention activities in schools, the task can be broadly divided into several major categories: (1) staff training and protocol, (2) gang prevention programs and other educational approaches for students, (3) dress and behavior codes, and (4) school safety plans, which include such components as perimeter security practices, physical building security (including physical barriers), controlled access, well-dispersed security personnel and coordination of building security practices with local law enforcement, and (5) model violence prevention programs.

Staff Training and Protocol

Prevention and intervention activities within a building require a solid educational foundation for both staff and students. New staff members should receive comprehensive training in dealing with gangs in the fall of each school year, and a refresher course with updates should be provided for veteran staffers. Initial training must include a review of current research on reasons for joining a gang; historical and current concepts of gangs among sociologists, law enforcement, and community groups; gang-facilitating and gang-maintaining structures and practices within a given community; basic gang identification signals (e.g., colors, hand signs, language, clothing modifications, and tattoos); and local gang-related activity and current trends as identified by local law enforcement.

The credentials of a person training others to deal with gangs must be verified by multiple sources as to that person's being (1) familiar with the current research, (2) experienced in conducting critical training programs, (3) directly experienced in dealing with gang-involved youths, (4) knowledgeable about current gang activity, and (5) experienced in coordination and collaboration (with schools, community groups, and juvenile justice agencies).

Following training, a staff member may be selected to receive further training at the school district or state department of education level. Such an individual may also be sent to specialized training sessions conducted by other agencies, such as local, state, or national law enforcement authorities. The individual may then be designated as the school's or school district's "gang resource person." The gang resource person should be prepared to make presentations to parent, student, and community groups regarding basic gang education and school prevention and intervention activities. Overhead projector illustrations or slides should be developed to facilitate such presentations. Basic handout materials may be useful for audience members, especially if they contain the names and telephone numbers of school building, school district, community, and local law enforcement personnel who can assist them with individual questions as they arise during the school year.

Teachers should receive a basic fact sheet to use as a ready reference during the school year. Such a sheet should list current gang names, numbers (which represent the gang, such as "5" for Vicelords), graffiti, and activity in or near the school. The school's gang resource person should maintain whatever professional materials are needed by a given school. This person can also act as a liaison between the school and either district security personnel or local law enforcement, with direct telephone access to the necessary parties.

Finally, each school should develop a protocol to follow for gang prevention education and development of a gang intervention policy. The following should be included in this protocol:

1. Published materials on gang prevention and intervention.
2. Brief flyers or brochures to send to parents regarding gang identification, community resources, and both school and law enforcement contacts.
3. A collection of sample letters. This should include a letter to send to parents in the fall of the year describing the school's gang prevention policies; a letter of notice to parents when their student is observed to be engaging in possible gang-related activity (see Figure 9.1); a letter of notice if increased gang-related activity is observed in or near the school (see Figure 9.2); a letter to accompany any disciplinary notice, if the discipline is a function of gang-related disruptive behavior in school; a letter to be sent home with students if a major gang-related violent event occurs on school grounds during the school day; and other letters as needed.
4. District-reviewed gang prevention education materials (see the next section, "Student Educational Approaches").
5. Perimeter and within-building emergency procedures (discussed in a following section, "School Safety Plans").
6. Recommendations for efficient and effective interactions with representatives of the electronic and print media.

Student Educational Approaches

Gang Prevention Education

Although the presence of gang-related activity in a school often leads to demands for gang prevention education, the literature is remarkably void of

Date _____

Dear parents or guardians of _____ :

As you are probably aware, gang violence is a problem in our city. Threats, intimidation, fights, beatings, and shootings are common when rival gang members meet. Unfortunately, many school-age youths find gangs fascinating. Some students regularly interact with older gang members. Some students are themselves involved in gangs. For others, it is popular to dress, talk, and act like active gang members, even when they are not. This can cause serious or even life-threatening problems when such "imitators" or marginal gang members encounter serious, sometimes armed, real gang members. Violent interactions have occurred around and in our school because of the display of gang colors, use of hand signs, and exchange of gang slang among students and others. To enhance student safety, we have a zero-tolerance policy regarding gang dress, talk, graffiti, and hand signing in our school.

This letter is written to inform you that your child has been engaging in some behavior in school that may be gang related. We have counseled your child to stop all such activity immediately. Further activity may lead to suspension from school if it constitutes a provable, immediate gang threat or gang intimidation. Criminal gang activity will be referred to the police.

Please speak with your child about the dangers of real or imagined gang involvement. Any of your child's teachers, the school social worker, or I would welcome a phone call from you. Please contact one of us as soon as possible.

Sincerely,

Principal

FIGURE 9.1. Sample letter to parents/guardians to inform them of a child's possible gang-related activity.

validated and replicated studies showing vigorous treatment effects for this type of education.

Caveat: A popular activity in schools is to employ former gang members as motivational speakers, who recite "cautionary tales" to dissuade young gang aspirants or entire student bodies from joining gangs. Some schools use such individuals as counselors for individual or groups of students. Unfortunately, little systematic study of such practices is available to guide educators. There is no research to suggest either the desirability or the necessity of employing such motivational speakers or counselors, but some reason to believe that such an approach may be counterproductive (Kodluboy & Evenrud, 1993). The recent experience of the New York City schools in hiring current gang members as school security officers resulted in major problems with the schools and in the community (Flamm, Keith, & Kleppel, 1997). In instances when it appears necessary to link a seriously gang-

Date _____

Dear parents or guardians of _____:

Providing a safe and respectable environment is our first and most important task when educating young people. Positive discipline and strong academic expectations can be achieved only when the physical environment is safe, clean, and presentable. We are requesting your active assistance in maintaining such an environment at our school.

Recently, we have begun experiencing significant problems with students writing graffiti in the building. Often the activity consists of students writing their names on walls, on posters, in the toilets, and on desks and textbooks. Increasingly, this graffiti also consists of gang logos, threats, and slogans. We remove all graffiti we see within minutes of discovery, but we need your help in reducing graffiti even further.

Your son or daughter does not need any indelible markers at school. Please do not allow your child to bring such markers to school unless specifically requested by letter from the classroom teacher. If your son or daughter has a folder, notebook, or books marked with writing that you do not understand, please ask your child the meaning of such writing. Call us if you have any specific concerns regarding graffiti.

In addition, please be aware that any graffiti that results in expense to the district through damage to school property may be recorded as vandalism and reported to the police department.

Thank you for your support. Please feel free to call if you have any suggestions, questions, or recommendations for making our school a safer place.

Sincerely,

Principal

FIGURE 9.2. Sample letter to parents/guardians to inform them of increased gang-related activity in school.

involved youth with a community-based mentor, a mentor with no history of gang involvement is desirable. If a former gang member is proffered as a mentor, it is preferable to select one who left the gang life years ago, who now has moved into a conventional life, and whose philosophy of mentorship is consistent with the mission of the school district. It is wise for the school to support only those mentors who reject gangs as a legitimate social structure in the community and who endorse conventional community and school values (Kodluboy & Evenrud, 1993). If the stated philosophy of the mentor is inconsistent with the policy and mission of the school district, it is unwise to allow the authority of the school to support the placement of a student with such a mentor.

Specific Gang Prevention Programs

Gang prevention programs are commonly associated with and frequently evolve from within existing drug prevention programs. In a national evaluation of the Youth Gang Drug Prevention Program, outcomes from 52 of these "combination" programs were reviewed. The programs were found to have "a positive influence on drug use and selling, delinquency behavior, involvement with the criminal justice system, school performance and peer relations. They had little or no apparent effect on gang membership" and did not appear to deter youths from gang membership (Development Services Group, 1993, p. 39).

Gang prevention programs per se, although lacking a firm database, nonetheless appear promising. A student gang prevention, gang resistance, or gang education program such as Gang Resistance Education and Training (GREAT), the Gang Risk Intervention Pilot Program (GRIPP), the Paramount Program, or the like may be considered for inclusion in the school's or district's comprehensive approach when (1) the critical mass of gang members within or near the school or school attendance area becomes significant or (2) parents, staff, or students indicate a need for gang education or gang resistance training for students.

The GREAT program was developed by the Bureau of Alcohol, Tobacco and Firearms in collaboration with the Phoenix, Arizona, police and other agencies in 1991 (Humphrey & Baker, 1994). Law enforcement officers teach school-age youths basic factual information and decision-making skills in regard to gang affiliation, over an 8-week period, with a summer follow-up component. Initial, short-term research findings were promising, with the results of the long-term follow-up assessment of GREAT revealing modest effects over time (Esbensen, 2000). The Bureau of Alcohol, Tobacco and Firearms, in a display of integrity, went back to the drawing board and developed a best-practice-enhanced revision of the GREAT program, utilizing published principles of social skills training, public health education, and cultural acceptability to recreate the program. The new curriculum was field tested in late 2000 and early 2001, with rigorous evaluation in small, medium, and large school districts to ascertain its effectiveness. Preliminary results are very encouraging, and the program now stands recommended as promising, pending further long-term follow up evaluation.

The specific objectives of GRIPP are to decrease gang affiliation, decrease gang crimes, link at-risk youths with community resources, provide positive youth programming and activities, facilitate a school–community linkage, provide counseling and job training, and promote positive interactions between youth and law enforcement. Results of a recent evaluation indicate that "the number of students arrested for gang-related crimes at GRIPP schools [has] been lower than [the number at] their non-GRIPP counterparts" (Hughes, 1994).

The Paramount Program, established by the school district in Paramount, California, also focuses on gang resistance training and demonstrates a positive impact on students' attitudes toward gangs. Further systematic replication of this program, when conducted, will, it is hoped, contribute to the schools' efforts to reduce gang involvement (Kodluboy & Evenrud, 1993).

Despite the lack of well-designed, clearly described, and research-validated gang prevention programs, it is apparent that schools cannot stand by and fail to educate students as to the risks of gang involvement. School districts may elect to effect one of the established programs now available and apply rigorous evaluation standards to the effort. Only through such evaluation efforts can a database be generated to guide school districts with varying degrees of the problem in making informed decisions about a proportional, efficient, and effective response.

Broad-Based Violence Prevention

Following a tragic shooting on a high school campus in Portland, Oregon, the school board began a full-scale gang prevention and intervention program. In addition to the establishment of "zero tolerance" for gang-related activities or displays of gang affiliation, a prosocial skills program was implemented, entitled Second Step—A Violence Prevention Curriculum (Gaustad, 1991; Prophet, 1990). Second Step, designed by the Seattle-based Committee for Children, has shown promising results in the Milwaukee public schools. The district reports a significant reduction in the number of incidents resulting in disciplinary action and referrals, as well as a marked improvement in school climate (Klonsky, 1995). A review of the program suggests that a well-thought-out program of social skills instruction might be used in the context of comprehensive violence prevention. An appropriate evaluation component should be developed before implementation of the program within a school district.

Gottfredson (2001) reports several sample programs with promising results in reducing school delinquency:

1. Rule setting and social control: Behavioral consultation to reduce violence, bullying prevention, and the senior high PATHE program
2. Organization of instruction: Classwide peer tutoring and the STATUS program
3. Management of the School Development Program and the PATHE program
4. Increasing school/community of caring adults: The STATUS program and the School Transitional Environment Project
5. Behavior management: playground aggression prevention, improving attendance, behavior modification and parent training, contingency management for truancy

6. Instruction in social skills for all students: PATHS curriculum, problems prevention group, positive youth development, life skills training, cognitive social skills training
7. Instruction in social skills for at risk students: interpersonal cognitive problem solving, fast track, anger coping program and social skills training, anger control training, moral reasoning development and decision making, and personal growth class (see Gottfredson, 2001, p. 270)

Conflict mediation programs are widely implemented in school systems as a supplement to social skills training, with the intent to decrease violent episodes and teach students how to resolve their own problems peacefully. Conflict resolution programs, which may include both peer mediation and adult-mediated problem solving, at first glance appear to be of some merit in reducing violent incidents within schools (Wilson-Brewer & Spivak, 1994; Goldstein & Huff, 1993). Sherman, et al. (1997) subjected conflict mediation program reports to independent meta-analysis. The findings suggest that mediation programs, when compared with rigorous evaluation criteria, have a low "effect size," that is, a low impact on reducing conflict. Nonetheless, such programs are, perhaps by their intuitive nature, highly popular and thus worthy of comment. When mediation programs are being considered, necessary modifications regarding the age of clients, availability of trainers, supervision of student mediators, and criteria for which behaviors are subject to peer versus adult mediation, must be made before the programs are implemented. Careful collection of outcomes can help a school district to establish the utility of such programs. Districts must be cautious to clearly define the program activities and to include all data, such as cases not subjected to mediation, cases in which mediation was not successful, and cases in which multiple strategies, in addition to mediation, were implemented.

Mediating Gang Disputes

Special problems may be encountered in mediating disputes between gang members. Mediators must (1) have basic fluency in the local gang culture, (2) be knowledgeable about issues of gang rank, if applicable, (3) be knowledgeable about words or actions that define respect within or between the gangs involved, (4) know whether the dispute is between two members of the same gang or members of different gangs, (5) know whether the individuals in mediation are speaking for their gang(s) or for themselves, and (6) determine whether allowing the mediation is likely to increase the status of a given gang member or increase the cohesion of a gang by granting the gang some legitimacy. If conflict mediation is used to prevent a gang-related violent incident on campus, it is necessary to counterbalance any status or legitimacy granted to a gang through the mediation process with a sustained effort to abate that legitimacy, both through individual intervention with the

participants and through vigorous attention to the district's zero-tolerance
policy toward gang-related activities or displays on campus (Kodluboy, 1994;
Kodluboy & Evenrud, 1993).

Aggression Replacement Training

In addition to violence prevention and conflict mediation, a new and research-validated approach called "aggression replacement training" has been
utilized not only with aggressive adolescents, but with aggressive juvenile
gang members as well. The approach focuses on social skills development
with rehearsal across settings, anger control training, and moral education.
This combination appears to address three important domains: social behavior, emotions or affect, and the social context in which behavior occurs. It
also provides reinforced practice of the newly acquired behavioral repertoire. Data on the results of this approach suggest a reduction in arrest rates
and other indices of gang-related delinquency among 10 aggressive youth
gangs in New York City. This most promising program warrants serious consideration by school districts experiencing gang-related aggression that affects student attendance, achievement, or safety (Goldstein, 1994; Goldstein,
Harootunian, & Conoley, 1994).

Alternative Schools

Alternative schools are often cited within a school district, not only as a viable means of educating youths who cannot or will not conform to more conventional types of schooling, but as a necessary form of relief for school administrators, who often place problem students in these schools. School
district personnel privately concede that alternative schools are a safety valve
for the district. Marginal and occasionally core gang members are sometimes
referred to alternative schools for one or both reasons. Although testimonials to their efficacy abound, little detailed research on alternative schools is
available for analysis. One meta-analysis of alternative schools suggests that
any enthusiasm for their role should be muted at best. Alternative schools appear to have a "small positive effect on school performance, school attitude
and self-esteem" (Cox, Davidson, & Bynum, 1995, p. 229). However, there
was a negative finding that alternative schools "have been unable to affect
delinquent behavior." The authors note that schools whose target
populations are carefully defined have a greater impact than less well
defined schools.

As a means of decreasing or preventing school gang violence, it may be
best to perceive placement of disruptive gang-involved youths in alternative
schools as a way of separating combatants, rather than as a healing intervention. In well-designed and well-supervised alternative schools, this separation
may allow disruptive gang members to concentrate more on their studies,
rather than worrying about and engaging in gang displays, challenges, or

"covering their backs" in a regular school setting. Alternative schools also offer students a smaller, less anonymous setting than a traditional setting, and thus they may more easily find a significant adult with whom to connect. Students who remain in conventional settings and those who leave the traditional setting for an alternative school both gain some relief from conflict. The lack of generalization of an alternative school's effects to abating delinquency in the community should be no more alarming than the similar failure of conventional schools to obtain generalization of effects with some resistant percentage of the school population.

Problem Displacement

Schools are cautioned to avoid dealing with gang problems by simply transferring students to "anywhere but here," whether the transfer is to an alternative school, another public school within the district, or to a new charter school. Such an approach is not in the best interests of the student, the student's family, or the community as a whole. It is equally unwise to allow a de facto designation of one school as "gang X school" and another as "gang Y school" and hope for the best. Such conditions and schools are identifiable within some school districts, having become so by circumstance rather than intentional district planning. It is recommended that school districts have a written plan for moving gang-involved students from school to school when necessary, to meet the short- and long-term academic and behavioral needs of the students, the school, and the community. Students who are moved for gang-related reasons should begin at the new school with written behavior plans that include weekly monitoring, academic progress monitoring weekly, or at least monthly, collaborative planning and programming with at least one community agency, and whatever else the team determines is necessary for a student to succeed. The common practice of simply warning the newly arrived gang-transfer student that it is "his or her decision" if he or she is to succeed, is unprofessional and counterproductive and denies the responsibility of the school to attempt to teach necessary social and academic skills to all students. Social skills must be directly taught, and if a school is to "fail" with a student, it should not be because best practice in academic and social instruction and community collaboration was not attempted.

Dress and Behavior Codes

When developing gang prevention policies, schools commonly implement restrictive dress and behavior codes in an attempt to reduce the disruption and violent episodes that can be directly related to gang apparel and actions (Kodluboy & Evenrud, 1993). Such codes generally prohibit certain dress articles, such as bandanas, specific jewelry (e.g., five-pointed stars worn on the left ear), shoelaces in gang colors and patterns (e.g., a yellow lace in the left shoe and a black lace in the right shoe), and the like; hand signs specific to gangs in the area of the school; and some gang language (e.g., "All's well" when students greet each other).

Limitations on gang-related dress and associated behaviors are controversial, despite the widespread implementation of such policies. Civil libertarians and many students feel that restricting these displays of affiliation is an unfair limitation on their free-speech rights. Indeed, some districts have overreacted to perceptions of gang-related activity and have imposed restrictions on broadly defined behaviors without sufficient cause for action. In areas where gang violence is endemic, however, little such debate is heard.

Basic issues to be addressed when limitations on gang-related behavior or dress are anticipated include the following: Is a behavior a particularized message? Is there provable fact of disruption caused by the behavior? Is the behavior otherwise protected speech? Is there a rational link between the anticipated limitations and the mission of the school? For a dress code to pass constitutional muster, each aspect of the issue must be addressed (*Olesen v. Board of Education*, 1987; *Bethel School District No. 403 v. Fraser*, 1986; Burke, 1993; Kodluboy & Evenrud, 1993). Each of these issues in discussed in turn.

In areas where gang-related messages are discernible by other students and staff, a particularized message to communicate may be construed when a student exhibits or expresses such a message (*United States v. O'Brien*, 1968). In order to restrict the message, the school must determine that such restriction is designed to protect the right of students to an education or to maintain an effective learning environment.

To determine that the gang-related display or expression is inimical to creating or maintaining an effective learning environment, it is necessary to demonstrate that it creates a material disruption to such an environment. There must be provable facts of disruptive behavior in the same or similar conditions to those defined as the occasion of the proposed sanction. When there is a history of assaults, mutual combat between gang members, absences from school by fearful students, or shootings at or near the school when gang-related displays are in evidence, it may be proposed that such displays advocate imminent lawlessness and thus create a material disruption to the school (*Olesen v. Board of Education*, 1987).

For speech to be protected, it must not "materially disrupt class work or involve substantial disorder or invasion of the rights of others" (*Tinker v. Des Moines Independent Community School District*, 1969, p. 513). In *Olesen v. Board of Education*, an Illinois district court supported the school district in prohibiting a student from wearing gang attire (i.e., gang-specific jewelry), stating that the district had a "clear and reasonable basis" for such prohibition (Burke, 1993, p. 525). The district presented evidence of gang activity that was not only disruptive to the school environment, but inimical to the rational purpose of providing students with an orderly learning environment. The court recognized that the right of the student to wear clearly discernible gang attire was limited by its impact on the school environment.

School districts are cautioned to be certain that any planned prohibitions on gang-related dress or behavior are thoughtfully and narrowly crafted. A careful review by school district attorneys should be part of this process. Collection of provable instances of fact, in which it can be shown that such displays have resulted in material disruption of the educational process, is necessary. The writing of the prohibition and proposed sanctions should emphasize overt items and behaviors, not classes of persons. The school's staff members should be educated to recognize that most often gang dress is merely "gangster chic" worn by youths who are more influenced by video and printed materials of the youth culture than by actual street gangs. Many youths who adopt gang attire or other symbolism do so simply because they grow up in such close proximity to public displays by actual gang members.

Sanctions should best follow this simple protocol: (1) educating all students about the importance of a prosocial demeanor, including dress, (2) educating students who engage in gang-related displays, (3) informing parents of the dangers of such displays and their disruptive effect on a school, and soliciting their understanding and support, (4) interviewing the offending students privately rather than in public, if possible, (5) utilizing discipline, such as exclusion or suspension, only if educational interventions fail or if an immediate threat is apparent, (6) remaining fair and consistent in the exercise of the policy, and (7) soliciting student body, parent, and community support for the policy.

SCHOOL SAFETY PLANS

Gang violence may occur before or after school; at bus pickup points or between these points and school; near campus or on campus; during school or after school; and in the building, on the grounds, or on adjacent property utilized by the school, such as city-run playgrounds. Each instance will require a discrete prevention and intervention strategy, and each strategy must be coordinated within a central school safety plan. School safety plans are at the heart of any gang prevention program. They are written documents developed by a committee of building staff members, with input by concerned parents, police, district-level school safety personnel, and building or community school leadership teams (when these exist). Such plans prescribe a discrete series of increasing and proportional responses to perceived threats to school safety. Best-case and worst-case scenarios are described that allow staff members to learn the broadest possible range of responses that can be reasonably expected of them, as well as what form and magnitude of response may be anticipated from the police, other community agencies, and district central staff. The school district's attorneys and loss prevention staff members should review all aspects of school safety plans. School safety plans are living documents that should be reviewed annually for major revision and more frequently by a standing school committee.

The standing committee, which should meet at least monthly, should be assigned the responsibility of developing and monitoring the building's safety plans. Other duties of the committee must include (1) developing a mechanism for gathering within-building information regarding gang-related activity, gang rumors, graffiti display and abatement, and shifts in indicators of gang membership or in affiliations with other gangs, (2) developing a mechanism for communicating such information to all staff members on a regular and "as-needed" basis, (3) conferring regularly with school district officials concerned with security and safety, including transportation officials, (4) conferring regularly with police officials from the district or from other local law enforcement agencies serving the school, and (5) distributing the written school safety plans to all staff members, parents, and appropriate community representatives (see Trump, 1998; Brock, Sandoval, & Lewis, 2001).

Personnel hired expressly to provide security should meet minimum requirements to ensure safe and professional conduct and to minimize liability resulting from misconduct. These minimum qualifications may include the following:

- Passing an unannounced preemployment drug screening test and remaining subject to random drug screening during employment
- Passing a criminal background check as defined by the district or local and state regulation, if applicable
- Completion of formal, supervised training in specific skill expectations
- Completion of a supervised probation period
- Qualifying for licensing and bonding as a security agent or for indemnification by the school district

The characteristics of the ideal security person will vary according to the needs of the district and the degree of apparent and provable risk. In situations of extreme risk, licensed and sworn off-duty police officers or on-duty city, county, or school police may be both necessary and desirable. In areas of emerging problems, a less rigorous standard may be appropriate. School district risk management personnel must carefully develop written guidelines for hiring, training, and supervising security personnel.

School safety plans should address a range of potential threats to school safety, as appropriate to the locale of the particular school. Schools in the Los Angeles area must address earthquake readiness, whereas Minneapolis-area schools must address tornado readiness. Each locale has its own specificity. All areas, however, must address problems such as natural disasters, intruders, lost or missing children, abduction threats, environmental hazards, and (most important for this discussion) violence, especially gang-related violence. Schools experiencing extreme risk should seek guidance on best practice regarding weapons interdiction and screening at the school entrance, use of off-duty police officers, and search procedures during school activities and during the school day (National Association of School Safety and Law Enforcement Officers [NASSLEO], 1994).

The development of school safety plans must also vary with the degree of threat posed by gangs in the area. Proportional and complete response is the goal of any safety plan. Even within a given school district, the range of responses will vary greatly. This is true of both heavily gang-infested cities and those that are only beginning to see gang-related problems within their boundaries.

School safety plans should address perimeter security (i.e., fences); parking lot access; building access procedures (including routine and emergency door-locking procedures); visitor identification and registration; patrol of the building and grounds by teaching, administrative, security, or police personnel; use of closed-circuit TV cameras, if needed; use of uniformed security or police personnel, as needed; lockdown procedures for emergencies, such as gang altercations or the presence of intruders; and similar matters. Figure 9.3 is a sample plan for dealing with gunfire and intruders.

Extra attention is needed for bus arrival and departure times, as these are prime times for visits from rival gang members. School assemblies, by their nature, force large numbers of students into a relatively small space; therefore, movement patterns must be considered if large numbers of rival gang members are present in the school. Evening activities that may be open to the community, such as school dances, require special precautions. Strict observance of rules as to who may attend, what forms of identification are required, and what form of dress is acceptable is necessary. For events that may be troublesome—such as dances, community festivals held on school grounds, or athletic competitions between schools—it may be necessary to present a strong visual deterrent to gang violence (e.g., the presence of several marked patrol cars, a high ratio of adults to students, and restricted access to the events).

SUMMARY AND CONCLUSIONS

The degree of gang impact on a school will vary with (1) the age range of the students served by the school, (2) the degree of social disorganization in the school's neighborhood, (3) the degree of social and economic disparity among students within the school complex, (4) current gang activities across the city, within the school's neighborhood, and within the school itself, (5) the degree and type of community concern and response to gang activities in the locale, and (6) the extent to which, and the way in which, the school district and school building recognize and conceptualize the status of gangs in the community.

To: All staff

From: Administration

Re: Protocol for gunfire and building intruders

When you hear the following over the loudspeaker, please do not leave the school building: "Attention all staff: All outdoor activities are canceled." This means that all exterior doors will be locked and monitored. Do not attempt to leave the building or use the playground or athletic field. Normal movement within the school building may continue.

When you hear "Attention all staff: Dr. Green is in the building," this means a total building lockdown is in effect. Do not leave your classroom. Lock your door, and while doing so, direct any passing staff members or students to enter your room immediately. Do not allow any staff member or student to leave your classroom until you hear the "All clear" message. Do not call the office for clarification. The office will call you or issue an "All staff" call to update you.

Begin outdoor security training for your classroom. You may wish to carry a whistle. One long blast of the whistle means "Look at me and do as I do." This may be dropping to the ground or remaining motionless. Three short blasts mean "Follow me now!" It is appropriate to do three successive bursts of three short blasts to be certain that all students and nearby adults can hear the directive. Do not use three whistle blasts for any other reason.

If a playground emergency occurs, follow the directions given by members of the security staff. They will be in touch with each other and the police officer on duty, so they may give you the best advice.

If you hear gunfire, do not automatically move to the school door. Stop, listen, and look! If you must act immediately, it may be best to drop to the ground until the direction and location of the gunfire are determined. We do not want students of three or four classrooms running to the door, serving as moving targets if the shooting is immediately next to where the students are playing or between the students and the school door.

If the shooting is away from your position, moving to the door briskly may be the best response. If the shooting is very close to your position, dropping to the ground may be the best response. When in doubt, drop! Also, when in doubt, look to security personnel if they are available.

As you can see, each incident will probably be different from any other and require a different response. When a police officer is present, the officer will direct the security staff and all within earshot as to the expected course of action. When only security personnel are present, they will make the call and advise you. When you will be alone on the playground, take a radio and take the initiative!

If a chaotic situation occurs, personal initiative and best judgment may be your only guide.

FIGURE 9.3. Sample plan for dealing with gunfire and building intruders.

Preventing and intervening in gang violence in schools require several discrete steps:

1. Identifying and defining the scope of gang activity in or near the school
2. Identifying gang members
3. Defining the scope of the problem
4. Training school staff members appropriately and developing a staff protocol
5. Developing student educational strategies, and establishing criteria for their implementation and evaluation
6. Developing dress and behavior codes as necessary
7. Developing and publishing school safety plans, to cover perimeter security, within-school security, bus and walking route security, liaison with law enforcement, and building and system response to emergencies

The necessity for schools to accept yet another burden resulting from the increasing social disorganization within our suburbs and cities is unfortunate but real. Gang violence is one more threat to the public order in our schools, and one that presents unique challenges. The social structures of gangs teach, reinforce, and reward antisocial behavior; as such, gangs always present a risk to their members, other students, and school staff. Only through careful education and systematic response can the likelihood of gang-related violence in our schools be reduced. No student should be denied access to public education because of gang membership. Yet no student or staff member should enter the school building in fear because of a gang presence. "Zero tolerance" means that no gang displays or activities are allowed in school, but it does not mean that gang members themselves are prohibited. Rather, it means that schools must find the common ground of conventional values and aspirations displayed by gang-involved youths and build upon that common ground. Gang members can be welcomed in school, but their gang-related behavior cannot be. This is the serious task of public education.

REFERENCES

Bastian, L. D., & Taylor, B. M. (1995, September). *School crime* (Report No. NJC-131645). Washington, DC: U.S. Department of Justice, Bureau of Justice Statistics.

Bethel School District No. 403 v. Fraser, 478 U.S. 675, 106 S. Ct. 3159, 92 L. Ed. 2d 549 (1986).

Brock, S. E., Sandoval, J., & Lewis, S. (2001). *Preparing for Crises in the Schools: A manual for building school crisis response teams.* New York: Wiley.

Burke, N. D. (1993). Commentary: Restricting gang clothing in the public school. *Education Law Reporter, 80,* 513–526.

Burnett, G., & Walz, G. (1994). Gangs in the schools. *ERIC Digest, 99*, 1–4.

Busch, K. G., Zagar, R., Hughes, J. R., Arbit, J., & Bussell, R. E. (1990). Adolescents who kill. *Journal of Clinical Psychology, 46*(4), 472–485.

Bushman, B. J., & Anderson, C. A. (2001). Media violence and the American public: Scientific facts versus media misinformation. *American Psychologist, 6/7*, 477–489.

Cox, S. M., Davidson, W. S., & Bynum, T. S. (1995). A meta-analytic assessment of delinquency-related outcomes of alternative education programs. *Crime and Delinquency, 41*(2), 219–234.

Cromwell, P., Taylor, D., & Palacios, W. (1992). Youth gangs: A 1990s perspective. *Juvenile and Family Court Journal, 3*, 25–31.

Curry, G. D., & Spergel, T. A. (1992). Gang involvement and delinquency among Hispanic and African-American adolescent males. *Journal of Research in Crime and Delinquency, 29*(3), 273–291.

Decker, S. H., & Van Winkle, B. (1996). *Life in the gang: Family, friends and violence.* Cambridge, UK: Cambridge University Press.

Development Services Group. (1993). *National evaluation of the Youth Gang Drug Prevention Program.* Bethesda, MD: Administration on Children, Youth and Families.

Esbensen, F.-A. (2000, September). *Preventing adolescent gang involvement.* Washington, DC: U.S. Department of Justice, Office of Justice Programs, Office of Juvenile Justice and Delinquency Prevention.

Fagan, J. (1989). The social organization of drug use and drug dealing among urban gangs. *Criminology, 27*(4), 633–667.

Fagan, J. (1990). Social process of delinquency and drug use among urban gangs. In C. R. Huff (Ed.), *Gangs in America* (pp. 183–222). Newbury Park, CA: Sage.

Felgar, M. A. (1992). Gangs and youth violence. *Journal of Emotional and Behavioral Problems, 1*(1), 9–12.

Flamm, S., Keith, L., & Kleppel, W. (1997). *An investigation into the Latin Kings: No tolerance for gangs in the public schools* (Report to the Special Commissioner of Investigations for New York City). New York: School District of the City of New York.

Gaustad, J. (1991). Schools attack the roots of violence. *ERIC Digest, 63*, 1–3.

Goldstein, A., Glick, B., Carthan, W., & Blancero, D. A. (1994). *The pro social gang: Implementing aggression replacement training.* Thousand Oaks, CA: Sage.

Goldstein, A., & Huff, C. R. (1993). *The gang intervention handbook.* Champaign, IL: Research Press.

Goldstein, A., & Kodluboy, D. W. (1998) *Gangs and Schools, Signs, Symbols and Solutions.* Champaign–Urbana, IL: Research Press.

Goldstein, A. P. (1994). Aggression toward persons and property in America's schools. *School Psychologist, 48*(1), 1, 6, 18, 21.

Goldstein, A. P., Harootunian, B., & Conoley, J. C. (1994). *Student aggression: Prevention, management, and replacement training.* New York: Guilford Press.

Gottfredson, D. (2001). *Schools and delinquency.* New York, New York: Cambridge University Press.

Gottfredson, G., & Gottfredson, D. (1999, July 29) *Survey of school-based prevention and intervention programs: Preliminary findings.* Paper presented at the National Youth Gang Symposium, Las Vegas, NV.

Graves, B. (1994, October). Antisocial traits show early. *The Oregonian*, p. A1.

Hagedorn, J. (1988). *People and folks: Gangs, crime and the underclass in a Rust Belt city.* Chicago: Lake View.

Holstrom, D. (1994, October 28). As youth murders rise, schools teach protection. *The Christian Science Monitor*, p. 6.

Howell, J. C., & Lynch, J. P. (2000, August). *Youth gangs in schools* (Juvenile Justice Bulletin). Washington, DC: U.S. Department of Justice, Office of Justice Programs, Institute of Intergovernmental Research from the Office of Juvenile Justice and Delinquency Prevention.

Huff, C. R. (1990). Denial, overreaction, and misidentification: A postscript on public policy. In C. R. Huff (Ed.), *Gangs in America* (pp. 310–317). Newbury Park, CA: Sage.

Hughes, H. C. (1994). *Gang Risk Intervention Pilot Program: Final evaluation report.* Sacramento: California Office of Criminal Justice Planning.

Humphrey, K. R., & Baker, P. R. (1994, September). GREAT program: Gang Resistance Education and Training. *FBI Law Enforcement Bulletin,* pp. 1–4.

Jankowski, M. S. (1991). *Islands in the street: Gangs in American urban society.* Berkeley: University of California Press.

Klein, M., & Maxson, C. L. (1989). Street gang violence. In N. A. Weiner & M. E. Wolfgang (Eds.), *Violent crime and violent criminals.* Newbury, CA: Sage.

Klein, M. W. (1995). *The American street gang: Its nature, prevalence, and control.* New York: Oxford University Press.

Klonsky, S. (1995, spring). To learn in peace: What schools are trying now. *City Schools,* pp. 18–25.

Kodluboy, D. (1994). Behavioral disorders and the culture of street gangs. In R. L. Peterson & S. Ishii-Jordan (Eds.), *Multicultural issues in the education of students with behavioral disorders* (pp. 233–250). Cambridge, MA: Brookline Books.

Kodluboy, D. W. (1996). Asian gangs: Basic issues for educators. *School Safety, 3,* 8–12.

Kodluboy, D., & Evenrud, L. (1993). School based interventions: Best practice and critical issues. In A. P. Goldstein & C. R. Huff (Eds.), *The gang intervention handbook* (pp. 257–300). Champaign, IL: Research Press.

Koklaranis, M. (1994, August 28). Area schools get set to open amid big increase in security. *The Washington Times,* p. A1.

Lane, J. R. (1991, spring). Schools caught in the crossfire. *School Safety,* p. 13.

Lantieri, L. (1995). Waging peace in our schools: Beginning with the children. *Phi Delta Kappan, 76,* 386–392.

Lyon, J. M., Henggeler, S. W., & Hall, J. A. (1992). The family relations, peer relations, and criminal activities of Caucasian and Hispanic-American gang members. *Journal of Abnormal Child Psychology, 20*(5), 439–449.

Maxson, C., & Klein, M. W. (1990). Street gang violence: Twice as great, or half as great? In C. R. Huff (Ed.), *Gangs in America* (pp. 71–102). Newbury Park, CA: Sage.

Mihalic, S., Irwin, K., Elliott, d., Fagan, A., & Hansen, D., (2001, July). *Blueprints for violence prevention.* Washington, DC: U.S. Department of Justice, Office of Justice Programs, Office of Juvenile Justice and Delinquency Prevention.

Miller, W. B. (2001). *The growth of youth gang problems in the United States: 1970–1998.* Washington, DC: Office of Juvenile Justice and Delinquency Preventsion, U. S. Department of Justice.

Morrow, L. (1992, March 9). Childhood's end. *Time,* pp. 22–23.

National Association of School Safety and Law Enforcement Officers (NASSLEO). (1994). *NASSLEO Quarterly, 3,* 7.

National League of Cities (NLC). (1994). *School violence in America's cities: NLC survey overview.* Washington, DC: Author.

National School Safety Center (NSSC). (1988). *Gangs in schools: Breaking up is hard to do.* Malibu, CA: Author.

National School Safety Center (NSSC). (1991, November). Gang membership crosses cultural, geographic bounds. *School Safety Update,* pp. 1–8.

Olesen v. Board of Education, 676 F. Supp. 820 (N.D. Ill. 1987).

Olweus, D. (1993). *Bullying at school: What we know and what we can do.* Cambridge, MA: Blackwell.

Prophet, M. (1990, October). Safe schools in Portland. *American School Board Journal,* pp. 28–30.

Resnick, M. D., & Blum, R. W. (1994). The association of consensual sexual intercourse during childhood with adolescent health risk and behaviors. *Pediatrics, 94*(6), 907–913.

Robson, B. (1990, May). Mean streets. *Mpls. St. Paul,* pp. 64–69, 84–100.

Sautter, R. C. (1993). Standing up to violence. *Phi Delta Kappan, 74,* K1–K12.

Spergel, I. A. (1990). Youth gangs: Continuity and change. In M. Tonry & N. Morris (Eds.), *Crime and justice: A review of research* (Vol. 12, pp. 171–273). Chicago: University of Chicago Press.

Spergel, I. A., & Curry, G. D. (1993). The National Youth Gang Survey: A research and development process. In A. P. Goldstein & C. R. Huff (Eds.), *The gang intervention handbook* (pp. 359–400). Champaign, IL: Research Press.

Spergel, I. A., Curry, D., Chance, R., Kane, C., Ross, R., Alexander, A., Simmons, E., & Oh, S. (1994, October). *Gang suppression and intervention: Problem and response.* Research summary. Washington, DC: Office of Juvenile Justice and Delinquency Prevention.

Stephens, R. J. (1989, Fall). Gangs, guns and drugs. *School Safety,* pp. 16–19.

Stephens, R. J. (1991, November). Gangs v. schools: Assessing the score in your community. *School Safety Update,* p. 8.

Thornberry, T. P., Krohn, M. D., Lizotte, A. J., & Chard-Wierschem, D. (1993). The role of juvenile gangs in facilitating delinquent behavior. *Journal of Research in Crime and Delinquency, 30*(1), 55–87.

Tinker v. Des Moines Independent Community School District, 393 U.S. 503, 89 S. Ct. 733, 21 L. Ed. 2d 731 (1969).

Trump, K. S. (1998). *Practical school security: Basic guidelines for safe and secure schools.* Thousand Oaks, CA: Corwin Press.

United States v. O'Brien, 391 U.S. 367, 376, 88 S. Ct. 1673, 1678, 20 L. Ed. 2d 672 (1968).

Wilson-Brewer, R., & Spivak, H. (1994). Violence prevention in schools and other community settings: The pediatrician as initiator, educator, collaborator, and advocate. *Pediatrics, 94*(4), 623–630.

Winfree, L. T., Jr., Fuller, K., Vigil, T., & Mays, G. L. (1992). The definition and measurement of "gang status": Policy implications for juvenile justice. *Juvenile and Family Court Journal, 43*(1), 29–38.

Zagar, R., Arbit, J., Sylvies, R., & Busch, K. G. (1990, December). Homicidal adolescents: A replication. *Psychological Reports,* pp. 1235–1242.

PART IV
School-Oriented Interventions

CHAPTER 10

Academic and Instructional Interventions with Aggressive Students

JEREMY R. SULLIVAN
JANE CLOSE CONOLEY

Since the previous version of this chapter was published (Gagnon & Conoley, 1997), school violence and student aggression have continued to receive substantial attention from the popular media and from scholarly researchers. In fact, several journals in the fields of school and clinical child psychology have devoted special issues to these topics, and numerous books have summarized the research in regard to possible causal factors of incidents of school violence, in addition to strategies for violence prevention and intervention. Despite all of this attention, however, there remains a relative paucity of research examining the application of academic and instructional interventions to aggressive students. Although recent efforts at extending research on instructional interventions to aggressive students are evident, research on these types of interventions has primarily used samples of learning disabled students, thereby leaving the applicability of these interventions to aggressive students largely unknown. Taking these limitations into account, this chapter reviews the current research literature on the effectiveness and implementation of such interventions, with emphasis on their practical utility. The chapter begins with a rationale for using academic and instructional interventions with aggressive students and continues with descriptions of some of the most widely used and empirically supported of these interventions. The chapter concludes with directions for future research.

RATIONALE FOR ACADEMIC INTERVENTIONS

Research suggests that students with emotional or behavioral problems are likely to experience concurrent difficulties in academic areas, and this likelihood increases as does the number of comorbid conditions experienced by students (Stahl & Clarizio, 1999). More specifically, research suggests that low academic performance and low educational aspirations are associated with violence in adolescence (Herrenkohl et al., 2000; Hinshaw, 1992; McEvoy & Welker, 2000; Saner & Ellickson, 1996) and that interventions that are successful at enhancing academic performance are simultaneously successful at reducing aggressive behaviors (Lalli, Kates, & Casey, 1999). Thus, interventions to improve the academic skills of underachieving aggressive students are vital. Hinshaw (1992) has noted, "Reducing problem behavior is not a sufficient intervention for youngsters with overlapping achievement and behavior problems; the promotion of academic success is critical for these children" (p. 899). Indeed, students with behavioral deficits are often doubly disadvantaged; they experience little success (and much frustration) during their school day because of their deviance from both behavioral and academic norms.

Academic and curriculum interventions represent a set of methods that may be especially useful in enhancing the psychosocial well-being of students. In delineating general principles of strong school-based interventions, Lentz, Allen, and Ehrhardt (1996) noted, "To the extent possible given the nature of a presenting problem, [strong] interventions are designed to build upon teacher's and student's natural interactions and realities of classroom environments; more radical changes in teacher roles or behavior are only considered as necessary" (p. 124). Academic and instructional interventions fulfill this principle by their very definitions, as they occur within the natural ecology and context of the classroom setting and take advantage of naturally occurring relationships between teachers and students. Thus, the nature of these interventions maximizes the likelihood that (1) teachers will accept the interventions and implement them with fidelity and (2) positive effects of the interventions will be maintained.

According to Lentz et al. (1996), academic and instructional interventions should (1) provide students with opportunities to respond, (2) provide positive contingencies following accurate performance, (3) provide immediate feedback regarding performance, (4) provide teachers with opportunities to make decisions based on progress monitoring, and (5) consider critical variables in the delivery of instruction, such as the pacing of instruction and appropriately timed fading of the use of prompts and models. Other researchers (e.g., Elliott, Busse, & Shapiro, 1999; Gettinger, 1995; Greenwood, 1996) have also noted the critical importance of maximizing students' academic engagement, academic learning time, and opportunities to respond and have emphasized that these variables can be influenced by academic and instructional interventions. Specific academic and instructional interventions that generally meet the criteria proposed by Lentz et al. (1996), and that appear to hold the greatest promise for improving the academic performance of aggressive students, include peer tutoring, time-delay procedures, mnemonic instruction, and self-monitoring. Each of these interventions is discussed separately in the following sections. For each intervention, a representative study, collection of studies, or summary of the methods with which numerous researchers have implemented it is described to provide recent examples of how these interventions have been implemented; it is our hope that these examples will be of some assistance to practitioners who may be considering implementing these techniques themselves.

PEER TUTORING

Peer tutoring involves the delivery of instruction by one student to another; it is one of the most widely studied academic interventions, and one for which much evidence of effectiveness has been gathered. Research has consistently shown that peer tutoring can be an effective intervention with nondisabled or normally achieving students (Greenwood, Carta, & Maheady 1991). Specifically, it has been found that after peer tutoring programs have been implemented, both tutees *and* tutors show improvements in social skills, cooperation, self-determination, and self-esteem, in addition to marked improvements in academic performance, thereby making this form of intervention both academically valuable and socially valid (Carpenter, Bloom, & Boat, 1999). Peer tutoring allows teachers to provide students with individual attention without wasting valuable class time or sacrificing the learning of other class members, thereby making this procedure broadly accepted by teachers, school administrators, parents, and students (Butler, 1999; DuPaul, Ervin, Hook, & McGoey, 1998; Greenwood et al., 1991; Scruggs & Richter, 1988; Sideridis et al., 1997). Furthermore, because peer tutoring is widely and broadly accepted, is cost-efficient relative to alternative practices, can be sustained over time, and can be implemented with minimal interference with general education classroom procedures, teachers appear willing to use it, thus making it a pragmatic and realistic intervention (Greenwood et al., 1991).

The efficacy of using peer tutoring as an intervention for students with learning disabilities has also been well established over the past several decades (see Arreaga-Mayer, 1998; Gordon, Vaughn, & Schumm, 1993; and Scruggs & Richter, 1988, for reviews). Indeed, peer tutoring seems to be an ideal intervention for these students, as it alleviates the pressure on teachers' time, allows children to work in one-to-one relationships, and helps develop cooperative attitudes and mutual self-respect among students (Scruggs & Richter, 1988). In addition, because learning deficits are often task specific and strategies appropriate to a given task can be taught, peer tutoring appears to be a viable instructional intervention for students with learning disabilities, as it provides the individualized instruction and additional practice necessary for skill improvement and academic achievement (Mastropieri, Leinart, & Scruggs, 1999; Prehm, 1976). Peer tutoring has also been implemented with students with behavioral disorders and students with attention-deficit/hyperactivity disorder (ADHD) with largely positive results (Cochran, Feng, Cartledge, & Hamilton, 1993; DuPaul & Eckert, 1998; DuPaul et al., 1998; Franca, Kerr, Reitz, & Lambert, 1990; Gardner et al., 2001; Scruggs, Mastropieri, Veit, & Osguthorpe, 1986).

The nature of peer tutoring interventions makes this method beneficial for several reasons. First, the interactive nature of the tutoring relationship provides students with numerous opportunities to respond, which, as mentioned earlier, is thought to be a critical element of any academic intervention. The interactive nature also provides a built-in social skills component, and peer tutoring programs also may have affective (in addition to academic and social) benefits for participants (Enright & Axelrod, 1995; Roswal et al., 1995). Similarly, tutoring provides immediate feedback in the form of either praise or correction. Maheady, Harper, and Mallette (2001) concluded that peer tutoring methods "established more favorable pupil–teacher ratios within the classroom, increased student on-task time and response opportunities, provided additional opportunities for pupils to receive positive and corrective feedback, and enhanced pupils' opportunities to receive individualized help and encouragement" (p. 7). Maheady et al. (2001) also noted that these methods may place additional demands on teachers' time, especially during initial phases of organization and material development; minor behavior problems among students (e.g., lack of cooperation) also may occur.

Some of the difficulties experienced in implementing peer tutoring programs include determining the optimal number of tutoring sessions per week, designing material that will be appropriately challenging to students, and consistent delivery of contingencies by the teacher (Enright & Axelrod, 1995; Greenwood, Terry, Arreaga-Mayer, & Finney, 1992). According to García-Vázquez and Ehly (1995), there are seven critical questions to consider before implementing a peer tutoring intervention: (1) What are the goals and objectives? (2) how will outcomes be assessed? (3) what materials and procedures will be used? (4) how will tutors be trained? (5) how will progress be monitored throughout the intervention? (6) should a pilot intervention be conducted before implementing a more large-scale intervention? and (7) how much time and additional resources will be necessary to effectively implement the intervention? Considering these questions well in advance will increase the likelihood that the intervention is implemented and evaluated successfully. A useful model for the conceptualization and implementation of peer tutoring programs is provided by Miller, Barbetta, and Heron (1994); the model includes steps for choosing a specific tutoring format, training tutors, structuring the environment and the tutoring sessions, implementing the program, and evaluating program effectiveness.

Rather than being thought of as a single intervention, peer tutoring may best be conceptualized as a constellation of interventions, as several types of peer tutoring have been described and evaluated empirically. Classwide peer tutoring, cross-age peer tutoring, and reverse-role peer tutoring are reviewed here.

Classwide Peer Tutoring

The work of Greenwood and his associates at the Juniper Gardens Children's Project, as well as that of others, has demonstrated the consistent effectiveness of classwide peer tutoring (CWPT) in improving the academic performance of diverse groups of students (i.e., students with and without disabilities) and across a variety of settings and academic subjects (Arreaga-Mayer, 1998; Bell, Young, Blair, & Nelson, 1990; Butler, 1999; Cheung & Winter, 1999; DuPaul et al., 1998; Greenwood, 1991; Greenwood, Delquadri, & Hall, 1989; Maheady, Harper, & Sacca, 1988; Malone & McLaughlin, 1997; Mastropieri et al., 1999; Sideridis et al., 1997). CWPT was developed as an instructional approach to increase students' active engagement in learning, and, as its name suggests, the method actively involves all of the students in a given classroom. CWPT utilizes a competing teams and games format, but also involves the use of an explicit format for the presentation of material, contingent point earning, systematic error correction strategies, and public posting of student performance. This format serves to motivate and engage the students while also facilitating progress monitoring at the individual, dyad, team, and class levels (Malone & McLaughlin, 1997).

The following discussion of the procedures involved in implementing CWPT programs is based on descriptions in the research literature provided by Arreaga-Mayer (1998), Cheung and Winter (1999), DuPaul et al. (1998), Enright and Axelrod (1995), Mastropieri et al. (1999), and Sideridis et al. (1997), who have described how CWPT interventions are typically implemented. First, students are assigned to dyads (either randomly or on the basis of ability level). These dyads are divided into two teams, so that a classroom of 20 students would have 10 dyads divided into two teams of 5 dyads each. The first week of the program can be used as training time for students, so they can learn (through modeling, supervised practice, and feedback) how to award points, provide correction and feedback to tutees, and other rules of the "game." Once the training is over and all students understand the procedures, the CWPT method can be used as often as the teacher sees fit (typically 3 or 4 class days per week). Ongoing teacher supervision and feedback on students' adherence to procedures is critical in order to maintain the integrity and consistency of the intervention. Within a tutoring session, each student typically spends 10 minutes as tutor and 10 minutes as tutee, with 5 or 10 additional minutes allowed to compute and post team scores. For each daily tutoring session, all students know what material to cover, how to provide feedback for both correct and incorrect responses, and how to award and keep track of points for each session and for the entire week. For example, the tutor provides an item, then the tutee responds. If the response is correct, a certain number of points are awarded (typically two). If the response is incorrect, the tutor provides the correct response, asks the tutee to write and say the correct response three times, and gives the tutee a certain number of points for the correction (typically one). If the tutee still does not provide a correct response, then no points are awarded and the next item is presented. If the tutee completes the daily unit and time remains, the tutor starts over and presents the unit again until time runs out. Daily scores are computed for each dyad, and then for each team, based on the number of points each student earned within the time limit. At the end of the week, points are totaled and the team with the highest score is the winner; this team is awarded praise (e.g., applause from the other team) and a previously agreed-upon special privilege or prize. To ensure that all students have an opportunity to be on a winning team, the tutoring dyads should be changed every week. The teacher's role in implementing the CWPT program includes (1) determining what academic content will be used in the program, (2) organizing this content into daily and weekly units, (3) preparing materials for the students to use during the tutoring sessions (e.g., flash cards, questions, worksheets, figures), (4) designing materials for record keeping and for the daily posting of team scores, and (5) developing and administering pre- and posttests to determine the extent to which students have improved in their mastery of the content (Arreaga-Mayer, 1998). The teacher also can award bonus points to on-task dyads and verbal praise to both teams.

Cross-Age Tutoring

Cross-age tutoring typically involves the pairing of an older student possessing relatively advanced skills with a younger student deficient in some skill area or areas, although differences in skill levels are not necessary (Miller et al., 1994; Rekrut, 1994). Unlike the roles in classwide peer tutoring interventions, the roles in cross-age tutoring are fixed, with the older student consistently acting as tutor throughout the intervention.

Maher (1982, 1984, 1986) employed students with conduct disorders and behavior disorders as cross-age tutors with students identified as educable mentally retarded (EMR). The tutors in Maher's studies had been classified as socially maladjusted or emotionally disturbed; problem behaviors of the tutors included verbal and physical aggression, noncompliance, truancy, verbal abuse of teachers, and low academic performance. In these studies, the cross-age tutoring intervention involved tutors providing instruction to EMR elementary school students in a variety of academic areas. Following a 1-day training workshop, tutors met with their tutees twice weekly for 30 minutes, as well as once weekly with the tutees' teachers to construct a weekly instructional plan. In one of the studies, three 2-hour tutoring support conferences also took place during the intervention in order to provide tutors with feedback and allow an opportunity for them to discuss questions or concerns. The tutoring interventions continued for 10 weeks. Overall findings of these investigations suggest that tutors demonstrated positive changes in academic and social performance, measured by course grades and disciplinary referrals, respectively.

More recently, Cochran et al. (1993) demonstrated the efficacy of cross-age peer tutoring using African American male students with behavioral disorders and low levels of reading achievement as both tutors and tutees. Thus, the difference between tutors and tutees was not in ability or skill level, but in age only (tutors were in fifth grade, tutees were in second grade). The intervention began with a 5-day tutor training procedure, followed by an 8-week tutoring program that sought to improve the sight word recognition of tutors and tutees; there were a total of 32 tutoring sessions. The sessions consisted of tutors' review of the day's instructional content, formal delivery of instruction by tutors, review and practice of newly learned words, and testing on the words for that session; each session lasted approximately 30 minutes. Tutors and tutees were reinforced with verbal praise and stickers for demonstrating appropriate behaviors. The authors found that tutees learned a greater number of new words than did students in the comparison group, and that tutors also increased the number of words that they could correctly identify to a greater extent than did comparison students. Both tutors and tutees also showed improvements based on teacher-rated social skills, and reported positive feelings about the tutoring program. Interestingly, the intervention did not appear to influence participants' self-perceptions of social skills.

Kamps, Dugan, Potucek, and Collins (1999) also examined the effect of cross-age peer tutoring on tutees' sight word recognition skills, but these authors employed students with autism as tutors and normally functioning but academically delayed first graders as tutees. The training and intervention were similar to those used by Cochran et al. (1993) and by researchers implementing CWPT as described earlier. Results of the evaluation suggest that the intervention resulted in gains in sight word recognition among the first graders. Further, the students with autism appeared to implement the tutoring procedures with acceptable levels of fidelity and seemed to increase their levels of social interaction during free time while the intervention was in effect (though much variability was noted).

Although the conclusions that can be drawn from these studies are limited by small sample sizes, the provision of cross-age tutoring by students with conduct disorders and students with disabilities appears to promote enhanced academic and behavioral performance.

Reverse-Role Tutoring

Reverse-role tutoring is another form of tutoring shown to have positive outcomes for students with behavior disorders (Shisler, Osguthorpe, & Eiserman, 1987; Top & Osguthorpe, 1987). In reverse-role tutoring, students with disabilities or with behavior disorders act as tutors to nondisabled students. Reverse-role tutoring gives special education students an unaccustomed experience: that of providing academic assistance to nondisabled students. Shisler et al. (1987) looked exclusively at social outcome in their investigation of reverse-role tutoring and found that nondisabled tutees viewed their behaviorally disordered tutors significantly more positively following the tutoring intervention.

In the Top and Osguthorpe (1987) study, fourth- through sixth-grade students with behavior disorders and students with learning disabilities were paired with first graders to tutor during four weekly 15–20-minute sessions. The intervention was implemented for a total of 14 weeks. Following the intervention, reading achievement scores were significantly higher for both tutors and tutees, as compared with pretest scores and the performance of controls. Impressively, tutors with the lowest reading achievement scores made the most gains, and results suggest that students with disabilities can be trained to be effective tutors. The effects of the tutoring intervention on the self-esteem of tutors, however, were not conclusive; tutors' scores on self-report measures of general self-concept and self-esteem were not significantly different from pre- to posttreatment and did not differ from the scores of controls. However, anecdotal evidence from parents and teachers suggest that tutors' self-esteem did benefit from their participation in the intervention.

It is important to recognize that any form or program of peer tutoring can be "reverse-role" if the tutors are students with disabilities and the tutees are nondisabled. Thus, for example, it would be possible to develop a cross-age, reverse-role intervention. Moreover, numerous examples of students with disabilities or emotional or behavior disorders providing tutoring to *other* students with disabilities, disorders, or academic challenges are present in the literature (e.g., Houghton & Bain, 1993, who examined the effectiveness of peer tutoring using students for whom English was a second language as tutees and students with reading disabilities as tutors). This may be a more common condition than students with disabilities providing tutoring to nondisabled students (i.e., reverse-role tutoring).

The family of tutoring interventions appears quite promising, although special attention must be given to choosing which aggressive children may be trained as tutors and allowed access to younger or nonaggressive children. The research gives little guidance on this issue, which is obviously quite critical to successful implementation.

TIME-DELAY PROCEDURES

Cybriwsky and Schuster (1990) have noted, "Time delay is a method for transferring stimulus control by changing the temporal interval between the natural cue and the teacher's prompt" (p. 54). In their study, for example, the question "What is 9 × 5?" (natural cue) was immediately followed by the teacher-provided correct answer, "45" (controlling prompt). Eventually, a time delay between the question and teacher presentation of the answer was inserted, giving the student an opportunity to respond. According to Cybriwsky and Schuster (1990), the use of time-delay procedures with students typically experiencing academic failure may be especially beneficial. Students are likely to make fewer errors, because they are repeatedly presented with the correct answer before they attempt to answer the question independently. Time-delay procedures allow for the systematic introduction of teacher assistance and provide initial opportunities for students to perform successfully without making errors (Koscinski & Gast, 1993). This initial error-free responding is important in providing the student with a positive academic experience, as more opportunities for reinforcement are present and more positive teacher–student interactions are facilitated, and because frequent incorrect responses may be associated with increases in disruptive behavior (Heckaman, Alber, Hooper, & Heward, 1998).

Two main forms of time-delay procedures include constant time delay and progressive time delay. With constant time delay, the temporal delay between the teacher's question or request and the teacher's presentation of the prompt remains constant; with progressive time delay, the temporal delay gradually increases. The following sections include separate discussions of these types of time-delay procedures.

Constant Time Delay

According to Telecsan, Slaton, and Stevens (1999), constant time delay (CTD) "is a response-prompting procedure in which stimulus control is transferred from a controlling prompt to a natural stimulus by systematically delaying the prompt on the basis of time" (p. 135). Thus, in the initial stages of the procedure, a question or item is presented to the student, immediately followed by a prompt (i.e., some form of hint or assistance) from the teacher. This is called a 0-second-delay trial, because no time elapses between the presentation of the question and the presentation of the prompt. These 0-second trials are followed by trials in which the teacher presents the prompt after a specified amount of time has passed; these typically are 3-, 4-, or 5-second trials. During these longer trials, the length of which remains constant throughout the intervention (hence *constant* time delay), students may provide a response either before or after the prompt is presented. Eventually, stimulus control is transferred from the prompt to the task request, question, or item provided by the teacher (Schuster et al., 1998).

In an innovative study, Telecsan et al. (1999) combined reciprocal peer tutoring and constant-time-delay procedures, such that students with learning disabilities ($n = 6$) tutored one another in written spelling using CTD. According to the authors, the combination of these individually effective methods provided students with frequent opportunities to respond and with feedback on performance, while also meeting individual student needs in regard to instructional content. Following a rigorous tutor training sequence to ensure tutor competence and treatment fidelity, the authors implemented the peer tutoring plus CTD intervention. Students took turns delivering and receiving instruction in a manner similar to that described in the earlier section on peer tutoring, only in this intervention, the instruction was delivered by means of the CTD procedure. The use of CTD involved the tutor immediately providing a prompt following the request to spell the target word (i.e., 0-second trial) for the first ten trials of the tutoring session, and then waiting for 3 seconds before providing the prompt (i.e., 3-second trial) for the rest of the session. Thus, for the first 10 words, the tutee did not have an opportunity to respond without the assistance of the prompt, thereby maximizing the likelihood that the words included in these initial trials would be spelled correctly. The prompt consisted of the target word printed on a slip of paper. After these 0-second trials (and during the 3-second trials), the prompt was shown to students only when they did not initiate a written response during the 3-second interval or when they provided an incorrect response. During the 3-second trials, correct spelling before the prompt earned two points; correct spelling after the prompt earned one point. Thus, students were reinforced for correct responses provided independently.

Results of the Telecsan et al. (1999) study suggest that students can be successfully trained to implement time-delay procedures and that the intervention can assist students with learning disabilities (both tutors and tutees) to learn academic content. Similar positive results were reported by Wolery, Werts, Snyder, and Caldwell (1994), who successfully trained nondisabled tutors to use CTD procedures to improve the academic skills of tutees with severe disabilities.

Constant time delay has also been used to teach multiplication facts to students with learning disabilities (Koscinski & Gast, 1993; Morton & Flynt, 1997). Caldwell, Wolery, Werts, and Caldwell (1996) embedded a CTD procedure into independent seat work activities and found it useful in teaching students information about states and vocations, though there was much variability in outcome among students. CTD has been used to teach a variety of students both discrete and chained tasks, such as those that may be taught within a task analysis, and has generally been successful in teaching these skills (Schuster et al., 1998). This intervention seems to be both efficient in terms of required preparation time, and effective in terms of student outcomes (Koscinski & Gast, 1993).

Progressive Time Delay

Progressive time delay (PTD) is another method that purports to maximize the probability of correct responses. The strategy is similar to constant time delay, but differs in that with PTD, the time between presentation of the item, question, or request and presentation of the prompt is gradually increased over the course of the intervention, so that students are given longer opportunities to respond as they progress. As explained earlier, this time be-tween presentation of the request and prompt remains fixed over trials with CTD once the criterion for the 0-second trials have been met.

Heckaman et al. (1998) examined the effectiveness of a PTD interven-tion in reducing the disruptive behaviors of students with autism during in-struction of difficult tasks. The teacher began the intervention using 0-second-delay trials, so that the prompt was presented immediately after the task request. Once the predetermined initial criterion was met (which varied across students), the intervention progressed to 0.5-second-delay trials. The students moved into 1-, 2-, 3-, 4-, and 5-second-delay trials as they met the cri-terion (i.e., for all students, 90% accuracy on unprompted responses for two consecutive sessions) for each trial. For all trials, correct responses were fol-lowed by verbal praise and presentation of the next item, whereas incorrect responses were followed by a negative feedback statement and presentation of the prompt, and the previous delay level was used as the item was pre-sented again. The prompt was also presented when students failed to re-spond to items or when they demonstrated disruptive behaviors during the delay. Results suggest that the PTD method was consistently more effective than an alternative least-to-most prompting procedure in minimizing both the number of errors that students committed and the rate of disruptive behaviors per minute during intervention sessions.

PTD procedures have also been effectively employed in teaching pur-chasing skills and calculator use to high school students with mental retarda-tion (Frederick-Dugan, Test, & Varn, 1991), teaching elementary students with mental retardation to identify different types of groceries (Doyle, Schuster, & Meyer, 1996), teaching words and abbreviations to elementary students with learning disabilities (Ault, Wolery, Gast, Doyle, & Martin, 1990), teaching students with mental retardation to read words commonly found on important signs within the community (Ault, Gast, & Wolery, 1988), and teaching high school students with mental retardation to read words found within recipes (Gast, Doyle, Wolery, Ault, & Farmer, 1991).

Studies have generally concluded that PTD represents both an effective and an efficient intervention strategy, and one that can be implemented reli-ably. Ault et al. (1988) compared CTD and PTD procedures and found that PTD required somewhat more instructional time and more sessions to meet the trial criterion than CTD; results were mixed in regard to which method re-sulted in a greater number of errors and a higher percentage of errors before reaching the criterion. These findings, however, should be seen as tentative, and both procedures appear to be more efficient than other interventions.

MNEMONIC INSTRUCTION

Mnemonic instruction represents a collection of very well established aca-demic interventions. Mnemonic strategies often are used to assist students with memorization of words and their meanings by constructing meaningful relationships between concepts or words; mnemonic instruction has also been used to teach historical, mathematical, and scientific facts. Scruggs and Mastropieri (1990) defined a mnemonic as "a specific reconstruction of target content intended to tie new information more closely to the learner's existing knowledge base and, therefore, facilitate retrieval" (pp. 271–272). For example, the keyword method teaches students to associate the word to be learned with an easily pictured keyword. According to Mastropieri and Scruggs (1989),

> The keyword reconstructs unfamiliar verbal stimuli into acoustically similar representations, and elaborates the reconstructed stimuli with response information. For example, to learn that the scientific root *ornith-* means "bird," an acoustically similar keyword for *ornith* (oar) can be shown interacting with the response; in this case, a picture of a *bird* carrying an *oar*. Learners are told, for example, when asked for the meaning of *ornith-*, to think of the keyword, think of the picture with the keyword in it, remember what else was happening in the picture, and provide the correct response: bird. (p. 86)

The keyword technique for creating meaningful relationships and learning and remembering words has proven to be more effective than drill-and-practice methods for students with a variety of disabilities. Further, materials for implementing the keyword method can be developed independently by teachers, and both teachers and students seem to like the method and perceive it as beneficial (Mastropieri, Sweda, & Scruggs, 2000). Although some of the pictures and prose passages created with the keyword strategy have been quite complex and may represent multiple attributes of the word or concept to be learned, students have still been able to use the strategy successfully (Mastropieri & Scruggs, 1989).

Meaningful relationships between words or concepts can also be established through the use of symbolic and mimetic reconstructions in the absence of keywords. For example, historical facts and events may be learned by studying pictures in which these events are symbolically reconstructed, and relationships between concepts may be learned by studying mimetic pictures in which these concepts interact with one another (Mastropieri & Scruggs, 1989).

Acronyms and acrostics are familiar mnemonic devices. An example of using an acronym is the use of "HOMES to retrieve the names of the Great Lakes: Huron, Ontario, Michigan, Erie, and Superior"; an acrostic is a special case of an acronym in which the letters of the acronym are in a specific order, such as "Every Good Boy Deserves Fudge, to retrieve the names of the notes on the lines of the treble clef" (Scruggs & Mastropieri, 1990, p. 274). Thus, with the acronym, the first letters of the lakes can be arranged in any order that makes the most sense, whereas with the acrostic, the notes are already in a fixed sequence and the mnemonic device must be constructed in a way that incorporates this sequence.

Other mnemonic strategies have been evaluated, but a discussion of these is beyond the scope of this chapter. For excellent examples of different mnemonic techniques, readers are referred to Mastropieri and Scruggs (1989) and Scruggs and Mastropieri (1990). These reviews suggest that mnemonic instruction is one of the most powerful instructional interventions currently in use, though initially much time may be required to develop the necessary materials.

Recently, Greene (1999) compared mnemonic with traditional instruction in teaching difficult-to-memorize multiplication facts to elementary and middle school students with learning disabilities. The 14 facts (e.g., 4 x 4 = _, 8 x 9 = _) to be taught were presented with flashcards in either mnemonic or traditional form. The mnemonic form consisted of a picture representing the multiplication fact, in addition to the fact and answer written out in numeric form; the traditional form consisted simply of the multiplication fact and its answer. All students received both forms of instruction. The mnemonic illustrations were based on a system of pegwords (e.g., 4 = *door*, 6 = *sticks*) and pegword phrases (e.g., 54 = *gifty door*, 36 = *dirty sticks*) that were taught to the students as an additional source of assistance in memorizing the material. Results of immediate and delayed posttests suggest that although both forms of instruction led to recall of the facts, mnemonic instruction contributed more to retention than did traditional instruction. Additional recent studies have examined the use of mnemonic instruction to teach academic content to a variety of students, including teaching college students to recall artists' names when presented with paintings (Carney & Levin, 2000), teaching computational skills to students with learning disabilities in mathematics (Manalo, Bunnell, & Stillman, 2000), teaching social studies content (i.e., states and capitals) to middle school students with mild mental retardation, and science content (i.e., parts of the body) to high school students with mild mental retardation (Mastropieri, Scruggs, Whittaker, & Bakken, 1994), and teaching science content to middle school students with learning disabilities (Scruggs & Mastropieri, 1992).

SELF-MONITORING

Self-monitoring is a method by which students keep track of their own feelings and behaviors, with the notion that monitoring and paying attention to feelings and behaviors will lead to the reduction of undesirable behaviors and an increase in appropriate behaviors. For example, students can record the amount of time they were on task during a certain class period, or record the number of times per day that they felt angry, anxious, or depressed. Although self-monitoring has been widely used in the assessment of children's internalizing and externalizing problems, the method has also been used as an intervention for a variety of concerns, including academic skill problems and medical conditions (see Peterson & Tremblay, 1999, and Shapiro & Cole, 1999, for reviews). Procedures for monitoring academic performance can be comprehensive and complex, as they may include students setting goals, determining how to meet these goals, and, following an attempt, determining whether they have met their goals (Shapiro & Cole, 1999).

Dunlap et al. (1995) examined the use and effectiveness of a self-monitoring intervention on the academic engagement and disruptive behaviors of two elementary school students with emotional disturbance and behavioral disorders. Before the intervention was initiated, the students were trained to use the self-monitoring procedures. This training included an explanation of the forms to be used, in addition to definitions and examples of behaviors. The students were also asked to demonstrate that they understood the procedures and definitions of behaviors by classifying sample behaviors provided by the investigators; this evaluation indicated that the students understood the content adequately. Next, practice sessions were held in which the students implemented procedures identical to those implemented during the intervention, but during the practice sessions the students' use of the procedures was closely supervised to determine whether they could implement the procedures with fidelity. Once this determination was made, the actual intervention was implemented. The intervention involved the students making checkmarks on their self-monitoring forms every minute (for 15 minutes per session), during reading class for one student and during several different activities for the other student. An audiotape player played soft sounds at 1-minute intervals to remind the students to mark their sheets. Every minute, the students marked either "yes" or "no," based on their compliance with target behaviors such as remaining on task, asking for assistance in an appropriate manner, remaining in seat, remaining quiet, and providing appropriate verbal responses. The investigators also conducted independent observations during much of the sessions and found that the students' ratings of their own behavior very closely matched the observers' ratings of their behavior. Further, the students were reinforced for accurate self-monitoring. Results suggest that for both students, academic engagement was higher and disruptive behavior was lower during the self-monitoring sessions than during baseline conditions. The students also endorsed the benefits of the intervention.

Self-monitoring has been employed and evaluated as an intervention with numerous student populations for a variety of problems; results of these evaluations suggest that self-monitoring procedures can be used to improve skills and productivity in mathematics for adolescent students with learning disabilities (Maccini & Hughes, 1997), written spelling skills of elementary students (Okyere, Heron, & Goddard, 1997), on-task behavior of elementary students with ADHD who were receiving concurrent pharmacological treatment (Mathes & Bender, 1997), on-task behavior of adolescent students with learning disabilities and attention deficits (Dalton, Martella, & Marchand-Martella, 1999), and social skills of high school students with emotional or behavioral disorders (Moore, Cartledge, & Heckaman, 1995). Solley and

Payne (1992) provided a detailed description of a self-talk intervention aimed at improving students' writing skills, in addition to their attitudes toward writing.

In sum, self-monitoring interventions can be effective in decreasing maladaptive behaviors while increasing more positive behaviors. Anecdotal support from students, teachers, and parents often accompanies quantitative support in the literature. General considerations in maximizing the effectiveness of self-monitoring interventions include adequately training students in the self-monitoring procedures, designing the self-monitoring system to be very easy for the student to use and to minimize interference with daily routines, reinforcing accurate reporting, taking time to develop an accurate operational definition of the behavior(s) to be monitored, and recording the behavior as it occurs rather than retrospectively (Peterson & Tremblay, 1999).

ADDITIONAL INSTRUCTIONAL MODIFICATIONS

Although the preceding discussion has focused on specific academic and instructional interventions with aggressive students, more general instructional modifications have been recommended that may also serve to decrease the occurrence of problem behaviors within the classroom. These modifications include giving students choices of tasks whenever possible, facilitating high levels of student participation and student–teacher interactions, presenting a variety of tasks rather than constantly repeating tasks, presenting instruction at an appropriately rapid pace, incorporating demands that students are unlikely to meet successfully within a series of demands that students are highly likely to meet successfully, minimizing opportunities for incorrect responding and maximizing opportunities for accurate responding, and maximizing opportunities for reinforcement (Gettinger, 1995; Munk & Repp, 1994). Clearly, the specific interventions described herein make use of many of these recommendations. In particular, providing students with choices may be especially effective in reducing off-task behaviors and increasing academic engagement (Foster-Johnson, Ferro, & Dunlap, 1994); activity preference represents a promising intervention, and one that recently has received much interest on the part of researchers. Finally, the use of functional assessment may be especially useful in constructing valid and effective academic interventions (Dunlap, White, Vera, Wilson, & Panacek, 1996; Lee, Sugai, & Horner, 1999).

SUMMARY AND CONCLUSIONS

It is vital that aggressive students with concomitant academic difficulties receive some form of academic or instructional intervention that maximizes opportunities for success and reinforcement. Researchers and practitioners have suggested a number of academic and instructional interventions that may facilitate increased academic engagement and reduced problem behaviors of aggressive students. This review briefly considered the application of peer tutoring, time-delay procedures, mnemonic instruction, and self-monitoring to the academic difficulties experienced by aggressive students. Each of these interventions appears to hold significant promise for enhancing the behavior and academic performance of aggressive students.

Unfortunately, there are numerous interacting etiological factors, in addition to academic problems, that contribute to the development of aggression in children and adolescents (i.e., there are aggressive students who do not experience academic difficulties, and students who do experience academic difficulties who are not aggressive). This reality helps us to understand that academic interventions are but one set of tools for the reduction of aggressive behavior. Behavioral strategies and interventions that focus on the development of prosocial skills and adaptive responses have also proliferated. Because aggressive students often have both academic and behavioral difficulties, the study of interventions that combine behavioral and academic components (and others, such as cognitive and family-based components, where appropriate) seem to be especially useful. Multicomponent, comprehensive interventions that address both students' aggression *and* academic difficulties across settings will likely be more powerful and effective than single, narrowly focused interventions (Dunlap et al., 1996; Hinshaw, 1992). Similarly, the combination of the academic and instructional interventions discussed here (e.g., time delay with peer tutoring) should be evaluated further, as this combination may lead to more effective interventions. An additional area of future investigation is research examining which methods work for whom (i.e., specific populations) and which methods may have to be modified (and in what way) in order to work for different populations.

Interestingly, McEvoy and Welker (2000) noted that "*any* academic intervention with antisocial students is likely to have prosocial effects if it functions to establish appropriate bonds between students and their mentors" (p. 131). Although the importance of positive student–teacher relationships to children's adjustment has been demonstrated (see Pianta, 1999), research examining the extent to which these relationships may be enhanced through academic and instructional interventions (i.e., as an "added benefit" of these interventions) would be helpful in making the rationale and justification for these interventions even stronger, and their value more undeniable.

REFERENCES

Arreaga-Mayer, C. (1998). Increasing active student responding and improving academic performance through classwide peer tutoring. *Intervention in School and Clinic, 34,* 89–94, 117.

Ault, M. J., Gast, D. L., & Wolery, M. (1988). Comparison of progressive and constant time-delay procedures in teaching community-sign word reading. *American Journal on Mental Retardation, 93,* 44–56.

Ault, M. J., Wolery, M., Gast, D. L., Doyle, P. M., & Martin, C. P. (1990). Comparison of predictable and unpredictable trial sequences during small-group instruction. *Learning Disability Quarterly, 13,* 12–29.

Bell, K., Young, K. R., Blair, M., & Nelson, R. (1990). Facilitating mainstreaming of students with behavioral disorders using classwide peer tutoring. *School Psychology Review, 19,* 564–573.

Butler, F. M. (1999). Reading partners: Students can help each other learn to read! *Education and Treatment of Children, 22,* 415–426.

Caldwell, N. K., Wolery, M., Werts, M. G., & Caldwell, Y. (1996). Embedding instructive feedback into teacher-student interactions during independent seat work. *Journal of Behavioral Education, 6,* 459–480.

Carney, R. N., & Levin, J. R. (2000). Mnemonic instruction, with a focus on transfer. *Journal of Educational Psychology, 92,* 783–790.

Carpenter, C. D., Bloom, L. A., & Boat, M. B. (1999). Guidelines for special educators: Achieving socially valid outcomes. *Intervention in School and Clinic, 34,* 143–149.

Cheung, C. C., & Winter, S. (1999). Classwide peer tutoring with or without reinforcement: Effects on academic responding, content coverage, achievement, intrinsic interest and reported project experiences. *Educational Psychology, 19,* 191–205.

Cochran, L., Feng, H., Cartledge, G., & Hamilton, S. (1993). The effects of cross-age tutoring on the academic achievement, social behaviors, and self-perceptions of low-achieving African-American males with behavioral disorders. *Behavioral Disorders, 18,* 292–302.

Cybriwsky, C., & Schuster, J. W. (1990). Using constant time delay procedures to teach multiplication facts. *Remedial and Special Education, 11,* 54–59.

Dalton, T., Martella, R. C., & Marchand-Martella, N. E. (1999). The effects of a self-management program in reducing off-task behavior. *Journal of Behavioral Education, 9,* 157–176.

Doyle, P. M., Schuster, J. W., & Meyer, S. (1996). Embedding extra stimuli in the task direction: Effects on learning of students with moderate mental retardation. *Journal of Special Education, 29,* 381–399.

Dunlap, G., Clarke, S., Jackson, M., Wright, S., Ramos, E., & Brinson, S. (1995). Self-monitoring of classroom behaviors with students exhibiting emotional and behavioral challenges. *School Psychology Quarterly, 10,* 165–177.

Dunlap, G., White, R., Vera, A., Wilson, D., & Panacek, L. (1996). The effects of multi-component, assessment-based curricular modifications on the classroom behavior of children with emotional and behavioral disorders. *Journal of Behavioral Education, 6,* 481–500.

DuPaul, G. J., & Eckert, T. L. (1998). Academic interventions for students with attention-deficit/hyperactivity disorder: A review of the literature. *Reading and Writing Quarterly: Overcoming Learning Difficulties, 14,* 59–82.

DuPaul, G. J., Ervin, R. A., Hook, C. L., & McGoey, K. E. (1998). Peer tutoring for children with attention deficit hyperactivity disorder: Effects on classroom behavior and academic performance. *Journal of Applied Behavior Analysis, 31,* 579–592.

Elliott, S. N., Busse, R. T., & Shapiro, E. S. (1999). Intervention techniques for academic performance problems. In C. R. Reynolds & T. B. Gutkin (Eds.), *Handbook of school psychology* (3rd ed., pp. 664–685). New York: Wiley.

Enright, S. M., & Axelrod, S. (1995). Peer-tutoring: Applied behavior analysis working in the classroom. *School Psychology Quarterly, 10,* 29–40.

Foster-Johnson, L., Ferro, J., & Dunlap, G. (1994). Preferred curricular activities and reduced problem behaviors in students with intellectual disabilities. *Journal of Applied Behavior Analysis, 27,* 493–504.

Franca, V. M., Kerr, M. M., Reitz, A. L., & Lambert, D. (1990). Peer tutoring among behaviorally disordered students: Academic and social benefits to tutor and tutee. *Education and Treatment of Children, 13,* 109–128.

Frederick-Dugan, A., Test, D. W., & Varn, L. (1991). Acquisition and generalization of purchasing skills using a calculator by students who are mentally retarded. *Education and Training in Mental Retardation, 26,* 381–387.

Gagnon, W. A., & Conoley, J. C. (1997). Academic and curriculum interventions with aggressive youths. In A. P. Goldstein & J. C. Conoley (Eds.), *School violence intervention: A practical handbook* (pp. 217–235). New York: Guilford Press.

García-Vázquez, E., & Ehly, S. (1995). Best practices in facilitating peer tutoring programs. In A. Thomas & J. Grimes (Eds.), *Best practices in school psychology—III* (pp. 403–411). Washington, DC: National Association of School Psychologists.

Gardner, R., Cartledge, G., Seidl, B., Woolsey, M. L., Schley, G. S., & Utley, C. A. (2001). Mt. Olivet after-school program: Peer-mediated interventions for at-risk students. *Remedial and Special Education, 22,* 22–33.

Gast, D. L., Doyle, P. M., Wolery, M., Ault, M. J., & Farmer, J. A. (1991). Assessing the acquisition of incidental information by secondary-age students with mental retardation: Comparison of response prompting strategies. *American Journal on Mental Retardation, 96,* 63–80.

Gettinger, M. (1995). Best practices for increasing academic learning time. In A. Thomas & J. Grimes (Eds.), *Best practices in school psychology—III* (pp. 943–954). Washington, DC: National Association of School Psychologists.

Gordon, J., Vaughn, S., & Schumm, J. S. (1993). Spelling interventions: A review of literature and implications for instruction for students with learning disabilities. *Learning Disabilities Research and Practice, 8,* 175–181.

Greene, G. (1999). Mnemonic multiplication fact instruction for students with learning disabilities. *Learning Disabilities Research and Practice, 14,* 141–148.

Greenwood, C. R. (1991). Classwide peer tutoring: Longitudinal effects on the reading, language, and mathematics achievement of at-risk students. *Reading, Writing, and Learning Disabilities, 7,* 105–123.

Greenwood, C. R. (1996). The case for performance-based instructional models. *School Psychology Quarterly, 11,* 283–296.

Greenwood, C. R., Carta, J. J., & Maheady, L. (1991). Peer tutoring programs in the regular education classroom. In G. Stoner, M. R. Shinn, & H. M. Walker (Eds.), *Interventions for achievement and behavior problems* (pp. 179–200). Washington, DC: National Association of School Psychologists.

Greenwood, C. R., Delquadri, J. C., & Hall, R. V. (1989). Longitudinal effects of classwide peer tutoring. *Journal of Educational Psychology, 81,* 371–383.

Greenwood, C. R., Terry, B., Arreaga-Mayer, C., & Finney, R. (1992). The classwide peer-tutoring program: Implementation factors moderating students' achievement. *Journal of Applied Behavior Analysis, 25,* 101–116.

Heckaman, K. A., Alber, S., Hooper, S., & Heward, W. L. (1998). A comparison of least-to-most prompts and progressive time delay on the disruptive behavior of students with autism. *Journal of Behavioral Education, 8,* 171–201.

Herrenkohl, T. I., Maguin, E., Hill, K. G., Hawkins, J. D., Abbott, R. D., & Catalano, R. F. (2000). Developmental risk factors for youth violence. *Journal of Adolescent Health, 26,* 176–186.

Hinshaw, S. P. (1992). Academic underachievement, attention deficits, and aggression: Comorbidity and implications for intervention. *Journal of Consulting and Clinical Psychology, 60,* 893–903.

Houghton, S., & Bain, A. (1993). Peer tutoring with ESL and below-average readers. *Journal of Behavioral Education, 3,* 125–142.

Kamps, D. M., Dugan, E., Potucek, J., & Collins, A. (1999). Effects of cross-age peer tutoring networks among students with autism and general education students. *Journal of Behavioral Education, 9,* 97–115.

Koscinski, S. T., & Gast, D. L. (1993). Use of constant time delay in teaching multiplication facts to students with learning disabilities. *Journal of Learning Disabilities, 26,* 533–544, 567.

Lalli, J. S., Kates, K., & Casey, S. D. (1999). Response covariation: The relationship between correct academic responding and problem behavior. *Behavior Modification, 23,* 339–357.

Lee, Y., Sugai, G., & Horner, R. H. (1999). Using an instructional intervention to reduce problem and off-task behaviors. *Journal of Positive Behavior Interventions, 1,* 195–204.

Lentz, F. E., Allen, S. J., & Ehrhardt, K. E. (1996). The conceptual elements of strong interventions in school settings. *School Psychology Quarterly, 11,* 118–136.

Maccini, P., & Hughes, C. A. (1997). Mathematics interventions for adolescents with learning disabilities. *Learning Disabilities Research and Practice, 12,* 168–176.

Maheady, L., Harper, G. F., & Mallette, B. (2001). Peer-mediated instruction and interventions and students with mild disabilities. *Remedial and Special Education, 22,* 4–14.

Maheady, L., Harper, G. F., & Sacca, K. (1988). A classwide peer tutoring system in a secondary resource room program for the mildly handicapped. *Journal of Research and Development in Education, 21,* 76–83.

Maher, C. A. (1982). Behavioral effects of using conduct problem adolescents as cross-age tutors. *Psychology in the Schools, 19,* 360–364.

Maher, C. A. (1984). Handicapped adolescents as cross-age tutors: Program description and evaluation. *Exceptional Children, 51,* 56–63.

Maher, C. A. (1986). Direct replication of a cross-age tutoring program involving handicapped adolescents and children. *School Psychology Review, 15,* 100–118.

Malone, R. A., & McLaughlin, T. F. (1997). The effects of reciprocal peer tutoring with a group contingency on quiz performance in vocabulary with seventh- and eighth-grade students. *Behavioral Interventions, 12,* 27–40.

Manalo, E., Bunnell, J. K., & Stillman, J. A. (2000). The use of process mnemonics in teaching students with mathematics learning disabilities. *Learning Disability Quarterly, 23,* 137–156.

Mastropieri, M. A., Leinart, A., & Scruggs, T. E. (1999). Strategies to increase reading fluency. *Intervention in School and Clinic, 34,* 278–283, 292.

Mastropieri, M. A., & Scruggs, T. E. (1989). Constructing more meaningful relationships: Mnemonic instruction for special populations. *Educational Psychology Review, 1,* 83–111.

Mastropieri, M. A., Scruggs, T. E., Whittaker, M. E. S., & Bakken, J. P. (1994). Applications of mnemonic strategies with students with mild mental disabilities. *Remedial and Special Education, 15,* 34–43.

Mastropieri, M. A., Sweda, J., & Scruggs, T. E. (2000). Putting mnemonic strategies to work in an inclusive classroom. *Learning Disabilities Research and Practice, 15,* 69–74.

Mathes, M. Y., & Bender, W. N. (1997). The effects of self-monitoring on children with attention-deficit/hyperactivity disorder who are receiving pharmacological interventions. *Remedial and Special Education, 18,* 121–128.

McEvoy, A., & Welker, R. (2000). Antisocial behavior, academic failure, and school climate: A critical review. *Journal of Emotional and Behavioral Disorders, 8,* 130–140.

Miller, A. D., Barbetta, P. M., & Heron, T. E. (1994). START tutoring: Designing, training, implementing, adapting, and evaluating tutoring programs for school and home settings. In R. Gardner, D. M. Sainato, J. O. Cooper, T. E. Heron, W. L. Heward, J. W. Eshleman, & T. A. Grossi (Eds.), *Behavior analysis in education: Focus on measurably superior instruction* (pp. 265–282). Pacific Grove, CA: Brooks/Cole.

Moore, R. J., Cartledge, G., & Heckaman, K. (1995). The effects of social skill instruction and self-monitoring on game-related behaviors of adolescents with emotional or behavioral disorders. *Behavioral Disorders, 20,* 253–266.

Morton, R. C., & Flynt, S. W. (1997). A comparison of constant time delay and prompt fading to teach multiplication facts to students with learning disabilities. *Journal of Instructional Psychology, 24,* 3–13.

Munk, D. D., & Repp, A. C. (1994). The relationship between instructional variables and problem behavior: A review. *Exceptional Children, 60,* 390–401.

Okyere, B. A., Heron, T. E., & Goddard, Y. (1997). Effects of self-correction on the acquisition, maintenance, and generalization of the written spelling of elementary school children. *Journal of Behavioral Education, 7,* 51–69.

Peterson, L., & Tremblay, G. (1999). Self-monitoring in behavioral medicine: Children. *Psychological Assessment, 11,* 458–465.

Pianta, R. C. (1999). *Enhancing relationships between children and teachers.* Washington, DC: American Psychological Association.

Prehm, H. J. (1976). Learning performance of handicapped students. *High School Journal, 59,* 275–281.

Rekrut, M. D. (1994). Peer and cross-age tutoring: The lessons of research. *Journal of Reading, 37,* 356–362.

Roswal, G. M., Mims, A. A., Evans, M. D., Smith, B., Young, M., Burch, M., Croce, R., Horvat, M. A., & Block, M. (1995). Effects of collaborative peer tutoring on urban seventh graders. *Journal of Educational Research, 88,* 275–279.

Saner, H., & Ellickson, P. (1996). Concurrent risk factors for adolescent violence. *Journal of Adolescent Health, 19,* 94–103.

Schuster, J. W., Morse, T. E., Ault, M. J., Doyle, P. M., Crawford, M. R., & Wolery, M. (1998). Constant time delay with chained tasks: A review of the literature. *Education and Treatment of Children, 21,* 74–106.

Scruggs, T. E., & Mastropieri, M. A. (1990). Mnemonic instruction for students with learning disabilities: What it is and what it does. *Learning Disability Quarterly, 13,* 271–280.

Scruggs, T. E., & Mastropieri, M. A. (1992). Classroom applications of mnemonic instruction: Acquisition, maintenance, and generalization. *Exceptional Children, 58,* 219–229.

Scruggs, T. E., Mastropieri, M. A., Veit, D. T., & Osguthorpe, R. T. (1986). Behaviorally disordered students as tutors: Effects on social behavior. *Behavioral Disorders, 12,* 36–44.

Scruggs, T. E., & Richter, L. (1988). Tutoring learning disabled students: A critical review. *Learning Disability Quarterly, 11,* 274–286.

Shapiro, E. S., & Cole, C. L. (1999). Self-monitoring in assessing children's problems. *Psychological Assessment, 11,* 448–457.

Shisler, L., Osguthorpe, R. T., & Eiserman, W. D. (1987). The effects of reverse-role tutoring on the social acceptance of students with behavioral disorders. *Behavioral Disorders, 13,* 35–44.

Sideridis, G. D., Utley, C., Greenwood, C. R., Delquadri, J., Dawson, H., Palmer, P., & Reddy, S. (1997). Classwide peer tutoring: Effects on the spelling performance and social interactions of students with mild disabilities and their typical peers in an integrated instructional setting. *Journal of Behavioral Education, 7,* 435–462.

Solley, B. A., & Payne, B. D. (1992). The use of self-talk to enhance children's writing. *Journal of Instructional Psychology, 19,* 205–213.

Stahl, N. D., & Clarizio, H. F. (1999). Conduct disorder and comorbidity. *Psychology in the Schools, 36,* 41–50.

Telecsan, B. L., Slaton, D. B., & Stevens, K. B. (1999). Peer tutoring: Teaching students with learning disabilities to deliver time delay instruction. *Journal of Behavioral Education, 9,* 133–154.

Top, B. L., & Osguthorpe, R. T. (1987). Reverse-role tutoring: The effects of handicapped students tutoring regular class students. *Elementary School Journal, 87,* 413–423.

Wolery, M., Werts, M. G., Snyder, E. D., & Caldwell, N. K. (1994). Efficacy of constant time delay implemented by peer tutors in general education classrooms. *Journal of Behavioral Education, 4,* 415–436.

CHAPTER 11

The Safe School

Integrating the School Reform Agenda
to Prevent Disruption and Violence at School

GALE M. MORRISON
MICHAEL J. FURLONG
BARBARA D'INCAU
RICHARD L. MORRISON

It is the goal of public schools to provide a safe environment where all students can be educated to their potential. In the late 1980s and through the mid-1990s, there was an increase in the level of lethal violence involving adolescents (see Furlong, Jimenez, & Saxton, 2003). Not coincidentally, it was during this time that the National School Safety Center and the United States Office of Education began to monitor news reports to document the number of violent deaths that occurred on school campuses and at school-related events. In 1992–1993, the first year that records were kept, there were 41 school-associated homicides involving students under the age of 19 (National School Safety Center, 2001). The time between 1993 and 2001 witnessed a series of shootings on school campuses by students that resulted in multiple deaths and injuries, most notably, of course, the 15 deaths that occurred at Columbine High School in 1999. What is less well recognized is that despite the increased public concern about youth violence generally, and specifically about school shooting tragedies, in more recent years student-involved school homicides actually decreased by 73% between 1993 and 2001 (from 41 to 11 homicides).

The occurrence of these notable events on school campuses has evoked responses from all sectors of society—for example, public health, law enforcement, politicians. Although the urge to react quickly to the perceived danger these events pose to school campuses is understandable, we argue that it is

also important to consider how these responses can be meaningfully integrated into the general mission of schools to promote student competence in
academic knowledge, personal-social skills, physical wellness, and vocational
preparation. Integrating school violence prevention and intervention efforts
into ongoing school improvement initiatives will ensure more seamless, long-
lasting violence prevention efforts (Furlong & Morrison, 2000).

This chapter provides a perspective for educators on ways to think about
and create safe school environments for all students within the context of the
overall school mission. We describe the process of reframing the issue of
school violence as one of school safety. As school safety is an educational issue, we link the critical risk, resilience, and safety concepts to the more common educational language of school effectiveness and reform. We emphasize
the premise that for lasting change toward safe schools, safety and prevention concepts must be integrated into the fabric of the primary school
mission.

HISTORICAL CONTEXT LEADING TO EDUCATORS' CONCERN ABOUT SCHOOL SAFETY

The past 30 years have seen an ebb and flow of concern and conceptualization about the issue of school violence. Ways of thinking about school violence depend on the origin of the perspective—for instance, its etiology and
preferred responses vary by perspectives given in the popular media or professional literatures (e.g., juvenile justice, law, and health professions;
Brener, Simon, Krug, & Lowry, 1999; Callahan & Rivara, 1992; Kann et al.,
1995). In the past the concerns of these groups and their particular brands
of solutions were imposed on the schooling institutions, often without much
thought to integrating education and violence prevention efforts into the
broader educational mission (Furlong & Morrison, 2000).

Although educators recognize that they must contribute to the public
discussion about school violence by advocating their unique perspective,
their overall efforts remain fragmented, often reactive to specific school
shootings, and may not be fully integrated into the high-priority school restructuring efforts that often focus primarily on academic reforms. Educators realize that schools are protective settings in many youths' lives. Schools
are quite safe when the levels of on-school-campus violence are compared
with the levels of violence occurring in the communities they serve (Hyman,
Weller, Shanock, & Britton, 1995; Morrison, Furlong, & Morrison, 1994;
United States Departments of Education and Justice, 2000). However, violence does occur on campuses, and educators must (1) first recognize that it
happens, (2) accept responsibility for it, and (3) then implement comprehensive programs to reduce its incidence. Part of education's response to school
violence is to recognize that the National Education Goals Panel (2001) and
the general public hold schools to a higher standard in matters involving vio-

lence. This concern about school violence does not necessarily reflect a lack of confidence in schools, but the public's desire that schools be places where no harm will come to any child—something that is expected in no other major social setting. Stated positively, schools are seen as places where children will be supported and nurtured, and where their development will be fostered.

In 1995, the California School Board Association acknowledged that school violence involves aggressive physical behavior accompanied with the intent to harm, as well as criminal acts of assault, battery, homicide, robbery, extortion, and weapons possession. More recently, state laws have acknowledged the seriousness of threats and less obvious forms of aggression as acts that merit disciplinary action (e.g., California Education Code includes offenses such as terrorist threats, sexual harassment, and intimidation of a witness of school rule breaking). A more inclusive definition of school violence has evolved, emphasizing that violence and disruption come from a variety of sources: Youth who engage in chronic antisocial behavior who often exhibit lifelong developmental trajectories, increasing in severity across time (e.g., Loeber, Farrington, & Waschbusch, 1993; Moffitt, 1993); perpetrators who have a history of being involved in school bullying (Fein & Vossekuil, 1995; Reddy et al., 2001); and incidents of low-level teasing, bullying, and other physical intimidation that limit the schools' capacity to build positive, supportive relationships with students (Furlong, Pavelski, & Morrison, 2000). This broader view of school violence is closely linked to national efforts to increase multilevel prevention programs that offer a continuum of prevention and intervention strategies (Dwyer & Osher, 2000).

Because extreme forms of violence occur infrequently on school campuses, there is sometimes a tendency to take a "wait-until-it-happens" approach. In contrast, the tragic events at Columbine High School have also spawned reactions that take an "it-can-happen-anywhere" approach, inappropriately resulting in the public's belief that school shootings are now "likely" to occur anywhere. A potential danger of this perspective is that it may also lead to the imposition of extremely harsh policies and discipline practices that can harm a school's climate (Morrison & D'Incau, 1997; Skiba & Peterson, 1999). This possibility is seen in the zero tolerance policies that have proliferated in schools since the passage of the Gun-Free School Act in 1994. Nonetheless, a benefit of this change in the school violence psychological landscape is that it has generated awareness and action. Federal and state governments have increased support significantly for safe and drug-free school activities. Perspectives that expand school violence to include various forms of psychological attacks, verbal assaults, and bullying behavior, better position educators to define the problem in ways that are preventive in schools, to implement programs that are consistent with the schools' educational mission (Furlong & Morrison, 2000; Morrison et al., 1994), and to cease simple reactions to broader juvenile justice and public health initiatives.

In summary, the history of professional orientations, assessments, and suggested solutions to school violence have historically been multidisciplinary, with the education profession slowly recognizing school safety as an educational problem. Nonetheless, there are benefits to this multidisciplinary approach because it enriches schools' efforts to act on crises as they occur and to protect students and school personnel from violent acts. It is critical that schools work with community law enforcement and justice systems to facilitate crisis prevention and intervention. Most important, however, the threat of violence to the disruption of schooling functions requires a comprehensive, educator-based response to ensure safe environments for learning.

SAFETY AS AN EDUCATIONAL ISSUE

School safety is more than the absence of violence—it is an educational right. A safe school limits the incidents of threat *and* curtails the incidence of violence and is one that allows for maximum growth and development of students. To understand this perspective, the meaning of safety needs exploration and application to professional perspectives that are familiar to educators in the schooling process. This topic has been discussed at greater length (Morrison et al., 1994); therefore, we provide two discussions of school violence "reframing" here: (1) an assessment of different kinds of safety and harm and (2) an examination of the frames provided by the developmental and educational perspectives on prevention and school effectiveness, respectively.

"Safety" is defined as freedom from danger, harm, or loss. A close companion term, "security" is defined as freedom from anxiety or apprehension of danger or risk. Although these terms are commonly associated with the physical harm resulting from violence, harm is also caused by anxiety or apprehension about impending harm, constituting *psychological* harm. Teachers and support personnel in schools are familiar with the disruption and harm caused by schoolyard bullies. Intimidation from bullies causes psychological harm not only to victims but also to bystanders (Batsche & Knoff, 1994; Besag, 1989).

In addition to psychological harm, bullying, or other situations in which there is a threat of harm, may also cause *developmental* harm; that is, anxiety about threats of harm can disrupt the educational process. Developmental harm has been defined as "harm that occurs due to events or conditions that prevent or inhibit children from achieving their maximum physical, social or academic potential" (Morrison et al., 1994, p. 241). Harm resulting in a disruption of the educational process places safety squarely in the realm of educational concerns. Educators cannot ignore developmental harm and should respond in ways to ensure that learning processes continue by understanding and acting to reduce the presence of such threats. Even verbal abuse and taunting threatens a school's capacity to provide positive, inclusive connections with students, thereby diminishing its role as a potential protective influence for its students.

SCHOOL VIOLENCE AND SCHOOL SAFETY IN THE CONTEXT OF DEVELOPMENTAL RISK AND RESILIENCE

An expanded view of safety—going beyond the absence of crime and violence and including the existence of factors that allow for psychological safety and developmental growth—is similar to concepts of *risk* and *resilience*. These are terms that, in the context of research and practice, were first attached to concepts in developmental psychopathology, based on early work by Garmezy and his colleagues (Garmezy, 1983; Garmezy, Masten, & Tellegen, 1984; Rutter, 1990). Garmezy (1983) defined *risk factors* as those associated with the increased likelihood of an individual's developing an emotional or behavioral disorder, in comparison with a randomly selected person from the general population. The constellation of risk factors includes characteristics of children themselves, as well as situations in their families, schools, and communities, that may act as stumbling blocks to their positive development and adjustment. In safety terms, the environment essentially imposes risk; that is, the risk of school violence increases the likelihood of negative educational outcomes for students. We (Morrison et al., 1994) have delineated a risk continuum that ranges from physical well-being threats to conditions in the school environment that impede maximum learning.

The schooling process can lead to significant risks that deter student development and adjustment. At the individual level, school failure is a strong correlate of later psychological disturbance, delinquency, substance abuse, and dropout (Cernkovich & Giordano, 1992; Gold & Osgood, 1992; Hawkins & Lishner, 1987; Roff, Sells, & Golden, 1972; Walker, Colvin, & Ramsey, 1995). In this chapter, we focus on specific aspects of schools that put students at risk above and beyond their individual, familial, and societal risk features, thus emphasizing the *school* component in school violence (Furlong & Morrison, 2000). For example, schools as institutions may negatively affect students. In its extreme, Epp and Watkinson (1997) have referred to this negative effect as "systemic violence": "Systemic violence has been defined as any institutional practice or procedure that adversely impacts on individuals or groups by burdening them psychologically, mentally, culturally, spiritually, economically, or physically. Applied to education, it means practices and procedures that prevent students from learning, thus harming them" (p. 1). Examples of systemic violence include, but are not limited to, exclusionary practices, overcompetitive learning environments, toleration of abuse, school disciplinary policies rooted in exclusion and punishment, discriminatory guidance policies, and the like.

The companion concept, *resilience*, captures the aspect of safety upon which educators must base their response to school violence. Garmezy and Masten (1991) define resilience as "a process of, or capacity for, or the outcome of successful adaptation despite challenging and threatening circumstances" (p. 159). A companion term for this concept is *protective factors*, indicating mechanisms that act as the counterparts to risk factors. Garmezy (1983) has categorized protective factors into (1) child characteristics, such as positive temperament and social competence, (2) a supportive family milieu, including supportive parent(s) and consistent rule setting, and (3) community factors, including positive relationships with significant adults and positive school environments.

In the case of the distinction between school violence and school safety, the challenge is to offset the risks of violence with the protective factors present in a "safe school." Knowing about general categories of protective factors can guide intervention efforts toward a safe school. The work of Hawkins and his colleagues (Hawkins, Catalano, & Miller, 1992; Hawkins, Lishner, Catalano, & Howard, 1985) has identified protective factors in the prevention of substance abuse, which include (1) bonding (attachment, commitment, and belief) to family, school, and community, (2) environments with norms opposed to substance abuse, (3) acquisition of skills to live according to these norms (such as resistance and refusal skills), and (4) the existence of opportunities to be successful in and rewarded for making positive contributions. Brown, D'Emidio-Caston, and Bernard (2001) have applied these concepts specifically to educational environments and have delineated the individual resilience categories as social competence, problem-solving skills, autonomy, and sense of purpose. In addition, they describe the protective mechanisms of schools, families, and communities as including the functions of caring and support, high/positive expectations, and opportunities for participation. Garbarino (1992) notes that schools are a major source of continuity for children and represent a secondary caregiving and learning environment that can play a vital protective role in their lives, particularly in regard to the provision of a predictable environment with consistently enforced standards, rules, and responsibilities and an overall positive school climate as a context for growth and development.

CONCEPTUAL DISTINCTIONS OF RISK AND RESILIENCE THAT INFORM SCHOOL SAFETY INTERVENTIONS

The mechanisms by which protective factors interact with or counteract risk factors are important to understand in relation to intervention efforts. Various models propose to explain the relationship between these two types of factors (Zimmerman & Arunkumar, 1994). Although some research supports each of these models, using a variety of factors and outcomes (Garmezy, 1983; Garmezy et al., 1984; Sameroff, Seifer, Baldwin, & Baldwin, 1993), how this relationship is defined determines the approach to intervention (Masten, 2001).

For example, Garmezy et al. (1984) describe a *compensatory model*, in which protective factors have the same effect at all levels of risk. For example, given a range of socioeconomic levels, intellectual competence should contribute equally to later academic outcomes. In the case of school violence and safety, interventions aimed at making the school "safe" should be equally beneficial to all children. The preferred approach, then, would be to target the entire population of students with safe school programming. Such programming would be considered a compensatory strategy in this model. This approach is referred to as "primary prevention." This level of intervention has been labeled "universal" intervention by professionals in the prevention area (Brock, 2000) and constitutes the schoolwide or Level I strategies discussed by Dwyer and Osher (2000) in the federal safe schools action guide.

Garmezy et al. (1984) also considered protective factors in interaction with risk factors. The *protective model* suggests that protective factors modulate or buffer the impact of stressors by improving coping, adaptation, and competence in individuals who are specifically at risk for negative outcomes. In this model, school safety interventions are restricted to those who are considered at risk for aggression or victimization. This approach is considered "secondary prevention" and encompasses "selected" interventions with fewer students, or Level II responses in Dwyer and Osher's (2000) discussion.

A more *intensive approach* would be used to intervene with a relatively small number of high-risk students and situations in which school violence has already occurred. In this case, schools must intervene with students who have already been victimized or were the perpetrators of the violence. This is "tertiary" or Level III (Dwyer & Osher, 2000) prevention, which involves broader, intensive school–community efforts to intervene with students and their families who are experiencing significant life troubles and challenges.

The most effective violence prevention programs are those that combine a number of strategies and approach the task in a comprehensive manner (Dwyer & Osher, 2000), including efforts made at the community, school, and individual levels. For example, Cunningham and Henggeler (2001) have built upon their *Multisystemic Therapy* model by integrating it into a school-based program that includes other prevention efforts such as a bullying prevention program. The original conceptualizations of the distinctions between primary, secondary, and tertiary prevention efforts have also been applied to interventions with students with emotional and behavior problems (Sugai, Sprague, Horner, & Walker, 2000; Walker & Sprague, 1999). The emphasis of this application is on the necessity of matching the intensity and nature of the intervention with the target population—all students, those who are at risk for behavioral and emotional problems, and those who display chronic and intense problem behavior. Furlong et al. (2000) outline the school relationship obligations for each of these target groups. For most students, schools need to *reaffirm* the students' relationship to the school by providing opportunities to participate and learn new skills. In addition, these efforts should be positively recognized by the school. For students who are at risk for academic and social problems, schools need to focus on *reconnecting*. These students may require different strategies for participation, skill acquisition, and recognition. Finally, for students whose relationship with the school is severely disrupted, the focus should be on *reconstructing* relationships through distinctly different and individualized opportunities and recognition.

Another conceptual argument with relevance for this application of prevention concepts to the school safety construct is the debate about whether to emphasize risk or resilience in the quest to create effective programs (Benard, 1993a, 1993b; Hawkins, Catalano, & Haggerty, 1993). One point of view argues that interventionists should abandon their focus on risk factors and aim most of their efforts at enhancing and developing resilience and protective factors. This focus on resilience is needed not only for the young people who are the targets of these efforts, but also for practitioners, who need to maintain positive and hopeful attitudes toward their work and toward the individuals whom they are attempting to help. In contrast, one could argue that practitioners would be shortsighted to ignore the risk factors that exist for young people, and that information about risk factors is necessary to tailor intervention efforts. This exchange mirrors the struggle between those educators who argue about whether to focus resources on defense strategies for school buildings (e.g., fences, metal detectors, and security guards) or on human resource capacity for both students and staff (e.g., conflict resolution, anger management, and the development of a positive school climate). As is the case with other prevention efforts, programs that are comprehensive in nature, designed to address specific problems, and enhance general resilience will enhance school safety efforts.

LINKING SCHOOL SAFETY, DEVELOPMENTAL RISK AND RESILIENCE, AND SCHOOLING RESEARCH

These prevention concepts provide a useful frame for viewing the problem of school violence and for constructing interventions to enhance school safety. Recently, the language of risk and resilience has been more thoroughly included in educational dialogue and practice (Kirby & Fraser, 1997). Programs that emphasize reducing risk and enhancing resilience have become more commonplace—for example, conflict resolution, substance abuse prevention, mentoring, and after-school programs. However, change oriented toward creating safe schools and based on developmental theories of prevention and intervention is not yet fully integrated with efforts at systems change led by mainstream educators. The latter change has been aimed at overall school reform and has maintained a primary focus on academic performance. In contrast, school violence prevention concepts are based in developmental psychology and still need translation into educationally based paradigms. Adelman and Taylor (2000) have identified this problem in the context of more general prevention efforts. They, too, recognize that prevention efforts have to be incorporated into the fabric of more general school mental health improvement efforts. The federal "Safeguarding" document (Dwyer & Osher, 2000) suggests that a "schoolwide team" focus on planning and implementing school safety programming. This document emphasizes the importance of representation by personnel who have credibility and expertise in the various areas such as prevention *and* school reform. However, the effectiveness of this type of team will depend on how representatives of each of these perspectives are able to understand, respect, and use each other's perspective in the program planning process.

Like any other challenge to schools, the creation of safe schools requires that change take place. A typical approach to challenges faced by schools is to "add on" new initiatives. Examples of adding on to established school practice include the use of technology, substance abuse prevention, child abuse prevention, and mainstreaming or inclusion of children with special needs. The challenge of school violence potentially requires yet another add-on. Although each of such add-ons has merit, when they are piled one on top of another, teachers and other educators, who rightfully ask, "How much more can we do?" often meet them with resistance. Fullan (1994) challenges educators not to consider innovations one at a time, but to engage in more comprehensive reforms that will address the complexity and immensity of the educational challenge.

Drawing from Fullan's perspective, it is our contention that significant strides toward safe schools can be made only when changes are introduced in the context of a wider, fuller effort toward school reform, in which the goals of safe schools are integrated with the goals of the school in general. Because school safety has physical, psychological, and developmental components, it is placed squarely in the territory of concern for all educators, from the individual classroom to the full school environment. In considering how the concepts of school safety can be incorporated into the central mission of the school, it is important to realize that its concepts fall naturally into the broader educational framework; thus, major retraining is unnecessary (Furlong, Babinski, Poland, Muqoz, & Boles, 1996; Furlong, Morrison, & Dear, 1994). Rather, educators need to take a fresh look at the proven educational practices they already use effectively, and recognize how these practices contribute to safe schools. In a sense, we are suggesting that the process of creating safe schools is partially a task of enabling and empowering school personnel to continue their effective practices (Furlong et al., 1994).

In the following section, we use the school effectiveness paradigm as a structure for examining what is known about school-based risk and protective mechanisms. We further note the parallels between school effectiveness indicators and schoolwide prevention (safety, discipline) components. We consider the essential school safety tasks, using school effectiveness components and highlighting school change principles.

SCHOOL EFFECTIVENESS: CONCEPTS AND TRADITIONS

The literature on school effectiveness has consistently identified the following factors that enhance or detract from school effectiveness: (1) clear school mission, (2) high expectations for students' learning and behavior, (3) instructional leadership, (4) a safe and orderly environment, (5) opportunity to learn and student time-on-task, (6) frequent monitoring and feedback in regard to student performance, and (7) positive home–school relationships (Block, Everson, & Guskey, 1995; Chrispeels, 1992; Edmonds, 1979; Purkey & Smith, 1983; Reynolds, Teddlie, Creemers, Scheerens, & Townsend, 2000). The literature on school *effectiveness* has been criticized for ignoring important contextual variables (e.g., socioeconomic status of the community and students and whether the school is urban, rural, or suburban) and lacking information on exactly how to effect change toward these school effectiveness (Bickel, 1999; Teddlie & Reynolds, 2000). School *improvement* approaches, in contrast, examine the processes by which schools can change. School improvement is also referred to as school restructuring, which involves changes in roles, rules, and relationships between and among students, teachers, and administrators at the building and district levels (Bickel, 1999). School change involves not only a consideration of the content of programs, but the involvement of school personnel and their strategic partners in a process that leads to the desired change.

A notable absence in the work described in the school effectiveness or school improvement literature is the incorporation of a broader view of student learning and behavior to include social and emotional outcomes. A similarly notable absence in the school improvement areas is the relative lack of attention to, and involvement of, support services personnel such as school counselors and school psychologists. Although a premise to school improvement approaches does include the importance of including multiple professional and constituent roles in the change process, much of the life and focus of the support services roles remains outside of school reform activity. In an attempt to show the parallel development of knowledge in school reform and safe schools movements, Table 11.1, Section A, uses the effective schools correlates suggested by Levine and Lezotte (1990) as a template for organization of the principles of safe and responsive schools (from the federal "Safeguarding" document; Dwyer & Osher, 2000) and orderly schools (from the "Opportunities Suspended" document; Advancement Project/Civil Rights, 2000).

The contents of Table 11.1 suggest that effective schools indicators roughly parallel those of safe schools. An obvious absence in the discussion of safety and discipline is the notion of effective leadership. We include a discussion of leadership later in this chapter, as this factor is critical to the success of safe school planning and implementation. It is also notable that the safe schools indicators add dimensions to the effective schools indicators that include safety and emphasis on more social/emotional developmental factors. Adelman and Taylor (2000) suggest that the missing piece in typical school reform efforts is the component that addresses barriers to learning (e.g., social and emotional difficulties). They propose adding an "enabling" component to the typical instructional and management components of school change efforts. One is left with the impression that these differences are those of emphasis, language, orientation, and focus but ones that retain the basic organizational framework. The important question is, to what extent are the professionals who work with basic school reform and those who work with safe schools/prevention programs talking to each other and collaborating in their efforts to achieve high-performing *and* safe schools? School improvement and reform efforts tend to be led by school administrators and teacher leaders relying on best practices generated from their respective orientations. School psychologists, mental health professionals, and special educators, capitalizing on their respective areas of expertise, have led safe school and prevention efforts. As their training traditions emanate from different disciplines, their practice and the roles they play in schools may not be well integrated with those of mainstream education.

In the following sections, we use the safety/effectiveness indicators as a structure to review the risk and resilience aspects of school safety, the tasks that can be undertaken to make any school safer. As we consider the tasks involved in improving relationships, we must remember that students vary in the nature of their connection to school; therefore, the nature and intensity of the intervention must vary (i.e., reaffirm, reconnect, reconstruct). Moreover, within each indicator section, where applicable, we speak to aspects of the process of school change that need to be addressed in moving toward safe and effective schools. Table 11.1, Sections A and B, represents the integration of the perspectives of school effectiveness, school improvement, and school safety that we discuss in the following section.

PRODUCTIVE SCHOOL CLIMATE

Levine and Lezotte (1990) include aspects of orderly environment, school relationships, and shared school mission in their effective schools correlates of productive school climate and culture.

Orderly Environment

Lack of an orderly school campus and disrupted school relationships have been noted as specific risks for poor student outcomes. Less adult supervision for troubled and troubling students can lead to an increase in delin-

TABLE 11.1. School Effectiveness, Reform, and Safety Indicators and Tips

Section A			Section B	
Effective schools correlates (Levine & Lezotte, 1990)	Schools with low discipline referrals (Advancement Project/Civil Rights Project, 2000)	*Safeguarding Our Children* (Dwyer & Osher, 2000)	School reform principles	School safety tasks
Productive school climate and culture Orderly environment Cohesion, collegiality Schoolwide emphasis on recognizing positive performance Commitment to shared mission	The school physical environment is a friendly and welcoming space. Administrators and teachers demonstrate ownership of discipline-related problems that students present. Opportunities exist to develop strong bonds between teachers and students. Explicit efforts are made to show students that they are valued and respected members of the school community and that they are expected to uphold high behavioral and academic standards.	Emphasize positive relationships among students and staff Discuss safety issues openly Treat students with equal respect Create ways for students to share concerns Help children feel safe expressing their feelings	Transform personal meaning and vision to a group mission Create a centering conviction with broad interest and appeal	*Orderly environment* Implement a firm, fair, and consistently enforced system of school rules and procedures Recognize positive behavior; catch students "being good" Implement classroom strategies for disruptive behavior Provide behavioral consultation Provide positive behavior support in settings where needed Maintain appropriate levels of campus supervision and security Make it a priority to supervise and properly support students at-risk of school failure Provide multiple alternatives for disciplinary consequences for rule breaking Engage in crisis and security planning (metal detectors, security cameras, school resource offices, staff IDs) Do a physical environment audit Increase supervision and contact Train all campus supervisors and security personnel in developmentally and educationally sound methods Acknowledge and recognize school safety problems *Relationships* Make adults available to listen to student safety concerns Engage in schoolwide discipline and behavior planning Commit to respectful, caring, nurturing relationships Make available buddies and mentors Know every child by name Celebrate diversity *Shared mission* Define the mission and vision to include academic, safety, and socioemotional outcomes Revisit the moral imperative of the right of students to safe schools Broaden the responsibility of all school personnel to include safety responsibilities Embed the safety mission within the broader academic mission Use symbols and ritual to highlight school safety aspects of school mission Allow variance in the mission for students with varied characteristics Strive for academic excellence and personal-social growth for all students Provide alternative routes to excellence for students who are at risk for negative outcomes Consider excellence in nontraditional areas Continually identify and publicize the major themes and commonly held hopes, wishes, and desires for the school

TABLE 11.1. School Effectiveness, Reform, and Safety Indicators and Tips

Section A			Section B	
Effective schools correlates (Levine & Lezotte, 1990)	Schools with low discipline referrals (Advancement Project/Civil Rights Project, 2000)	*Safeguarding Our Children* (Dwyer & Osher, 2000)	School reform principles	School safety tasks
Effective instructional arrangements and implementation Effective teaching *Successful grouping and organizational arrangements* Classroom adaptation	A process, location, and plan for students who need to "cool off" is available so that more severe outbursts cam be prevented. Student sanctions are considered on a case-by-case basis with input from students and parents.	Have a system in place for referring children who are suspected of being abused or neglected Offer extended day programs for children		Provide a high-quality enrollment and new student orientation and welcoming program Integrate personal and social skills instruction into the academic program—acknowledge as a basic school skill Build talents in arts and music Encourage responsibility; develop leadership in all student groups Seek out effective and culturally appropriate programs Primary prevention—safety awareness, character traits curriculum, classroom discussions, social skills, friendships Secondary prevention—conflict resolution, peer mediators, mentors Tertiary prevention—functional assessment and individual behavior plans, wraparound services, anger management, counseling Provide alternative education options Provide a variety of clubs—especially for marginalized groups
Focus on student acquisition of central learning skills Time for learning Focus on central learning skills	A wide variety of prevention and intervention support programs are available for students.	Focus on academic achievement Promote good citizenship and character Support students in making the transition to adult life and the workplace	Encourage collaboration Build effective teams	Build a collaborative approach to program and service choices and delivery Recruit well-informed people and build their skills Explain the scope of responsibility Provide good "tools" for the task Plan structure and document meetings Acknowledge contributions Make the process safe
High operationalized expectations and requirements for students	A schoolwide code of conduct and expectations is promoted.			
Appropriate monitoring of student progress		Identify problems and assess progress toward solutions		Keep track of school crime and school rule violations Survey students, staff, and parents about their perceptions of school safety Be receptive, sensitive, and responsive when students express fears and concerns Implement early behavior screening Use functional behavioral assessment Conduct informal classroom behavior assessment Utilize and document student support team actions Use multiple-gate behavioral screening Track and monitor discipline incidents (office referrals, suspensions, expulsions)

TABLE 11.1. School Effectiveness, Reform, and Safety Indicators and Tips

Section A			Section B	
Effective schools correlates (Levine & Lezotte, 1990)	Schools with low discipline referrals (Advancement Project/Civil Rights Project, 2000)	*Safeguarding Our Children* (Dwyer & Osher, 2000)	School reform principles	School safety tasks

Practice-oriented staff development at the school site	Ongoing staff development is conducted about "best practices" in handling student misconduct.		Develop skills and practices
			
			 Use empowerment principles
				Discuss during professional development:
				   Infusing social, emotional, behavioral, character, and safety content into standards and curriculum
				   Using teachable moments throughout the day
				   Using positive, proactive behavioral and discipline methods
				 Encourage listening and relationship building
				 Provide training in prevention programming

Outstanding leadership Monitoring of activities and vision Instructional leadership Support for teachers Resource acquisition Effective utilization of instructional support personnel			Leaders provide vision, guidance, challenge, support, recognition, and resources; monitor speed and depth of change Disperse leadership among a wide range of personnel and community members	Encourage high visibility by the administration Involve all school personnel in leadership functions Encourage staff to feel ownership for all schooling tasks (i.e., academic, social, emotional) Reach out to student leadership in all campus subgroups Involve more students in the student power structure. Don't always give the "best" kids the privileges Involve students and cultivate ownership of school safety planning
Salient parental and community involvement	Community participants are welcomed into the school, including parents, mental health and juvenile justice professionals, business leaders, etc.	Involve families in meaningful ways; develop links to the community		Cultivate the support of parents Inform parents regarding what you are doing and why Inform and involve parents so they will back you and support you when policies and actions are put in place Reach out to all parents to encourage involvement and responsibility for solving campus problems Involve parents in school decision making Provide educational programs for parents (literacy, parenting, etc.) Know your community and its changing conditions Be alert to media twisting and distorting (this has a great effect on community perceptions of the school and can make good things look bad) Develop interagency agreements with the juvenile justice systems to monitor, supervise, and properly support youthful offenders on campus (truancy, probation)

quent associations and behaviors (Barr & Parrett, 2001). In terms of the physical environment, The National Research Council's report notes that the following characteristics of schools may contribute to violence: (1) relatively high numbers of students occupy a limited amount of space, (2) the capacity to avoid confrontations is somewhat reduced, and (3) poor building design features may facilitate the commission of violent acts. Zwier and Vaughan (1984) report that the derelict appearance of a school is associated with higher rates of vandalism.

Common conceptualization of school safety focuses on an orderly school environment; for example, California's required comprehensive school safety plan (CA.E.C.35294.2) includes child abuse reporting procedures, disaster plans, disciplinary policies (suspension, expulsion), sexual harassment policies, dress code, safe ingress and egress, and a safe and orderly school environment. Ensuring a safe physical environment is an important part of school safety and entails attending to three areas: (1) *access control* (control of entrance/exit areas with the ability to lock these areas), (2) *surveillance measures*, and (3) *security practices* (guards, metal detectors, and landscape control; Barton, 2000). Green, Travis, and Downs (1999) have delineated basic guidelines for deciding, in collaboration with law enforcement agencies, what, if any, security technologies should be considered as schools develop safe school strategies. Figure 11.1 displays a form that can be used for a physical environment audit.

An important part of a positive, orderly school climate is the fair implementation of a strong discipline policy. A school protective function is the provision of a predictable environment with consistently enforced standards, rules, and responsibilities (Garbarino, 1992). In effective schools, discipline practices are clear, respectful, and fair, and teachers model and teach desired behaviors (Bear, Webster-Stratton, Furlong, & Rhee, 2000). Where students display challenging behaviors that go beyond the classroom discipline and feedback structure, support personnel should be available to assess the antecedents, the communicative intent of the behavior, and the consequences that often reinforce and sustain the problem behavior. Principals can help teachers and staff put into place positive behavioral and disciplinary programs to teach prosocial behaviors, intervene early in troublesome behavior, and respond effectively to serious transgressions (Horner & Sugai, 2000; Skiba et al., 2001; Walker et al., 1996).

Comprehensive schoolwide discipline plans are a foundation of an orderly school campus. Skiba (1999) describes effective responses to school disruption as one of the three cornerstones of effective violence prevention strategies. Sugai et al. (2000) present a multilevel system of schoolwide discipline strategies, noting that students who exhibit different types and different levels of severity of antisocial behavior will necessitate different types and intensities of intervention to arrest and prevent such behavior in the future. In addition, a number of other researchers have proposed preventive models that focus on schoolwide reform (Knoff & Batsche, 1985) and a comprehensive combination of program components with documented effectiveness, such as skill training (conflict resolution/social skills), parent involvement, classroom and schoolwide behavior management, functional assessment and individual behavior plans, school safety planning, and school and district data management systems (Skiba & Peterson, 2000).

Relationships

Lack of attachment, commitment, or bonding to school, which often accompanies school failure, is a predictor of negative student outcomes (Cernkovich & Giordano, 1992; Wehlage, Rutter, Smith, Lesko, & Fernandez, 1989). In terms of the social environment, peer rejection or association with a peer culture whose norms are not conducive to academic achievement or rule compliance are school-related risk factors (Walker et al., 1995). From the whole-school perspective, negative school climate, teacher apathy, and authoritarian leadership without teacher or student participation are negative indicators for effective schools (Zwier & Vaughan, 1984). Zwier and Vaughan also note a similar association at the community level in regard to disinterest in school affairs.

Although crisis planning is essential, having a disaster–response frame of reference does nothing to address the small, day-to-day aversive aspects of interpersonal relationships (such as bullying) that build over time and may ultimately fuel tragic situations. Sheerens and Bosker (1997) suggest that effective and safe schools emphasize the well being of all individuals within the system: students and staff members alike. An institutional climate of interpersonal respect and open communication is vital to the safe school mission. Possibilities for resilience arise from opportunities to develop strong relationships with adult role models (Garbarino, 1992). Relationships contribute to a positive school climate in which students value teachers' opinions, teacher–student interactions are evident, and informal teacher–teacher and teacher–principal interactions are productive (Garbarino, 1992). Wehlage et al. (1989) emphasize the importance of school membership or social bonding in attempting to keep students in school who are at risk for dropping out. Brendtro, Brokenleg, and Van Bockern (1990) refer to creating empowering environments that "reclaim" youths at risk. That is, through developing belonging, mastery, independence, and generosity in youths, we ensure that they become contributing members of schools and society.

Maehr and Midgley (1996) suggest that both schools and *schooling* must be redesigned in terms of students' developmental stage, sociocultural experience, and emotional and behavioral characteristics. Complicating this agenda, most schools today are culturally, ethnically, and linguistically diverse. School-based programs must foster norms against bullying, aggression, and violence, while maintaining sensitivity to the different cultural norms of constituent families (Bear et al., 2000). Establishing and promoting caring relationships with *all* students is foundational in any district mission.

Shared Mission and Vision

Although most of the risk and resilience applications for schools have focused on the order and relationships aspects of climate, the nature of the school mission and vision is a critical guide for the nature and emphasis of school programs. The extent to which the focus of the school mission is exclusively on academic achievement may have implications for school safety outcomes (Mayer & Leone, 1999). For example, a narrow view of acceptable behavior and limited responsibility of educators for the behavioral development of students combined with a singular focus on academic performance, may lead to strategies that exclude students who struggle with academic competence and break school rules. In contrast, the school may choose to broaden the mission and vision for schooling, providing alternative methods and routes for students to follow toward success in school. Students would experience schools with missions that differed along these lines as negative or positive influences in their lives, depending on their individual talents and abilities.

A mission statement is like an introductory paragraph. It provides a statement of purpose (what is to be accomplished), the method of accomplishment (activities), and the principles and beliefs that are behind the purpose and methods. A vision statement provides an image of what success will look like. Fullan (1994) discusses the importance of building a personal vision—specifically, reexamining why we entered the field of education and what we hoped to accomplish. We (Furlong, Morrison, & Clontz, 1993) have noted that a school safety planning process starts with creating a vision, and that the beginning of this vision making starts as a private experience (i.e., thinking about personal feelings of safety and what enhances or detracts from these feelings of safety).

Change Principle: Tapping into Personal Vision and Beliefs
to Fuel and Articulate a Group Vision

Transforming personal visions and individual thinking into a group vision is a challenge. Snyder, Morrison, and Smith (1996) note that there is no single path from personal beliefs and convictions to engaging others in a larger group vision. In the school reform projects they describe, some educators were "on board" from the beginning with their beliefs about student potential and educators' responsibility to develop that potential; other educators, though they may not have "believed" at first, were brought along through their observations and experience of success in working with students and other educators in a different way.

For change to even begin, school personnel, whether as individuals or as a group, must see the need to change and be motivated to take on the risks and tasks that change will entail. Engaging in a visioning process helps educators see new potential in their work, which then energizes and motivates

School _____ Principal _____ Phone _____

Address _____

               #   Street   Zip

GENERAL DESCRIPTION

Enrollment_____Grade Levels_____School Calendar ❏ Traditional ❏ Year Round

Staffing _____ _____ _____ _____ _____
      # Teacher   # Classified   # Specialists   # Campus Supervisors   # Administrators

Site Acreage _____ Facilities _____

School Location

❏ Entrances, access, visitor entrance clearly indicated
❏ Traffic, parking
❏ Public information signs, regulations
❏ Neighboring homes, businesses, roadways
❏ Adverse commercial activities
❏ Attractive nuisances, any notable "location" concerns?

Comment:

_____

_____

_____

_____

_____

_____

School Grounds

❏ Fencing, gates
❏ Blacktop, sidewalks, grass areas
❏ Shrubs, trees, grass
❏ Field areas, playground equipment
❏ Clean, attractive, appropriate lighting
❏ Gravel, rocks, sand, glass, graffiti
❏ Supervision concerns
❏ Comment:

_____

_____

_____

_____

_____

_____

School Buildings & Classrooms

❏ Appearance
❏ Roof access
❏ Blind areas
❏ Trash disposal
❏ Fire safety
❏ Lighting
❏ Door, windows, locks
❏ Communication systems, security alarms, police security
❏ Stairs, ramps, floors, aisles (clean, dry, tripping hazards, etc.)
❏ Notable storage dangers in classrooms
❏ Student work displays
❏ Evidence of character traits education
❏ Classroom & school rules posted/ uniform
❏ Notable noise, odor
❏ Condition, appearance of furniture & equipment
Comment:

_____

_____

_____

Campus Supervision & Emergency Response

❏ Current, written School Rules & Procedures Plan?
❏ Supervision strategies are discussed & reviewed?
❏ Current, written Emergency Response Plan?
❏ Staff is trained and plan is practiced?

Comment:

_____

_____

_____

_____

FIGURE 11.1.   *(continued)*

FIGURE 11.1. *continued*

Specifically Mentioned Problems
Concerns mentioned by the Principal or
other site staff member? (Write name of
the person who expresses the concern)

Summary Comments

Most notable concerns?

Most notable strengths?

Recommendations?

_____   _____   _____
   Safety Observer   Safety Observer   Safety Observer

FIGURE 11.1. School physical environment audit. From R. L. Morrison, Ventura Unified School District, Ventura, CA

their future efforts. However, a crisis is often the precipitating event for change. In the case of school violence, its visibility and potential for gruesome scenarios can act as a natural mobilizer for change. This type of crisis must also be put in the context of other crises experienced by the public education system. For example, the publication of A Nation at Risk (Herr, 1991) served as a notice to educators and their public that "business as usual" was failing a large number of children throughout the nation.

A number of researchers describe the importance of motivating change efforts by helping the change agents to revisit or develop a moral/philosophical "origin" for professional actions (Block et al., 1995; Comer, 1988; Fullan, 1994; Sergiovanni, 1994; Snyder et al., 1996). Greenfield (1991) used the notion of "moral orientation" for the point of view on which actions, influence, and decisions are anchored. Sergiovanni (1994) has stated, "Real change can only come as a result of the commitments of both the minds and the hearts of the total school community. . . [It] should be based on careful identification of deeply and commonly held values" (p. 1). We, too, have highlighted the notion of responsibility in regard to school safety (Weis, Morrison, Furlong, & Morrison, 1993), in emphasizing that the "first responsibility of educators is therefore to systematically create a school environment where all forms of harm to its students and staff are minimized" (p. 8).

A beginning point for school safety planning is the recognition that although school violence necessitates the use of law enforcement strategies at some level, the core interest of educators is in the provision of a nurturing and supportive school environment. The reframing of the school violence issue as one of school safety is the starting point for this planning process. Although this reframing is critical, the experience of others involved in crafting schools' responses to violence is that it is important, up front, to acknowledge the possibility of violence on school campuses and to take protective measures as may be indicated (e.g., increased supervision during breaks, restrictions on off-campus visitors, and close relationships with law enforcement). Allowing for and responding to concern about school violence then paves the way for the participants in school safety activities to take more productive steps toward creating safe school environments.

Change Principle: Deciding on a Centering Conviction

Another major challenge for the school safety movement is to decide on a centering conviction associated with the vision that will allow the safe school notion to be incorporated into a central mission or effort in the "mainstream" of schooling efforts. Although the end product may be safe schools, the interim efforts may be tied to efforts such as "success for all." In other words, the safe school vision may be seen as a facilitator of the academic mission of the school. It is the challenge for personnel who see the importance of safe schools to relate that importance to ongoing schooling efforts that have the attention of most educators.

Often, the centering convictions chosen by reform efforts can serve as an "umbrella" for organizing the understandings, interpretations, and implementation guidelines associated with change activities. The effective use of such an umbrella in one project was described by Snyder et al. (1996). The leader of this effort chose "Partners for Excellence" as the title for an original project aimed at increasing the postsecondary options for students graduating from the school system. However, as this title became a recognizable entity in both the school and the community, it was used for a variety of efforts that were loosely connected with the original theme of the project—the inclusion of children with severe disabilities in regular education elementary school classrooms, a peer counseling program, and an academic recognition program, among others. Although these various efforts did not directly address the school safety question, they improved the overall climate for student achievement and progress in these schools and thus resulted in a safer, more positive school climate for all (Snyder et al., 1996).

Centering convictions can be used as a base for public rituals and symbols. The functions of rituals and the symbols around which they are built are to provide personal and collective meaning and to serve as guiding themes that allow connections to be made among seemingly disparate phenomena (Roberts, 1988). Fullan and Miles (1992) note that symbols can provide personal and collective meaning in situations of change, where complex situations and unclear goals foster confusion. Symbols can serve to crystallize images. An example of this in the Partners for Excellence project was "sweatshirt day." To reinforce the importance of postsecondary education, once a year faculty and staff wore sweatshirts depicting the college from which they graduated. At another school, teachers from a variety of disciplines, such as history, art, and math, displayed career possibilities for each of their professions on their classroom bulletin boards (Snyder et al., 1996). Symbols may provide galvanizing themes around which political support and financial resources can be generated (Fullan & Miles, 1992).

For this discussion of safe schools, the obvious centering conviction is that all children have a right to learn in a safe school environment, and that schools should be a place where children are not harmed. However, in terms of relating this right to that of a central and dominant mission of education, it can be easily reasoned that the rock-bottom belief is that all children have an equal right to an education. For all children to exercise this right, they must be provided with school environments that maximize their chances for learning and positive development. A critical characteristic of such environments is safety. Two related convictions that also have implications for educators' approach to change in educating children are that all children are innately resilient and that they deserve respect.

Specific school safety tasks related to and extending this discussion (and that those in the following sections) are shown in Table 11.1, Section B.

HIGH EXPECTATIONS, EFFECTIVE INSTRUCTION, AND STUDENT ACQUISITION OF CENTRAL LEARNING SKILLS

In this section, we combine the indicators of high expectations, effective instruction, and student acquisition—these all target "what" and "how" instruction is delivered and, subsequently, what students learn. Negative expectations for students, as communicated by school staff members, have been noted as risk factors for students (Elliott & Voss, 1974; Montague & Rinaldi, 2001). In contrast, in high-achieving schools, teachers hold high expectations for all students and a belief that all students can learn (Reynolds et al., 2000). Students are given choice, responsibility, and support; then they are held accountable for achievement of age-appropriate standards.

Expectations for students accompany "what" and "how" instruction is delivered. The "what" consists of academic content, social skills, personal competence skills (self-esteem and coping), and vocational skills. Each district may wish to adopt a strategic plan to guide, review, and revise the academic and social mission of its schools. In addition to high academic standards, the social and emotional climate is critical. Districts and schools have to develop systematic and sustainable programs that promote social and emotional learning in addition to cognitive-academic learning. Prevention of violence goes hand-in-hand with promotion of student health behaviors in four curricular areas: life skills and social competencies, health promotion and problem prevention, coping skills and social support, and positive and contributory service (Zins, Elias, Greenberg, & Weissberg, 2000). As an addition or alternative to emphasizing the installation of metal detectors and establishing police presence on campus, districts can adopt programs that focus on students' emotional intelligence, or "EQ," instituting programs to develop character, citizenship, and resiliency. Enhancing students' growth through community service requirements helps them to develop personal and social skills, connect to their community, gain positive recognition, and enhance self-esteem through responsibility, accountability, and contribution. Districts may also create positive alternatives to suspension and expulsion that keep students connected to schools and teach prosocial behaviors (Indiana Education Policy Center, 2000).

Research on prevention and intervention programs in schools has indicated that empirically effective programs are (1) comprehensive, (2) broad based, (3) intensive and sustainable over time, (4) developmentally appropriate, (5) provided early—before problems are exacerbated, and (6) employ ongoing and summative evaluation (Bear et al., 2000; Zins et al., 2000). A National Institute on Drug Abuse report also noted that effective prevention practices should include family, school, and community interventions that target information, skills, and resilience-building aspects (*www.nida.nih.gov/Prevention/PREVPRINC.html*, 4/4/1997). The National Mental Health Association adds, (1) "Effective programs are holistic, and focus on reducing risk factors and supporting healthy development by addressing multiple aspects of a child's life and environment" and (2) "Effective programs are replicable in a variety of settings, which are accessible, community-friendly and culturally sensitive" (*http://www.nmha.org/children/prevent/effective.cfm*, 1/23/04). Cohen (1998) refers to the comprehensive nature of the aforementioned prevention programs as the "Spectrum of Prevention" and adds that changing organizational practices and influencing policy legislation are also important aspects of prevention programming (*http://www.preventioninstitute.org/conflict.html*, 7/30/01).

The "how" of instructional delivery consists of methods such as classroom instruction (cooperative learning, small-group work), support services (counseling and guidance, consultation), alternative structures (block scheduling, school-within-a-school models, homerooms or student advisory classes, year-round schools), alternative programs (classes for at-risk students, continuation schools, independent study, in-school disciplinary options), special education programs, and prevention programs. The risk and protective factors associated with these practices are associated with the extent to which these practices are available, comprehensive, and coordinated with a unifying programmatic philosophy (Garbarino, 1992). Schooling practices associated with risk include grade retention, tracking, and zero tolerance (Epp & Watkinson, 1997; Morrison et al., 2001). Resilient and effective practices include the utilization of a variety of teaching and service delivery methods (*http://www.hec.ohio-state.edu/famlife/bulletin/volume.1/bullet12.htm*, 1/23/04).

Change Principle: Collaboration and Team Building

Implementation of these programs and services requires the contributions of a variety of school personnel (teachers, support service personnel) who will need to collaborate in the delivery of services to students. We (Furlong et al., 1993) have emphasized the importance of working collaboratively in the safe school planning process as well as creating a "climate for action" that signals the importance of the work and ensures a safe working environment for participants. Collaboration among school professionals has received much attention in the past decade as a mechanism for dealing with the complexities of educating a diverse population of students because it is one mechanism for sharing specialized knowledge and skill areas across professional boundaries. Furthermore, it can also lead to the development of a school community, in which the bonds between people facilitate the accomplishment of their shared goals (Sergiovanni, 1994). Sizer and others (Keller, 1995; O'Neil, 1995) emphasize the importance of including the entire educational community in this collaboration—teachers and support staff, students and their families, administrators, central and district office representatives, and community members. The accelerated schooling philosophy labels this process "empowerment through responsibility"; the entire school community assists in educational decision making and takes responsibility for the results (Keller, 1995). School safety is an issue that demands input from a variety of professional perspectives; therefore, collaboration is critical for effective progress.

The "team" or the group is an important unit of change for school reform. Comer's (1980) model of school reform refers to this group as the "stakeholders." The individuals on a team involved in school change provide support and encouragement for enacting personal and team visions. Snyder et al. (1996) delineate several aspects of effective team building and implementation of goals:

1. *Continuity of membership is critical.* Teams will suffer in cohesion, performance, and accomplishment if the turnover in membership is too high.

2. *Team members share centering convictions.* At the core of every change effort is a group (more than one) of educators who believe in and act on the centering convictions behind the change effort. These individuals gradually expand their efforts by (a) bringing other educators with similar convictions on board or (b) involving others who may not initially believe in the centering convictions, but who may come to believe through their successful efforts in the reform project.

3. *Team members need to share ownership of tasks.* Rigid role and professional boundaries work against getting the job done. At least some redefinition of what each educator does may be needed. More important than role boundaries is the guarantee that the functions of the change will be accomplished (e.g., providing guidance to students, creating safe classroom and school environments).

4. *Team members support each other.* Team members need support from within the team to bolster their resolve when the going gets difficult. Support and recognition from others outside the team also helps to maintain their work.

APPROPRIATE MONITORING OF STUDENT PROGRESS

In effective schools, student progress is monitored closely and students receive regular and constructive feedback about their learning (Levine & Lezotte, 1990). If the school mission is broadened to incorporate skills in other than academic domains, the assessment and monitoring of these skills should be tracked as well. Schools that do not monitor the ebb and flow of behavioral and discipline data, for example, are at risk of failing to modify policies and interventions that are ineffective in changing behavior and making schools safer for all participants. For example, students who exhibit chronic patterns of misbehavior at school are highly likely to experience future adjustment problems in school (Sprague & Walker, 2000). Walker and Sprague (1999) found that the number of discipline contacts during the school year for an individual child was one of three salient predictors of arrest status in the fifth and again in the tenth grades. Early and continued behavioral assessment contributes to the school's ability to provide support for students who are at risk for aggressive or disruptive behavior. Kazdin's (1987) research suggests that for the small number of students whose behavior problems are particularly entrenched, aggressive conduct patterns are present by age 3 and fairly well established by age 8, making early and effective intervention necessary. In recent school practice, however, most students with academic or behavioral difficulties are not referred to student study or intervention teams until the third grade (Duncan, Forness, & Hartsoough, 1995).

Three areas to consider in monitoring school progress beyond the academic arena include (1) monitoring of individual aggressive and antisocial behavior, (2) monitoring behavior and discipline on a schoolwide basis, and (3) assessing student and staff perceptions of school safety.

Sugai et al. (2000) have noted the importance of establishing a system for tracking office referrals and other disciplinary actions, as these are "red flags" signaling the possibility of future acts of disruption. The *Early Warning, Timely Response* document (Dwyer, Osher, & Warger, 1998) provides guidelines for assessing students who are at risk for aggressive and violent behavior. In addition, multiple screening approaches have shown promise in early identification of students with emotional and behavior problems (Walker & Severson, 1990). It should be noted that *Psychology in the Schools* (Furlong, Kingery, & Bates, 2001) recently published a special issue on threat assessment, containing analysis and appropriate cautions about our ability to predict future violent behavior. In addition to facilitating early intervention, functional assessment methods have provided an excellent resource for educators to understand, assess, and monitor the effectiveness of ongoing interventions designed to change behavior (Dwyer & Osher, 2000; Gresham, Watson, & Skinner, 2001).

In addition to a focus on students' contribution to school violence, there is concern about the systemic contribution of high levels of overall disciplinary reactions in a school to acts of more serious violence (Skiba & Peterson, 2000). Skiba et al. (2001) suggest that school- and districtwide data systems be established to monitor and assess the patterns of office referrals, suspensions, and expulsions. The patterns that are evident from this type of data collection and analysis must be interpreted in light of important system variations such as school administrator philosophy and the existence of schoolwide planning and agreement with regard to discipline procedures and processes (Morrison & Skiba, 2001).

On a schoolwide level, there is also a need to attend to general perceptions of school safety. A comprehensive assessment may raise awareness about the multifaceted nature of school safety—that it includes physical, psychological, and developmental components. A determination of needs in relationship to school safety must include consideration of a full range of needs and risks that may operate in the school environment. Of course, it must also include a focus on resilience/protective dimensions that may exist in the environment to counteract the risk factors. We have encouraged the collection of this type of data, the primary objective being to understand the "current reality" of the personal characteristics of students and staff, the school's physical environment, the school's social environment, and the school culture (Cornell & Loper, 1998; Furlong, Casas, Corral, Chung, & Bates, 1997; Furlong, Chung, Bates, & Morrison, 1995). We have developed and refined survey instruments for students and staff members that can be utilized to capture the major components of school safety. Students are a particularly important source of information, as their experience of safety is an important target for change in addition to the more obvious aspects of the physical environment. The data collected through such efforts can also be used as an impetus for change. Knowing about staff and student perceptions of safety may motivate changes in schooling structures, curriculum, and personnel functions. Knowing how to utilize this assessment information is

TABLE 11.2. Tips for School Safety Assessment

- *Do assessments within a planning process.* All assessments should be done in the context of a careful, local school climate and safety planning process. Data collected without a purpose serves no useful function.

- *Build consensus for doing a survey.* The school community should be involved in planning the logistics of completing the survey. Surveys are usually completed by students and staff during a prespecified class period. The quality of the data is enhanced when teachers and students understand why the survey is being conducted and what the expected use of the data will be.

- *Ask about everyone's experiences.* School site planners should ask for the views of as many students, teachers, and parents as possible. Asking for opinions increases awareness and helps to make school safety a top priority.

- *Talk about the survey results.* Surveys are most informative when they include procedures for discussing reactions immediately after a survey is completed. Classroom lessons, focus groups, and community meetings are means of obtaining more personal views of what is behind the numbers and graphs.

- *Use the survey information responsibly.* A number of ethical questions and related responsibilities are raised when a survey is conducted. Make sure that privacy and anonymity of individuals are maintained. Try to anticipate potential adverse reactions, especially among individuals who may have been previously victimized on campus. Make sure there is commitment to use the information in helpful and productive ways. This should not be a fault-finding enterprise.

Note. From R. L. Morrison, Ventura Unified School District, Ventura, CA and M. J. Furlong, University of California, Santa Barbara.

as important as collecting and analyzing it. Table 11.2 contains tips for school safety assessment.

PRACTICE-ORIENTED STAFF DEVELOPMENT AT THE SCHOOL SITE

Staff members who are unhappy and alienated contribute to an unsafe and ineffective school (Zwier & Vaughan, 1984). It is interesting to note that much of the school effectiveness literature refers to school-level and staff characteristics that mirror the individual resilience mechanisms of bonding, opportunities, and recognition. That is, for adult educators, it is important to have opportunities to participate in decision making, acquire new skills, and be recognized for good performance. Garbarino (1992) refers to this as the "parallel experience for the staff." If these factors are in place, members of the staff are more likely to be "bonded" or committed to their place of work—the school. Therefore, resilience dimensions are important for both students and educators to ensure satisfactory school environments.

Effective schools have ongoing mechanisms to support school personnel and provide them with professional development opportunities. If school safety concepts are to be integrated into the mission of the school, a shift will be needed not only in terms of roles and responsibilities, but also in the way that these personnel do their jobs. For example, if the acquisition of social and emotional skills is part of the school mission, all personnel need to know strategies for "infusing" this content into the curriculum or capitalizing on "teachable" moments as pertinent situations arise (Skiba, 1999). Changes in personnel, new developments in best practices, changes in the student and community demographics of the school are indicators that personnel development may be needed (Barton, 2000). Fullan (1994) makes the point that this process of professional development should be viewed as a continuous process. It is likely that as one problem is solved, others will arise. The safety issue is one that—when defined in physical, psychological, and developmental terms—provides an infinite number of possibilities and challenges that require as many different approaches.

Change Principles: Developing Skills and Practices

A key part of any change effort is learning new skills and implementing new practices. Part of working together is learning together (Sergiovanni, 1994). This is the "how" of change efforts. Skill development should take place according to the "laws" of empowerment. That is, professional development is likely to be most effective if (1) it begins with and capitalizes on strengths, (2) the professionals are given a choice in and collaborate in the direction of the professional development activities, and (3) acquisition and performance of new skills are valued and recognized.

The development of new skills serves a recursive function; that is, as educators learn new skills, they become more confident in their ability to effect change and therefore increase their efforts toward that end. Snyder et al. (1996) found that those educators who were involved in successful reform efforts felt more assured about their ability to help students. Their feelings of efficacy were related to how much responsibility they felt they "owned" for helping students in their schools take the next step toward their future education. This factor is particularly important, for school safety research has shown that educators express a low sense of efficacy about their skills for addressing school violence (Dear, 1995; Furlong et al., 1996), in part because they perceive its solution as falling outside their areas of expertise.

Empowerment Principles Applied to School Safety Reform

As educators are asked to change the way they do their jobs, it is necessary to understand the conditions under which this change will be facilitated. We have found empowerment concepts particularly useful in framing the process of change in a way that makes it accessible and approachable. The literature that discusses the core components of enabling and empowering (see Dunst, Trivette, & Deal, 1988) provides a framework for outlining actions that follow from our reframing of school violence. Whitmore and Kerans (1988, as cited in Dunst, Trivette, & Deal, 1994) define empowerment as "an interactive process through which people experience personal and social change, enabling them to take action to achieve influence over the organizations and institutions which affect their lives and the communities in which they live." Dunst et al. (1988) emphasize three important concepts in empowerment: (1) People either are already competent or have the capacity to become competent, (2) the failure to display competence is not attributable to personal deficits, but to the failure of the system in which people operate to provide opportunities for competencies to be displayed, and (3) people seeking help or new areas of competence must attribute behavior change to their own actions, in order to gain the sense of control necessary to maintain changes.

An application of these principles to educational change and reform implies the following: (1) Educators already do many things that help students develop, and nurture skills that will help them to be safe in their schools and other environments, (2) school systems that concentrate on defensive and control strategies to prevent school violence (e.g., higher walls, metal detectors) may fail to recognize the actual and potential contributions of teachers and educators to the development of students into nonviolent, contributing members of society, and (3) the ongoing actions of educators and their efforts toward safe schools must be recognized by themselves as well as others. Hyman et al. (1995) have reinforced two of these points in their commentary about schools as a safe haven; they noted that schools should "congratulate themselves for creating a relatively safe haven for youths" (p. 37). This recognition then provides the base for thinking through constructive plans and actions toward safer schools.

EFFECTIVE LEADERSHIP

We (Furlong et al., 1993) have stated that a crucial issue with regard to ensuring safe schools is what actions by staff (and others) will produce the desired school environment. We emphasize, as do other reformers, that involving students, parents, and faculty members in prioritizing and determining actions is critical to the process of ensuring safe and effective schools. On the basis of the literature reviewed earlier in this chapter, we further suggest that consideration be given to including a variety of educational staff members (faculty, administrators, school counselors, school psychologists, other specialists, and noncertificated personnel) in this process and the actions that follow. As the plan unfolds, dispersing leadership functions throughout this group will facilitate the implementation efforts. Also during this stage of selecting actions, the empowerment principles of deemphasizing blame and emphasizing actions and choice will be important principles for leaders to employ.

Change Principle: Leadership Functions

Much has been written about the characteristics and styles of effective school leaders (Blumberg & Greenfield, 1986; Fink, 2000; VanBerkum, 1997). Regardless of leaders' personal characteristics, most reform efforts recognize the importance of having key "power brokers" involved and committed to the change that is being attempted; in the case of the local school, the principal is a key individual. Although this point is seemingly obvious, it may be overlooked when the change originates in sectors other than instruction (e.g., guidance and counseling, school psychology, or other support services). The principal's support (not control) is key to "mainstreaming" proposed changes and incorporating them into everyday schooling practice. The originators of one of the guidance and counseling reform projects described by Snyder et al. (1996) failed to involve school principals in their early efforts and experienced slower and more frustrating efforts toward change. As an adjustment to the original plan, principals were later incorporated as critical team members in the change efforts. Fullan and Miles (1992) note that such power can also be found in a cross-role group (e.g., teachers, administrators, parents, and students working collaboratively) that has been authorized by other school personnel to make decisions and take action.

Perhaps more important than personal characteristics of leaders are the "functions" of leadership and how those functions are carried out. Greenfield (1991) refers to these as the behaviors, tactics, and strategies undertaken to encourage leadership in others. For example, one function of leadership is to maintain a clear focus on goals (Sergiovanni, 1994). Participants in reforms need to know where they are going and why (Schlechty, 1993). In addressing this type of leadership, Sergiovanni (1994, p. 190) quotes Chavez (1992): "My role isn't so much to make things happen but to make sense of things, to show how things fit together."

The understandings about goals and directions are most potent when their meaning is developed by the participants themselves, rather than simply dictated by leaders of the process (Fullan & Miles, 1992). Reform efforts have recognized that positive and lasting changes occur when change is neither highly centralized nor highly decentralized—that is, when there is a productive tension between individualism and collectivism (Fullan, 1994).

A critical function of effective leadership is to provide strong guidance and vision, while dispersing leadership functions widely enough to ensure ownership and enthusiastic participation. Giving up centralized control and encouraging the involvement and leadership of others may seem like risky business to some leaders. Fullan (1994) highlights this quotation from Pascale (1990): "Productive educational change roams somewhere between over control and chaos" (p. 19).

As students need guidance and support, so do educators who are involved in their own process of changing and learning (Comer, 1980). Snyder et al. (1996) isolated the concepts of challenge, support, and recognition as critical processes that were provided by effective school change leaders. The challenge involves raising awareness of the problem and pushing toward some kind of solution. The leadership challenge is the centering conviction or the moral "bottom line" that provides the impetus for change. Support, which involves creating a solution through increasing skills and changing practices, is a key function that needs to be provided by change leaders. This support may include time, resources, professional training, coordination of efforts, and/or communications implying value and recognition. One aspect of support is ensuring that what is being asked of change participants is based on their existing strengths—building on strengths is a critical ingredient of empowerment (Keller, 1995). As Lao-tsu noted in the sixth century B.C., "Start with what they know; build with what they have." Any "stretch" beyond these strengths should be thoroughly supported through professional development and follow-up intervention. Finally, recognition, appreciation, and public valuing of change efforts is critical to those involved.

In addition to keeping the vision of change in focus, a critical leadership function is to monitor the speed and depth of change. Fullan (1994) refers to the "Ready—Fire—Aim" sequence. This sequence emphasizes the need to get the change process going and to do the fine-tuning in the midst of change, rather than waiting until people and conditions are perfectly in line. This process was seen clearly in the guidance-centered change projects described by Snyder et al. (1996). A key factor in programs that experienced early success was that they "did something," however small. The early success of small

286   SCHOOL-ORIENTED INTERVENTIONS

efforts fed the energy of participants and helped to bring on other participants or to "widen the circle" of change efforts.

Change Principle: The Importance of Broad Participation

Change involves the cooperation and participation of all educators. Too often, one professional group or another is targeted separately for one reform
or another; for example, teachers and administrators are often targeted for
reforms in school restructuring, often with little input or involvement from
support personnel such as school counselors or school psychologists. These
support personnel were conspicuously absent from discussions stemming
from the reforms suggested by *A Nation at Risk* (Herr, 1991). Most school effectiveness studies tend to look at the structural aspects of schools, rather
than the personal connections (Fink, 2000). The culture of schools, the roles,
philosophies, norms, habits, and meanings that are made around these practices, all involving individual actors, is extremely resistant to change (Fink,
2000; Fullan, 1994; Maehr & Midgley, 1996).

Snyder et al. (1996) found that in schools where reform projects were
particularly successful, all educators, parents, and community members, regardless of their role, title, or professional identification, were considered
important participants and contributors to reform activities. In one case described by these authors, a media specialist was critical in spearheading
changes related to career planning and college entrance exam availability. Although these are tasks typically left to the purview of school counselors, the
leadership of this particular project was highly effective in including and
empowering all school staff to participate.

Snyder et al. (1996) have documented the wide distribution of change
activities, especially leadership functions, across entire school staffs. Although such dispersal did not take away the importance of the vision and
guidance provided by the leaders of the change, it did get more people involved in implementing desired changes—more specifically, in reaching out
to more students and providing them with guidance and support.
Sergiovanni (1994) concludes, "No one person can pull it off"; school personnel must "share together in the obligations of leadership" (p. 202).

SALIENT PARENTAL AND COMMUNITY INVOLVEMENT

Parents are the first teachers of their children. Children learn language, socialization, values, reasoning, and a sense of self from their home environment. Parents have a life-long personal investment in their child's social, intellectual, and academic development. As such, parents as well as schools
have the responsibility to foster collaborative working relationships. Most
parents want to be involved in the moral, social, and psychological development of their children that is shaped by the schooling process (Chrispeels,

1992; Comer, 1988). In some schools, parents and community members are seen as stakeholders and partners in the strategic planning process and are empowered to shape school policy, attend school events, and contribute expertise to daily school activities. Where schools serve racial, ethnic, and culturally diverse populations, all voices need to be included. The Committee on Policy for Racial Justice (1989) suggested that minority churches, social groups, and fraternities must enter into partnerships with schools to strengthen and emphasize human relations and personalization and reduce the social and psychological distance that exists between some parents and their child's school. Parents can help schools to select and develop culturally sensitive and values-oriented curricula that contribute to positive civic outcomes.

School effectiveness research, as well as best practices in prevention and intervention, documents the importance of involving parents in the educational process of their children (Committee on Policy for Racial Justice, 1989; Epstein, 1996; Henderson & Berla, 1996). School effectiveness and improvement literature notes the importance of parent support, assistance, and communication about the academic work of their children (Reynolds et al., 2000). These functions not only involve the tasks themselves, but the creation of a norm of importance about school performance. In parallel, parental participation in the norming of appropriate behavior supports a school's effort toward safe and effective practices (Hawkins, Farrington, & Catalano, 1998).

Home discipline practices that teach skills and help the child to reason about actions and consequences support the development of a sense of responsibility and foster cause-and-effect thinking. To the extent appropriate, parents should support the discipline practices of the school or work with the principal and staff to create fair and effective policies and procedures. Where children's behavior is excessive or dangerous, parents, school officials, and community agencies work together to support the child and family in receiving appropriate assessment and targeted intervention. Parents can encourage and support one another in attending school conferences, and employers and employment policies should provide time off from work for parents to meaningfully participate in their child's school experience (Henderson, Benard, & Sharp-Light, 2000). Figure 11.2 contains a set of suggestions for how parents can help foster safe schools.

Safe and effective schools incorporate the input and assistance of the community at large (Dwyer & Osher, 2000). Parents may provide an important structural function for schools by mobilizing community and political resources to address families' needs (Comer, Ben-Avie, Haynes, & Joyner, 1999; Committee on Policy for Racial Justice, 1989). Unemployment; lack of health care; dissolution of the family structure; cultural, linguistic, or geographic isolation; and illiteracy are all barriers to families' participation in their children's schooling that can be overcome with targeted community resources. Where community violence threatens the well-being of children and

MAKING SCHOOLS SAFE
SOME WAYS PARENTS CAN HELP

One of the most important priorities of the Ventura Unified School District is keeping children safe from any kind of physical harm or violence. This is a natural concern for parents, so we encourage you to be involved in helping make our schools safe by doing the following:

1. *EMERGENCY CARDS MUST BE CURRENT*
Make sure correct and up-to-date information is provided at the beginning of each school year and forward new information throughout the school year.

2. *KNOW THE EMERGENCY RESPONSE PLAN*
Make sure you understand your school's emergency response plan. Make donations of money and/or supplies and volunteer to help.

3. *SUPPORT THE SCHOOL RULES AND PROCEDURES*
Help your child/children comply with the school rules. If you own firearms, make sure they are all secure and out of reach. No type of weapon, even a small pocket knife, is allowed on campus.

4. *BE AN EXAMPLE OF NONVIOLENCE*
Talk with your child/children about solving problems with words. Resolve disagreements through open, caring communication.

5. *REPORT POTENTIAL DANGERS OR THREATS*
Impress upon your child/children the importance of notifying school staff if they feel threatened or unsafe. If they see someone with a weapon, make a confidential report to an administrator immediately.

6. *LIMIT YOUR CHILD'S EXPOSURE TO VIOLENCE*
Exposure to violence of any kind—media, music, video games, etc.—can desensitize children. Please make informed choices with your child to limit and supervise use of such material.

7. *INVOLVE YOUR CHILDREN IN SUPERVISED ACTIVITIES*
After-school programs and activities will help them be safe and productive. Contact the school for suggestions. Know where your child is and whom he or she is with.

8. *SHOW YOUR INTEREST IN SCHOOLWORK*
Talk to your child/children about the importance of school. Make homework a priority and monitor school progress. Maintain positive relationships with teachers and other school staff. Become active in school events, field trips, and PTA/PTO.

9. *OBSERVE AND LISTEN TO YOUR CHILDREN*
Be alert to any signs of personal difficulties. If your child is experiencing a serious personal loss or concern, be sure to notify a school staff member.

10. *WATCH FOR AND REPORT NEIGHBORHOOD CONCERNS*
Contact the school immediately or report to city police any safety concerns or criminal activity. Be on alert for neighborhood intruders and notify the school. Drive cautiously and observe the speed limit near school. STOP when school buses are stopped!

THANK YOU FOR YOUR SUPPORT

FIGURE 11.2. Tips for parents. From R. L. Morrison, Ventura Unified School District, Ventura, CA.

families, neighbors can band together to support one another and exert political pressure on governance, police, and health and human services to address the unmet needs from which violence stems. Collaboration efforts among community teams—education, mental health, welfare, and law enforcement—are directed at the prevention of crime and poverty in addition to intervention for identified problems (Indiana Education Policy Center, 2000).

Two primary models of collaboration have been used to this end: *school-based services* and *community-based models* (Adelman, 1996; Rigsby, Reynolds, & Wang, 1995). The California Healthy Start collaborative programs constitute an example of school-based programs that bring community health, welfare, educational, and social services and resources into the schools to facilitate parent access. Community-based approaches involve businesses and organizations in extending the school walls by providing training and education to parents and students *in situ*. A critical task of school support staff is the building, strengthening, and coordination of interagency partnerships and collaboratives that come together to meet the needs of students.

CONCLUSIONS

For any institution, change is bound to be an arduous and sometimes trying process. Public schools, in particular, base established routines, policy, and practice on years of knowledge building and shared meaning (Maehr & Midgley, 1996). One of the most important approaches to change is to understand it and recognize the difficulties while in the midst of it. "The term 'lasting change' is an oxymoron. Something that is changing cannot be lasting, and yet the quest is to establish an effective direction for an organization that remains true across time" (Wheatley, 1994, in Grimes & Tilly, 1996, p. 465). A key factor in maintaining the energy and trajectory of change is the understanding by key personnel that the nature of change is an up-and-down process and that support and understanding for everyone involved are needed throughout the process.

A safe school is one that prevents physical, psychological, and developmental harm to its students. The fact that an unsafe school can cause developmental or educational harm mandates that educators integrate the traditions of safe schools and school reform. The challenge of ensuring safe schools requires that education professionals, trained in a variety of disciplines, be able to work together in an ongoing, continual process of school change. This challenge will require that these professionals clearly communicate their vision and understand the perspectives that others bring to the work process. In this chapter we have attempted to draw parallels between the developmental psychology tradition of prevention, risk, and resiliency and the educational traditions of school effectiveness and school reform, aligning the principles of change with the mission of safeguarding schools. The case has been advanced that academic reforms cannot be fully realized without a broader vision that considers the physical, contextual, interpersonal, emotional, and developmental factors inherent in establishing and maintaining safe schools. The parallels are evident; however, the change process will require continual efforts to create shared understanding of the different ways of talking about critical issues.

To the school safety planning process, educators bring intimate knowledge of curriculum, instructional techniques, how students learn, and how schools work. Support personnel such as school psychologists and school counselors bring a different perspective about how students develop and can contribute a broader view of the effects that the contexts of community, home, and school may have on students. Both perspectives are necessary in the challenge of creating safe schools. Further, we have argued that these efforts are most likely to have pervasive and lasting effects if the mission of safe schools is incorporated into the more general mission of excellence in education.

REFERENCES

Adelman, H. S. (1996). Restructuring education support services and integrating community resources: Beyond the full service school model. *School Psychology Review, 25,* 431–445.

Adelman, H. S., & Taylor, L. (2000). Moving prevention from the fringes into the fabric of school improvement. *Journal of Educational and Psychological Consultation, 11,* 7–36.

Advancement Project/Civil Rights Project (2000). *Opportunities suspended: The devastating consequences of zero tolerance and school discipline policies.* Cambridge, MA: Harvard University Press.

American Psychological Association. (1993). *Youth and violence: Psychology's response. Vol. 1: Summary report of the American Psychological Association Commission on Violence and Youth.* Washington, DC: Author.

Barr, R. D., & Parrett, W. H. (2001). *Hope fulfilled for at-risk and violent youth: K–12 programs that work* (2nd ed.). Needham Heights, MA: Allyn & Bacon.

Barton, E. A. (2000). *Leadership strategies for safe schools.* Arlington Heights, IL: Skylight Professional Development.

Batsche, G. M., & Knoff, H. M. (1994). Bullies and their victims: Understanding a pervasive problem in the schools. *School Psychology Review, 23,* 165–174.

Bear, G. C., Webster-Stratton, C., Furlong, M. J., & Rhee, S. (2000). Preventing aggression and violence. In K. L. Minke & G. C. Bear (Eds.), *Preventing school problems–promoting school success: Strategies and programs that work* (pp. 1–69). Bethesda, MD: National Association of School Psychologists.

Benard, B. (1993a, September). Resiliency paradigm validates craft knowledge. *Western Center News,* pp. 5–6.

Benard, B. (1993b, March). Resiliency requires changing hearts and minds. *Western Center News,* pp. 4–5.

Besag, V. E. (1989). *Bullies and victims in schools.* Milton Keynes, UK: Open University Press.

Bickel, W. (1999). The implications of the effective schools literature for school restructuring. In C. R. Reynolds & T. B. Gutkin (Eds.), *The handbook of school psychology* (3rd ed., pp. 959–983). New York: Wiley.

Block, J. H., Everson, S. T., & Guskey, T. R. (Eds.). (1995). *School improvement programs: A handbook for educational leaders.* New York: Scholastic Leadership Policy Research.

Blumberg, A., & Greenfield, W. (1986). *The effective principal* (2nd ed.). Boston: Allyn & Bacon.

Brendtro, L. K., Brokenleg, M., & Van Bockern, S. (1990). *Reclaiming youth at risk: Our hope for the future.* Bloomington, IN: National Educational Service.

Brener, N. D., Simon, T. R., Krug, E. G., & Lowry, R. (1999). Recent trends in violence-related behaviors among high school students in the United States. *Journal of the American Medical Association, 282,* 440–446.

Brock, S. E. (2000). Development of school district crisis intervention policy. *California School Psychologist, 5,* 53–64.

Brown, J. H., D'Emidio-Caston, M., & Benard, B. (2001). *Resilience education.* Thousand Oaks, CA: Sage.

Callahan, C. M., & Rivara, F. P. (1992). Urban high school youth and handguns: A school-based survey. *Journal of the American Medical Association, 267,* 3038–3042.

Cernkovich, S. A., & Giordano, P. G. (1992). School bonding, race, and delinquency. *Criminology, 30,* 261–290.

Cohen, L. (1998). *The spectrum of prevention.* Berkeley, CA: The Prevention Institute.

Comer, J. (1980). *School power.* New York: Free Press.

Comer, J. P. (1988). Educating poor minority children. *Scientific American, 259*(5), 42–48.

Comer, J. P., Ben-Avie, M., Haynes, N. M., & Joyner, E. T. (Eds.). (1999). *Child by child: The Comer process for change in education.* New York: Teachers College Press.

Committee on Policy for Racial Justice. (1989). Visions for a better way: Improving schools for black children. *Equity and Choice, 6,* 5–9, 49–54.

Cornell, D. G., & Loper, A. B. (1998). Assessment of violence and other high-risk behaviors with a school survey. *School Psychology Review, 27,* 317–330.

Cunningham, P. B., & Henggeler, S. W. (2001). Implementation of an empirically based drug and violence prevention and intervention program in public school settings. *Journal of Child Clinical Psychology, 30,* 221–232.

Dear, J. D. (1995). *Creating caring relationships to foster academic excellence: Recommendations for reducing violence in California schools.* Sacramento: California Commission on Teacher Credentialing.

Duncan, B. B., Forness, S. R., & Hartsough, C. (1995). Students identified as seriously emotionally disturbed in school-based day treatment: Cognitive, psychiatric, and special education characteristics. *Behavioral Disorders, 30,* 238–252.

Dunst, C. J., Trivette, C. M., & Deal, A. G. (1988). *Enabling and empowering families: Principles and guidelines for practice.* Cambridge, MA: Brookline.

Dunst, C. J., Trivette, C. M., & Deal, A. G.(1994). *Supporting and strengthening families, Vol. 1: Methods, strategies and practices.* Cambridge, MA: Brookline.

Dwyer, K., & Osher, D. (2000). *Safeguarding our children: An action guide.* Washington, DC: United Sates Departments of Education and Justice, American Institute for Research.

Dwyer, K., Osher, D., & Warger, C. (1998). *Early warning, timely response: A guide to safe schools.* Washington, DC: U.S. Department of Education.

Edmonds, R. R. (1979). Effective schools for the urban poor. *Educational Leadership, 37,* 15–24.

Elliott, D. S., & Voss, H. L. (1974). *Delinquency and dropout.* Lexington, MA: Lexington Books.

Epp, J. R., & Watkinson, A. M. (Eds.). (1997). *Systemic violence in education: Promise broken.* Albany: State University of New York Press.

Epstein, J. L. (Ed.). (1996). *Perspectives and previews on research and policy for school, family, and community partnerships.* Hillsdale, NJ: Erlbaum.

Fein, R. A., & Vossekuil, B. V. (1995, September). Threat assessment: An approach to prevent targeted violence. *National Institute of Justice: Research in Action,* pp. 1–7.

Fink, D. (2000). *Good schools/real schools: Why school reform doesn't last.* New York: Teachers College Press.

Fullan, M. (1994). *Change forces: Probing the depths of educational reform.* New York: Falmer Press.

Fullan, M. G., & Miles, M. B. (1992). Getting reform right: What works and what doesn't. *Phi Delta Kappan, 73,* 744–752.

Furlong, M., Casas, J. M., Corral, C., Chung, A., & Bates, M. (1997). Drugs and school violence. *Education and Treatment of Children, 20,* 263–280.

Furlong, M., & Morrison, G. (2000). The school in school violence: Definitions and facts. *Journal of Emotional and Behavioral Disorders, 8,* 71–82.

Furlong, M., Morrison, R., & Clontz, D. (1993, spring). Planning principles for safe, secure, and peaceful schools. *School Safety,* pp. 23–27.

Furlong, M., Pavelski, R., & Morrison, G. (2000). Trends in school psychology for the 21st century: Influences of school violence on professional change. *Psychology in the Schools, 37,* 81–90.

Furlong, M. J., Babinski, L., Poland, S., Muqoz, J., & Boles, S. (1996). Factors associated with school psychologists' perceptions of campus violence. *Psychology in the Schools, 33,* 29–38.

Furlong, M. J., Chung, A., Bates, M., & Morrison, R. (1995). Who are the victims of school violence? A comparison of student non-victims and multi-victims. *Education and Treatment of Children, 18,* 1–17.

Furlong, M. J., Jimenez, T., C., & Saxton, J. D. (Eds.). (2003). The prevention of adolescent homicide. In T. Gullotta & M. Bloom (Eds.), The encyclopedia of primary prevention and health promotion (pp. 575–582). New London, CT: Kluwer Academic/Plenum.

Furlong, M. J., Kingery, P. E., & Bates, M. P. (2001). Introduction to special issue on the appraisal and prediction of school violence. *Psychology in the Schools, 38,* 89–92.

Furlong, M. J., Morrison, G., & Dear, J. (1994). Addressing school violence as part of the school's educational mission. *Preventing School Failure, 38*(3), 10–17.

Garbarino, J. (1992). *Children in danger: Coping with the consequences of community violence.* San Francisco: Jossey-Bass.

Garmezy, N. (Ed.). (1983). *Stressors of childhood.* Minneapolis: McGraw-Hill.

Garmezy, N., & Masten, A. S. (1991). The protective role of competence indicators in children at risk. In E. M. Cummings, A. L. Greene, & K. H. Karraker (Eds.), *Life-span developmental psychology: Perspectives on stress and coping* (pp. 151–174). Hillsdale, NJ: Erlbaum.

Garmezy, N., Masten, A. S., & Tellegen, A. (1984). The study of stress and competence in children: A building block for developmental psychopathology. *Child Development, 55,* 97–111.

Gold, M., & Osgood, D. (1992). *Personality and peer influence in juvenile corrections.* Westport, CT: Greenwood Press.

Green, M. W., Travis, J., & Downs, R. (1999). *The appropriate and effective use of security technologies in U.S. schools: A guide for schools and law enforcement agencies.* Washington, DC: U.S. Department of Justice, Office of Justice Programs, National Institute of Justice.

Greenfield, W. D. (1991). *The micropolitics of leadership in an urban elementary school: A research study* (#4). Portland, OR: Center for Urban Research in Education, Portland State University.

Gresham, F. M., Watson, T. S., & Skinner, C. H. (2001). Functional behavioral assessment: Principles, procedures, and future directions. *School Psychology Review, 30,* 156–172.

Grimes, J., & Tilly, W. D. (1996). Policy and process: Means to lasting educational change. *School Psychology Review, 25,* 465–476.

Hawkins, J. D., Catalano, R. F., & Haggerty, K. (1993, September). Risks and protective factors are interdependent. *Western Center News,* p. 7.

Hawkins, J. D., Catalano, R. F., & Miller, J. Y. (1992). Risk and protective factors for alcohol and other drug problems in adolescence and early adulthood: Implications for substance abuse prevention. *Psychological Bulletin, 112,* 64–105.

Hawkins, J. D., Farrington, D. P., & Catalano, R. F. (1998). Reducing violence through the schools. In D. S. Elliott, B. A. Hamburg, & K. R. Williams (Eds.), *Violence in American schools* (pp. 188–216). New York: Cambridge University Press.

Hawkins, J. D., & Lishner, D. (1987). Etiology and prevention of antisocial behavior in children and adolescents. In D. H. Crowell, I. M. Evans Clifford, & R. O. O'Donnell (Eds.), *Childhood aggression and violence: Sources of influence, prevention, and control. Applied clinical psychology* (pp. 263–282). New York: Plenum Press.

Hawkins, J. D., Lishner, D. M., Catalano, R. F., & Howard, M. O. (1985). Childhood predictors of adolescent substance abuse: Toward an empirically grounded theory [Special issue]. Childhood and Chemical Abuse: Prevention and Intervention. *Journal of Children in Contemporary Society, 18*(1–2), 11–48.

Henderson, A. T., & Berla, N. (1996). *A new generation of evidence: The family is critical to student achievement.* Washington, DC: Center for Law and Education.

Henderson, N., Benard, B., & Sharp-Light, N. (Eds.). (2000). *Schoolwide approaches for fostering resiliency.* Rio Rancho, NM: Resiliency in Action.

Herr, E. (1991). *Guidance and Counseling: A Shared Responsibility.* Alexandria, VA: National Association of College Admission Counselors.

Horner, R. H., & Sugai, G. (2000). School-wide behavior support: an emerging initiative. *Journal of Positive Behavioral Interventions, 2*(4), 231.

Hyman, I. A., Weller, E., Shanock, A., & Britton, G. (1995, March 1). Schools as a safe haven: The politics of punitiveness and its effect on educators. *Education Week,* pp. 37, 48.

Indiana Education Policy Center. (2000, September). *Understanding school violence.* Available online at: *www.indiana.edu/~safeschl/guide.html*

Kann, L., Warren, C. W., Harris, W. A., Collins, J. L., Douglas, K. A., Collins, M. E., Williams, B. I., Ross, J. G., & Kolbe, L. J. (1995). Youth risk behavior surveillance—United States, 1993. *Morbidity and Mortality Weekly Reports, 44*(SS-1), 1–55.

Kazdin, A. (1987). *Conduct disorders in childhood and adolescence.* London: Sage.

Keller, B. M. (1995). Accelerated schools: Hands-on learning in a unified community. *Educational Leadership, 52*(5), 10–13.

Kirby, L. D., & Fraser, M. W. (1997). Risk and resilience in childhood. In M. W. Fraser (Ed.), *Risk and resilience in childhood: An ecological perspective* (pp. 10–33). Washington, DC: NASW Press.

Knoff, H. M., & Batsche, G. M. (1985). Project ACHIEVE: Analyzing a school reform process for at-risk and underachieving students. *School Psychology Review, 24,* 579–603.

Levine, D. U., & Lezotte, L. W. (1990). *Unusually effective schools: A review and analysis of unusually effective schools.* Madison, WI: National Center for Effective Schools Research and Development.

Loeber, R., Farrington, D. A., & Waschbusch, D. A. (1993). Serious and violent juvenile offenders. In R. Loeber & D. P. Farrington (Eds.), *Serious and violent juvenile offenders: Risk factors and successful interventions* (pp. 13–29). Thousand Oaks, CA: Sage.

Maehr, M. L., & Midgley, C. (1996). *Transforming school cultures.* Boulder, CO: Westview Press.

Masten, A. S. (2001). Ordinary magic: Resilience processes in development. *American Psychologist, 56,* 227–238.

Mayer, M. J., & Leone, P. E. (1999). A structural analysis of school violence and disruption: Implications for creating safer schools. *Education and Treatment of Children, 22,* 333–356.

Moffitt, T. E. (1993). Adolescence-limited and life-course persistent antisocial behavior: A developmental taxonomy. *Psychological Review, 100,* 674–701.

Montague, M., & Rinaldi, C. (2001). Classroom dynamics and children at risk: A followup. *Learning Disability Quarterly, 24,* 75–83.

Morrison, G. M., Anthony, S., Storino, M., Cheng, J., Furlong, M. F., & Morrison, R. L. (2001). School expulsion as a process and an event: Before and after effects on children at-risk for school discipline. *New Directions for Youth Development, 92,* 45–72.

Morrison, G. M., & D'Incau, B. (1997). The web of zero-tolerance: Characteristics of students who are recommended for expulsion from school. *Education and Treatment of Children, 20,* 316–335.

Morrison, G. M., Furlong, M. J., & Morrison, R. L. (1994). School violence to school safety: Reframing the issue for school psychologists. *School Psychology Review, 23,* 236–256.

Morrison, G. M., & Skiba, R. (2001). Predicting violence from school misbehavior. *Psychology in the Schools, 38,* 173–184.

National Education Goals Panel. (2001). Safe school climate becomes focus of state policies. *NEGP Monthly, 2*(23), 1–8.

National School Safety Center (2001). *School-associated violent deaths report.* Available: www.nssc1.org.

O'Neil, J. (1995). On lasting school reform: A conversation with Ted Sizer. *Educational Leadership, 52*(5), 4–9.

Purkey, S. C., & Smith, M. S. (1983). Effective schools: A review. *The Elementary School Journal, 83,* 427–452.

Reddy, M., Borum, R., Berglund, J., Vossekuil, B., Fein, R., & Modzeleski, W. (2001). Evaluating risk for targeted violence in schools: Comparing risk assessment, threat assessment, and other approaches. *Psychology in the Schools, 38,* 157–172.

Reynolds, D., Teddlie, C., Creemers, B., Scheerens, J., & Townsend, T. (2000). An introduction to school effectiveness research. In C. Teddlie & D. Reynolds (Eds.), *The international handbook of school effectiveness research* (pp. 3–25). London: Falmer Press.

Rigsby, L. C., Reynolds, M. C., & Wang, M. C. (Eds.). (1995). *School-community connections.* San Francisco: Jossey-Bass.

Roberts, J. (1988). Setting the frame: Definition, functions, and typology of rituals. In E. Imber-Black & J. Roberts (Eds.), *Rituals in families and family therapy* (pp. 3–46). New York: Norton.

Roff, M., Sells, S. B., & Golden, M. M. (1972). *Social adjustment and personality development in children.* Minneapolis: University of Minnesota Press.

Rutter, M. (1990). Psychosocial resilience and protective mechanisms. In A. S. Masten, J. Rolf, D. Cicchetti, K. N. Nuechterlein, & S. Weintraub (Eds.), *Risk and protective factors in the development of psychopathology* (pp. 181–214). Cambridge, UK: Cambridge University Press.

Sameroff, A. J., Seifer, R., Baldwin, A., & Baldwin, C. (1993). Stability of intelligence from preschool to adolescence: The influence of social and family risk factors. *Child Development, 64,* 80–97.

Schlechty, P. C. (1993). On the frontier of school reform with trailblazers, pioneers, and settlers. *Journal of Staff Development, 14*(4), 46–50.

Sergiovanni, T. J. (1994). *Building community in schools.* San Francisco: Jossey-Bass.

Sheerens, J., & Bosker, R. (1997). *The foundations of educational effectiveness.* New York: Elsevier Science.

Skiba, R. (1999). *Preventing school violence: A practical guide to comprehensive planning.* Bloomington: Indiana School Safety Specialist Academy.

Skiba, R., & Peterson, R. (1999). Zero-tolerance: Can punishment lead to safe schools? *Phi Delta Kappan, 80,* 372–376, 381–382.

Skiba, R., & Peterson, R. (2000). School discipline at a crossroads: From zero tolerance to early response. *Exceptional Children, 66,* 335–346.

Skiba, R., Peterson, R., Miller, C., Boone, K., McKelvey, J., Fontanini, A., Strom, T., & Simmons, A. (2001). The safe and responsive schools project: Comprehensive planning for school violence prevention. *Communique, 29*(7), 16.

Snyder, J., Morrison, G. M., & Smith, R. C. (1996). *Dare to dream: Educational guidance for excellence.* Indianapolis, IN: Lilly Endowment.

Sprague, J., & Walker, H. (2000). Early identification and intervention for youth with antisocial and violent behavior. *Exceptional Children, 66,* 367–379.

Sugai, G., Sprague, J. R., Horner, R. H., & Walker, H. M. (2000). Preventing school violence: The use of office discipline referrals to assess and monitor school-wide discipline interventions. *Journal of Emotional and Behavioral Disorders, 8,* 94–101.

Teddlie, C., & Reynolds, D. (Eds.). (2000). *The international handbook of school effectiveness research.* London: Falmer Press.

United States Department of Justice. (2000). *Indicators of school crime and safety, 2000.* Washington, DC: Author. Retrieved January 22, 2004, from *http://nces.ed.gov/pubsearch/pubsinfo.asp.pubid-2001017*

United States Departments of Education and Justice. (1989). Visions for a better way: Improving schools for black children. *Equity and Choice, 6,* 5–9, 49–54.

VanBerkum, D. W. (1997). The quality principal. In M. Richardson, R. Blackbourn, C. Ruth-Smith, & J. Haynes (Eds.), *The pursuit of continuous improvement in educational organizations* (pp. 153–173). Lanham, MD: University Press of America.

Walker, H. M., Colvin, G., & Ramsey, E. (1995). *Antisocial behavior in school: Strategies and best practices.* Pacific Grove, CA: Brooks/Cole.

Walker, H. M., Horner, R. H., Sugai, G., Bullis, M., Sprague, J. R., Bricker, D., & Kaufman, M. (1996). Integrated approaches to preventing antisocial behavior patterns among school-age children and youth. *Journal of Emotional and Behavioral Disorders, 4,* 194–209.

Walker, H. M., & Severson, H. H. (1990). *Systematic screening for behavior disorders.* Longmont, CO: Sopris West.

Walker, H. M., & Sprague, J. R. (1999). The path to school failure, delinquency, and violence: Causal factors and some potential solutions. *Intervention in School and Clinic, 35*(2), 67–73.

Wehlage, G. G., Rutter, R. A., Smith, G. A., Lesko, N., & Fernandez, R. (1989). *Reducing the risk: Schools and communities of support.* New York: Falmer Press.

Weis, C., Morrison, R. L., Furlong, M. J., & Morrison, G. M. (1993). Creating safe schools. *Healthy Kids Connection, 4*(1), 1, 8–9.

Zimmerman, M. A., & Arunkumar, R. (1994). Resiliency research: Implications for schools and policy. *Social Policy Report: Society for Research in Child Development, 8*(4), 1–17.

Zins, J. E., Elias, M. J., Greenberg, M. T., & Weissberg, R. P. (2000). Promoting social and emotional competence in children. In K. L. Minke & G. C. Bear (Eds.), *Preventing school problems–promoting school success: Strategies and programs that work* (pp. 71–99). Bethesda, MD: National Association of School Psychologists.

Zwier, G., & Vaughan, G. M. (1984). Three ideological orientations in school vandalism research. *Review of Educational Research, 54,* 263–292.

CHAPTER 12

Security Policy, Personnel, and Operations

KENNETH S. TRUMP

School leaders are increasingly faced with pressure to enhance school security measures. Such pressures often stem from high-profile incidents, media coverage of school violence, and/or political influences. Pressure sources may include faculty and staff, students, parents, the media, community members, and elected officials. A growing number of educators are looking to improve security simply to be proactive before a crisis strikes their school.

Comprehensive school safety programming involves many issues, including security operations, sound discipline policies and practices, crisis preparedness, intervention services, a violence prevention curriculum, and much more. This chapter provides a starting point for school officials wanting to professionalize the security component of their school safety programs. It begins with an honest look at the issue most critical to having professional, effective school security: shifting from a traditional framework influenced by denial, image concerns, and politics, to a new framework in which school security efforts are viewed as proactive measures performed consistently and unapologetically.

Within this new framework, readers are presented with various security personnel options; the choice of options should be based on the needs of the school or district. Some basic organization and operational considerations are also offered to help build solid security operations, regardless of the type of personnel used in the program. Components of a thorough safety assessment are highlighted, along with a discussion of crisis preparedness guidelines and cautionary warnings to districts seeking outside resources to help in developing security and crisis programs.

FRAMING SECURITY POLICY

Awareness and Response Continuum

Elsewhere (Trump, 1996), I have described a continuum of positions that may be held by individuals, organizations, and communities in recognizing and responding to gang violence. This continuum ranges from lack of awareness at one extreme, through denial, qualified admittance, and a balanced and rational response, to overreaction at the other extreme. The same continuum can be applied to understanding how school crimes and security threats have been viewed both within and outside the educational environment.

Lack of awareness may be defined as simply not recognizing a problem or not knowing how to address a problem that is recognized. Most educators sorely lack a substantive understanding of youth violence, current street crime trends, basic criminal law, security procedures, and crisis planning; through no fault of the educators, teacher and administrator preparation programs rarely require courses covering the details of these subjects, and in-service programs are often not offered on an ongoing basis. Although many educators will argue that they chose to be teachers, not cops, the current reality is that to be successful teachers, they need an orderly, crime-free environment where the focus is on what is being taught, not on personal survival for those teaching or learning. To achieve such a setting, educators must have a basic understanding of what to look for and how to handle what they may encounter in their classrooms, hallways, and grounds.

Denial occurs when officials are aware of a problem, and possibly even know an appropriate response to the problem, but refuse to admit that the problem exists. For example, Huff (1988) has identified denial as a major obstacle to effectively managing the youth gang problem and has particularly noted the impact of denial on schools:

> It is probable that the official denial of gang problems actually facilitates victimization by gangs, especially in the public schools. School principals in several Ohio cities are reluctant to acknowledge "gang-related" assaults for fear that such "problems" may be interpreted as negative reflections of their management ability. This "paralysis" may actually encourage gang-related assaults and may send the wrong signals to gang members, implying that they can operate within the vacuum created by this "political paralysis." (p. 9)

The denial illustrated in Huff's observations on gang issues can be applied to the overall issue of school crime and disruptions, because many administrators historically refused to admit that they faced security problems in school and on school grounds.

Why would educators deny problems with school crime and serious incidents? As Huff has noted, principals often perceive that they will be viewed as poor managers if they publicly acknowledge ongoing problems with crime in their schools. In some cases, this perception has become a reality, but a reality created by the school system—not by actual problems or by the students, parents, or community members who support crime-free schools. Some districts have used the number of suspensions, expulsions, and criminal incidents reported as formal evaluation measurements for principals, creating a situation in which the salaries and careers of those administrators who acknowledge and deal with crime and discipline problems are negatively affected. Meanwhile, administrators who have problems, but do not report or address them, are rewarded with positive evaluations and promotions.

Another reason for denial centers on the distorted school image created by an unbalanced focus on isolated occurrences or a limited number of incidents. Schools receiving an inordinate amount of media coverage or other public attention for violent incidents or threats to student safety are often inaccurately characterized by the perceptions created by such disproportionate attention. For example, a high school in which 10 students are arrested for possession of drugs may be labeled a "drug school" after several news stories on the arrests. Such unfair labeling, which fails to account for the larger percentage of achievements accomplished in most schools, also drives school administrators to deny and suppress security-related concerns.

Furthermore, denial is often encouraged by superintendents, cabinet-level officials, and school board members who are concerned that public discussions of security issues may create an image not conducive to obtaining successful public support for additional funding. This is particularly true in districts that are dependent on public approval of school levies. One school board president was overheard saying, "Public discussions of gangs, drugs, and other security matters have political ramifications. These issues do not sell levies or get board members reelected." Although some parents and community residents may agree with this position, the majority are less supportive of denial and more supportive of districts where officials tackle difficult security issues head-on in a rational manner.

Finally, for some officials, denial is often (at least initially) an easier option than directly attacking security problems. If a school leader admits to having a problem with crimes in a school, then others generally look to this leader to solve the problem. Although a principal can solve the problem of a lost lunch card, he or she will most likely be unable to "solve" the problem of juvenile crime, disruptive behavior, and other factors threatening school security. Efforts to minimize security threats must involve the entire school community, not one individual. However, the leaders (i.e., the principal, the superintendent, school board members) can set the tone for improving school safety by acknowledging the problem, or potential for a problem, and taking the lead in organizing a proactive strategy to minimize the threat.

What happens when security problems are so prevalent that officials can no longer deny them? Torok (personal interview, November 7, 1994), a now-retired veteran Cleveland (Ohio) police lieutenant, describes the next position on the continuum as "qualified admittance." This position exists when the problem is partially recognized and confronted, but only in a limited manner and not to the actual degree to which it needs to be addressed. Efforts are often made to convince target populations (e.g., parents, community residents, and the media) that the maximum efforts are being made to deal with security problems in order to reduce public pressure. In reality, the efforts made frequently involve "smoke and mirrors" rather than concrete, ongoing, proactive measures.

Among the more familiar examples of the smoke-and-mirrors approach are press conferences or public announcements of "new" zero-tolerance programs. Board members and superintendents, responding to public pressure, have created a significant amount of hype in recent years by announcing that they will take a new stance of zero tolerance for weapons or drugs brought to school by students. One might simply ask how much tolerance the officials have previously had for weapons and drugs: 25% tolerance? 50% tolerance? 100% tolerance? Simply put, a one-shot public announcement consisting of popular rhetoric is generally nothing more than qualified admittance unless it is backed by comprehensive plans for ongoing prevention, intervention, and enforcement strategies related to school security.

A balanced and rational strategy incorporates all three components—prevention, intervention, and enforcement. Pointing fingers, placing blame, and implementing single-strategy solutions accomplish little in actually dealing with school security. It is often thought that violence can be solved with just one solution, such as unplugging television, teaching parenting skills, or giving kids jobs, when experience illustrates that any single approach alone will probably not cure any of our social and economic ills.

The potential for overreaction, the final point on the continuum, grows as security threats continue to appear in our schools. Schools have traditionally been perceived as the safe havens of society. When violence appears in the home and in the community, children are thought to be protected in schools. But during the last decade, when violence has increasingly crossed the playground and entered into the classrooms and hallways, these traditional safe havens have been violated; unfortunately, they are no longer places of guaranteed safety.

School violence has reached a point where many people perceive most schools as being filled with gun-toting, drug-dealing gang members who spend their entire school day committing crimes on campus. This misconception, fueled by the high-profile crimes that actually do occur in schools, can easily create an overreaction as counterproductive as denial. The resulting tension and hysteria can lead to increased violence by students and to progressively harsher reactions by adults, who respond more to the perception of fear than to the reality of the threats that may actually exist.

The five possible positions on the awareness and response continuum are more complicated than they may appear. The initial tendency is to categorize particular individuals as falling into one of the four less preferable positions, and to attempt to move a group of these individuals to the balanced and rational position in order to address security concerns effectively. Although this task may appear manageable, it is more difficult when an individual is at one point on the continuum, but the person's organization as a whole is at another point (e.g., a balanced and rational response vs. denial). The picture becomes even more complex as attempts are made to coordinate multiple agencies and their key representatives; such attempts can create endless opportunities for mixed positions and conflicting agendas, which need to be resolved before the problem itself can be addressed honestly. In many communities, this clarity and the subsequent results are not achieved for several years after the problem gets a foothold or until after a crisis occurs.

All hope is not lost. Lack of awareness can be overcome through education. Denial, qualified admittance, and overreaction can be overcome through balanced and rational programming. Most important, balanced and rational programming can be reached by shifting from the old to the new school of thought in conceptualizing school security.

Changing Schools of Thought

Summarized in Table 12.1 are five shifts in thinking that are needed for a better conceptualization of critical school security issues. By adopting the new school of thought, educators and security authorities will be better equipped to implement practical measures for improving school security effectively. The five views that need to be adopted are as follows:

1. *Law enforcement and schools have similar, not competing, goals.* Behind closed doors in years past, school officials often characterized law enforcement and security personnel as alarmist, punitive, insensitive, and untrained for dealing with youths. Yet law enforcers and security officers frequently described educators as excessively liberal, hypersensitive, and conspirators in the concealment of criminal offenses occurring in buildings and on school grounds. These characterizations have caused both groups to feel that they have opposing goals, although high-profile incidents of nationwide school violence have brought the two professions closer together than ever before in history.

In reality, the two groups have a shared goal: providing crime-free environments in which children can learn and teachers can teach. School leaders and law enforcers must recognize this unified goal and work sincerely to develop acceptable objectives for reaching it. Issues that are of high priority, sensitivity, and controversy in terms of organizational needs and political agendas should be openly identified from the onset, so that a workable understanding is created prior to the time when school officials and law enforcers must jointly address specific incidents and security threats.

2. *Crimes must be handled both administratively and criminally.* Many school administrators mistakenly believe that if a student misbehavior is pro-

TABLE 12.1. Schools of Thought on School Security Issues

Old school	New school
Police and schools have competing philosophical beliefs on school safety.	Police and schools have similar, if not identical, goals; they need to develop objectives cooperatively to reach common goals.
Student misbehaviors constituting crimes should be handled only "administratively."	Crimes should be distinguished from violations of school rules and processed accordingly; school officials must be trained in criminal law and police procedures; written guidelines should be formulated for crime reporting.
The reporting of school-based crime should be avoided or minimized.	There should be mandatory, standardized, and consistent crime-reporting laws, policies, and procedures; the data should be used for analyzing, preventing, and intervening in school-based crimes.
Security is reactive and is a public relations disaster.	Security is proactive and is a positive public relations tool.
School safety should be based largely on prevention-oriented curriculum and traditional administrative discipline.	School safety requires a multifaceted, balanced approach consisting of prevention, intervention, and enforcement strategies.

cessed administratively (i.e., through detention, suspension, or expulsion), no further action is required. Although this is appropriate for such misbehaviors as class cutting and insubordination, such acts as assault, theft, and extortion are also criminal offenses and must be handled as such with the involvement of the police. In some jurisdictions, the failure to report certain offenses is an offense in itself, and a school administrator who fails to report such an incident to police can be criminally charged.

Principals and other administrators must realize that there are two separate systems working simultaneously on school-based crimes—a school administrative (disciplinary) system and a criminal system. The actions and consequences associated with the school disciplinary system are not contingent upon those associated with the criminal system, or vice versa. There is no "double jeopardy" involved in taking school disciplinary action for a crime and in reporting the same offense to police for criminal charges. In fact, failure to report crimes actually creates an environment in which students perceive that they can commit crimes with few, if any, consequences; this results in the potential for additional and more serious offenses.

Concerns about negative publicity or political pressures from central office administrators can encourage principals to process criminal incidents only administratively. However, failure to involve the police is often the result of administrators' being inadequately trained in criminal law and police procedures. Most educators receive little or no training in defining basic criminal offenses, distinguishing felonies from misdemeanors, or knowing the steps taken in the criminal justice process (from making the police report to the final court disposition).

Security programs should include training for school personnel in relevant laws and reporting procedures, to minimize potential discrepancies. Consideration should be given to having local juvenile detectives and juvenile court prosecutors work with school security officials to conduct basic in-service training and annual updates for all administrators in identifying and reporting crimes occurring on school grounds and in school buildings. Police and court officials may also consider providing school administrators with written summaries of key laws and reporting guidelines, so that they will have a reference available in their offices.

In addition to training, school boards and superintendents should develop policies and procedures to ensure that all employees report crimes and serious incidents occurring under school jurisdiction. Reporting procedures should include directions for internal reporting from staff members to principals to the central office, and external reporting from principals and administrators to law enforcement agencies. When clear internal and external reporting procedures exist, school officials ensure that law enforcement agencies are properly notified about specific incidents, while such reporting method also provide a mechanism within the district to monitor, track, intervene in, and prevent school crime and serious incidents from a systemwide perspective.

School districts with their own security personnel, school police departments, or School Resource Officers (SROs) have an in-house resource to consult when questions arise about the potential criminality of a situation. Districts should form ongoing relationships with police and court officials so that they may contact a representative of one of these agencies when a reporting question arises. In the best interests of student safety and their own personal liability, administrators should consult any available resource to ensure that crimes occurring within their jurisdictions are properly reported to police.

3. *Crime reporting is a positive safety tool.* Regardless of the reasons for the failure of school officials to report campus crimes, these concealed incidents eventually come to light, and usually in a more negative light than if they had been officially reported at the onset. Many times this intensified publicity is viewed as so damaging to the school image that school officials think it would be better not to have reported the incident or to have no reporting system whatsoever.

In reality, mandatory, standardized, and consistent crime reporting provides data for school officials to use in analyzing, intervening in, and preventing school-based crime and violence. Officially collected data may help, not hinder, the district's public relations position by dispelling myths, rumors, and perceptions that the number of violent crimes occurring in schools is higher than it actually is. The documentation of incidents also provides school districts with written details about incidents and official responses, which can actually help educators in the event that they need to provide evidence of their affirmative action in response to liability claims months or years after an incident occurs. In the long run, crime reporting is a positive tool for accurately identifying, preventing, and managing school safety threats.

4. *Security is a public relations tool, not a public relations disaster.* Many officials traditionally viewed discussions of school security as a public relations nightmare: "If we talk about the need for improved school security, parents will think we are unable to control our school." However, by publicly framing security improvements as a prevention mechanism rather than as a reactive measure, educators can enhance their school security posture, as well as their public image with parents and the community. Honest discussions and proactive, up-front action will win out over hindsight reaction following a crisis.

This is not to say that there will be no resistance to improving security measures. Something as simple as reducing the number of entrance points to an elementary school can cause some initial controversy. Parents who have used a back door for several years may now have to walk to the front door. Teachers and staff members may have to walk an additional walkway to get to the designated entrance from where they park.

The best way to minimize the rumblings that may occur in situations like these is to involve key stakeholders in the planning of security improvements and to publicize these improvements and the reasons for them to parents, staff, and students. Reasonable modifications, made with reasonable notice, will generally be understood by reasonable people. Most school administrators are experienced and prepared to deal with those few unreasonable people who always complain about everything, and safety should be a topic on which these administrators are willing to stand their ground.

5. *School safety requires a multipronged approach.* School safety concerns have traditionally manifested themselves in the form of antidrug, antiviolence, or other curriculum-based prevention measures. Although prevention is unquestionably the desired focus and outcome, school safety efforts must be framed in a multipronged approach consisting of prevention, intervention, and enforcement. One or two of these components alone will not suffice.

For example, enforcement strategies may be employed through administrative discipline and security or police involvement. However, it is commonly agreed that such strategies will be effective in addressing only short-term problems. Although enforcement is necessary and serves an important role in securing the immediate situation, longer-term approaches are also needed to prevent such occurrences in the future; thus a prevention-oriented curriculum becomes important. At the same time, these prevention programs will be effective only if they are administered in a secure setting, the maintenance of which requires enforcement and intervention services.

Examples of the prevention component include such programs as Project DARE (Drug Abuse Resistance Education), Gang Resistance Education and Training (GREAT), social skills training, and other violence prevention instruction programs. The intervention component may include counseling, peer mediation, crisis intervention, peer courts, and similar strategies. The enforcement component includes administrative disciplinary action and, when appropriate, specialized school security or police services available in-house to address school-specific needs.

Educators have traditionally relied on a prevention-oriented curriculum, intervention services, and administrative discipline as their primary resources in school safety programming. More recently, because of an increased number of threats to the security of students, staff, and facilities, districts are turning to specialized security or school police departments, and to School Resource Officer (SRO) programs, to enhance school safety within their district. By proactively, consistently, and unapologetically integrating professional school security and school policing programs into their overall safety plans, educators can move one step closer to ensuring safer schools.

SECURITY AND POLICE PERSONNEL

Traditional Practices

Schools have generally used available staff members to address security needs both within and outside schools. Teachers have traditionally been scheduled during their nonteaching periods to monitor hallways for class cutters and to guard isolated areas against intruders. Particularly in light of the budgetary constraints facing most districts and the minimal security threats to teachers and schools as a whole, this system has worked until recent years. As security threats and incidents have increased, along with the number of classes to be taught in a workday, so have the efforts made by teachers (including those undertaken through union contracts) to reduce or eliminate such nonteaching assignments.

It has been customary for schools to fill this gap by employing hall monitors, teachers' aides, or other nonteaching individuals to support the regular faculty and staff by monitoring hallways and restrooms, checking passes, assisting in cafeteria supervision, and escorting unruly students to the office for disciplinary action. These hall monitors or "hall guards" have been (and in most cases still are) without degrees, poorly paid, and often elderly individuals employed under generic job descriptions, with little or no training in dealing with aggressive, violent youths. Although many hall monitors have been successful in dealing with average students, they often pose little threat to the smaller percentage of more disruptive, chronic offenders they are likely to encounter on a daily basis.

The Need to Professionalize

These descriptions of traditional practices are in no way intended as criticisms of teachers, hall monitors, or others who have dutifully attempted to fulfill their responsibilities in these unrefined security capacities. However, individuals in these personnel classifications have not been trained or experienced in professional security. Traditionally, individuals responsible for school security have been placed in these positions without the background, knowledge, and training needed to deal with youth violence, drugs, weapons, gangs, and other threats to school safety and security.

Having a custodian perform school legal work, a curriculum director repair boilers, or a person without a teaching certificate teach second grade would be unacceptable to almost all school board members and superintendents. Just as custodians, curriculum directors, and teachers are expected to have specialized knowledge and experience in their particular fields, so should school security officials. Yet, for decades, individuals have repeatedly been put in positions of responsibility for school security with minimal or no training or experience. Ironically, this trend has continued through the last decade, which has experienced the greatest public concern and outcry for school safety in the history of the United States.

Educators must recognize school security as a profession and treat its representatives as professional support service specialists and as integral members of the school staff. In turn, security personnel must set and adhere to professional standards in such areas as education and training, appearance, and job performance. Once educators and security officials are "on the same page" in accepting and performing security functions as a profession, expectations and outcomes related to security services can be held to a higher level.

Program Options

School security departments, school resource officers, and school police departments are the three most popular means of providing specialized safety services in districts seeking regular in-house resources beyond the traditional approaches. Which model is the best? Each model can be the best, depending on who is asked this question. The more objective answer is that the "best" model will depend on the needs and desires of the particular school system seeking to establish a program.

Each program option has both positive features and drawbacks. Brief descriptions of these options and their key features are provided in the following sections.

School Security Departments

School security departments usually consist of in-house, noncertified support staffers who are responsible for general security functions inside schools and on school grounds. These functions may vary from the traditional hall monitor duties previously described to more professional security services, including investigative responsibilities, physical security assessments, crisis preparedness planning, and related tasks. Depending upon state and local laws, these individuals may be commissioned with limited arrest authority within the school's specific jurisdiction.

In larger districts, security officers may be assigned to specific schools under the direction of a principal or his or her designee. They may also have primary or secondary reporting responsibilities to a districtwide security director or coordinator, depending on the district. In smaller districts with fewer needs, a districtwide security official, possibly with a staff of mobile security specialists available to serve all schools, is another popular option.

A positive aspect of school security departments is that the district has control over personnel selection, responsibilities, assignment, and supervision. In some jurisdictions security personnel may be commissioned with arrest authority through the city or the courts. As long as the security personnel are properly trained and supervised, this arrest authority is another positive feature for educators, because the school-based security staff has the legal authority to directly enforce pertinent laws on the school campus and is available on-site throughout the school day.

Another positive feature of having a full-time school security department is that the individuals employed in such departments often remain with the school system for a lengthy period of time, gathering a unique history of knowledge and experience in effectively dealing with and preventing disruptions and crime in schools. Many professional school security officials can successfully defuse potentially violent or disruptive situations with the skills gained from working extensively in schools. School security departments are also exceptionally different from other law enforcement and security agencies, and individuals who are knowledgeable and experienced in dealing with school bureaucracies, politics, and discipline systems are much better equipped for survival and effectiveness in an educational setting.

The negative side of a school security department is that it is often tucked away in other major school departments, frequently getting lost in the school system bureaucracy and having minimal status and input as a professional support service. Security personnel are often poorly paid and undertrained and are frequently required to perform non-security-related duties that are more appropriate for administrative assistants to school principals and staff than for professional security officials. The failure to have security personnel under the direction and supervision of a professional security administration contributes significantly to the ambiguity of the role of the school security staff, as well as to inconsistencies in job tasks, inadequate or improper training, and an overall lack of professionalism in school security departments. Unfortunately, control struggles frequently occur between principals and centralized security administrators when a strong security administrator attempts to professionalize school security operations.

School Resource Officers

School resource officers (SROs) have quickly gained in popularity since the late 1980s. SROs are usually city or county law enforcement officers assigned by their departments to work in one or more schools on a regular basis. Their responsibilities may vary, but generally include the "Triad Model" functions of law enforcement officer, classroom instructor, and counselor on issues related to appropriate behavior and the law.

A positive aspect of SRO programs for educators is having a sworn law enforcement officer with full arrest authority on-site on a regular basis. This is particularly helpful in communities that may have longer police response times. A related benefit is that these officers come to the school with training and, in most cases, with experience in other areas of law enforcement.

An even more positive aspect is that SROs provide the school staff with an in-house resource not only for law enforcement and security purposes, but also for prevention services as instructors and counselors to students. The street experience of SROs is often a unique qualification among professionals in the school setting. The SRO program also benefits the police department and community, because crime information and activity in the broader community and in the school are often interrelated.

Difficulties with SRO programs that arise often focus on financial issues. In some locations, SROs are funded completely by the law enforcement agency; in other areas, completely by the school district; and in still other areas, with a mixture of funds from the two agencies. Although there may be no problems as long as local funding exists or grants are intact, difficulties may arise when funds run short—particularly in a law enforcement agency, where personnel and funding shortages may dictate removing the officers from schools and placing them back on the streets. Management changes and political shifts can also result in program changes.

Difficulties can also arise with personnel assignments and reporting procedures if programs are implemented haphazardly, rather than professionally. If the criteria for selection as an SRO do not focus on the desire of an officer to perform in this capacity—that is, if the SRO assignment is involuntary or is used to avoid placing the officer in a regular capacity within the police department—problems may occur. If roles and procedures are clearly defined prior to the implementation of the program, questions and conflicts over the responsibilities of the SRO in the school and the authority for supervision of the SRO can be prevented from the outset.

One of the more absurd arguments that tends to arise prior to assignment of police officers in schools (SROs or school police, for that matter) centers on the issue of whether officers who work in schools should carry firearms. A firearm is a standard tool of the trade for a properly trained, commissioned police officer and should be a part of the equipment carried by any such police officers, including those who work in schools. To disarm an otherwise trained and certified police officer not only puts at risk the safety of the officer and those whom he or she is hired to protect, but also increases the potential liability of the school district should an incident occur that could have been prevented or minimized if the officer had been armed.

The National Association of School Resource Officers (*www.nasro.org*) is the nation's largest, highly credible training and technical assistance provider for SRO programs. It strongly recommends specialized and ongoing training for SROs, because of the unique nature of policing in school environments, as well as the arming of appropriately trained and certified peace officers. The Association also stresses the importance of having a balanced SRO program that follows the Triad Model, which makes SRO programs much more preventative in nature than they are often perceived to be by outside observers unfamiliar with the SRO approach to school safety. School and police organizations should give serious consideration to consulting with this organization for professional guidance before implementing SRO or other school-based policing programs.

School Police Departments

School police departments are certified law enforcement agencies like regular city or county police departments. Similar departments operate in many colleges and universities. Personnel generally have full police authority and are full-time employees of the school district.

Among the positive features of a school police department are that the school district has full control over a department, including personnel selection, responsibilities, assignments, and supervision. As full-time district employees, the officers' primary responsibility is to serve the schools. Moreover, provided that their pay and benefits are comparable to those offered by other police departments, so that they remain on the job for a longer term, their longevity with the district can provide a wealth of knowledge and experience in school-specific policing.

Difficulties with this type of program can center on financial resources. A great deal of ongoing training for school police officers is likely to be mandatory under state law. Costs for vehicles, equipment, and related items may also tend to be higher than the costs associated with school security departments or SRO programs, and school politics can adversely impact the operations of such departments.

Other Options

The aforementioned program options are the three most popular, but they are not the only options. Some districts hire off-duty local police officers to work on a part-day or full-day basis at select schools. This generally requires a pool of officers to fill these daily slots, because of rotating shifts, court time, and other contingencies associated with the full-time responsibilities of the police officers. Although the officers are familiar with crimi-

nal activity and trends in the broader community, the rotation of the officers at the school, combined with potential fatigue and conflicts with their
primary employment duties, frequently makes this a less than desirable
model for districts wishing to develop comprehensive and consistent
security programming.

One of the least popular options is the use of contracted security personnel. Private security agencies exist in most metropolitan areas of the
United States and, at least in financial terms, may appear attractive to districts wishing to save money on security. Unfortunately, contracted security
companies are known for their high turnover rate, their low pay, and often
the limited training of their personnel. School districts have little if any control over the selection of personnel who work with students and staff, not to
mention the inconsistencies resulting from frequent changes in these personnel. Some districts, however, are content with this approach.

Broadly speaking, school police departments are more common in Western and Southern states, whereas security departments are more common in
the Midwest and in Eastern states. SRO programs are growing across the
country, with no exclusive concentration in any particular region. It is also
not unusual to see a combination of these options used in some districts,
particularly larger school systems with intense problems and varying security
needs. For example, some districts may employ their own in-house school security departments, but may also supplement these personnel with off-duty
city police officers to cover high-priority or problem areas. Other districts
may have their own SROs or school police departments, as well as personnel
working in a nonsworn, security capacity to handle noncriminal incidents or
security-related service calls.

Basic Requirements

Regardless of the model a district chooses, serious attention must be given to
the qualifications of personnel who make up a program. The success of any
model depends not only on its structure, organization, and operational
guidelines, but more importantly on the quality of its personnel. Key considerations for review include education and training, experience, and pay.

Education and Training

Although one might expect the education and training of potential school
security personnel to be the area that is first and most stringently reviewed
by educators, it is often the area with the *lowest* standards in school personnel
selection. The qualifications required for other professionals providing direct service to students and staff generally include an undergraduate degree
and specialized training or certification. Security positions—particularly
those on the front line and in the field providing direct service—frequently
require only a high school diploma or the equivalent, and little to no educa-

tion or training in working with violent and disruptive juveniles or in providing professional security services.

In addition to the notable absence of requirements for preemployment education and training, there is little training provided by most school districts for new security personnel employed by their systems. New employees are often given the general orientation provided to any new school employee, without any security-specific training whatsoever. In some cases, security personnel have been hired, assigned to a school, handed keys and a walkie-talkie, and told, "Go get 'em."

More progressive districts will develop formal training programs, as well as on-the-job training requirements, for new security employees. Larger districts employing a substantial number of security personnel should consider establishing a program similar to an in-house academy for new recruits. Districts using school police forces will most likely require police certification as a mandatory qualification for applicants or will provide a specific certification program (i.e., a police academy) upon their being hired.

Districts employing an SRO program almost always have officers with the same certified training required for all police officers within their jurisdictions, although many may not have the specialized SRO training recommended for officers assigned to SRO programs. They may or may not have officers with college degrees or extensive specialized training in working specifically with juveniles, depending upon the police department in which they work and the prerequisites for SRO assignments. All districts employing security or police personnel should establish on-the-job training programs, in which new personnel complete a predetermined period of field training under the direction of experienced officers.

Professional development does not stop with prerequisite and initial employee education and training. Ongoing training programs in many school districts, however, are often geared toward certified teaching and administrative personnel. Nonteaching support staff often receive limited training provided by the district, often in a one-shot annual meeting ranging from 1 to 3 days prior to the opening of school. Funds are rarely available, even in the larger and better-established school security or police departments, to send personnel to seminars, workshops, conferences, or related programs during the course of the school year.

Surprisingly, education and training requirements for the leaders of many school security or police departments are also at the lower end of the scale, as compared with those for other department heads in school systems. School security directors or police chiefs are often recently retired city, county, state, or federal law enforcement officers, selected on the basis of their years of experience in traditional police agencies. A good number of these individuals may not have college degrees or specialized education in working with juveniles or schools, although this appears to be changing over time. Individuals tapped to head school security offices who are not former law enforcement officers may include heads of other school divisions (e.g., business, transportation, pupil services, other support service departments) or even former principals and educators, who are assigned for various logistical, political, or organizational reasons. Although these individuals may hold degrees and be knowledgeable about working in a school system, they frequently do not have a solid foundation of education and training in the security field.

It is ironic that for security personnel requirements, school systems do not place a greater emphasis on the issue they represent and stress with students: education. Security department heads, frequently on pay scales ranging from $40,000 to $80,000 in medium-sized to larger districts, should be required to have a minimum of an undergraduate degree, specialized training in juvenile crime and school security issues, and any police commission or security certification required in their particular city or state. Districts employing leaders of larger or more complex school security programs should consider requiring graduate degrees and extensive specialized training.

Education requirements for midlevel and front-line security personnel should vary, depending on the duties and responsibilities of the job position. Supervisory staff, investigators, specialized support staff, and patrol or stationary officers should have advanced education and training requirements commensurate with their areas of responsibility and expertise. Two- and 4-year college degrees should not be uncommon expectations for security personnel providing direct services to students and staff.

In lawsuits related to safety and security, one of the first topics scrutinized by attorneys is the education and training of the defendants—in this case, the individuals responsible for providing safety services. Poor or inadequate training and educational standards for security and police personnel open the doors for potential liability. They also increase the chances of having less-than-professional school safety services.

Experience

As previously noted, school systems typically turn to retired law enforcement officers to head their school security or police programs. Although the amount of law enforcement experience these individuals have after 20–30 years on the job cannot be questioned, some concerns may be raised about this approach as the only option. For some officers who go this route, the school system becomes a postretirement home for 5–10 years, during which time they take a status-quo approach to developing school security programs. In fairness, it should be noted that there are also numerous retired individuals from law enforcement agencies who aggressively pursue the development and growth of professional, efficient school security programs.

When educators choose to hire a retired police official, less consideration should be given to the person's rank in the police department and to the number of years on the job, and more to the responsibilities, accomplishments, and performance history of the individual under consideration. An officer with juvenile crime and administrative experience close to the time of the school district's hiring would certainly be a more viable candidate than a 25-year captain who is retiring after working the past 10 years in the police record room. The ideas, specific plans, and ambitions of the applicant should be discussed openly and honestly during the interview process, so that neither the school district nor the applicant will experience surprises down the line if he or she is employed.

If school security or school policing is ever to be professionalized, its leaders must become established as career-oriented professionals. The positions of school security directors and police chiefs should be viewed as career positions. Although change is a part of any organization or department, the longevity of individuals in these positions must be extended beyond the current 5–10-year period seen in many school systems. This revolving-door practice does little toward establishing continuity, professionalism, and high-quality security services in school districts.

The same concept must be applied to field and front-line school security positions. These positions must be incorporated into the organizational structure and culture of the school system as career-oriented, professional support service employment positions. A balance between past experience and future plans to continue in school security should be the focus of current hiring efforts. Because the field is in a relatively early stage of development, especially as a professional field, school officials cannot expect to find a significantly large pool of applicants with extensive school-specific experience in security. However, higher standards should be set; these should include a combination of professional security service and experience in performing tasks directly related to working with juveniles in crisis, conflict, and security-oriented situations. Once the field becomes more stable as a profession, a larger pool of school-experienced security professionals will become available and experience requirements can be adjusted accordingly.

Pay

Although SRO pay is typically based upon the standard pay scale of the officer's law enforcement agency, most school systems currently pay their security personnel at the lowest levels within their districts, and yet they expect the security staff to handle the most difficult students and threatening situations—those that, despite their higher pay scales, most teachers, administrators, and central office executives are not equipped or prepared to handle. If security personnel are expected to be qualified and to perform as professionals, then school districts must offer professional-level pay and benefits. Districts seeking to establish and maintain a solid in-house school security or police program must structure their employee pay scales so that the pay and benefits are comparable to those for similar positions in local, county, state, or university-based security or police departments.

SECURITY ORGANIZATION AND OPERATIONS

The foregoing description of program options illustrates the varying preferences and nature of school security programs across the United States. It
also depicts the underlying problem in professionalizing the school security
field. Educators, most of whom are unfamiliar with the security profession,
receive conflicting messages as to which model is "the best" and assume that
because no model has been determined to be unquestionably the best, they
can implement a program on their own by trial and error. Without the necessary training and experience in the security field, they proceed with trial and
error until a program is implemented that they deem to be adequate, with
school politics often interfering along the way. Unfortunately, such programs
often reflect policies, procedures, and practices of lower standards than
those directed by experienced security professionals.

There is far too much work to be done in designing, implementing, and
evaluating professional school security programs before anyone can pro-
claim one approach as the perfect model. In fact, most school security and
police administrators themselves agree that this field is in the early stages of
being recognized and fine-tuned as a profession. Still, school leaders who
want to establish new security programs or to raise existing programs to a
greater level of professionalism must address some basic issues and
considerations.

Mission

The school and community culture will largely dictate what structure and
form a security program should take within a school system. A school police
department may be too bold a step for some communities; others may find it
to be completely necessary and appropriate to address the problems the district currently faces and is likely to face in the future. Budgetary boundaries,
logistical issues, and political concerns are also likely to influence decisions
in this area.

School boards and superintendents must first determine the mission of
the department providing security services. Will the department be addressing ongoing criminal offenses on a daily basis; will it deal mostly with serious
disciplinary incidents and only periodically with criminal cases; or will it address both? Are the schools experiencing entrenched crime problems that
will require a more reactive department, or is the number of incidents small
enough that departments will focus on a more preventative, proactive approach? What roles do budgetary considerations, public demand, and political issues play as to whether the district wants to create one type of program
over another? These types of questions—and many, many more—will have to
be openly and honestly addressed by board members and administrators
prior to taking any action.

Several underlying conditions must be met as these issues are being studied and debated. First and foremost, all efforts must be exerted to set political and personal agendas aside when decisions are being made about safety and security issues. Although security issues are loaded with potential political implications (image, public perception, etc.), rational minds must prevail if school officials expect to have an end product that is logical, reasonable, professional, and appropriate for meeting the security needs of the school system.

Decisions related to school security or police operations must also be made with regard to current and long-term projected trends in safety issues facing the district. If problems are currently entrenched, they are not likely to go away, so educators should plan on developing a more sophisticated security operation. But what if the school system has a moderate or smaller amount of problems, or even no specific concerns at all, but wants to be proactive in addressing its security needs? Should the decision be made to set up a full-scale security operation? Should the decision be made to hire only one security professional? Two professionals? Three?

These are questions, of course, that can be answered only on the basis of specific knowledge of the particular school district and community in question. However, board members and superintendents are encouraged to consider in their analysis these long-term questions: Where are we likely to be in 5 years with this issue? Where will we be in 10 years? Once acceptable answers are found to these and related questions, strategic planning for a security program should begin. Although school leaders may believe that they do not need officers today, it may very well be more prudent to hire an officer now to prevent problems than to hire 10 officers 5 years from now to do nothing but respond to problems.

Board Policies

Regardless of the security program selected, school boards should establish clear policies reflecting a commitment to the safety and security of students, staff members, and facilities. In fact, every school board should adopt policies specifically articulating a pledge to the school community: Although it is impossible to guarantee 100% safety to all, the board should commit itself to undertaking policies, procedures, and programs promoting safe and secure schools. This commitment should be openly communicated on an ongoing basis and reflected in the actions and decisions of board members, administrators, students, and other stakeholders in the school community.

Board policies should, at a minimum, also address such specific security threats as drug use, possession, and sales; gang activity; and possession or use of weapons. Boards need to formulate policies directing and supporting all school personnel to report crimes and serious incidents to the appropriate law enforcement officials, as well as internally to a designated security administrator for the purpose of tracking, handling, and preventing ever-

changing crimes and disruptive activities. Related issues, such as creating visitation and building access procedures, should be clearly incorporated into
the district security operations through board-initiated policies.

The commitment cannot stop with the creation of policies. Policies must
be reflected in standard procedures. More important, policies and procedures must be consistently reflected in daily practice. Although school security may not initially be foremost in the mind of every staff member, it seems
to move more closely to that importance when it is a high priority of the
board, superintendent, top administrators, and principals. In short, school
safety and security must become a part of the school system's organizational
culture.

Organization

The organization and lines of authority for departments providing school security services vary across the United States, depending on the model used
and the overall organization of the school district. Generally, departments
with centralized administrations and districtwide staffs are placed under the
direction of a deputy or assistant superintendent responsible for support services, rather than for curriculum-related services. Depending on the size of
the security program and the nature of its services, the person responsible
for school security may be subordinate to the head of a broader department,
such as business or pupil services.

Educators seeking to establish a professional security or police department should make the department equal to and independent of other departments within the school administration and should establish a director-
level position with sole responsibility for a districtwide security program.
This position should be an advanced managerial position, with duties, responsibilities, and qualifications requiring administrative and leadership
skills, technical expertise, and program development and oversight functions
comparable to those of any other department head within the school administration. Because school security issues involve the protection of life and
property, often require immediate or quick decisions from top school officials, and are frequently confidential, sensitive, and high-profile in nature,
the security or police department head should report directly to the superintendent or to the ranking administrator for support services immediately
under the superintendent, in order to facilitate timely and efficient decisions
on these matters.

Problems arise when educational administrators who lack training and
experience in the security and police professions are responsible for such
programs, especially when this is only one of their many responsibilities.
Problems also occur when departments are tucked away so far down the organization chart that they have no access to the key decision makers in the
organization, or there are multiple obstacles between them. If safety is truly

a high priority within the school system, this priority must be reflected in the organizational position of the department and its leader.

Another problem area encountered in many security programs involves the authority and supervision of security personnel assigned to specific school buildings. The main issue centers on who is directly responsible for the school-based security staff members—the principal or the centralized security administrator. The decentralized school-based management process that is being adopted in many districts, combined with the likelihood of turf conflicts, multiplies the potential for major battles on this issue.

The critical point in this case is not who is in charge, but rather who can provide the best direction and support of a professional school security program. This returns us to the analogy of having a custodian perform the legal work of a school, a curriculum director repair boilers, or a noncertified individual teach second grade. These individuals are not incompetent employees; they are simply performing tasks for which they most likely have no education, training, or experience. This is also the case when principals, assistant principals, or even central office administrators without any background in security are solely responsible for security policy, personnel, and operations.

Therefore, the primary authority for personnel selection, assignment, and deployment; for development of job function parameters; and for implementation of training, supervision, evaluation, and discipline for school security personnel should rest with the professional security administrator. This is not to say, however, that the building principal should be left out in the cold, with no input or involvement in managing security personnel assigned to the principal's school. On the contrary, the principal should work actively with the centralized security administrator to develop written work plans for the school-based security staff that are specific to the needs of the particular school, but not unduly restrictive.

If an open relationship exists between the security administrator and the principal, and if egos are set aside in the best interests of the safety of students and staff, there should be minimal problems with this type of organization. When problems do occur with school-based security personnel, the principal should be able to work collaboratively with the security administrator to correct the problems or, if necessary, to initiate disciplinary action. Meanwhile, during most of the time when there are no conflicts, the security administrator has the time and authority to provide the necessary staff and program development to professionalize security services. Most principals or other school administrators with broader areas of responsibility simply do not have this amount of available time or the necessary exposure to the security field.

Functions and Services

The nature and extent of services provided in a school security or police program will depend on the demands made on the department and the resources available to provide the services. Some of the basic functions that should be included in programs offering comprehensive services are included in the list that follows. However, programs facing high demands for addressing crimes and serious incidents on a regular basis, particularly with limited personnel, will have to prioritize their responses to these incidents and to adjust the amount of time allocated to nonurgent needs.

1. *Enforcement and investigation.* The primary responsibility of safety service providers must be to enforce all criminal laws, as well as school policies and procedures regarding the appropriate conduct of persons on school property. The staff should be responsible for investigating and documenting all violations of these laws and regulations in cooperation with school administrators. Safety officials may use a variety of techniques for preventing personal injury, property loss or damage, and disruptions of the educational process—including, but not limited to, building and mobile patrol (where applicable), surveillance and investigation, support in controlling emergency situations, and application of crime prevention strategies. Enforcement and investigation functions include providing support to district administrators in conducting sensitive and confidential internal investigations involving allegations of staff misconduct. Personnel can also play a key role in monitoring and advising students on appropriate behavior expectations.

2. *Crisis preparedness.* Security and police officials should actively participate in the development of crisis preparedness guidelines. Both district-level and building-level guidelines should be prepared. Safety staff should serve as the primary resource for drafting guidelines for the prevention of and response to criminally oriented crisis situations, such as abductions, removal of students by noncustodial parents, large-scale riots or altercations, bomb threats and actual bomb placement, gunfire in or around schools, hostage situations, trespassers and suspicious persons, and weapons threats. Safety officials should also be consulted as a resource related to the development of protocol for handling noncriminal crises, such as large-scale accidents, serious illnesses or deaths on or off school grounds, environmental emergencies, and other possible concerns.

3. *Security assessments.* The school security or police staff should serve as an in-house resource for conducting periodic assessments of security procedures, physical security conditions, crime prevention measures, and related matters.

4. *Technical assistance with security equipment.* School systems are increasingly turning to mechanical devices to improve school security. These devices may include such items as alarm systems, metal detectors, and surveillance cameras. Security or school police officials can typically serve as a source of technical assistance to educators in determining equipment needs, use, and effectiveness. It is important to remember, however, that equipment should be a supplement to, not a substitute for, professional security personnel, policies, and procedures.

5. *Education and training.* To raise awareness and enhance the prevention capacity of key players, school security or police personnel should be included in board and administrative briefings and planning, in-service training for teachers and support personnel, parent meetings, and student classes, as appropriate. Presentation topics may include security procedures, crisis preparedness guidelines, crime prevention, and awareness of specific issues associated with school security (e.g., gangs, drugs, weapons, and other "hot topics").

6. *Liaison with other entities.* School security or police personnel should take the lead in establishing contacts and regular communication with outside law enforcement agencies, court staff, probation officers, social service providers, other youth service providers, and parents. These contacts can provide critical information on activity in the community that may have an impact on school safety. They can also serve as excellent resources in preventing and responding to crisis situations within the school system. In turn, in-house personnel can be equally valuable to the outside entities, inasmuch as they gather a significant amount of information and insight from working with students and security problems within the schools on a regular basis.

The internal organization of school security or police departments will vary, based on the staffing and functions of these departments. Boards and superintendents should give serious consideration to providing services on a districtwide basis, rather than only at selected sites. Depending on the extent of problems within a system, specialized units may have to be developed to address gang activity, weapons detection, or similar chronic problems.

One of the most common problems associated with school security programs pertains more to the functions performed by security personnel than to the actual organization or structure of the department. Although job descriptions may clearly delineate security-specific functions to be performed by department personnel, there is a tendency for security personnel to be improperly used for non-security-related duties. This appears at both the building and district levels.

At the school level, security personnel are misused in many districts to perform non-security-related functions for principals, assistant principals, and the school staff. Some of the more common tasks have included supervising classes and internal suspension rooms, cleaning cafeteria tables, logging in tardy students, looking up student schedules and serving as a student escort service for building administrators dealing with nonthreatening discipline matters, transporting ill students home, and running errands to stores, banks, post offices, or other schools. By performing these administrative assistant functions, school security officials are placing themselves, their supervisors, and their district in a position of questionable liability. If a serious incident should occur that could have been prevented (or that others believe could have been prevented) had a security official been performing security-specific duties, a major lawsuit may be the result.

Similar examples of the inappropriate use of security personnel occur at the district level, but less frequently. Numerous school security directors can cite examples of having been called upon routinely to deliver mail to the homes of board members, distribute items to multiple schools, or perform other menial tasks that do not fit into the job descriptions of any other staff members. Like the school-based security staff, the district-level staff should adhere to security-specific duties and should not be approached by upper-level school administrators to perform non-security-related chores.

SAFETY AND SECURITY ASSESSMENTS

How should educators assess their safety and security posture and needs? Again, the analogy of consulting a lawyer to perform a plumbing repair can be applied to the question of who should be consulted regarding security concerns. If a school system currently employs security personnel, then they should be the first source for assessing school security. If the current security staff cannot provide an adequate assessment, or if the district has no security program in place, then educators should look to outside professional school security resources to evaluate their needs and to recommend the appropriate steps toward establishing a professional security program.

School security assessments provide educators with an audit of existing conditions within their school district and with recommendations for improving these conditions at the building and district levels. The benefits of conducting an assessment include completion of a review of school conditions and operations to identify areas for improvement from a professional security standpoint (a standpoint that may otherwise be lacking within the district). Assessments often identify practical strategies, such as procedural changes, that require only minimal costs for better safeguarding of students, staff, and facilities. Assessments also demonstrate a commitment to safety and security through a professional and methodical review without overreaction, panic, or other negative response following a crisis situation.

Many districts historically responded to safety concerns with a curriculum-only approach or an enforcement-only approach, without considering the entire range of issues involved in providing safe and secure schools, although many more are balancing such approaches with security and crisis preparedness measures following high-profile tragedies of school violence. Areas for assessment should include security operations and procedures, crisis preparedness, physical security, special event management, personnel security, education and training, intervention services, and community coordination. The assessment process should include a review of policies and procedures, an analysis of crime and discipline data, an examination of the physical design and structure of facilities, and structured interviews with administrators, teachers, support staff members, students, parents, law enforcement officials, and other key individuals in the school community (Trump, 1998).

Public and private organizations faced increasing vulnerability in the last decade. Although no plans or guarantees for absolute safety are possible, an assessment of a district and its operations by school security professionals can help educators shape and focus their program implementation and other planning for preventing and minimizing safety and security threats. Such proactive efforts serve as a positive risk management tool and communicate to staff, students, parents, and the overall community that the district is sincere in its commitment to their safety.

CRISIS PREPAREDNESS PLANNING

Crisis preparedness planning should be an integral part of any school security or school police department's operation. Prior to the recent national tragedies, school crisis plans largely focused on managing disasters caused by weather and other natural forces, suicides and other deaths, and dealing with the media when they come on campus. Today, crisis guidelines have expanded to include crises related to crime and violence, including, but not limited to, abductions, gunfire, hostage situations, homemade bombs and bomb threats, and a host of similar concerns.

Merely having crisis guideline documents is not enough, however. Following high-profile incidents of school violence in the news, many districts moved to create crisis documents in order to be able to say that they existed if anyone asked. School crisis guidelines must be developed by school personnel in cooperation with their public safety agencies, and they must be tested and exercised so that everyone involved in the process knows that what is written on paper may actually work in the event of a real crisis incident (Trump, 2000).

Some individuals may argue that the testing and exercising of crisis guidelines will unnecessarily traumatize students. Although this makes good theory, the reality is that tested crisis guidelines stand a much better chance of working properly in a real crisis situation than documents that are neatly packaged, containing guidelines that are never actually exercised. The key rests in how school and safety officials communicate to students why the plans are important and why they must be tested. (Perhaps the best existing example that this approach works is the use of fire drills—we never hear anyone object to conducting them because they traumatize schoolchildren.)

OUTSIDE RESOURCES AND EXPERTS

In considering who should conduct assessments, training, and services related to professional school security, educators may turn to individuals or groups outside the school districts. Unfortunately, the growth of school security problems has generated a corresponding increase in school security "experts" across the United States. Less than a decade ago, it was taboo for many school officials even to publicly discuss crimes, gang activity, drug offenses, weapon concerns, and security procedures. Today, with dollar signs in their eyes, former educators, retired law enforcement officers, drug abuse prevention specialists, and individuals from totally unrelated professions are now professing to have school security expertise that can be purchased by school officials.

Educators should exercise caution in purchasing books, audiotapes, videotapes, and other products that claim to have "the" solution to school safety problems. Organizations and associations offering school safety and security programs are cropping up annually across the country. Unfortunately, the majority of these agencies offer either single-solution programs or broad generalities as the answer to school security woes.

Likewise, caution should be exercised in selecting individuals to provide consultation services on school safety and security. The background of such individuals should be examined in detail to determine their actual level of expertise in providing security services to school systems and in working with youthful offenders, security services, and other areas specifically related to school security and school crisis preparedness. It would be very appropriate to look at their demonstrated performance, related job experience, education, and training, and especially to determine whether they had such experience and training prior to the series of school violence tragedies that has stimulated the exploitation of this field. Biographical information that is sketchy, incomplete, or questionable should make educators leery when they are considering a consultant or trainer.

FUTURE DIRECTIONS

This chapter has presented a candid look at critical issues surrounding school security policy, personnel, and operations. In view of the continuing growth of the school security profession, readers are encouraged to consult with in-house school security staff, bona fide outside security professionals, and district legal counsel for opinions on specific policies, procedures, and programs developed by individual schools or school districts. The concepts presented here describe the school security field as a whole. Each district must avoid looking for "the" panacea or "the" checklist for perfect school security, and instead conduct an in-depth review of its own beliefs, policies, procedures, and practices related to school security today and in the future.

Regardless of the model adopted, all school systems should strive to ensure that their programs are based on professional security principles and standards and that these programs are staffed with professional employees.

REFERENCES

Huff, C. R. (1988). *Youth gangs and public policy in Ohio: Findings and recommendations*. Paper presented at the Ohio Conference on Youth Gangs and the Urban Underclass, Ohio State University, Columbus.

Trump, K. S. (1996). Youth gangs and school safety. In A. M. Hoffman (Ed.), *Schools, violence, and society* (pp. 45–58). Westport, CT: Praeger.

Trump, K. S. (1998). *Practical school security: Basic guidelines for safe and secure schools*. Thousand Oaks, CA: Corwin Press.

Trump, K. S. (2000). *Classroom Killers? Hallway Hostages? How Schools Can Prevent and Manage School Crises*. Thousand Oaks, CA: Corwin Press.

CHAPTER 13

Controlling Vandalism

The Person–Environment Duet

ARNOLD P. GOLDSTEIN

Most efforts to understand and reduce human aggressive behavior—toward other persons or toward property—focus on the perpetrator. Regardless of whether the persons making these efforts are specialists or members of the general public; teachers, psychologists, sociologists, or criminologists; theoreticians, researchers, or practitioners; or individuals concerned with prediction, prevention, rehabilitation, or public policy, the person or persons actually committing an aggressive act are almost always the primary target(s) of attention. Who he or she is, the person's relevant background experiences, history of similar behaviors, mood and rationality at the time the act occurred, and related intraindividual matters are the typical issues addressed. The abuser's parenting, the delinquent's early temperament, the student offender's personality traits, the vandal's hormonal levels or television viewing habits, and other in-the-person markers are posited, examined, and held responsible. In most attempts at explaining aggression, aggression is viewed as in the perpetrator, by the perpetrator, and from the perpetrator. This chapter presents an alternative view.

The present perspective is responsive to one of the most significant developments in the study of human behavior in recent decades: the ascendance of "interactionism." Broadly defined, the interactionist approach to understanding and predicting human behavior maintains that such efforts should reflect both intraindividual (e.g., trait) qualities *and* relevant characteristics of the individual's environment. These latter ecological features may be other people (e.g., victims, fellow students) or qualities of the immediate or larger physical location in which the behavior occurs (e.g., school size, disrepair). In recent years this interactionist perspective has been brought to bear on a wide range of behaviors, and aggression is certainly among them.

This body of aggression-relevant knowledge, as it bears on student aggression toward property, is the central focus of this chapter.

AGGRESSION TOWARD PROPERTY

Vandalism, whether it takes place in schools or in other settings, has been defined with varying degrees of inclusiveness. However, each of the 10 definitions I have located highlights at least to some degree the perpetrator's intentionality, the destructiveness of the behavior, and property ownership (Goldstein, 1995). The definition employed by the Federal Bureau of Investigation (FBI) for its annual uniform crime report seems quite fitting for a school context:

> The willful or malicious destruction, injury, disfigurement, or defacement of property without the consent of the owner or person having custody or control by cutting, tearing, breaking, marking, painting, drawing, covering with filth, or any such means as may be specified by local law. (FBI, 1978, p. 217)

There were approximately 136,500 arrests in the United States in 1997 of persons under age 18 for vandalism. These juvenile arrests were 44% of all arrests for vandalism. Eighty-eight percent of these juveniles were males. Paralleling the decline between 1994 and 1997 of all crime by juveniles, vandalism incidence reached a high of 496 per 100,000 youths in 1994 and progressively declined to 426 per 100,000 in 1997. Thus, as again is true for juvenile crime in general, although relative rates have diminished, absolute levels remain quite high. Juvenile arrest rates for vandalism, 1980–1997, are depicted in Figure 13.1 (U.S. Department of Justice, 2000).

Motivational typologies seeking to specify subtypes of vandalistic behavior have varied greatly in the degree to which they employ person-centered versus environment-centered perspectives. Viewing vandalism causation as essentially an in-the-person phenomenon, Cohen (1971) offers acquisitive, tactical, ideological, vindictive, play, and malicious subtypes. In full contrast, holding that vandalism "resides" not in persons but in the nature of buildings, school or park equipment, or other public facilities, Weinmayer (1969) categorizes the following vandalism subtypes: overuse, conflict, curiosity, leverage, deleterious, irresistible temptation, and "no-other-way-to-do-it" vandalism.

Across the several typologies that have been suggested, school (and other) vandalism is an expensive fact of U.S. life. Comprehensive monetary cost estimates of vandalism have been put forth; these collectively illustrate that the expense of vandalism, like its incidence, is both absolutely high and increasing. In the approximately 90,000 schools in the United States, for example, monetary vandalism cost estimates over the past 25 years show a clear upward trend, peaking at $600 million in the available data (Stoner, Shinn, &

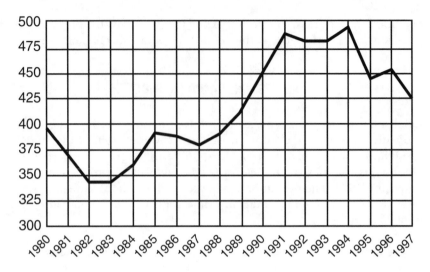

FIGURE 13.1. Juvenile arrest rates for vandalism, 1980–1997: Arrests per 100,000 youth ages 10–17.

Walker, 1991). Even this substantial cost figure may, however, be a serious underestimate. Kempt, Skok, and McLaughlin (1996) suggest that because of fear of increased insurance costs as well as reprisals against the school, many school administrators may avoid reporting much of the vandalism that occurs in their schools.

Arson, a particularly dangerous form of vandalism, perhaps deserves special comment. Whereas window breaking is the most frequent single act of aggression toward property in schools, arson is clearly the most costly, typically accounting for approximately 40% of total vandalism costs annually (Mathie & Schmidt, 1977).

The costs of school vandalism are not only monetary but social, as perhaps explicated best by Vestermark and Blauvelt (1978):

> By limiting criteria of vandalism's impact to only monetary costs, we overlook those incidents which have low monetary cost but, nevertheless, tremendous impact upon the school. The impact of a seventy-nine cent can of spray paint, used to paint racial epithets on a hallway wall, far exceeds the monetary cost of removing the paint. A racial confrontation could result, which might force the closing of the school for an indefinite period. How does one calculate that type of expense: confrontation and subsequent closing of a school? (p. 138)

In addition to the several reports of high levels of in-school violence and vandalism, data are now emerging on a parallel pattern of near-school aggression. In both San Diego (Roncek & Lobosco, 1983) and Cleveland (Roncek & Faggiani, 1985), residences on blocks adjacent to public high schools had significantly higher crime victimization rates than did residences in areas even a single block farther away from the schools. This was found to be so even after the investigators controlled for an array of demographic, social, and housing characteristics of the residential areas compared.

CAUSES AND CORRELATES

In a school context, the vandal may be a youngster who feels particularly alienated from the school, believes that he or she has been unjustly placed in detention, or is the recipient of what he or she deems an unfair grade. According to Tygert (1988) and Zweig and Ducey (1978), vandalism reaches its peak frequency in seventh grade and then progressively decreases with each succeeding grade. Socioeconomically, the typical school vandal is as likely to be a middle-class youth as one from a low-income background (Howard, 1978); emotionally, he or she is no more disturbed than are youngsters less prone to vandalize (Richards, 1976). However, vandals are more likely to have been retained (Nowakowski, 1966), to have often been truant (Greenberg, 1969), or to have been suspended from school altogether (Yankelovitch, 1975).

Youngsters prone to vandalism also often appear to have a poor understanding of the impact of their behavior on others and are primarily concerned with the consequences of such behavior for themselves, such as getting caught. In their view, public property in a real sense belongs to no one. In contrast, for youngsters less prone to vandalism, such property belongs to everyone; this view reflects their greater sense of themselves as part of a larger community ("Vandals," 1978). As is true for all forms of aggression, the single best predictor of future vandalistic behavior is similar past behavior (Tygert, 1988).

To turn from individual to environmental correlates, vandalism has been shown to be associated with autocratic or laissez-faire versus "firm but fair" school administration; inconsistent or weak administrative support and follow-through (Casserly, Bass, & Garrett, 1980); school governance that is too impersonal, unresponsive, nonparticipatory, overregulated, oppressive, arbitrary, or inconsistent (Greenberg, 1969; Ianni, 1979); high teacher turnover rates (Leftwich, 1977); such teacher inadequacies as disrespectfulness, callousness, lack of interest, and middle-class bias (Bayh, 1978; Rubel, 1977); overuse of punitive control methods; and inadequate clarity of school and classroom rules and discipline procedures (Mayer & Sulzer-Azaroff, 1991). In contrast, aggression toward property in schools is lower in those venues whose social ecology is characterized by high levels of teacher identification with the school, evenhanded rule enforcement, parental support of school disciplinary policies, teacher avoidance of the use of grades as disciplinary tools, and teacher avoidance of hostile or authoritarian behavior toward students (Bayh, 1978; Goldstein, 1992).

The school's physical ecology also bears importantly on its frequency as a context for vandalism. Noteworthy here are its age, as reflected in the obsoleteness of its facilities and equipment (Greenberg, 1969; Howard, 1978), its size, with larger schools having more incidents per capita (Garbarino, 1978; Goldman, 1961; Kingston & Gentry, 1977; Stefanko, 1989), its physical appearance (DeBunza, 1974; Pablant & Baxter, 1975), its density (little space per student) (Stefanko, 1989), and the general facts that it is often unoccupied, is easily accessible, and is a public place owned by no one in particular (Vestermark & Blauvelt, 1978). In an attempt to determine physical ecological correlates of *low* school vandalism levels, Pablant and Baxter (1975) studied 16 pairs of schools. One school in each pair had a high vandalism rate and the other had a low rate; the two schools were matched for similarity in other respects (size, ethnic composition, grade level, and location). The schools with lower rates, as the authors had predicted, (1) were characterized by better aesthetic quality and maintenance of school property, (2) were located in more densely populated areas with higher activity levels, (3) furnished a less obstructed view of school property to surrounding residents, and (4) were located in better-illuminated neighborhood areas.

A school is thus a prime ecological context for vandalism, not only because of the presence of large number of youths at a highly vandalism-prone age (the person component), but also because of a number of real and symbolic qualities of the school itself (the environmental component). Size, age, aesthetic appearance, public ownership, maintenance level, and location vis-à-vis possible sources of surveillance have been mentioned. Community characteristics are also often important influences on in-school events: School vandalism tends to be correlated with community crime level and the degree of nonstudent (intruder) presence in the school (Casserly et al., 1980; Irwin, 1978; Skelton, 1996). Furthermore, several of the vandalism-relevant physical ecological characteristics of the school site and its community location appear to constitute relevant contexts for vandalism elsewhere—libraries, museums, highway signs, trains, buses, mass transit stations, public telephones. All of these are easily accessible public sites; many have low levels of formal or informal surveillance; and many, because of low maintenance efforts, display the already vandalized "releaser cues" that permit and encourage further destruction. In addition, they are all "symbols of the social order" (Zimbardo, 1973, p. 73), and hence handy targets of dissatisfaction or frustration.

The ecology of vandalism has a temporal dimension as well. When does it occur? For many of the same contextual reasons that contribute to site determination—especially accessibility and the presence or absence of surveillance—a high proportion of vandalism (of schools and elsewhere) occurs before and after school hours, at night, on weekends, during vacation periods, later in the school week, and later in the school year (Anderson, 1977;

Casserly et al., 1980; Massucci, 1984; McPherson & Carpenter, 1981; Rautaheimo, 1989). Kempt et al. (1996) have noted that several of these high-vandalism times of occurrence mean that its perpetration is often un-witnessed, thus making more difficult the identification and apprehension of its perpetrators.

THE PERSON–ENVIRONMENT DUET

The central tenet of the interactionist perspective on human behavior is cap-tured well in the following quotation from two of its energetic proponents:

> The trait model and the psychodynamic model propose that actual behav-ior is primarily determined by latent, stable dispositions. Both assume that the sources for the initiation and direction of behavior come primarily from within the organism. The situational model assumes that the sources for the initiation and direction of behavior come primarily from factors ex-ternal to the organism. The interactional model assumes that the sources for the initiation and direction of behavior come primarily from the con-tinuous interactions between the person and the situations that he or she encounters. (Endler & Magnusson, 1976, p. 960)

Person–environment interactionism had its early roots in the works of Lewin (1935, 1936) and Murray (1938). In Lewin's well-known formula, $B = f(p,e)$, not only was behavior considered a function of both the person and the environment, but the environment most influential in its behavioral con-sequences was seen as subjective in nature—that is, the "environment-as-perceived" (also termed the "phenomenal field" or the "psychological situa-tion"). Murray (1938) took a similar position in his description of behavior as a joint outcome of both the individual's needs (the person variable) and environmental "press" or need-satisfying potential (the situation variable). Others followed Lewin's (1935, 1936) and Murray's (1938) early theorizing. Murphy's (1947) organism–field perspective, Rotter's (1954) and Mischel's (1968) social learning positions, and Angyal's (1959) phenomenological theory—all of which emphasize the inseparability of organism and environ-ment, and the subjectivity of environment in shaping human behavior—are major examples of this interactionist theme in psychological theory.

In addition to the phenomenologists and social learning theorists, a third view advancing interactionism emerged, variously called "ecological psychology" and "environmental psychology." Roger Barker and his research group's studies of the "stream of behavior" in a variety of field settings were the pioneering works in this context (Barker & Gump, 1964; Barker & Wright, 1954). Their investigations were a major clarification of the effects of diverse real-world "behavior settings" on behavior, as well as a significant step forward in determining how environments might be optimally defined, classified, and measured. Both the spirit and substance of the interactionist perspective have continued to grow and find empirical support in modern psychological theory and research (e.g., Altman, Brown, Staples, & Werner, 1992; Goldstein, 1994, 1995; Little, 1987; Pervin, 1986; Stokols & Altman, 1987). Furthermore, and directly to the point of this chapter, investigative support for a person–environment view of the sources and reduction of aggressive behavior has been amply forthcoming (Campbell, 1986; Cordilia, 1986; Forgas, 1986; Gibbs, 1986; Goldstein, 1994; Page & Moss, 1976; Rausch, 1967, 1972).

I have termed this section "The Person–Environment Duet" as a means of proposing that the person–context interactions at the heart of the interactionist position taken here are both probabalistic and reciprocal. "Probabilism" contrasts with both "determinism" and "possibilism." Determinism views the environment as the shaper of human behavior and the individual as the passive responder, inexorably led, with little ability or opportunity to select or alter his or her environment. In contrast, possibilism sees the person as acting on an environment that provides opportunities to grasp but that does little or no selecting or shaping of its own. Probabilism views the environment as neither determining nor merely providing possibilities. Instead, it makes certain choices more likely, enlarges them, and reinforces them. Moreover, in Krupat's (1985) view,

> the relationship of person to environment is dynamic, rather than static. There is a give and take, with each part of the system providing reciprocal influences on each other. We shape our environments and in turn are shaped by them in a never-ending cycle of mutual influence. (p. 12)

As the chapter now turns to consideration of vandalism intervention strategies, it will become clear that some are deterministic in their orientation, holding that the physical and social environment determines vandalistic behavior, and hence that environmental changes will reduce it. Other strategies are possibilistic, asserting person qualities as the predominant influences upon vandalistic behavior and its remediation. Still others are probabilistic and interactionistic, calling for both person- and environment-related means for altering vandalistic behavior.

VANDALISM INTERVENTION STRATEGIES

Changing the Ecology of the School

The deterministic perspective on vandalism control and reduction has appeared and reappeared under a variety of rubrics: "utilitarian prevention" (Cohen, 1973), "deopportunizing design" (Wiesenthal, 1990), "architectural determinism" (Zweig & Ducey, 1978), "crime prevention through environmental design" (Angel, 1968; Wood, 1991), "situational crime prevention"

(Clarke, 1992), and "environmental criminology" (Brantingham & Brantingham, 1991). Unlike the person-oriented strategies, all of which in a variety of ways seek to reduce the potential or actual vandal's *motivation* to perpetrate such behavior, the environment-oriented strategies seek to alter the physical setting, context, or situation in which vandalism might occur, so that the potential or actual vandal's *opportunity* to perpetrate such behavior is reduced. This ecological strategy, of altering the physical or social environment to prevent or reduce the occurrence of vandalism, has been an especially popular choice, particularly in a society as technologically oriented as the United States. Thus, venues as diverse as school districts, mass transit systems, museums, shopping malls, national and state parks, and many others have time and again opted for target hardening, access controlling, offender deflecting, entry–exit screening, surveillance increasing, inducement removing, and similar environment-altering intervention strategies as their first, and often only, means of defense against vandalism. Later in this chapter, the several dozen strategies of this sort that have been implemented are enumerated and cataloged. I suspect the reader will respond (correctly) to this lengthy, technology-oriented enumeration with the sense that we Americans certainly love our hardware.

Yet, paradoxically, very little other than anecdotal, impressionistic, or testimonial "evidence" exists for the actual effectiveness of these widely used strategies in controlling vandalism. Furthermore, the very scope of their implementation—in their most extreme form, the "Bastille response" (Ward, 1973) or the "crimeproof fortress" (Zweig & Ducey, 1978)—has in some settings had a quite negative impact on the very mission for which the setting was created in the first place. For example, "More and more high schools are becoming mechanical systems ruled by constraints on timing, location, and behavior. The similarity between schools and jails is becoming ever more pronounced" (Csikszentmihalyi & Larsen, 1978, p. 25).

Not only may the setting's mission be compromised, but as a sort of paradoxical self-fulfilling prophecy, the environmental alterations put in place to *reduce* vandalism may be experienced by a vandal-to-be as an inviting, potentially enjoyment-providing challenge to his or her vandalistic skills, and thus may actually serve to *increase* such behavior (Wise, 1982; Zweig & Ducey, 1978). The fence around the school, the graffiti-resistant wall surface, the theftproof parking meter, the slashproof bus seat, the toughened glass, the camera in the store's aisle—each is a possible opportunity-reducing deterrent; as such, each is also a challenging invitation to vandalism.

Thus, the downside of reliance on alterations to the physical environment as *the* means of vandalism control and reduction is not inconsiderable. Yet an important upside also exists. First, without concurring with a position as extreme as Weinmayer's (1969) assertion that "ninety percent of what is labeled vandalism can be prevented through design" (p. 286), one may still accept and act on the belief that venue changes can be significant components of effective person–environment interventions. First, design innovations may be relevant to "deopportunizing" vandalism in more than one way. Wiesenthal (1990), for example, observes that "property damage can be avoided by design elements that do more than resist attack; design can be used to subtly steer the user away from destruction or defacement" (p. 289). Wise (1982) suggests that design may be employed to channel attention away from potentially damaging activities, to reduce the effects of natural processes (e.g., erosion, weathering) that vandals may augment, and to eliminate or reduce the type of environmental feedback that may serve to reinforce vandalistic behavior.

Levy-Leboyer (1984) augments the case for design-as-intervention by noting that some locations are more prone to vandalism than others—a view also put forth by Christensen, Mabery, McAllister, and McCormick (1988) in their call for a predictive framework for identifying various degrees of site vulnerability. The public sites, the newer sites, the ones previously vandalized, the ones previously damaged by something other than vandalism, the ones located in "low-status" institutions, and the venues providing inadequate service are all common targets, and thus desirable sites for environmental alteration. Wilson (1977), writing as an architect, summarizes the case for design-as-intervention succinctly:

> The shape of buildings can dictate patterns of use and the circulation of people around them and hence help to structure the networks of social relationships that develop. In addition, buildings, by the amount of surveillance they afford, may prevent or offer opportunities for certain activities to take place unobserved. Finally, attrition and damage to buildings can be prevented to an extent by careful use of materials and finishes. It is eminently sensible to suppose that there is some connection between design and behavior, including vandalism. (p. 795)

Those taking a deterministic view believe that individuals choose to engage in vandalistic behavior in response to characteristics not only of their physical environment, but also of their social environment. This is purported to be the case on both micro- and macrolevels. At the micro-, immediate, level, the central social-ecological intervention concept is perceived and actual surveillance. Vandalism, it is held, is less likely to occur if the potential perpetrator believes he or she will be observed and perhaps apprehended. Thus, for example, Blauvelt (1980) urges making the school "occupied." He claims:

> The key to controlling vandalism is to make the school a place that in some sense is continuously occupied by some form of human or mechanical presence, which will deter or respond to the vandal. The heart of any effective approach to controlling vandalism will be establishing that sense of "presence" which defines the building as no longer being an inert target. (p. 47)

Added bus conductors, real and dummy TV cameras in stores, Neighborhood Watch programs, improved neighborhood lighting, and increased number of store employees are all examples of opportunity-reducing, surveillance-increasing social-ecological interventions.

Blauvelt (1980) extends the notion of "presence" in his emphasis on shared responsibility. The broader the responsibility within an institution for deopportunizing vandalism, the more likely such an approach is to succeed. Thus, in a school setting, such matters are ideally the concern not only of security personnel or administration, but also of all teachers, secretaries, custodians, kitchen personnel, and fellow students. Porter's (1980) "place defense model" suggests a taxonomy of means for citizens in general, and not only institutional personnel, to join the social-ecological intervention effort against vandalism. Included are incident-specific personal confrontations, in which citizens are urged when appropriate to threaten transgressors and physically stop vandalistic behavior; incident-specific appeals to authority, in which police or other authorities are requested to confront transgressors; and non-incident-specific social interventions, such as forming a crime watch group or hiring security personnel. Ducey's (1976) call for heightening citizen involvement via antivandalism public relations efforts, and Yambert and Donow's (1984) highlighting of the need for enhanced "community instincts" and "ecological commandments," are further citizen-oriented social-ecological calls for intervention.

Finally, and in quite a different manner, Shaw (1973) also accords the vandal's social ecology a central intervention role with this macrolevel observation:

> Vandalism is a rebellion with a cause. To prevent it, we must combat social indifference, apathy, isolation and the loss of community, neighborhood and family values. We must reaffirm the principle that human rights are more important than property rights, and property rights are acknowledged by all only when all have a share in them. (p. 18)

Changing the Vandal

The other half of the person–environment duet is now considered. In contrast to intervention efforts directed toward the actual or potential vandal's physical or social environment, here the intervention target is the vandal him- or herself. Cohen (1974) suggests three such person-oriented strategies:

1. *Education.* Here the effort is made to increase the potential vandal's awareness of the costs and other consequences of vandalistic behavior. These interventions assume that once this awareness is increased, the person will consider the possible consequences and choose to refrain from perpetrating vandalism.

2. *Deterrence and retribution.* These strategies rely on threat, punishment, or forcing those committing vandalistic acts to make restitution. Punishment strategies are especially widely employed. Ward (1973) comments:

The most frequent public reaction to vandalism is "Hit them hard": all that is needed is better detection by the police and stiffer sentences by the court. The general tendency is to support heavier fines, custodial sentences. . . . Other, extra-legal sanctions include banning offenders from swimming baths, sports fields, youth clubs or play centers. Some local authorities have suggested the evicting of tenants whose children are responsible for vandalism. (p. 256)

3. *Deflection.* Strategies of deflection "attempt to understand and redirect the motivational causes of vandalism into non-damaging means of expression" (Cohen, 1974, p. 54). They include allowing controlled destruction, providing substitute targets, or furnishing alternative outlets for energetic activity.

Koch (1975) describes a parallel array of person-oriented strategies employing coercive controls, the indoctrination of information, legal regulations, or the substitution of functional equivalents:

The first model has as its goal the total prohibition or elimination of some objectionable behavior. It implies strict enforcement and punishment of offenders. The second is an educational and/or propagandistic strategy. It has as its major goal the objective of changing behavior and attitudes. The third model is a regulative approach which utilizes rules or laws and prescribes allocations of time, space, age groupings, and monetary costs, in order to influence behavior. . . . The final alternative involves the substitution of some functional equivalent for an identified objectionable behavior. (p. 61)

To repeat an earlier-mentioned distinction, environment-focused interventions target opportunity reduction; person-oriented efforts seek to alter motivation. Although punishment, as noted earlier, appears to be an especially frequently used person-oriented strategy (Heller & White, 1975; Stoner et al., 1991), there is evidence that heavy reliance on it may often actually result in an increase, not a decrease, in the frequency of vandalism (Greenberg, 1969; Scrimger & Elder, 1981). Vandalism decreases as punitiveness decreases. Interventions such as increased use of teacher approval for desirable student behaviors are also related to lower levels of vandalism (Mayer & Butterworth, 1979; Mayer, Butterworth, Nafpaktitis, & Sulzer-Azaroff, 1983; Mayer, Nafpaktitis, Butterworth, & Hollingsworth, 1987).

In contrast to such use of extrinsic rewards (e.g., teacher approval) targeted toward altering vandalistic behavior, Csikszentmihalyi and Larsen (1978) focus more directly on a strategy calling for enhancement of intrinsic processes. Reliance on extrinsically provided rewards or reinforcement, they propose, is cumbersome and cost-ineffective; most significantly, in their view, it functions to diminish the individual's intrinsic motivation not to engage in vandalistic behavior. A second vandal-oriented strategy, of which they are similarly critical on these very same grounds of diminished intrinsic motivation, is that of "strengthening the means–ends connection between adherence to school constraints and achievement of desired future goals" (p. 29). This is a difficult strategy to implement, as it requires a considerably closer correspondence between school performance and future rewards. For many youths and in many schools, such a connection is not easy to perceive. And when it is perceived, it is yet a second instance of training youths to guide their behavior on the basis of extrinsic rather than intrinsic motivations. As their recommended alternative strategy, Csikszentmihalyi and Larsen (1978) suggest reorientation of school procedures and curriculum in a manner designed to stimulate and respond to youths' intrinsic motivation for challenge, for extension of their skills, for mastery, for growth, and for (in their terms) the experience of "flow." In their view,

> the state of enjoyment occurs when a person is challenged at a level matched by his or her level of skill. . . . Ideally, learning should involve systemic involvement in sequences of challenges internalized by students. . . . In the absence of such opportunities, antisocial behavior provides an alternative framework of challenges for bored students. Disruption of classes, vandalism, and violence in schools are, in part, attempts of adolescents to obtain enjoyment in otherwise lifeless schools. Restructuring education in terms of intrinsic motivation would not only reduce school crime, but also accomplish the goal of teaching youth how to enjoy life in an affirmative way. (p. 1)

My own strategic perspective regarding vandal-oriented intervention suggests that both externally imposed incentives *and* intrinsic motivators serve the cause of vandalism reduction well. Vandalism is a domain of interest that has a remarkably meager research base. When rigorous and relevant studies on aspects of this topic do exist, they need to be attended to especially closely. Mayer and colleagues' extrinsic-reward studies (Mayer & Butterworth, 1979; Mayer et al., 1983, 1987), and relevant intrinsic-motivation studies (deCharms, 1968, 1976; Deci, 1975), stand in support of the value of both orientations in enhancing vandals' prosocial motivation.

One final point needs to be offered regarding vandal-oriented intervention strategies. I urge the desirability of a prescriptive intervention response plan. Ideally, both who the vandal is (Griffiths & Shapland, 1979) and the level his or her vandalistic behavior has reached (Hauber, 1989) will in part determine the nature of the intervention implemented. Griffiths and Shapland (1979) correctly assert that the vandal's motives and the very meaning of the act itself change with age and context, and that strategies have to vary accordingly:

The preventive measures that need to be taken to make any given environment vandal-proof may be different according to the nature of the vandal. . . . As an example of this, look at how a window in a deserted house may be broken. This may have been done by kids getting in to play; by older children as a game of skill; by adolescents or adults in order to remove the remaining furniture or fittings; by someone with a grudge against the present or previous landlord; by a pressure group to advertise the dereliction of empty property; or by [a vagrant] to gain attention or to [get in to spend] the night. (pp. 17–18)

Person–Environment Strategies

Earlier, I offered a rationale for my preferred intervention strategy. Every act of vandalism, I hold, springs from *both* person and environment sources—a dualism that must similarly characterize efforts at its prevention and remediation. The separate person–oriented and environment–oriented vandalism intervention strategies I have now explored—in addition to their several strengths and shortcomings—will optimally be implemented in diverse, prescriptively appropriate combinations. Casserly et al. (1980), Cohen (1973), Geason and Wilson (1990), Kulka (1978), Vestermark and Blauvelt (1978), and Wilson (1979) are among the several vandalism theorists and researchers also championing multilevel, multimodal, person–environment intervention strategies. Several practitioners have already put in place such joint strategies and, at least impressionistically, report having done so to good advantage (Hendrick & Murfin, 1974; Jamieson, 1987; Levy-Leboyer, 1984; Mason, 1979; Panko, 1978; Scrimger & Elder, 1981; Stover, 1990; Weeks, 1976; White & Fallis, 1980). The section that follows provides a comprehensive listing and cataloging of the many environment-oriented and person-oriented tactics that have been employed in an array of commonly vandalized settings as means of enacting the strategies considered here.

INTERVENTION: IMPLEMENTATION TACTICS

This section catalogs the various vandalism intervention tactics that have been employed in school settings. In arranging this listing, I have incorporated and built upon Clarke's (1992) taxonomy for categorizing methods of situational crime prevention. I have employed his taxonomic system elsewhere to good advantage in an ecological analysis of aggression interventions targeted more broadly than just at vandalism (Goldstein, 1994), and I believe that with the modifications and new categories I have added to it, it will serve the current purposes well. It should be noted that Clarke's (1992) categories (I–XI) list vandalism interventions directed at the physical and social environments, and that my own categories (XII–XVII) are directly or indirectly targeted toward changing the potential or actual vandal him- or herself.

I. *Target hardening*. This situational crime prevention approach involves the use of devices or materials designed to obstruct the vandal by physical barriers:

1. Toughened glass (acrylic, polycarbon, etc.)
2. Latticework or screens to cover windows
3. Fire-retardant paint
4. High-impact plastic or steel fixtures
5. Hardened rubber or plastic swing seats
6. Concrete or steel picnic tables, benches, bleachers
7. Trash receptacles bolted to concrete bases
8. Rough-play-tolerant adventure playgrounds
9. Original planting of large-diameter trees
10. Slashproof transit vehicle seats
11. Steel-framed bus seats
12. Antigraffiti repellent spray on bus seats
13. Tamperproof sign hardware and fasteners
14. Door anchor hinges with nonremovable pins

II. *Access control*. This approach involves architectural features, mechanical and electronic devices, and related means for maintaining prerogatives over the ability to gain entry:

15. Key control systems
16. Locked gates, doors, windows
17. Electromagnetic doors unopenable from outside
18. Deadbolt and vertical-bolt locks
19. Metal door/window shutters
20. Protective grilles over roof access openings
21. Fenced yards
22. Vertical metal or small-mesh (unclimbable) fencing
23. Reduced number of building entrances
24. Unclimbable trees/bushes planted next to building
25. Prickly bushes planted next to site to be protected
26. Sloped windowsills
27. Elimination of crank-and-gear window mechanisms
28. Steeply angled roofs with parapets and ridges
29. Use of guard dogs
30. Use of student photo identification
31. Partitioning off of selected areas during "downtime" hours
32. High curbs along areas to be protected

III. *Deflecting offenders*. This is the channeling of potentially criminal or aggressive behavior in more prosocial directions by means of architectural, equipment, and related alterations:

33. Graffiti boards, mural programs
34. Schools/studios to give graffiti writers exposure and recognition
35. Interesting wallpaper, daily newspaper, chalkboard on bathroom wall
36. Litter bins
37. Wash fountains and towel dispensers in school hallways
38. Steering of pathway circulation:
    • Paving the shortest walk between connecting points
    • Avoiding sharp changes in direction
    • Paving natural shortcuts after demonstrated use
    • Installing or landscaping traffic barriers (e.g., benches, bushes)

39. "Next steps" to repair posters on broken equipment

IV. *Controlling facilitators*. This is the alteration of the means to criminal or aggressive behavior by making such means less available, less accessible, or less potentially injurious:

40. Control over sales of spray paint and indelible markers
41. Removal of debris from construction/demolition sites
42. Removal of waste paper, rubbish, and other combustibles
43. Use of tamperproof screws
44. Placement of permanent signs, building names, and decorative hardware out of reach from ground
45. Placement of school thermostats, fire alarms, and light switches far from "hang-out" areas

V. *Exit–entry screening*. Instead of seeking to exclude potential perpetrators (as in access control), this set of tactics seeks to increase the likelihood of detecting persons who are not in conformity with entry requirements (entry screening) or detecting the attempted removal of objects that should not be removed from protected areas (exit screening):

46. Closed-circuit TV
47. Metal detectors
48. Vibration detectors
49. Motion detectors
50. Perimeter alarm system
51. Library book tags

VI. *Formal surveillance*. This is surveillance by police, guards, monitors, citizen groups, or other paid or volunteer security personnel:

52. Police, citizen, senior citizen, tenant, parent patrols
53. Neighborhood Watch, School Watch, Block Watch, Rail/Bus Watch groups
54. Provision of on-site living quarters for citizens or security personnel (e.g., "school sitters," "campground hosts")
55. Informant hotlines (e.g., "rat-on-a-rat program," "secret witness program")
56. Crime Solvers Anonymous reward program
57. Mechanical, ultrasonic, infrared, electronic intruder alarm systems
58. Automatic fire detection systems
59. After-hours use of school public address system for monitoring

VII. *Natural surveillance*. This is surveillance provided by employees, home owners, pedestrians, and others going about their regular daily activities:

60. Community after-school use
61. Reduced teacher–student ratio
62. Increased number of employees (e.g., playground supervisors, bus conductors, teachers)
63. Round-the-clock custodial staffing
64. Live-in custodian/caretaker
65. Distribution of faculty/staff offices throughout the school
66. Assignment of additional faculty/staff members to hall, cafeteria duty
67. "Youth vacation vigil" student surveillance program
68. Use of bus/train employees to report vandalism on their routes
69. Improved exterior and interior lighting
70. Low trimming of shrubbery and plants

VIII. *Target removal*. This is the physical removal or enhanced inaccessibility of potential vandalism targets:

71. Use of graffiti dissuaders
    - Teflon, plastic laminate, fiberglass, or melamine covering
    - Rock cement, slanted siding, or deeply grooved surfaces
    - "Paint-outs" or use of contrasting colors in patterned surfaces
    - Fast-growing wall vines or shrubbery, or construction of wall barriers

72. Removal of pay phones from high-loitering areas

73. Removal of corner bus seats, hidden from driver's view
74. Removal of outside plant bulbs
75. Windowless school or other buildings
76. Omission of ground-level windows
77. Concealed school door closers
78. Concealed pipework
79. Fittings moved out of reach (e.g., from wall to ceiling)
80. Signs/fixtures made flush with wall or ceiling
81. Key-controlled light fixtures in public areas
82. Removal of (or no replanting of) easily damaged trees/bushes

IX. *Identifying property.* This is the physical identification marking of potential vandalism targets:

83. Property marking with school district identification
84. Property marking with business logo
85. Property marking with identification seals
86. Property marking with organization stencil
87. Property marking with individual's Social Security number

X. Removing inducements. This is the physical alteration of potential vandalism targets:

88. Rapid repair of damaged property
89. Rapid removal of graffiti
90. Use of small windowpanes
91. Elimination of school washroom and toilet stall doors
92. Elimination of bars over toilet stall doorways
93. School restroom thermostats kept at 62°F
94. Removal of gates and fences
95. Repainting of playground equipment in bright colors
96. Beautification programs (e.g., landscaping, painting, maintenance)

XI. *Rule setting.* This is the making of explicit prior statements about acceptable and unacceptable behaviors, as well as about penalties for noncompliance:

97. Model "hate crime" bill
98. Antivandalism laws
99. Building design specifications
100. Building security codes
101. Parental liability statutes
102. Prohibition of sale of spray paint and indelible markers
103. Codes of rights and responsibilities
104. School rules of student conduct

105. Rigorous, irregular, no-warning fire drills

XII. *Education*. These are direct efforts to dissuade potential and actual vandals by informing them about vandalism costs, consequences, and alternatives:

106. Vandalism education programs
107. Arson education programs
108. Vandalism awareness walks
109. Vandalism case study classroom discussions
110. Classroom brainstorming on vandalism reduction
111. School cleanup days
112. Year-round education
113. Student orientation handbook and meetings
114. Multicultural sensitivity training
115. Antivandalism lectures by older students to younger ones
116. Antivandalism films
117. Antivandalism games
118. Antivandalism slide or tape program
119. Antivandalism brochures
120. "Ride with pride" antivandalism transit program

XIII. *Publicity*. These are indirect efforts to inform potential and actual vandals, as well as the general public, about vandalism costs, consequences, and alternatives:

121. Antivandalism advertising
122. Antivandalism news releases
123. Milk carton/grocery bag antivandalism messages
124. Antivandalism decals on mass transit vehicles
125. Antivandalism slogan contests
126. "Sign amnesty" day (a day of no fines or other penalties for those who return stolen signs)
127. "Help the playground" campaigns
128. Antivandalism buttons, T-shirts, rulers, bookmarks, posters

XIV. *Punishment*. These are negative experiences directed to perpetrators consequent to their vandalistic behavior:

129. Suspension from school
130. Monetary fines
131. Restitution
132. Student vandalism account
133. Group billing for residence hall damage

XV. *Counseling*. These are remedial experiences directed to perpetrators consequent to their vandalistic behavior:

134. Student counseling programs
135. Conflict negotiation skills training
136. Moral reasoning training
137. Interpersonal skills training
138. Aggression replacement training
139. Behavior modification treatment for arson
    • Stimulus satiation
    • Contingency management
    • Assertion training

XVI. *Involvement*. These are efforts to increase the sense of involvement with and ownership of potential vandalism targets:

140. Encouraging students in residence halls to personalize (paint, furnish) their rooms
141. Permitting students in residence halls to retain same room for several semesters
142. Student participation in school decision making
143. School administration collaboration with student organizations
144. School–home collaboration
145. Hiring of unemployed youths as subway vandalism inspectors
146. "Adopt-a-station" antivandalism program

XVII. *Organizational climate*. These are procedures for enhancing the quality of the potential or actual vandal's social/educational/daily living context:

147. Teacher/staff approval/reward for student prosocial behaviors
148. Teacher respect toward students
149. Teacher/parent modeling of respect for others and for property
150. Regular, visible presence of school principal
151. Involvement of school principal in community activities
152. School curriculum revision
153. Improved student–custodian relationships
154. Improved school–community relationships
155. Reorganization of large schools into schools-within-a-school or house plans

This extended list of context-oriented and vandal-oriented interventions forms a substantial pool of diverse means for seeking to prevent, control, and reduce vandalistic behavior. In the next section, I propose and examine meaningful rationales for selecting wisely from this intervention pool, in order to put together synergistic sets or programs of vandalism interventions that are likely to have significant impacts on such behaviors.

INTERVENTION: COMBINATIONS AND EVALUATION

Viewed collectively, the array of preventive and remedial tactics employed in the schools and in other venues frequently targeted for vandalism is diverse and creative; it reflects the substantial energy that a wide variety of professionals continue to expend in their attempt to control and reduce such costly antisocial behavior. This array of *potentially* effective interventions is the good news. The bad news is that anything approaching hard evidence (or even "soft evidence" in most instances) that would aid potential users in sorting through and selecting among these numerous interventions simply does not exist.

One intervention issue that can be addressed with certainty at this point, however, is the need to identify potent *combinations* of interventions. Vandalism, like all instances of aggression, is a complexly determined behavior. Every act of vandalism derives from several causes and therefore is best combated with equally complex interventions. In this section, I examine and elaborate these assertions regarding complexity of causes and the parallel need for complexity of interventions.

Complexity of Causes

Suppose a teacher walking down a school corridor turns a corner and comes upon one of her students spray-painting his initials across the doors of several other students' lockers. Later that day, the teacher meets with the assistant principal to discuss the incident—both its causes and its consequences. In my experience, it is quite common that in discussions such as this, both teacher and administrator focus their attention *exclusively* on the perpetrator. "Johnny is a chronically bad kid [or a good kid]. He is angry [or aggressive, or misunderstood, or abused, or sleepy, or whatever]. We should caution him [or deny him certain privileges, discipline him, detain him, or suspend him]."

Is something missing here? Are the teacher's and the assistant principal's views of both causality and cure too limited? I do not want to belabor the central theme of earlier chapters of this book; I simply wish to reiterate that every act of aggression, including vandalistic acts, is a person–environment event. This perspective on complexity of causes is elaborated in Table 13.1. If the table's assertion of complex causality for all acts of aggression is correct, then it logically follows that such complexity must also optimally characterize intervention attempts. Cure must follow cause. In a related context, I have sought to describe this perspective more specifically:

TABLE 13.1. Multiple Causes of Aggressive Behavior

General category	Specific factors
Person variables	
Physiological predisposition	Male gender and associated testosterone and temperament levels
Cognitive–affective patterns	Attribution of hostile intent; projection of blame; mislabeling; low level of moral reasoning
Interpersonal skills	Absence of self-control, anger management, prosocial skill alternatives
Environmental variables	
Cultural context	Societal traditions and mores that encourage aggression
Immediate interpersonal environment	Parental/peer criminality; peer pressure; video, film, live models of aggression
Immediate physical environment	Temperature; crowding; low probability of surveillance; incivilities
Presence of disinhibitors	Alcohol, drugs; successful aggressive models
Presence of means	Weapons, tools (spray paint, markers, bricks, etc.)
Presence of targets	Windows, walls, transit vehicles, fencing, etc.

The call for complexity of solution has been heard before, from the community psychologist (Heller et al., 1984), the ecological psychologist (Moos & Insel, 1974), the environmental designer (Krasner, 1980) and the systems analyst (Plas, 1986). . . . [To] have even [a] modest chance of enduring success, interventions designed to reduce aggression towards persons or property in school contexts must be oriented not only towards the aggressor himself, but also at the levels of the teacher, school administration and organization, and the larger community context. Furthermore . . . an optimally complex intervention designed to reduce school violence ought to seek to do so via a variety of modes or channels. The first requisite, therefore, which we propose as necessary for the effective planning of a successful aggression reduction intervention is multilevel, multichannel complexity. (Goldstein, 1988, p. 294)

In the following discussion, I draw upon the pool of vandalism interventions presented earlier in order to illustratively reorganize samples of these interventions into just such multilevel, multichannel configurations. In the absence of efficacy evaluations, no particular interventions or intervention

TABLE 13.2. A Multilevel, Multichannel Schema for the Reduction of School Vandalism

Level of intervention	Mode of intervention				
	Psychological	Educational	Administrative	Legal	Physical
Community	"Youth vacation vigil" program	Arson education programs	"Adopt-a-school" programs	Monetary fines	Citizen, police, parent patrols
School	Conflict negotiation programs	Year-round education	Schools-within-a-school	Codes of rights and responsibilities	Lighting, painting, paving programs
Teacher	School–home collaboration	Multicultural sensitivity training	Reduced teacher–student ratio	Property marking with school ID	Distribution of faculty offices throughout school
Student	Interpersonal skills training	Vandalism awareness walks	School detention, suspension	Restitution, student vandalism accounts	Graffiti boards, mural walls

345

configurations can be singled out for recommended use at this time. However, I believe that this emphasis on the selection and implementation of meaningful intervention *combinations* is likely to prove a major step toward truly effective vandalism prevention, control, and reduction.

Complexity of Interventions

Table 13.2 presents a level x channel intervention schema targeted to the reduction of vandalism in school contexts. My intent here is to urge both practitioners and evaluators of vandalism prevention/reduction efforts to make sure that interventions at all levels and through all channels are included in their packages or sets of interventions.

A second factorial schema seeking to reflect in its particulars the desirable complexity of vandalism intervention programming is that offered by Harootunian (1986). Instead of mode or channel of intervention, Harootunian's proposal crosses level of intervention with intended goal. In a later publication (Goldstein, Harootunian, & Conoley, 1994, p. 204), he observes:

> Various actions taken against aggression are initiated to prevent or discourage hostile acts directed against persons or school property. Such measures as 24-hour custodial service and better lighting are designed to prevent aggression. The use of Plexiglas windows may not prevent aggressive acts, but

TABLE 13.3. A Multilevel, Multigoal Schema for the Reduction of School Vandalism

| Level of intervention | Goal of intervention | | |
	Prevention	Compensatory	Remediation
Community	Adopt-a-school programs	Less restrictive child labor laws Short-term treatment centers	Family support services
School	24-hour custodial service	Use of Plexiglas windows	Prescriptively tailored courses
Teacher	Programs to enhance knowledge of ethnic and minority milieu	Better teacher–pupil ratio	Acquisition of new training techniques in psychological skills (e.g., structured learning)
Student	Identification cards	School transfers Part-time programs	Interpersonal training Behavior modification

Note. From Harootunian (1986, p. 131). Copyright 1986 by Pergamon Press, Inc. Reprinted by permission.

it will certainly reduce the incidence of broken windows. Compensatory interventions do not in themselves change aggressive or disruptive students, but they do offset the consequences of their actions. Remedial interventions, on the other hand, are aimed at changing students, not simply providing them with ways of circumventing their aggressive acts.

Table 13.3 illustrates this levels x goals perspective.

Beyond the multilevel, multigoal vandalism intervention combinations derivable from Table 13.3, the schemas of Tables 13.2 and 14.3 may be combined in the actual practice of planning and implementing vandalism prevention/reduction programs. Such a three-dimensional schema based simultaneously on intervention levels, channels, and goals may be a bit complex to conceptualize, but it is no more complex than the multiply determined behavior it seeks to alter—vandalism. Furthermore, as Harootunian (Goldstein et al., 1994, p. 206) notes,

> any one strategy in isolation often has resulted in confusion, if not contradictory findings. A multiple perspective strategy makes it possible to determine where a suggested intervention or approach fits and how it may influence or be influenced by adjacent solutions. Also, a comprehensive view of school aggression may reveal gaps and overloads in the system. There is evidence, for example (Zwier & Vaughan, 1984), that almost one-half of the literature on school vandalism focuses on the physical dimensions of the school.

In quite the same factorial spirit as Tables 13.2 and 13.3, Zwier and Vaughan (1984) propose a schema for combining vandalism interventions—one that crosses level of intervention (defined differently than it is defined earlier) with ideological orientation. Educational practices in U.S. public schools have long been fair game for broad and often intense public concern and debate. This spotlight of attention most certainly includes disciplinary practices. Harootunian (Goldstein et al., 1994) quite correctly notes that in order for a specific intervention to be accepted, to be implemented, and to have a chance of succeeding, the values it elicits must overlap to an appreciable degree with the values or ideologies of those who are asked to accept and participate in its implementation. Table 13.4 details this level x ideology perspective.

As noted earlier, the different ideological perspectives included in this table have generated considerable historical and current debate and contentiousness in the United States. My own belief is that the appropriate position at this point is an empirical one. Whether a set of vandalism interventions reflecting one or another ideological orientation (crossed with levels) proves most efficacious, or a mixing of ideological implementations is to be preferred, is a matter for yet-to-be-conducted efficacy evaluations. Whichever ideological stance or stances guide the selection and implementation of interventions, and whichever levels, channels, or goals are also reflected

TABLE 13.4. The Relationship between Ideological Orientations and Assumptions Concerning the Cause of School Vandalism, and Types of Solutions Offered

Ideological orientation and assumption of cause	Type of solution		
	Specific Physical environment	School system	Diffuse Community at large
Conservative Vandals are deviant. They must be caught and punished.	Protection of school and school grounds, employment of security officers and security officers and caretakers[a]	Encouragement and enforcement of school rules, use of contingency contracts	Involvement of community in antivandalism patrols and (parent) restitution programs, dependence on judicial system
Liberal The school system is malfunctioning. Vandals capitalize on this.	(Superficial) improvement of the design, appearance, and layout of the school grounds	Modifications in school climate, curriculum, and use of special conflict management programs[a]	Extension of recreational activities, use of school after hours for health and social services
Radical The school system is debilitating. Vandalism is a response of normal individuals to abnormal conditions.	Promotion of radical changes in the structure and appearance of the school, approval of policy to decrease the size of large schools and maintain small schools	Provision of student involvement in decision-making process, adoption of changes in assessment procedures, and exploration of alternative schooling methods	Involvement of the whole community in school affairs, installment of community education programs, improvement of social situation in society at large[a]

Note. From Zwier and Vaughan (1984, p. 269). Copyright 1984 by the American Education Research Association. Reprinted by permission.
[a]The solution considered most favorably by the particular ideological orientation.

therein, I believe that three qualities of such programming are essential to success: Vandalism interventions must be comprehensive, prescriptive, and appreciative.

OPTIMAL INTERVENTION CHARACTERISTICS

Comprehensive Programming

As quite directly implied in the presentation and discussion of Tables 13.1–13.4, I view vandalism as a complexly determined phenomenon requiring equally complex intervention responses. The notions of the person–environment duet, levels of intervention, multiple channels or modes of response, diverse intervention goals, and varied intervention ideologies all call, in their different ways, for comprehensive intervention combinations.

Prescriptive Programming

The second highly desirable quality of interventions offered is that they be differential, tailored, individualized, or prescriptive interventions. "Vandalism" is a term identifying a very wide array of behaviors that express exceedingly diverse motivations, are carried out in a great variety of settings, and are enacted by persons differing widely in age, experience, past antisocial behavior, peer group affiliation, system support, and numerous other characteristics possibly relevant to intervention effectiveness. One size does not fit all.

Understandably, most discussions of differential or prescriptive intervention programming, whether directed toward vandalism or other problem behaviors, have focused on examining which type(s) of interventions should be employed with which type(s) of perpetrators. There is, however, an important third aspect of optimal prescriptions:

> . . . optimal prescriptions should be tridifferential, specifying type of intervention by type of client by type of change agent. This last class of variable merits attention. Interventions as received by youths to whom they are directed are never identical to the [intervention] procedures as specified in a textbook or treatment manual. In actual practice, the intervention specified in a manual is interpreted and implemented by the change agent and perceived and experienced by the youths. The change agent looms large in this sequence. . . . Who administers the intervention does make a difference. (Goldstein, 1978, pp. 479–480)

Appreciative Programming

Vandalism is committed by European American, African American, Latino, Asian, Native American, and other children, adolescents, and adults. Such diversity among perpetrators has implications not only for how a given intervention is best presented and by whom, but also for the very structure and content of the intervention itself. A prime route to maximizing the impact of intervention structure and content is to involve persons representative of the ultimate target group(s) in the intervention's development. Effective interventions cannot be developed only "from the outside in." The very meaning of vandalistic behavior; the perception and potency of its consequences; the role of peer pressure, neighborhood incivility, and other external influences; and the apparent appropriateness and utility of alternative interventions must all be viewed through the age-graded, gender-associated, and cultural lenses of its likely perpetrators and intervention targets. Whether such "inside information" is obtained by means of formal or informal "consumer consultants," through focus groups, or in other ways, it is likely to prove highly useful in the effort to enhance intervention efficacy.

I have urged that rationally composed vandalism intervention combinations be planned comprehensively, prescriptively, and appreciatively. When such interventions are implemented, I further encourage their users to pay adequate attention to intervention integrity, intensity, and coordination.

Intervention Integrity

Intervention "integrity" is the degree to which an intervention as actually implemented corresponds to the intervention as planned. Intervention integrity may be problematic for a number of reasons. An adequately detailed plan may never have been developed. Ideally, interventions to be carried out will first be described in full, sequential, user-friendly detail in "treatment manuals" that can be widely distributed to serve as concrete, step-by-step, systematic guides for intervenors. Even when such a manual has been developed, distributed, and read, intervention monitoring will often reveal substantial discrepancies between plan and reality (i.e., low intervention integrity). Other responsibilities, large teaching loads, extra bus routes to drive, and larger areas to keep under surveillance may all lead to overburdened, tired, or lazy intervenors. Distractions, emergencies, exigencies, or other realities may detour the practitioner from the intervention plan. Supervision or monitoring of intervenors, intended to "keep interventions on track," may be inadequate or may fail to materialize altogether. Even if a plan is appropriately described, detailed, and exemplified in a vandalism intervention procedures manual, it may fail to anticipate an array of significant circumstances. For interventions to succeed in their intended purpose, integrity is a crucial prerequisite.

Intervention Intensity

"Intensity" means the amount, quantity, or dosage of the intervention provided. Vandalism, as but one expression of aggression, is often a chronic, overlearned, well-reinforced behavior. One-shot, short-term, or otherwise limited interventions will rarely if ever be potent enough to prevent or remediate such behavior on anything approaching a sustained basis. Consider a small sampling of the intervention tactics listed earlier in this chapter—locks, tamperproof hardware, steering of pathway circulation, control of spray paint sales, use of closed-circuit TV, hiring citizens for watch patrols, collecting restitution, curriculum revision, and antivandalism education and publicity. In each instance, the intervenor must ask: Is this enough, or strong enough, or numerous enough, or sustained enough? These are questions about intervention intensity.

Intervention Coordination

I have placed a great emphasis in this chapter on intervention combinations or sets as a necessary requirement for successful vandalism prevention and reduction; moreover, person–environment targeting, multiple levels of intervention, and multichannel interventions all mean that a variety of persons and agencies may be offering parts of an intervention combination. Accordingly, the coordination of effort rises to become a significant concern, as I have observed elsewhere:

> Society's agents often work in splendid isolation from one another. Their efforts are sometimes conflicting or at cross purposes, often quite independent, and infrequently additive. Not unlike the far too specialized physician who has not a "whole patient" but "an interesting liver" on his ward, agency personnel often fail to see and respond to . . . youth as a gestalt. Instead, they concern themselves exclusively with their own segmented, limited domain, or mandated agency focus. When this occurs, the potential for uncoordinated, nonadditive, and conflicting interventions is high. Major attention to intervention coordination is crucial, especially in the context of comprehensive intervention programming, in which a number of diversely targeted agencies may be simultaneously involved with the same youth. (Goldstein, 1993, p. 484)

CONCLUSION

Vandalism in U.S. schools is a frequent, costly, and persistent fact of educational life. Like its counterpart, aggression toward persons, it is causally a person–environment event; thus, parallel interactionist strategies and tactics are required for its reduction and control. I have sought in this chapter to provide such rationales and means, as well as to propose meaningful bases for selecting among and grouping these several alternatives in order to constitute intervention programs that are likely to be effective. Supportive research has not yet been accomplished. The monetary, social, and educational costs of contemporary vandalistic behavior are, however, quite major; so too must be efforts at its prevention and reduction.

REFERENCES

Altman, I., Brown, B. B., Staples, B., & Werner, C. M. (1992). A transactional approach to close relationships: Courtship, weddings, and placemaking. In W. B. Walsh, K. H. Craik, & R. H. Price (Eds.), *Person–environment psychology: Models and perspectives* (pp. 193–241). Hillsdale, NJ: Erlbaum.

Anderson, J. (1977). *Vandalism in the Unified School District of Los Angeles County.* Unpublished doctoral dissertation, University of Southern California.

Angel, S. (1968). *Discouraging crime through city planning.* Berkeley: University of California Press.

Angyal, A. (1959). *Foundations for a science of personality.* Cambridge, MA: Harvard University Press.

Barker, R. G., & Gump, P. (1964). *Big school, small school.* Stanford, CA: Stanford University Press.

Barker, R. G., & Wright, H. F. (1954). *The Midwest and its children.* New York: Harper & Row.

Bayh, B. (1978). School discipline, violence and vandalism: Implications for teacher preparation. *Action in Teacher Education, 1,* 3–10.

Blauvelt, P. D. (1980). School security doesn't have to break the bank. *Independent School, 40,* 47–50.

Brantingham, P. J., & Brantingham, P. L. (1991). *Environmental criminology.* Newbury Park, CA: Sage.

Campbell, A. (1986). The streets and violence. In A. Campbell & J. J. Gibbs (Eds.), *Violent transactions: The limits of personality* (pp. 115–132). Oxford, UK: Blackwell.

Casserly, M. D., Bass, S. A., & Garrett, J. R. (1980). *School vandalism: Strategies for prevention.* Lexington, MA: Lexington Books.

Christensen, H. H., Mabery, K., McAllister, M. E., & McCormick, D. P. (1988). *Cultural resource protection.* Denver, CO: Rocky Mountain Forest and Range Experiment Station.

Clarke, R. V. (Ed.). (1992). *Situational crime prevention: Successful case studies.* New York: Harrow & Heston.

Cohen, S. (1971). Direction for research on adolescent school violence and vandalism. *British Journal of Criminology, 9,* 319–340.

Cohen, S. (1973). Campaigning against vandalism. In C. Ward (Ed.), *Vandalism* (pp. 215–257). London: Architectural Press.

Cohen, S. (1974). Breaking out, smashing up and the social context of aspiration. *Working Papers in Cultural Studies, 5,* 37–63.

Cordilia, A. T. (1986). Robbery arising out of a group drinking-context. In A. Campbell & J. J. Gibbs (Eds.), *Violent transactions: The limits of personality* (pp. 167–180). Oxford, UK: Blackwell.

Csikszentmihalyi, M., & Larsen, R. (1978). *Intrinsic rewards in school crime.* Hackensack, NJ: National Council on Crime and Delinquency.

DeBunza, C. (1974). *A study of school vandalism: Causes and prevention measures currently found in selected secondary schools throughout Alabama.* Unpublished doctoral dissertation, Alabama State University.

deCharms, R. (1968). *Personal causation.* New York: Academic Press.

deCharms, R. (1976). *Enhancing motivation: Change in the classroom.* New York: Irvington.

Deci, E. L. (1975). *Intrinsic motivation*. New York: Plenum Press.

Ducey, M. (1976). *Vandalism in high schools: An exploratory discussion*. Chicago: Institute for Juvenile Research.

Endler, N. S., & Magnusson, D. (1976). Toward an interactional psychology of personality. *Psychological Bulletin, 83*, 956–974.

Federal Bureau of Investigation (FBI). (1978). *Crime in the United States*. Washington, DC: U.S. Government Printing Office.

Forgas, J. P. (1986). Cognitive representations of aggressive situations. In A. Campbell & J. Gibbs (Eds.), *Violent transactions: The limits of personality* (pp. 41–58). Oxford, UK: Blackwell.

Garbarino, J. (1978). *The human ecology of school crime*. Hackensack, NJ: National Council on Crime and Delinquency.

Geason, S., & Wilson, P. R. (1990). *Preventing graffiti and vandalism*. Canberra: Australian Institute of Criminology.

Gibbs, J. J. (1986). Alcohol consumption, cognition and context: Examining tavern violence. In A. Campbell & J. J. Gibbs (Eds.), *Violent transactions: The limits of personality* (pp. 133–151). Oxford, UK: Blackwell.

Goldman, N. (1961). Socio-psychological study of school vandalism. *Crime and Delinquency, 7*, 221–230.

Goldstein, A. P. (1978). *Prescriptions for child mental health and education*. Elmsford, NY: Pergamon Press.

Goldstein, A. P. (1988). *The Prepare curriculum*. Champaign, IL: Research Press.

Goldstein, A. P. (1992, May 4). *School violence: Its community context and potential solutions*. Testimony presented to Subcommittee on Elementary, Secondary and Vocational Education, Committee on Education and Labor, U.S. House of Representatives.

Goldstein, A. P. (1993). Gang intervention: Issues and opportunities. In A. P. Goldstein & C. R. Huff (Eds.), *The gang intervention handbook* (pp. 477–493). Champaign, IL: Research Press.

Goldstein, A. P. (1994). *The ecology of aggression*. New York: Research Press.

Goldstein, A. P. (1995). *The psychology of vandalism*. New York: Plenum Press.

Goldstein, A. P., Harootunian, B., & Conoley, J. C. (1994). *Student aggression: Prevention, management, and replacement training*. New York: Guilford Press.

Greenberg, B. (1969). *School vandalism: A national dilemma*. Menlo Park, CA: Stanford Research Institute.

Griffiths, R., & Shapland, J. M. (1979). The vandal's perspective: Meanings and motives. In P. Bural (Ed.), *Designing against vandalism* (pp. 11–18). New York: Van Nostrand Reinhold.

Harootunian, B. (1986). School violence and vandalism. In S. J. Apter & A. P. Goldstein (Eds.), *Youth violence: Programs and prospects* (pp. 120–139). Elmsford, NY: Pergamon Press.

Hauber, A. R. (1989). Influencing juvenile offenders by way of alternative sanctions in community settings. In H. Wegener (Ed.), *Criminal behavior and the justice system* (pp. 382–398). New York: Springer-Verlag.

Heller, K., Price, R. H., Reinharz, S., Riger, S., Wandersman, A., & D'Aunno, T. A. (1984). *Psychology and community change*. Homewood, IL: Dorsey Press.

Heller, M. C., & White, M. A. (1975). Rates of teacher verbal approval and disapproval to higher and lower ability classes. *Journal of Educational Psychology, 67*, 796–800.

Hendrick, C., & Murfin, M. (1974). Project library ripoff: A study of periodical mutilation in a university library. *College and Research Libraries, 35*, 402–411.

Howard, E. R. (1978). *School discipline desk book*. West Nyack, NY: Parker.

Ianni, F. A. J. (1979). The social organization of the high school: School-specific aspects of school crime. In E. Wenk & N. Harlow (Eds.), *School crime and disruption* (pp. 21–36). Davis, CA: Responsible Action.

Irwin, F. G. (1978). Planning vandalism resistant educational facilities. *Journal of Research and Development in Education, 11,* 42–52.

Jamieson, B. (1987). Public telephone vandalism. In D. Challinger (Ed.), *Preventing property crime* (pp. 31–34). Canberra: Australian Institute of Criminology.

Kempt, D. L., Skok, R. L. & McLaughlin, T. F. (1996). Programs and procedures that reduce school vandalism. *Corrective and Social Psychiatry, 42,* 12–19.

Kingston, A. J., & Gentry, H. W. (1977). Discipline problems: Then and now. *National Association of Secondary School Principals Bulletin, 61,* 94–99.

Koch, E. L. (1975). School vandalism and strategies of social control. *Urban Education, 10,* 54–72.

Krasner, L. (1980). *Environmental design and human behavior.* Elmsford, NY: Pergamon Press.

Krupat, E. (1985). *People in cities: The urban environment and its effects.* Cambridge, MA: Harvard University Press.

Kulka, R. A. (1978). School crime as a function of person–environment fit. *Theoretical Perspectives on School Crime, 1,* 17–24.

Leftwich, D. (1977). *A study of vandalism in selected public schools in Alabama.* Unpublished doctoral dissertation, University of Alabama–Birmingham.

Levy-Leboyer, C. (Ed.). (1984). *Vandalism: Behavior and motivations.* Amsterdam: North-Holland.

Lewin, K. (1935). *A dynamic theory of personality.* New York: McGraw-Hill.

Lewin, K. (1936). *Principles of topological psychology.* New York: McGraw-Hill.

Little, B. R. (1987). Personality and the environment. In D. Stokols & I. Altman (Eds.), *Handbook of environmental psychology* (pp. 205–244). Malabar, FL: Krieger.

Mason, D. L. (1979). *Fine art of art security: Protecting public and private collections against theft, fire, and vandalism.* New York: Van Nostrand Reinhold.

Massucci, J. (1984). School vandalism: A plan of action. *National Association of Secondary School Principals Bulletin, 68,* 18–20.

Mathie, J. P., & Schmidt, R. E. (1977). Rehabilitation and one type of arsonist. *Fire and Arson Investigator, 28,* 53–56.

Mayer, G. R., & Butterworth, T. W. (1979). A preventive approach to school violence and vandalism: An experimental study. *Personnel and Guidance Journal, 57,* 436–441.

Mayer, G. R., Butterworth, T. W., Nafpaktitis, M., & Sulzer-Azaroff, B. (1983). Preventing school vandalism and improving discipline: A three-year study. *Journal of Applied Behavior Analysis, 16,* 355–369.

Mayer, G. R., Nafpaktitis, M., Butterworth, T. W., & Hollingsworth, P. (1987). A search for the elusive setting events of school vandalism: A correlational study. *Education and Treatment of Children, 10,* 259–270.

Mayer, G. R., & Sulzer-Azaroff, B. (1991). Interventions for vandalism. In G. Stoner, M. R. Shinn, & H. M. Walker (Eds.), *Interventions for achievement and behavior problems* (pp. 559–580). Silver Spring, MD: National Association of School Psychologists.

McPherson, M., & Carpenter, J. (1981). *Rural youth vandalism in four Minnesota counties.* Minneapolis: Minnesota Crime Prevention Center.

Mischel, W. (1968). *Personality and assessment.* New York: Wiley.

Moos, R. H., & Insel, P. M. (1974). *Issues in social ecology.* Palo Alto, CA: National Press Books.

Murphy, G. (1947). *Personality: A biosocial approach to origins and structure.* New York: Harper.

Murray, H. (1938). *Explorations in personality*. New York: Oxford University Press.

Nowakowski, R. (1966). *Vandals and vandalism in the schools: An analysis of vandalism in large school systems and a description of 93 vandals in Dade County schools*. Unpublished doctoral dissertation, University of Miami.

Pablant, P., & Baxter, J. C. (1975). Environmental correlates of school vandalism. *Journal of the American Institute of Planners, 41*, 270–279.

Page, R. A., & Moss, M. K. (1976). Environmental influences on aggression. The effects of darkness and proximity of victim. *Journal of Applied Social Psychology, 6*, 126–133.

Panko, W. L. (1978). *Taxonomy of school vandalism*. Unpublished doctoral dissertation, University of Pittsburgh.

Pervin, L. (1986). Persons, situations, interactions: Perspectives on a recurrent issue. In A. Campbell & J. J. Gibbs (Eds.), *Violent transactions: The limits of personality* (pp. 15–26). Oxford, UK: Blackwell.

Plas, J. M. (1986). *Systems psychology in the schools*. Elmsford, NY: Pergamon Press.

Porter, G. V. (1980). *The control of vandalism in urban recreation facilities: A revision of the defensible space model*. Unpublished doctoral dissertation, Boston University.

Rausch, H. L. (1967). Interaction sequence. *Journal of Personality and Social Psychology, 2*, 487–499.

Rausch, H. L. (1972). Process and change. *Family Processes, 11*, 275–298.

Rautaheimo, J. (1989). The making of an arsonist. *Fire Prevention, 223*, 30–35.

Richards, P. (1976). *Patterns of middle class vandalism: A case study of suburban adolescence*. Unpublished doctoral dissertation, Northwestern University.

Roncek, D. W., & Faggiani, D. (1985). High schools and crime: A replication. *Sociological Quarterly, 26*, 491–505.

Roncek, D. W., & Lobosco, A. (1983). The effect of high schools on crime in their neighborhoods. *Social Science Quarterly, 64*, 598–613.

Rotter, J. B. (1954). *Social learning and clinical psychology*. Englewood Cliffs, NJ: Prentice-Hall.

Rubel, R. J. (1977). *Unruly schools: Disorders, disruptions, and crimes*. Lexington, MA: D. C. Heath.

Scrimger, G. C., & Elder, R. (1981). *Alternative to vandalism–"Cooperation or wreckreation."* Sacramento: California Office of the Attorney General School Safety Center.

Shaw, W. (1973). Vandalism is not senseless. *Law and Order, 12*, 14–19.

Skelton, C. (1996). Learning to be "tough": The fostering of maleness in one primary school. *Gender and Education, 8*, 185-197.

Stefanko, M. S. (1989). *Rates of secondary school vandalism and violence: Trends, demographic differences, and the effects of the attitudes and behaviors of principals*. Unpublished doctoral dissertation, Claremont College.

Stokols, D., & Altman, I. (1987). *Handbook of environmental psychology*. New York: Wiley.

Stoner, G., Shinn, M. R., & Walker, H. M. (Eds.). (1991). *Interventions for achievement and behavior problems*. Silver Spring, MD: National Association of School Psychologists.

Stover, D. (1990, November). How to be safe and secure against school vandalism. *Executive Educator*, pp. 20–30.

Tygert, C. (1988). Public school vandalism: Toward a synthesis of theories and transition to paradigm analysis. *Adolescence, 23*, 187–199.

U.S. Department of Justice. (2000, July). *Juvenile vandalism, 1997* [Fact Sheet #10]. Washington, DC: Office of Juvenile Justice and Delinquency Prevention.

Vandals. (1978, March). *Justice of the Peace*, pp. 169–172.

Vestermark, S. D., & Blauvelt, P. D. (1978). *Controlling crime in the school: A complete security handbook for administrators*. West Nyack, NY: Parker.

Ward, C. (1973). *Vandalism*. New York: Van Nostrand Reinhold.

Weeks, S. (1976). Security against vandalism: It takes facts, feelings and facilities. *American School and University, 48*, 36–46.

Weinmayer, V. M. (1969). Vandalism by design: A critique. *Landscape Architecture, 59*, 286.

White, J., & Fallis, A. (1980). *Vandalism prevention programs used in Ontario schools.* Toronto: Ontario Ministry of Education.

Wiesenthal, D. L. (1990). Psychological aspects of vandalism. In P. J. D. Drenth, J. A. Sergeant, & R. J. Takens (Eds.), *European perspectives in psychology* (Vol. 3). New York: Wiley.

Wilson, S. (1977). Vandalism and design. *Architect's Journal, 166*, 795–798.

Wilson, S. (1979). Observations on the nature of vandalism. In P. Bural (Ed.), *Designing against vandalism* (pp. 19–29). New York: Van Nostrand Reinhold.

Wise, J. (1982, September). A gentle deterrent to vandalism. *Psychology Today*, pp. 28–31.

Wood, D. (1991). In defense of indefensible space. In P. J. Brantingham & P. L. Brantingham (Eds.), *Environmental criminology* (pp. 77–95). Prospect Heights, IL: Waveland Press.

Yambert, P. A., & Donow, C. F. (1984). Are we ready for ecological commandments? *Journal of Environmental Education, 3*, 13–16.

Yankelovitch, D. (1975, April). How students control their drug crisis. *Psychology Today*, pp. 39–42.

Zimbardo, P. G. (1973). A field experiment in auto shaping. In C. Ward (Ed.), *Vandalism* (pp. 85–90). London: Architectural Press.

Zweig, A., & Ducey, M. H. (1978). *A paradigmatic field: A review of research on school vandalism.* Hackensack, NJ: National Council on Crime and Delinquency.

Zwier, G., & Vaughan, G. M. (1984). Three ideological orientations in school vandalism research. *Review of Educational Research, 54*, 263–292.

PART V
System-Oriented Interventions

CHAPTER 14

Families with Aggressive Children and Adolescents

SANDRA L. CHRISTENSON
AMY R. ANDERSON
JULIE A. HIRSCH

Educators routinely encounter a small percentage of children and adolescents who exhibit persistent patterns of antisocial and externalizing behaviors in school settings. Frequently, the relationship between educators and the families of these students is strained and intense—not only because of the students' extremely disruptive behavior and low academic performance, but because of the specific relationship between home and school, which contributes to either blaming or diffuse responsibility for resolving the problematic situation. Elsewhere, we (Christenson & Hirsch, 1998) have described five conditions that contribute to blaming between families and educators: (1) social distance in the family–school relationship, (2) attitudes and beliefs held by families about school environments and by educators about home environments, (3) quantity and quality of communication between families and educators, (4) lack of clarity in the socialization roles for the school and family, and (5) the institutional nature of many school policies and practices. These conditions, at a minimum, serve to reinforce stereotypes about families with aggressive children and adolescents; worse, and all too frequently, they block prevention and intervention efforts for students.

This chapter proposes guidelines for school-based professionals to work effectively with families of aggressive children and adolescents. We have based these guidelines, which are organized into the categories "approach," "attitude," and "action," on a review of the intervention-oriented literature for working with families of children who display externalizing behaviors. We think of these guidelines as a road map to change psychological and educational service delivery targeted at addressing violence and aggression in

359

schools. We believe that the role of school-based professionals is to make a difference in children's lives; the goal is not simply to predict or understand child behavior and performance. In this chapter, we review background information about child and family characteristics related to aggression, summarize the efficacy of interventions for families with children and adolescents who are aggressive in school contexts, and describe guidelines for working with families to increase the school success of aggressive children and adolescents.

BACKGROUND INFORMATION

A critical challenge facing professionals in educational settings today is to create and maintain safe, violence-free school environments. The significance of this goal is reflected in the sixth National Education Goal: "By the year 2000, every school in the United States will be free of drugs, violence, and the unauthorized presence of firearms and alcohol, and will offer a disciplined environment conducive to learning" (National Education Goals Panel, 1995, p. 15). The passage of the Improving America's Schools Act of 1994 by President Clinton and Congress, Title IV of which provides funding and technical assistance for the development of safe school plans, reinforces the importance of this goal in contemporary U.S. society.

Although estimates of the amount and intensity of school violence vary, concern about the level of violence and aggression occurring in U.S. schools appears to be warranted. The U.S. Department of Justice (1993) reports that nearly 3 million crimes occur on or near school campuses each year. This translates into 16,000 incidents per school day, or one every 6 seconds. In their review of school violence research over the last two decades, Furlong and Morrison (1994) noted that in the 1970s, approximately 20% of students reported feeling "afraid of being hurt or bothered" at school (National Institute of Education, 1978). In a more recent survey of primarily African American students in urban settings, approximately 15% of students reported "often feeling afraid" at school, although 38% indicated that there was "a lot" of violence in their schools (Sheley, McGee, & White, 1992). With respect to teachers' views on aggression, Mansfield, Alexander, and Farris (1991) found in a national survey of teachers that 51% of the respondents had been verbally abused by a student at some point in their teaching careers.

Fortunately, aggression and other acts of violence in schools are not perpetrated by many students in every school. Rather, violent and aggressive acts are typically committed by a very small percentage of students. For example, the Centers for Disease Control and Prevention (1990) conducted a national study of self-reported fighting behavior of high school students; of all serious fights reported, nearly half were accounted for by only 1.6% of the students. Understanding these students, their families, and promising practices for prevention and intervention is the focus of this chapter.

A comment regarding terminology is in order. Aggressive behaviors cut across several diagnostic categories and labels—most notably conduct disorder (CD), oppositional defiant disorder (ODD), antisocial personality disorder (APD), attention-deficit/hyperactivity disorder (ADHD), and other problem behaviors that have traditionally been labeled "externalizing" or "disruptive" behavior disorders. Although the differentiations among these disorders are becoming better understood, the comorbidity of these problem behaviors and labels is well documented (Kazdin, 1987a). Moreover, interventions designed to assist families with aggressive children have common elements that appear to be useful for children and adolescents with different diagnostic labels but similar constellations of problems. Therefore, our focus in this chapter is on family interventions for aggressive child and youth behaviors, regardless of diagnostic labels.

Prevalence

One way to determine the amount of aggression and violence among children and adolescents is to examine the prevalence rates of the disorders associated with aggressive behavior. For example, it is estimated that approximately 4–10%, or from 1.3 to 1.8 million children in the United States, meet the diagnostic criteria for ODD and CD (Webster-Stratton, 1993). In the educational domain, more than 400,000 children and adolescents ages 6–21 were identified as having a serious emotional disturbance (SED) in the 1992–1993 school year, accounting for approximately 9% of all children who received special education services (U.S. Department of Education, 1994). Although the number of students identified with SED continues to increase each year, only a small proportion of the estimated 6–10% of all school-age children who have emotional or behavioral disorders receive services (Kauffman, 1985; U.S. Department of Education, 1994).

CD and other aggressive disorders occur more frequently in males than in females, although there are indications both in the literature and anecdotally that female aggression is rising (Loeber, 1990). A more troubling picture of youthful aggression emerges when adolescents themselves are surveyed. For example, in several studies of adolescents 13–18 years old, more than 35% admitted to committing assault, and more than 60% reported involvement in more than one type of antisocial behavior, including aggression, vandalism, substance abuse, and arson (Feldman, Caplinger, & Wodarski, 1983; Williams & Gold, 1972). Referral rates for mental health services provide another indicator; approximately one-third to one-half of all child and adolescent clinic referrals are made for children exhibiting aggressiveness, conduct problems, or other antisocial behaviors (Herbert, 1987; Kazdin, 1987b; Robins, 1981).

Continuity over Time

The importance of knowing how many young people are affected by CD and other aggressive disorders becomes clear when we consider the developmental outcomes associated with these disorders. CD and other externalizing behavior disorders are among the most stable of all childhood disorders (Kazdin, 1987a; Kolko, 1994). Although other disorders often remit with maturation, childhood antisocial disorders tend to be enduring, to intensify over time without treatment, and to become more resistant to change with age (Kazdin, 1987b; Robins, 1981). Researchers have shown that even for very young children, high rates of aggression are stable over time. For example, Richman, Stevenson, and Graham (1982) reported that of those children with externalizing behavior problems at age 3, 67% continued to be aggressive at age 8. Similarly, Campbell, Ewing, Breaux, and Szumowski (1986) found that more than half of preschoolers who had been labeled "hard to manage" continued to exhibit problem behaviors at age 6. The implications of this developmental stability are profound. Currently, a large body of research indicates that children and adolescents who exhibit ongoing aggression and other antisocial behaviors are at risk for a variety of negative developmental outcomes.

In general, persistent aggressive behavior and related disorders in childhood and adolescence have been associated with peer rejection, substance abuse, social skills deficits, criminal behavior, interpersonal problems, marital disruptions, unemployment, and pervasive academic problems (Coie, 1990; Coie, Dodge, & Coppotelli, 1982; Dodge, 1980; Farrington, 1991; Kazdin, 1985; Loeber & Stouthamer-Loeber, 1987; Patterson, DeBaryshe, & Ramsey, 1989; Robins, 1978; Robins & Ratcliff, 1980). In studies that specifically examined aggression in school settings, researchers found that adolescents who are aggressive in school have higher dropout rates than average; poorer overall school adjustment; higher rates of juvenile delinquency, particularly for males; and higher than average rates of referral for mental health services (Cox & Gunn, 1980; Kuperschmidt & Coie, 1990; Loeber & Stouthamer-Loeber, 1987; for a review, see Hudley, 1994). Furthermore, the costs associated with aggression and other related disorders are immense. For example, the costs of vandalism and arson among juvenile delinquents in a single year in the mid-1970s totaled approximately $1.3 billion, and the cost of educating a student with SED is estimated to be three times the cost of educating a student in regular education (Kauffman, 1985; Kazdin, 1987b).

Because of the seriousness of childhood aggression for young people themselves and for society, the need for effective prevention and intervention efforts is great. As we turn to what is currently known about the causes of aggression in children and adolescents, the need to work closely with both family members and school personnel to address the early onset and stability of aggression in young people becomes evident.

Risk Factors Associated with Child Aggression

A review of the empirical literature indicates that various factors are related to the development and maintenance of CD and other externalizing behavior problems (Conduct Problems Prevention Research Group [CPPRG], 1992; Kazdin, 1985; Patterson, Capaldi, & Bank, 1991). The CPPRG asserts, "Although the debate continues about the relative importance of genetic and environmental factors in determining CD, the dominant perspective is that individual characteristics interact with family and environmental conditions to place some children at identifiable high risk for CD by the time they enter school" (p. 511). It is our belief that this assertion also applies to the development of other externalizing behavior disorders, and specifically to the development of aggression in young people.

Webster-Stratton's (1993, 1994) organizational framework for conceptualizing factors related to CD is useful for describing the development and maintenance of child aggression. We use her delineation of child-related, parent- and family-related, and school-related factors to summarize predictors for child aggression.

Child-Related Factors

Five child-related risk factors associated with the development and maintenance of CD in children and adolescents are identified in reviews by Webster-Stratton (1993, 1994): (1) a difficult temperament in infancy and/or as a toddler (Bates, 1990; Thomas & Chess, 1977), (2) neurological difficulties, such as frontal lobe and limbic system problems, (3) cognitive and social skills deficits, including the attribution of hostile intent to neutral stimuli (Milich & Dodge, 1984), social problem-solving skills deficits (Asarnow & Callan, 1985) and low levels of empathy for others (Feshbach, 1989), (4) academic deficits, primarily low academic achievement and reading problems/disabilities (Kazdin, 1987a; Sturge, 1982; Rutter, Tizard, Yule, Graham, & Whitmore, 1976), and (5) genetic factors/contributions, some evidence for which has been found through twin and adoption research studies (Kazdin, 1987a). As is true of any contributing factor for CD, these child factors are not thought to exist in isolation, and the evidence to support each of these factors has often been correlational in nature.

Parent- and Family-Related Factors

Extensive research has examined the relationship between parent- and family-related factors and the development of aggression, CD, and other behavior disorders. Overall, results indicate that such factors are strongly related to the development and maintenance of externalizing problems (e.g., Loeber & Dishion, 1983; Patterson, 1982). In fact, Reid and Patterson (1991) have suggested that parent and family variables—specifically, parenting factors related to the parent–child relationship—are the "most proximal determinants underlying the early development of antisocial behavior" (p. 719). Webster-Stratton (1993, 1994) has labeled parent-related factors as skill deficits, interpersonal factors and interparental factors, and has conceptualized family-related factors as those related to environmental stress.

Parenting skill deficits are well known. Arguably the best-known and widely accepted theory of parent–child interaction with aggressive children has been advanced by Patterson and his colleagues (Patterson, 1982, 1986). Patterson's work suggests that aggressive behavior in young children is developed through a coercive style of day-to-day interactions between the children and their parents. Parents whose resources may already be stretched by life stresses or by having children with irritable temperaments may find themselves struggling to set consistent limits with their children. Children eventually learn that if they escalate their level of negative behavior when they are asked to comply with a request, their parents will yield. For the parents, "giving in" leads to temporary relief from the aversive child behavior. At the next parental request, parents are determined for children to comply; however, the children boost the level of negative behavior up another notch until the parents again yield. This bidirectional and truly interactive process between parents and children is described by Reid and Patterson (1991) as follows:

> To the extent that parents are ineffective, noncontingent, and irritable in their attempts to manage aggressive and noncompliant children's behavior on a moment-by-moment basis, that behavior will become stronger over time. And as the children's aggressive patterns increase in frequency and intensity, the parents' attempts to deal with the children become even less effective, which further exacerbates the children's aggressiveness, and so on. (p. 719)

As these interactions continue and the behaviors grow stronger through mutual parent–child reinforcement, the children internalize this style of interaction and generalize it to other settings.

Additional research suggests that some parents of aggressive and conduct disordered children lack two essential parenting skills (Webster-Stratton & Herbert, 1994a)—(1) poor supervision and ineffective monitoring and (2) harsh and inconsistent punishment practices—both of which are strongly associated with CD (Eron, Huesmann, & Zelli, 1991; Kazdin, 1987a; Reid & Patterson, 1991; Rutter & Giller, 1983). In their meta-analysis of 29 studies examining the relationships of family factors to delinquency and juvenile conduct problems, Loeber and Stouthamer-Loeber (1986) found that insufficient parental supervision and parental involvement in children's lives were consistent predictors of conduct problems. Reid and Patterson (1991) assert that poor monitoring stems from parents' earlier failures in dealing with their children's aggressive or noncompliant behaviors. With repeated failures, parents become both unable and less likely to monitor their children, because they feel powerless to alter their children's behavior. Moreover, it appears that parents of antisocial children may be less able to differentiate positive and aversive child behaviors than parents whose children are not exhibiting problem behaviors (Holleran, Littman, Freund, & Schmaling, 1982).

The importance of the quality of parent–child relationships for children with CD has been underscored (e.g., Webster-Stratton & Herbert, 1994a). Children and adolescents who exhibit aggressive behaviors are often members of family systems characterized by instability, high conflict, criticism, low levels of warmth, and few positive interactions (CPPRG, 1992; Kazdin, 1987a; Haddad, Barocas, & Hollenbeck, 1991; Pettit, Bates, & Dodge, 1993; Vostanis, Nicholls, & Harrington, 1994). In related research, children with CD have been found to exhibit fewer positive and more negative verbal and nonverbal behaviors (e.g., gestures, expressions, and tones of voice) in their interactions with both their mothers and their fathers than children without CD (Webster-Stratton & Herbert, 1994a).

Interpersonal factors are the effects of parental psychopathology on the development of CD (Webster-Stratton, 1993, 1994). Research suggests that the presence of aggressive or antisocial behaviors in either parent increases the risk of childhood CD, although paternal alcoholism and criminal behavior appear to be the most strongly related (Frick et al., 1992; Kazdin, 1987a; Rutter & Giller, 1983). Moreover, studies examining the antisocial behavior of both grandparents and parents indicate that in addition to current parental antisocial behaviors, "a previous history of antisocial or aggressive behavior in one's family places children at-risk for these behaviors" (Kazdin, 1987a, p. 58). One question that has not yet been fully answered is whether parental antisocial behavior increases children's risk by means of a genetic predisposition or as the result of social learning processes between parents and children (Frick, 1994).

Beyond parental antisocial behavior, the relationship between other forms of parental psychopathology and child outcomes is not as clear. For example, although maternal depression is associated with behavior problems and childhood CD, some researchers have concluded that it is a nonspecific risk factor for a multitude of childhood problems (e.g., Frick, 1994). Others view maternal depression as relevant to the discussion of CD, because depression distorts maternal interpretations of child behavior and subsequently influences mothers' ability to be effective parents (Webster-Stratton & Herbert, 1994a).

Interparental factors are the effects of the parental relationship (or caregiver relationship) on the development of aggressive behaviors in children. Research on the effects of interparental factors focused initially on investigations of conflict and events surrounding separation and/or divorce (e.g., Rutter, Graham, & Yule, 1970, cited in Frick, 1994). What has emerged from this evolving research is the conclusion that the amount of interparental conflict in the home, not the actual act of separation or divorce, is most influential for child behavioral outcomes (Amato & Keith, 1991; Loeber & Stouthamer-Loeber, 1986; O'Leary & Emery, 1982). For example, in a meta-analysis of 92 studies of the impact of divorce on children's psychological well-being, Amato and Keith (1991) found that although children living in divorced families tended to show poorer adjustment than children living in intact families characterized by low levels of conflict, the children who showed on average the poorest adjustment of all groups were children living in two-parent families with high levels of conflict.

The exact nature of the relationship between marital conflict and the development of aggressive disorders is still being explored. In one study of both preschoolers and early adolescents, Miller, Cowan, Cowan, Hetherington, and Clingempeel (1993) examined the relationships between parental depression, marital quality, parenting style, and children's externalizing behaviors. Their results indicated that parental depression is related to higher rates of marital conflict, that positive affect in the parental relationship is associated with parental warmth in the parent–child relationship, and that parental warmth contributes to lower levels of externalizing behavior in both preschoolers and adolescents. They assert that the link between parental relationship and externalizing behaviors is indirect: When the parental relationship is positive, parents' relationships with their children are warmer, resulting in fewer acting-out behaviors by children. Other research supports this assertion. Several researchers have found that the stresses associated with marital conflict interfere with parents' abilities to interact positively with their children and to discipline them effectively (Frick, 1994; Loeber & Stouthamer-Loeber, 1986; Patterson, 1986).

Environmental stress, the family-related component of Webster-Stratton's (1993) organizational framework, consists of extrafamilial factors that contribute to the development and maintenance of aggression: unemployment, illness, and poverty (including issues related to low socioeconomic status (SES), such as crowded living conditions and unsafe neighborhoods). Although these more distal factors do not necessarily lend themselves directly to intervention, they contribute to our understanding of the lives of aggressive children and adolescents.

In her studies of families with children or adolescents with CD, Webster-Stratton (1990b) reported that these families experienced two to three times more major life stresses, as well as more day-to-day life hassles, than families whose children were not conduct disordered. The mechanism through which child behavior is affected by environmental stresses appears to be similar to that of marital conflict. It is hypothesized that environmental stresses contribute indirectly to child conduct problems through the interruption of parenting practices (McLoyd, 1990; Patterson, 1983; Reid & Patterson, 1991; Webster-Stratton, 1990b). Environmental stresses influence parents' views of their children, their behaviors, and the ways they respond to them. Mothers who have experienced high levels of negative life stress perceive their children's behavior to be more deviant than mothers reporting low stress perceive their offspring's behavior to be (Middlebrook & Forehand, 1985; Webster-Stratton, 1990b). Other studies found that high rates of stressful life events are related to more punitive and controlling parenting behaviors, attachment problems, and more aversive maternal interactions (McLoyd, 1990; Patterson, 1982; Vaughn, Egeland, Sroufe, & Waters, 1979). The extent to which parents are affected by these extrafamilial stresses appears to be mediated by several factors, including their own psychological well-being, the amount of family and social support, the parents' gender, and their level of substance use (Webster-Stratton, 1990b).

School-Related Factors

Research has focused on interactions with peers, teacher–child interactions, home–school connections, and characteristics of the school; all have been shown to be associated with the development and maintenance of child aggression.

Reid and Patterson (1991) suggest three reasons why children who are aggressive and coercive at home are at significant risk for exhibiting similar problems at school. First, given that they have developed strong behavior patterns at home, children are "primed" to demonstrate these same patterns when confrontations or problems with teachers or peers arise. Second, for school-age children whose home lives continue to be characterized by coercive interaction patterns, any attempts by the school to socialize the children are likely to compete with continued reinforcement of aggression in the home. Third, the authors assert that a child's aggressive behavior will induce interactions with teachers and peers that are much like the interactions that take place at home. In other words, "the coercive process will likely be recreated with each person who must deal with the child on a daily basis" (p. 734). Their explanations underscore the importance of working with families to reduce aggression in school settings.

The implications of coercive interactions with teachers and peers are significant. Aggressive children are quickly rejected by nonaggressive peers, and it is likely that this rejection may be fairly permanent (Ladd, 1990). Rejection has been shown to influence the way aggressive or disruptive children interact with peers on an ongoing basis. Over time, peers become more and more mistrustful of aggressive children and react to them in ways that actually increase the likelihood of reactive aggression (Dodge & Coie, 1987; Dodge & Somberg, 1987). These rejecting interactions are often made worse by the fact that aggressive children tend to attribute hostile intent incorrectly to even neutral personal interactions (Dodge & Frame, 1982; Dodge, Murphy, & Buchsbaum, 1984; Lochman, 1987). The same types of relationships have been shown to develop between teachers and aggressive students, with one result being that aggressive students receive less nurturance and support than students who behave appropriately (Campbell & Ewing, 1990).

Given the previous discussion, it is not surprising to find that the connections between home and school for young people who are aggressive are often strained, fraught with tension, and uncomfortable for both parents and teachers. Reports of negative encounters with teachers are commonplace among parents of children with externalizing behavior problems. These encounters contribute to "parents' feelings of incompetence, their sense of helplessness regarding strategies to address school problems, and their alienation from school" (Webster-Stratton & Herbert, 1994b, p. 23). The authors describe these phenomena as "a spiraling pattern of child negative behavior, parent demoralization and withdrawal, and teacher reactivity, which can ultimately lead to a lack of coordination and support between the socialization activities of school and home" (p. 23). With respect to school factors, it appears that "once they enter school—be it preschool or grade school—negative school experiences and social experiences further exacerbate the adjustment difficulties of children with conduct problems" (Webster-Stratton & Herbert, 1994b, p. 21).

Summary

In this section, we have reviewed relevant background information on aggressive children and adolescents and their families. In particular, we have described a multicausal model of the development and maintenance of aggressive behavior in children that includes child-related, parent- and family-related, and school-related factors. Although the notion of multiple risk factors influencing children may seem overwhelming in the face of trying to assist aggressive students in school each day, we believe that change and successful prevention and intervention efforts are possible. Reid and Patterson (1991) have suggested that the key to finding effective strategies is to focus on those variables that are malleable to prevention and intervention efforts. In other words, it is important to focus on those variables that are within the power of school personnel and others to help change (e.g., monitoring and supervision practices, interaction styles between caregiver and child, discipline practices, positive reinforcement of appropriate behaviors, behavior referrals in school, and failing grades). This stands in contrast to focusing only on more distal or static variables, such as SES, parental marital status, or education level. These factors, although associated with CD and other aggressive disorders, are generally not within the power of school personnel to influence or change. Other critical strategies are to intervene early, over time, and across contexts (namely, family and school) in order to address generalization and intervention. As Webster-Stratton (1993) states, "by the time the child manifests conduct disorders, it is likely that these child, family, and school factors are inextricably interconnected" (p. 443). In the following section, we review the literature on prevention and intervention programs.

SCHOOL-BASED FAMILY INTERVENTIONS

The need for early intervention is clear. If left untreated, aggressive children are at increased risk for peer rejection (Coie, 1990), abuse (Reid, Taplin, & Loeber, 1981), and the development of problems in later life, such as school dropout, alcoholism and other substance abuse, criminal activity, antisocial personality, marital disruption, interpersonal problems, and poor physical health (Kazdin, 1985; Loeber & Dishion, 1983). In addition, aggressive and antisocial children cost society a great deal because of their heavy use of mental health services and criminal justice systems (Webster-Stratton & Herbert, 1994b).

The value of family-focused intervention is supported by "strong links between family antecedent factors and prevalence of childhood conduct problems" (Miller, 1994, p. 85). Kazdin (1987b) outlined three major classes of treatment for antisocial behavior—child-focused, family-focused, and community-based—and delineated the following types of treatment within classes: individual and group psychotherapy, behavior therapy, problem-solving skills training, residential treatment, pharmacotherapy, parent management training, family therapy, and communitywide interventions. Although the majority of approaches Kazdin reviewed focus on the individual child, he considered family-focused interventions based on social learning principles the most promising.

In this section, we describe examples of parent- and family-focused interventions that have demonstrated success in reducing childhood aggression: parent management training, expanded parent management training, family therapy, and multisystemic approaches. The criteria used to select the interventions described herein include clarity of program definition, delineation of intervention components, and availability of positive outcome data. The description of each intervention is followed by efficacy data, factors affecting treatment outcomes (when these are known), and the merits and limitations of implementing the intervention in school settings.

Parent Management Training

Parent management training (PMT), the most commonly used family intervention in schools, teaches parents to alter the contingencies and communication processes occurring within the family (Miller, 1994; Miller & Prinz, 1990). The underlying assumption for PMT is that aggression and antisocial behavior are acquired and maintained through social learning processes in the family. Research indicates that parents of aggressive children have deficits in parenting skills (Webster-Stratton & Herbert, 1994b) and have inadvertently developed maladaptive parent–child interactions (Kazdin, 1987b). Parents of antisocial children engage in practices that promote aggressive behavior and suppress prosocial behavior, such as use of punitive discipline or permissiveness, low levels of monitoring, reinforcement of aggressive behaviors, and punishment of prosocial behaviors (Patterson, 1982). PMT targets changes in the family social environment and places parents in the role of therapeutic change agents. Parents learn to modify the antecedents and consequences that elicit and maintain child aggression and to improve family communication and problem solving. PMT alters parent–child interaction patterns so that prosocial behavior, rather than coercive behavior, is reinforced.

Program Description

Miller (1994) has identified six critical areas of parental competence emphasized in structured PMT programs: (1) tracking, labeling, and pinpointing problematic behavior, (2) emphasizing positive behavior, (3) using appropriate commands, (4) using effective discipline, (5) communicating clearly, and (6) troubleshooting and generalization to other settings. Most programs teach child behavior management skills to families by means of such techniques as role play, discussion, modeling, *in vivo* practice, homework assignments, and guided feedback. The content and pace of the training are matched to each family's competence and needs.

The contents of three frequently cited PMT programs are described. The first parent training program was developed by Patterson, Reid, and their colleagues at the Oregon Social Learning Center (Patterson, 1982; Patterson, Reid, Jones, & Conger, 1975). In this program for parents of children ages 3–12 with overt CD, parents read a programmed text, which provides a conceptual background for the content of therapy, and are tested on the material. Parents are taught a step-by-step approach for implementing five family management practices: (1) identifying and tracking problem behavior at home, (2) social and tangible reinforcement techniques, (3) nonpunitive discipline procedures, (4) monitoring children's time, and (5) problem-solving and negotiation strategies. The program requires 20 hours of one-to-one therapy and includes home visits and homework assignments to foster generalization. This program has been modified for use with families of delinquent adolescents; the adolescent program requires 45 hours of therapy and greater participation by the adolescent.

A second program, developed by Forehand and McMahon (1981), provides training to parents of children ages 3–8 who are noncompliant. In the first phase of training, parents are taught to play with their children in a nondirective way and to use positive reinforcement of prosocial behaviors via praise and attention. In the second phase, parents are taught to use effective commands and time-out procedures for noncompliance. Progression to each new skill is dependent on a parent's successful acquisition of the preceding skill. Parents and children work individually with a therapist, and methods of treatment include role playing, modeling, and coaching. The use of one-way mirrors and "bug-in-the-ear" instruments allows a therapist to observe and coach a parent without being physically present. In addition, homework is assigned daily to provide parents with opportunities to practice skills at home with their children.

The third PMT program, BASIC, designed by Webster-Stratton (1984), is for parents of children ages 3–8 with CD. BASIC teaches parents problem-solving and communication strategies, and it incorporates components from the Patterson program (discipline and monitoring) and the Forehand and McMahon program (child-directed play, differential attention, and effective commands). Relying on principles derived from social learning theory, the program utilizes modeling via videotape demonstrations, in which models display "right" and "wrong" behaviors with children. The videotape modeling is viewed by a group of parents and followed by a group discussion with a therapist. BASIC parent training requires 26 hours. Children are not involved in the training, but parents are given weekly assignments to practice the skills with their children at home.

Efficacy Data

Extensive evaluations of PMT have revealed positive results. There is substantial evidence of a reduction in children's aggressive behaviors, often to the normative levels exhibited by their peers (McMahon & Forehand, 1984; Patterson, 1974; Webster-Stratton, 1984); there is also evidence of long-term child behavior change, lasting from 1 to 4 years after PMT (Baum & Forehand, 1981; Patterson & Fleischman, 1979; Webster-Stratton, 1990a). PMT's effectiveness, which is documented both by parent and teacher reports and by direct observation of children in home and school settings, exceeds the effectiveness of family-based psychotherapy and discussion (Patterson, Chamberlain, & Reid, 1982). In addition, PMT has been found to alter untreated behaviors, such as destructiveness (Arnold, Levine, & Patterson, 1975; Forehand & Long, 1986; Webster-Stratton, 1982), sibling behavior, and maternal psychopathology (Patterson & Fleischman, 1985).

Although the aforementioned studies identified treatment generalization across settings, other studies do not support generalization. For example, Forehand et al. (1979) did not find that program effects generalized to the school setting. Furthermore, some families, especially multistressed families, do not experience favorable outcomes (Miller & Prinz, 1990). Families with extremely conduct-disordered children show little improvement (McMahon & Forehand, 1984), primarily because of coercion into treatment by public agencies, as well as other family problems that exacerbate child aggression (Miller & Prinz, 1990).

Factors Affecting Treatment Outcomes

Treatment and family factors serve to maximize or mitigate the effects of PMT. Treatment factors include duration of treatment, training components, and characteristics of the therapist (Kazdin, 1987b; Webster-Stratton & Herbert, 1994a). Time-limited treatments, especially those lasting less than 10 hours, are less likely to produce positive results than time-unlimited programs, which can last from 50 to 60 hours (Kazdin, 1987b). Specific training components also affect treatment outcome. For example, the teaching of social learning principles and time-out procedures for reinforcement improves treatment effects (McMahon, Forehand, & Greist, 1981). Furthermore, therapist training and skill correlate with longer-lasting and more intense family changes (Patterson, 1974). Patterson and Forgatch (1985) found that supportive therapists decreased noncompliance with treatment procedures, whereas directive and confronting therapists increased parental resistance and uncooperativeness.

Family factors that predict treatment outcomes include structural characteristics and personal and marital problems. Unemployment, poverty, low levels of education, and single parenting are structural factors associated with poorer treatment outcomes (Wahler & Afton, 1980). Marital distress, spousal abuse, parental depression, poor problem-solving skills, and high life stress are associated with fewer treatment gains (Kazdin, 1987b; Webster-Stratton, 1993). Similarly, Dumas and Wahler (1983) reported that mothers insulated from supports outside the home are less likely to benefit from treatment. Moreover, negative life stress, such as a family's move or a death following PMT, affects the family's ability to maintain treatment effects (Webster-Stratton, 1985). Families with these characteristics are more likely to drop out or fail to maintain treatment effects (McMahon, Forehand, Greist, & Wells, 1981; Reid & Patterson, 1976).

Merits and Limitations

There is evidence to support PMT's effectiveness in reducing children's aggressive behavior. PMT has also been successful in altering disruptive behaviors not directly targeted by the intervention and in improving sibling behavior and parental psychopathology. The use of PMT in school settings is appealing because of its structured and prescriptive approach. Programs are "prepackaged" and require less planning and training than other interventions. In addition, PMT programs are short-term and efficient (most utilize a group format as opposed to an individual one), thus making them ideal for use in school settings.

Unfortunately, the effectiveness of PMT is limited by family and treatment factors. Research indicates that simply ameliorating a deficit in parenting skills is insufficient to reduce children's aggressive behavior, especially when parents confront such problems as isolation, lack of support, and high levels of stress and depression (Webster-Stratton & Herbert, 1994b). It is not uncommon for PMT therapists to experience high levels of resistance when working with families of antisocial children (Miller & Prinz, 1990). Furthermore, Webster-Stratton and Herbert (1994b) note that, ironically, the most promising and commonly used approach to treating childhood aggression is a practice that places blame on the parents for a deficit in parenting skills. Despite these limitations, the potential strengths of PMT have led program developers to modify their programs. These modified programs are referred to as "expanded PMT."

Expanded Parent Management Training

The limitations associated with PMT have led to a broader conceptualization of parent-focused services. Expanded PMT seeks to alter the external and internal conditions that interfere with parents' ability to interact effectively with their children (Miller & Prinz, 1990). The underlying assumption in expanded PMT is that stress reduction in the family environment will increase parental use of PMT strategies. Expanded programs have incorporated therapy for stress and marital discordance, as well as training to address multiple effects of insularity and other socioeconomic disadvantages (McMahon, Forehand, & Griest, 1981; Webster-Stratton, 1985).

Program Descriptions

Several varieties of expanded PMT have been developed. First are the expansions of the three PMT programs described earlier. Patterson and colleagues have adapted their PMT program so that 30% of therapy time focuses on parental adjustment problems such as marital discordance and depression (Patterson & Chamberlain, 1988). Forehand and colleagues have expanded the Forehand and McMahon program to include training of mothers and children in self-control procedures (McMahon et al., 1981; Wells, Forehand, & Greist, 1980). Webster-Stratton has expanded the BASIC program, referred to as ADVANCE, to focus on personal parent issues such as anger management, ways to give and get support, and problem solving between adults (Webster-Stratton & Herbert, 1994b).

The second group of expanded PMT programs consists of programs that focus on parental adjustment factors. An example is an intervention by Greist and colleagues (Greist et al., 1982; Greist & Wells, 1983) that addressed parental perceptions of child behavior, personal and marital adjustment, and extrafamilial relationships in addition to PMT. Another example is described by Dadds, Schwartz, and Sanders (1987), who provided discordant couples with partner support training in conjunction with PMT.

A third group of expanded PMT programs consists of programs that provide synthesis and self-sufficiency training. As a supplement to PMT, these models emphasize enhancing parental awareness and sensibility to broad-based events that interfere with successful parenting. Synthesis training, a molar approach, trains parents to identify personal, general reactions to stressful events (Wahler & Dumas, 1984). Wahler and Dumas used synthesis training to increase the parental monitoring and supervision of parents who were socioeconomically disadvantaged and had few social resources and supports. Parents were taught to understand their ecosystem and the contextual influences that contributed to coercive interactions with their children. The training format was a discussion of parents' coercive interactions, facilitated by a therapist whose role was to reflect upon the parents' global descriptions of events. As training progressed, the therapist systematically taught the parents more detailed recognition of contextual influences and encouraged comparisons between the parents' interpretations of extrafamilial events and specific interactions with their children.

Similar to synthesis training, self-sufficiency training, developed by Blechman (1984, 1987), has a more molecular focus in working with families. Parents of children with CD are taught a structured problem-solving strategy to identify practical solutions to specific stressful events. Extrafamilial problems that contribute to poor parenting are broken down into smaller units, to allow parents to develop a plan of action for resolution more readily. Intensive discussions of the antecedents and consequences of problems characterize self-sufficiency training.

Efficacy Data

The use of expanded PMT has been shown to improve treatment maintenance over that of basic PMT (Webster-Stratton & Herbert, 1994b). Greist et al. (1982) reported that noncompliant children showed greater changes in decreased deviant behavior and increased compliance after a 2-month follow-up when parents were involved in expanded PMT, as opposed to basic PMT. Similarly, Dadds et al. (1987) reported greater long-term maintenance of positive parenting and child behavior changes at a 6-month follow-up for maritally discordant couples who received PMT plus marital communication training, as compared with parents who received PMT only. With regard to the third group of expanded PMT programs, Wahler and Dumas (1984) reported greater improvements for insular and noninsular mothers in tracking of child behavior when PMT was combined with synthesis training. Blechman (1984) reported that treatment gains were maintained at a 6-month follow-up for a highly stressed mother with several problem children who received self-sufficiency training adjunctive to PMT. The effects of the ADVANCE program are currently being studied (Webster-Stratton & Herbert, 1994b). We found no discussion of factors contributing to treatment outcomes.

Merits and Limitations

Expanded PMT interventions have demonstrated improved success over basic PMT programs. Specifically, children have shown more significant improvements and longer-term maintenance of treatment effects when parents were involved in expanded PMT than when parents were involved in PMT only. However, because of methodological problems (e.g., no long-term follow-up data, nonspecific measures), Miller and Prinz (1990) concluded that it remains unclear whether long-term effectiveness in improving childhood aggression is really achieved with this family intervention. In addition, Wahler and Dumas (1984) suggested that expanded PMT programs focusing exclusively on reduced parental distress may be inadequate to promote significant change in child behavior for families facing multiple problems.

Expanded PMT programs are less suitable for some school settings because they require more time and highly skilled professionals to work with families. Fortunately, many schools employ school psychologists capable of initiating integrated service delivery models (Hooper-Briar & Lawson, 1994; Paavola, 1994).

We now turn to another common intervention used with families of aggressive children: family therapy, in which the focus of intervention shifts from the parents to the family as a whole. Although generally not used in schools, family therapy techniques inform us about successful methods for families with aggressive children.

Family Therapy

The short-term and ungeneralizable results of PMT concerned researchers, who have concluded that the problem lies in its narrow focus on remedying parenting skill deficits (Webster-Stratton & Herbert, 1994b). Like expanded PMT, family therapy considers other factors, such as marital discord and parental cognitions, that affect family functioning. Rather than focusing solely on child-only or parent-only factors, family therapy focuses on the interrelationships among family members in relation to the target child's aggressive behavior (Gordon & Arbuthnot, 1987). Family systems theorists view a child or adolescent's acting-out behavior as a contributor to family tension and marital conflict. Much of the work of family therapists involves helping family members overcome their resistance to change. Types of family therapy include "analytic," "strategic," "structural," and "functional" (also referred to as "behavioral systems"). Of these, we discuss structural and functional family therapy approaches, which have been used with some success to intervene with families of aggressive and/or delinquent children (Kazdin, 1987b; Webster-Stratton & Herbert, 1994b).

Program Description

Minuchin (1981, cited in Horne, 1993) is credited with the development and use of structural family therapy (SFT) in his work with delinquent adolescents. The goal of SFT is a restructuring of family patterns, which are defined by boundaries of the entire family and family subsystems (e.g., husband–wife, parent–child). In dysfunctional families, family patterns are often characterized by either enmeshment (overinvolvement of family members) or disengagement (underinvolvement of family members). Overinvolved families prevent children from achieving autonomy, whereas underinvolved families prevent them from receiving adequate support. For example, when enmeshed parents do not teach their children to obey rules and respect authority, this leaves the children ill prepared to negotiate successful entrance into school. The children may be used to getting their own way and become disruptive and aggressive.

For the therapist, SFT includes three overlapping phases: (1) joining the family as an accepted member, to help overcome the family's resistance to change, (2) mapping the underlying structure, and (3) intervening to transform the structure. Restructuring involves directive maneuvers, enactments, and reframing to disrupt dysfunctional structure by strengthening diffuse boundaries and softening rigid ones. The therapist asks the family members to demonstrate or enact how they solve a problem, to allow the therapist to observe dysfunctional patterns. Reframing is then used to shift the focus from the target child's problem to a family problem. The structural therapist's overall aim is to help the family modify its functioning so that family members learn to solve their problems.

Developed by Alexander and colleagues specifically for treating juvenile delinquents (Alexander & Parsons, 1973), functional family therapy (FFT) is based on systems theory and behaviorism and also includes a focus on cognitive processes (Alexander & Parsons, 1982; Kazdin, 1987b). Problems are conceptualized according to the functions they serve for the family system and for individual family members. FFT was based on research indicating that families of delinquent children show higher levels of defensiveness and lower levels of mutual support than do families of nondelinquent children (Alexander, 1973).

The main goal of FFT is to change family interactions and communication patterns to promote adaptive functioning (Kazdin, 1987b). As in Patterson's PMT program, families are asked to read a manual describing social learning principles and are taught behavioral management strategies, including behavioral contracting and contingency management. Therapists using FFT help family members increase reciprocity and positive reinforcement, establish clear communication, identify desirable behaviors, develop constructive negotiations, and identify solutions to interpersonal problems. Family members are taught to relabel problems to reduce blaming. Direct alteration of family communication patterns occurs in the treatment sessions, as the therapist provides immediate social reinforcement for solution-oriented statements. Family members are asked to identify desired behaviors for one another and to use a home reinforcement system to promote the desired behaviors. Families typically receive a total of eight 90-minute sessions over a 4-week period.

Efficacy Data

Very few studies have evaluated SFT's impact on reducing children's disruptive behavior; most evaluations of SFT have focused on evaluating structural changes in families. Readers are encouraged to see Horne (1993) for a more comprehensive review.

The few studies that have evaluated the effectiveness of FFT have obtained positive results. For example, Alexander and Parsons (1973) reported that positive family interactions and lower recidivism rates from involvement with juvenile court were maintained up to 18 months after treatment. Delinquents and members of their families who received FFT increased family discussions, equalized speaking among themselves, and produced more spontaneous speech than did those in attention placebo and no-treatment conditions. Family changes were also shown to be greater than those of families in a control group, in client-centered counseling, or in psychodynamic therapy. In another study, Klein, Alexander, and Parsons (1977) demonstrated that the delinquents' siblings showed significantly lower rates of referral to juvenile courts more than 2 years later. Fifteen months after treatment, delinquent adolescents exposed to FFT were less likely to be charged with an offense than were adolescents who received standard mental health services or who were placed in group homes (Barton, Alexander, Waldron, Turner, & Warburton, 1985).

Gordon and colleagues (Gordon & Arbuthnot, 1987) used FFT with delinquent adolescents in the home setting (instead of a clinic) and compared recidivism rates for these adolescents with those for delinquents receiving probation only. More than 2 years later, recidivism rates for the adolescents receiving probation only exceeded those of the FFT treatment group by more than 50%. Adolescents in the FFT treatment group also showed a decrease in the severity of their offenses.

Factors Affecting Treatment Outcomes

As in PMT, the efficacy of family therapy is mediated by the therapist's skill in developing relationships (Alexander, Barton, Schiavo, & Parsons, 1976). Warmth and directiveness were associated with improved outcomes and longer participation in therapy. In a replicated study by Gordon and colleagues (Gordon & Arbuthnot, 1987), time-unlimited treatment (an average of 16 sessions) resulted in greater improvement in recidivism rates.

Merits and Limitations

The few studies that have evaluated the effectiveness of family therapy have indicated some positive results. An emphasis on the entire family's functioning and a shift to altering family interactions have improved family communication patterns and decreased the juvenile offenses and recidivism of target children and siblings. However, the minimal number of studies make it difficult to conclude confidently that family therapy is effective in treating aggressive children. When compared to PMT or expanded PMT, family systems therapy and eclectic family therapy have been shown to be less effective

(Webster-Stratton & Herbert, 1994b; Wells & Egan, 1988). Furthermore, reliance on additional training and supervision of the therapist is an obstacle to use in the school setting.

Multisystemic Model

The limitations of both parent training and family therapy in addressing multiple factors that contribute to childhood aggression have led to a broader conceptualization of family-focused treatment, represented by the multisystemic model (Miller & Prinz, 1990). Although the aim of this chapter is to discuss interventions with families, we would be remiss if we ignored other treatment settings. For example, the school setting is an important target for intervention, as aggression generalizes from home to school, negatively affecting both teacher and peer relationships (Patterson et al., 1991; Webster-Stratton, 1993). In addition, many parents of children with conduct disorders experience negative interactions with teachers concerning their children's behavior problems (Webster-Stratton, 1993). This only exacerbates the parents' feelings of incompetence and helplessness, as well as alienation from the school (Hawkins & Weis, 1985). As previously noted, by the time a child manifests CD, it is likely that "child, family, and school factors are inextricably connected" (Webster-Stratton, 1993, p. 443). This lends support for an intervention model that targets the skills of both parents and children, in addition to building positive relationships between families and the schools. Although school professionals have not always worked directly with families to improve students' behavior, they are in a unique position to provide or facilitate family-based services (Miller, 1994).

The multisystemic model views childhood aggression within the broader social context (Miller & Prinz, 1990); family, school, and peer contexts are considered. Webster-Stratton and Herbert (1994b) hypothesize that child treatment plus family treatment will improve generalization and long-term outcomes for children with CD. Research indicates that PMT plus child problem-solving training is more effective in treating antisocial adolescent males than is PMT alone (Kazdin, 1987b). This finding has led to the development of more ecological approaches to treating childhood aggression.

A "multisystemic" model is one in which separate treatment components are combined to form an overall treatment program. Kazdin (1987b) has cautioned that the components included in such a program must be selected carefully. The purpose of multiple treatments is to address the different predictors or risk factors for antisocial behavior. Treatments should not serve as a collection of techniques implemented in a diluted fashion. Therefore, the approach should be "guided by initial evidence that the constituent techniques produce some change and that the domain of the focus is relevant to the problem" (Kazdin, 1987b, p. 199).

Program Descriptions

Multisystemic approaches take varying forms and have different names. We discuss three such approaches: ecological, collaborative, and prevention/promotion.

According to Miller and Prinz (1990), the ecological intervention approach to childhood aggression views child maladjustment as a problem that extends across multiple ecosystems and views the child's aggression as embedded within multiple, interconnected systems and subsystems. It stresses the importance of interactions between the individual and the environment and views intervention as maintaining a balance between them (Apter & Propper, 1986). Ecological treatments emphasize improving the person– environment fit; changing negative processes and relevant contingencies within home, school, and community settings; and maintaining a balance among the child's multiple ecosystems.

Miller (1994) has outlined seven principles that characterize most ecological programs. These principles reflect attempts to address limitations of the parent training and family therapy approaches. The first principle, adopting a multisystemic orientation, involves using an array of approaches to link family, peer, school, and community environments to ameliorate the stressors contributing to a child's maladaptive behaviors. The second principle, attending to consumers' expectations and social cognitions, addresses personal belief systems and expectations. Because much noncompliance with treatment and poor maintenance of behavioral outcomes is attributed to a mismatch of expectations, efforts are made to openly discuss family or school concerns regarding intervention (e.g., "What are your thoughts about seeking help?" "Tell me how you think this plan might work"). The third ecological principle, building on family strengths and adaptive coping, emphasizes strengthening families' internal (e.g., decision-making skills) and external (e.g., social support networks) support systems. The fourth principle, considering family circumstances, suggests responsiveness to family values, needs, and routines. The fifth principle, fostering a collaborative environment, involves a partnership approach in which trust, mutual respect, and positive communication pervade the family–school relationship. The sixth ecological principle, designing culturally sensitive interventions, suggests that intervention goals and the behavioral targets of change must be jointly decided to ensure that the cultural perspectives of all individuals are considered. The final principle, initiating interagency coordination and follow-up services, involves linking families to community agencies to meet basic needs. Family progress is monitored through routine contact.

An example of an ecological program is family-ecological treatment (FET) for juvenile offenders (Henggeler et al., 1986). Based on family systems, behavioral, and ecological theories, FET attempts to alter interactions within and among those systems that maintain, or are maintained by, child deviance. Instead of focusing on the linear cause–effect relationship between parent and child, FET emphasizes circular causality—that is, the impact of the interaction of multiple systems on child behavior. This multidimensional focus is reflected in FET's four domains: individual adjustment (social, cognitive, and interpersonal functioning), family interactions (e.g., child-rearing strategies, marital issues), extrafamilial systems (e.g., peers, school, parents' workplaces), and cultural/community systems. Family strengths are used to elicit change in family problems. The length of FET varies (the average is 60 hours over a 4-month period), depending on family needs (Family Services Research Center, 1995). It is conducted in both home and community settings (e.g., schools, recreation centers).

A few examples of the collaborative approach for addressing the needs of aggressive young people are emerging in the literature. Short and Shapiro (1993) have recommended that school personnel expand traditional service delivery boundaries (within the school) by providing PMT and other family interventions in coordination with community agencies. This approach includes collaborative problem solving between parents and school personnel, as well as joint decision making about school activities (Short & Shapiro, 1993). Similarly, Hawkins and Fraser (1983) have suggested that interventions must focus on replacing negative social networks with positive social networks to prevent delinquency. Families, schools, and communities are encouraged to develop partnerships for supporting at-risk adolescents. Social support to families, development of supportive relationships for identified adolescents, and strengthening of home–school linkages are the strategies that make up this social-support-centered approach (Hawkins & Fraser, 1983).

In their book, *Troubled Families–Problem Children*, Webster-Stratton and Herbert (1994b) describe a collaborative model in which school professionals intervene concurrently with parents and teachers. Based on a combination of problem-oriented and humanistic therapy models, their collaborative model emphasizes a reciprocal relationship, in which parents and professionals share their knowledge and perspectives in designing an intervention. It is not a hierarchical relationship, in which a parent is seen as having deficits requiring intervention by an expert, a therapist (Webster-Stratton & Herbert, 1993). The collaborative relationship is characterized by trust, an absence of blaming, and open communication. As a collaborator, the role of the professional is to listen to the parent, clarify issues, and teach and suggest alternatives. This model is intended to promote self-efficacy for parents, especially at a time when they may be most vulnerable. Specifically, parents are assisted in gaining knowledge and competence to cope effectively with the stress of having a child with conduct disorder. Although the roles and strategies used by the therapist are listed in Table 14.1, we encourage readers to consult Webster-Stratton and Herbert (1994b) for more detailed information on the specifics of the therapeutic process.

Finally, a third multisystemic approach is characterized by a focus on health promotion. Health promotion efforts promote psychological wellness

TABLE 14.1. Roles and Strategies of the Therapist

Therapist's role	Strategies
Building a supportive relationship	Use of self-disclosure Use of humor Optimism Advocating for parents
Empowering parents	Reinforcing and validating parents' insights Modifying powerless thoughts Promoting self-empowerment Building family/group support systems
Teaching	Persuading, explaining, suggesting, and adapting Giving assignments Reviewing and summarizing Ensuring generalization Using videotape modeling examples Role play and rehearsal Evaluating
Interpreting	Use of analogies and metaphors Reframing
Leading and challenging	Setting limits Pacing the group Dealing with resistance
Prophesying	Anticipating problems and setbacks Predicting parent resistance to change Predicting positive change/success

and enhance areas of personal competence, which act as protective factors by buffering the risks associated with psychopathology. Two school-based health promotion programs are described.

First, a competence enhancement program for children with ADHD is relevant, because some children with ADHD develop problems of aggression (Braswell & Bloomquist, 1991). Derived from ecological, developmental, and cognitive-behavioral theories, this competence enhancement program consists of multiple training components for children, as well as for parents, teachers, and peers who serve as resources for children. Training provides parents with information about ADHD and about appropriate parental expectations; recognition of dysfunctional cognitions and beliefs; and specific behavior management, problem-solving, communication, and anger management skills. The intervention seeks to modify a child's cognitive processes and social interactions, as well as the interactional patterns within the child's home, school, and community. This occurs in six stages: (1) assessment, (2) preparation for change, (3) cognitive-behavioral skills training, (4) school consultation, (5) termination, and (6) follow-up. Intervention occurs over 9 weeks, with 18 child group training sessions, 9 parent group meetings, and 9 teacher group meetings. The entire school is involved in the intervention, because every teacher participates in the training. Training includes the use of didactic instruction, videotaped role-play examples, and homework assignments. The therapist forms a collaborative relationship with each family and emphasizes joint decision making. Teachers are trained to prompt and reinforce all children's problem-solving and self-instructional strategies. The therapist monitors children's and families' progress and provides booster sessions by phone or in person to maintain generalization.

Another example is the FAST (Families and Schools Together) Track program (CPPRG, 1992), which aims to prevent the development of CD by promoting competence in children, families, and educators. Based on a developmental and clinical model of CD, the intervention program targets multiple domains: children's adaptive personal relationships with peers, family members, and teachers, as well as their academic achievement. It is also responsive to developmental, cultural, and individual differences in socialization processes. FAST Track integrates five components: parent training, home visiting/case management, social skills training, academic tutoring, and teacher-based classroom intervention. Our discussion focuses on the first two components of the program.

FAST Track targets the entire school population, as well as high-risk kindergartners identified via a multistage process. It is a time-unlimited intervention that begins in first grade and extends through sixth grade. Intervention occurs in two intensive periods: at school entry (first and second grades) and at transition to middle school (fifth and sixth grades). The first period of intervention includes a parent group, parent–child sharing time, and home visiting (McMahon, Slough, & CPPRG, 1996). The parent group occurs weekly (during first grade) or biweekly (during second grade) in a group of five to seven parents. A family coordinator and coleader conduct the parent group in 60- to 90-minute sessions. The goals of the parent group are to create positive family–school relationships, to increase parental self-control, to establish developmentally appropriate parental expectations for children's behavior, and to develop parenting skills in order to enhance positive parent–child interactions and reduce children's acting-out behaviors. Training methods include didactic techniques, group discussion, skill demonstration, and role play. During the parent group, children meet in a friendship group. Following both groups, the parents and children join for parent– child sharing time for 30 minutes, the purpose of which is to promote positive parent–child relations through cooperative activities. This time provides opportunities for parents to practice newly acquired skills with immediate support from the FAST Track staff. The home visiting component, which occurs biweekly and is supplemented with weekly phone contact, aims to develop trust and promote generalization, parental support, and problem solving.

Efficacy Data

Evaluations of the ecological approach for reducing childhood aggression reveal some positive results. Henggeler et al. (1986) reported a greater decline in conduct problems, anxious/withdrawn behaviors, and associations with delinquent peers for antisocial adolescents whose families participated in FET than for adolescents whose families who received a variety of other mental health services (recreational activities and traditional psychotherapy). FET families also exhibited warmer family interactions with increased adolescent involvement. Moreover, Brunk, Henggeler, and Whelan (1987) reported greater improvements in family interactions (parental control of child behavior, parental responsiveness to child behavior, and children's compliance with parental commands) for FET families than for families receiving PMT.

Program evaluations for the two competence enhancement programs are in process. Braswell and Bloomquist (1991) emphasize that their program is based on empirically validated approaches of PMT, FFT, and cognitive-behavioral therapy. The FAST Track program is a long-term, multisite research project that is still in progress; thus, efficacy data are not yet available. Preliminary evidence indicates success in recruitment and participation of families during first grade. At the end of the first year, the CPPRG found a high level of family participation (94%) and satisfaction (93%) (cited in McMahon et al., 1996). We found no discussion of factors affecting treatment outcomes for multisystemic models.

Merits and Limitations

An advantage of the ecological model is that it addresses influences from the multiple contexts in which children develop. Although the impact of intervening across systems is difficult to measure, and such an intervention requires considerable planning and the ongoing involvement of many people, the collaborative model helps to reduce parents' feelings of helplessness because it encourages joint ownership of solutions and outcomes (Webster-Stratton & Herbert, 1994a). It also offers an opportunity to improve the home–school relationship, but it is more dependent on professionals' having a variety of clinical skills than are other models of family intervention. Health promotion programs offer promise for reducing violence by targeting interventions early. Such programs undoubtedly require intervention across grades K–12. Finally, the multisystemic models were specifically designed for use in school settings; however, each is time-

TABLE 14.2. Differences among Family Interventions for Treating Childhood Aggression

	PMT	Expanded PMT	Family therapy	Multisystemic approaches
Assumptions	Parenting skill deficits exist	High level of stress affects effective parenting	Dysfunctional relationships within family exist	Negative interactions among broad social contexts take place
Target of intervention	Parent	Parent and extrafamilial factors	Family	Child, family, school, peers, and community
Intervention modality	Individual or group	Individual or group	Family	Individual, family, and group
Procedure	Didactic Role play Modeling Homework	Discussion Training Role play Homework	Discussion Training Relabeling/reframing	Ecological Collaborative Early intervention Promotional
Intervention content	Behavior management skills	Anger control Problem solving Marital adjustment	Communication Behavioral management	Child training Parent training Peer training Teacher training
Treatment outcome	Reduced problem behavior Poor generalization	Reduced problem behavior Longer-term maintenance of treatment effects	Reduced offenses and recidivism Improved family interactions	Reduced problem behavior Reduced offenses and recidivism Improved family interactions
Merits	Suitable for school Prescriptive procedures	Targets extrafamilial factors that interfere with parenting	Long-term maintenance of treatment effects	Suitable for school setting Parents treated as equals
Limitations	Less effective with multistressed parents Blames parents	Methodological problems Requires skilled professional	Few studies Requires skilled professional	Few studies Requires skilled professional Requires planning and multiple players Long-term intervention

intensive and has nontraditional components for school-based interventions for families.

Summary

Four approaches to intervening with families with children who are aggressive have been described: PMT, expanded PMT, family therapy, and multisystemic models. Table 14.2 provides a summary of differences in family intervention approaches across eight domains. Horne (1993) has provided a helpful framework by placing the interventions on a continuum. PMT, the most structured intervention, requires the least therapist training, whereas family therapy, the least structured, requires the most training. Multisystemic approaches fall in the middle of the continuum. To deliver multisystemic interventions, school professionals will need administrative support, reduced caseloads, more flexible role expectations, supportive supervision, and continued professional training (Conoley, 1989).

Whichever interventions are adopted, most researchers are in agreement that aggression and conduct problems require long-term monitoring, evaluation, and intervention (Kazdin, 1987b; Offord & Bennett, 1994; Webster-Stratton & Herbert, 1994b). Intervention requires frequent training and support provided at critical points throughout a child's and family's development. In addition, intervention must target not only the family, but also the child, peers, school, and community settings. Key socializing agents must work together to promote prosocial behavior and prevent the learning of aggression (Dubow & Cappas, 1990).

In the final section of this chapter, we discuss guidelines for intervening with families of aggressive children. On the basis of lessons we have learned from family interventions, we recommend that school professionals build positive, trusting relationships with parents; intervene early to identify and resolve the factors that predict antisocial outcomes; and adopt health promotion strategies that build competence in children and families.

GUIDELINES FOR INTERVENTION

In this section, intervention guidelines for working with families who have children and adolescents demonstrating externalizing behaviors are described. In the introduction of this chapter, we have referred to our guidelines as a road map to change psychological and educational service delivery for aggressive children and adolescents. The analogy of a road map is relevant for working with families of aggressive children and youths, because there are several routes available to reach the desired destination—in this case, improved outcomes for these young people. The specific route chosen, or exactly what is implemented, is dependent on the unique contextual factors present in a child's or adolescent's home, school, and community settings. Although we acknowledge that there is no exact prescription for working with families to improve educational and developmental outcomes for aggressive young people, we underscore that the undisputed role of the school professional is to make a positive difference in young people's lives, even the lives of those who are aggressive and disruptive in school settings. To implement an intervention without consideration of these guidelines would compromise the effectiveness of the intervention. Inherent in this role is a positive way to connect with families.

An overarching principle for working with families to improve outcomes for aggressive children and adolescents is early, sustained intervention across the contexts in which these young people live and learn, most notably home and school. The failure of parent training programs to generalize improvements in child outcomes from the home to peer and school contexts is the single most important reason for intervening across contexts. Educators observe child behavior continually and therefore are in an ideal position to intervene early in the development of aggression. The guidelines, all of which are influenced by this overarching principle, are organized into three categories: approach, attitude, and action. We hope that school-based professionals will find these guidelines a useful road map as they design particular intervention strategies to implement in their schools.

Approach

The approach to working with families should be based on an ecological and systemic understanding of children's development and behavior (e.g., Bronfenbrenner, 1979; Christenson & Hirsch, 1998). Therefore, the focus is on improving child outcomes by developing mesosystemic interventions, which focus on the relationships between contexts for children's development (e.g., home and school). Thus, we recommend establishing partnerships with families of children and youths who are aggressive.

In addition, the approach should be based predominantly in primary prevention and health promotion, rather than in the traditional service delivery model of tertiary prevention (i.e., treatment). The objective of primary prevention is to affect correlates of the problem behavior (Short & Shapiro, 1993), and we suggest that competence enhancement approaches offer the greatest promise for achieving this objective. This change in service delivery requires new roles for school-based mental health professionals, who will serve as resources or information synthesizers for all families and educators about the environmental influences that promote competence in children and adolescents. Secondary prevention efforts, described as immediate interventions for the predictors or warning signs of aggression, antisocial behavior, or externalizing disorders in children and adolescents, offer promise for building a partnership with families. Educators who monitor the warning signs regularly and systematically will be able to intervene early and more effectively with families, because there is a lower probability that the relationship between families and school personnel will have escalated to the point of extreme contentiousness.

Finally, the approach adopted should recognize that both primary prevention and secondary prevention need to extend beyond school bounds (Short & Shapiro, 1993). Because school-based professionals are interested in promoting the development of young people, factors in family contexts (e.g., maternal depression) that influence positive parenting practices cannot be ignored. Although we are strong advocates of interventions for proximal factors, as suggested by Reid and Patterson (1991), we also recognize that integrated services are implicated. Integrated services are particularly important for young people experiencing multiple risks. A mesosystemic, preventive approach that builds partnerships with families to enhance child and adolescent outcomes is beneficial, primarily because it facilitates coordinating socialization opportunities for children and adolescents and planning for generalization of expected behavior across contexts.

Attitude

The attitude of families and educators toward each other when students are aggressive and disruptive in educational settings has been well described; too often, it is characterized by alienation and blaming (Christenson & Hirsch, 1998). In the worst situations, families, scapegoated by school professionals, are labeled as the explanation for children's behavior; similarly, school professionals (most often teachers) are singled out by families as the reason for children's unsuccessful experience in school. In some cases, a total lack of contact between families and educators results in unfounded assumptions about the behavior of parents, educators, and students. In other cases, documented extenuating circumstances in families, such as alcoholism, serve to reinforce the belief that families are the single cause of aggressive, disruptive behavior in children and adolescents. School practices, such as contacting parents only when their children have engaged in aggressive, disruptive behavior, and family behaviors, such as limited follow-through on school requests, may be understandable and adaptive responses; however, they also maintain blaming. Such practices do not allow for opportunities to share information about the children in one context or the other, or about specific constraints faced by families and educators. Regardless of the specifics of the situation, these attitudes do not lend themselves to positive family–school partnerships to enhance child outcomes.

Both a change in attitude toward the role played by families and educators in the socialization of children and adolescents, and the active involvement of children and adolescents in planning interventions, are necessary. We suggest that the presence of five attitudes will help to ensure the development of mesosystemic, collaborative interventions for children and adolescents demonstrating aggressive and antisocial behaviors. First, we believe that working with families of aggressive children requires a belief by educators that a partnership with families is essential—not just desirable, but essential. Both family and school environments, conceived of as the curriculum of the school and the curriculum of the home, contribute to child competence (Christenson & Buerkle, 1999).

Second, the focus of the partnership across home and school should be solution oriented. To this extent, educators are encouraged to invite parents to help resolve school-based concerns for their children, and to develop plans directed toward academic and behavioral skill acquisition for the children. Third, the task facing the partners in each case is to alter the environmental influences on a child or adolescent, to produce more favorable outcomes and place the student on a better developmental trajectory. To this end, the partners must suspend judgment about the cause of the student's problem and engage in nonblaming interactions as parents and educators coconstruct a picture of the student's needs. Rather than searching for who is the source of the problem, the partners discuss who is a source for solving the problem and enhancing the student's competence. Thus, the partners' attitude should be that parents, educators, and the student are facing a problematic situation (not a problematic parent, student, or educator), and that the input of all parties is needed to plan an intervention that meets the needs of all parties.

Fourth, conflict across family and school environments should be viewed as natural, not as something to be feared and avoided (Christenson & Hirsch, 1998). Finally, there is an assumption that the problematic situation can be improved with support and resources tailored to the specific situation. There is recognition that parents and educators vary in their need for information and support to address children's aggressive behavior, and that persistence will be required (particularly by educators) in working to create partnerships and outreach activities with some families.

Action

Seven broad-based actions are recommended for the consideration of school professionals who work with families of aggressive children and adolescents. First, a system must be created to disseminate information and educate school personnel and families—the key stakeholders in children's lives—about ways to promote academic, social, and behavioral competence for students in grades K–12. Information about school, family, and community influences on child outcomes should be disseminated to all families and school personnel on a regular and routine basis. This approach creates a climate for sharing information on the healthy development of children and adolescents. Information on predictors of psychological disorders (e.g., CD, ODD, ADHD) should also be routinely disseminated. The information must be presented in multiple formats, including print media, nonprint media, home visits, didactic presentations and discussions (workshops), and consultations; it should also be accompanied with information about specific strategies, such as alternatives to punishment and childhood management, and ways for families to learn more about their children's development. This is admittedly a schoolwide dissemination strategy that creates opportunities for nonblaming discussions of the factors that lead to aggression in children.

Second, supportive opportunities for parents to develop parenting skills also need to be created. However, in keeping with the vein of partnership, we suggest that parents be asked what they want to learn and discuss so that they can assist their children's or adolescents' development and competence. Successful family workshops are responsive to parents' needs (Goodman, Sutton, & Harkavy, 1995). It may be helpful to generate a list of specific topics and ask parents to prioritize and add to the list of desired topics. Given the database on parent correlates of childhood aggression, such topics as using positive reinforcement, alternatives to physical punishment, monitoring and supervising adolescents' behavior, problem-solving and negotiation strategies, defining problems in nonhostile ways, and helping children make friendships are relevant to include on the list. PMT programs provide helpful content to share with parents; however, parents' preferences should be assessed. Creating opportunities for parents sharing with parents what works in difficult situations has also been found to be an effective strategy in involving families who often feel alienated from schools (Goodman et al., 1995).

Third, early identification across grade levels of students who are demonstrating aggressive behaviors, paired with immediate outreach for family involvement, is necessary. Helpful strategies include asking parents to help address the school-based concern, maintaining a focus on what both parents and educators can do to improve a student's performance, and building a relationship around promoting a more successful adaptation for the child or adolescent in the school environment. Fortunately, several problem-solving models that focus on creating shared responsibility for student success are available. The reader is referred to Carlson, Hickman, and Horton (1992), Christenson (1995), Sheridan and Kratochwill (1992), and Weiss and Edwards (1992) for specific details about procedures to be used in family–school problem-solving consultation. The benefits of these models include coordination between home and school in setting social and academic goals; clarification of roles and responsibilities for parents, educators, and students; and increased contact between families and educators about children's behavior in multiple contexts.

Fourth, effective home–school communication strategies that reach all families must be developed and maintained. Communication strategies that facilitate partnership and reduce the probability of blaming between home and school include (1) maintaining a positive orientation for communication, rather than a deficit-based or crisis orientation, (2) developing and publicizing a regular, reliable home–school communication system that increases the potential for two-way communication, (3) focusing communication and dialogue between parents and educators on their shared vested interest, the progress of the students, and (4) ensuring that parents have the information they need to support their children's educational progress (Christenson & Hirsch, 1998). With respect to parents of aggressive children, we emphasize the need to communicate regularly, in order to keep them informed of their children's progress and to enlist their help in developing a plan of action; to call parents on a regular basis, not only when there are problems; and to be a resource for parents (Evelo, Sinclair, Hurley, Christenson, & Thurlow, 1996). We encourage educators to establish one school contact for parents. Parents of families with aggressive children often feel isolated and therefore may find it helpful when asked whether they desire suggestions, resources, or support for handling their children's behavior. If anything is desired, educators should facilitate ways to address the request.

Fifth, to maintain participation in treatment (especially for those families most likely to drop out), program developers must pay careful attention to the characteristics of the children and families, as well as to the design of the program. Attrition rates and the reasons for attrition must be considered in designing programs for families of aggressive children. Family factors associated with dropping out of treatment include greater socioeconomic disadvantage; greater stress and higher number of adverse life events; and child-rearing practices associated with a long-term prognosis for child antisocial behavior, such as punitive and inconsistent discipline, and poor monitoring and supervision. Other specific characteristics linked with premature treatment termination are as follows: multiple child diagnoses and high levels of child contact with antisocial peers, single-parent or minority status of families, and a maternal history of antisocial behavior (Kazdin, Mazurick, & Bass, 1993).

Treatment factors to consider in designing a family intervention program include the setting and structure of the intervention. For example, J. Hughes (personal communication, November 1995) found that only 20% of families completed half of a voluntary school-based parent training program that included child care and monetary compensation. In contrast, 93% of families completed 18 months of treatment when the program was conducted in the home setting and the structure of the treatment was responsive rather than prescriptive.

Sixth, connections with community agencies must be developed to supplement services for families. School-linked services are needed to address issues related to marital conflict, maternal depression, and environmental stresses such as poverty and unemployment. The timing of referral for these services is crucial, as follow-through by families for mental health services is generally low (Zins, 1981). From our experience in working with families of adolescents at risk of dropping out of school, many of whom demonstrate aggressive and violent behaviors, we speculate that referral for these services should be made only after a trusting relationship between a school and family is formed. Moreover, referral to community agencies for family services should be made only after family–school problem-solving consultation has occurred. This takes time and persistence.

Finally, staff development workshops should be provided for educators on positive strategies for communicating with families; conflict resolution and structured problem solving, and ways of handling angry parents. Furthermore, if parents and educators attend the same workshops on topics related to aggression in young people, there is an opportunity for them to be colearners and coteachers. This strategy has been used with success in reducing suspensions and behavior referrals (Comer & Haynes, 1992).

CLOSING COMMENTS

In closing, we believe that a partnership approach is essential in working with families of aggressive children and adolescents. It is our contention that intervention with these families will be most efficacious if two conditions are met. First, school-based efforts with families should strive to maintain the partnership by focusing on positive outcomes for children, or ways for educators and families working in tandem to enhance children's competence by helping the children to make a more successful match to the task demands of the school environment.

The second condition relates to the distinction between content and process. We assert that our content knowledge surpasses our process knowledge. The predictors of aggressive behavior in young people, and the components of effective parent education programs, are well documented. Process, or how this knowledge base is implemented to support families, is the key for successful intervention. Building trust between home and school is a prerequisite for working effectively with families of aggressive children. Trust cannot be mandated; trust is built piece by piece, interaction by interaction, communication by communication. We recognize that the aggression of some children and adolescents is intense and intractable, and that persistence is needed to involve some families even minimally. Alternative approaches for creating collaborative partnerships with families are evolving (e.g., Webster-Stratton & Herbert, 1994b). An essential feature of creating healthy connections between home and school to enhance outcomes for aggressive children is dealing systematically with conditions that contribute to blame between these systems. Our sense is that a partnership orientation that increases communication, contact, problem solving, conflict resolution, and clarity in socialization roles between home and school will reflect a welcome change in psychological and educational service delivery to aggressive children and adolescents.

REFERENCES

Alexander, J. F. (1973). Defensive and supportive communications in normal and deviant families. *Journal of Consulting and Clinical Psychology, 40*, 223–231.

Alexander, J. F., Barton, C., Schiavo, R. S., & Parsons, B. V. (1976). Systems-behavioral intervention with families of delinquents: Therapist characteristics, family behavior, and outcome. *Journal of Consulting and Clinical Psychology, 44*, 656–664.

Alexander, J. F., & Parsons, B. V. (1973). Short-term behavioral intervention with delinquent families: Impact on family process and recidivism. *Journal of Abnormal Psychology, 81,* 219–225.

Alexander, J. F., & Parsons, B. V. (1982). *Functional family therapy.* Pacific Grove, CA: Brooks/Cole.

Amato, P. R., & Keith, B. (1991). Parental divorce and the well-being of children: A meta-analysis. *Psychological Bulletin, 110,* 26–46.

Apter, S. J., & Propper, C. A. (1986). Ecological perspectives on youth violence. In S. J. Apter & A. P. Goldstein (Eds.), *Youth violence: Programs and prospects* (pp. 140–159). New York: Plenum Press.

Arnold, J. E., Levine, A. G., & Patterson, G. R. (1975). Changes in sibling behavior following family intervention. *Journal of Consulting and Clinical Psychology, 43,* 683–688.

Asarnow, J., & Callan, J. (1985). Boys with peer adjustment problems: Social cognitive processes. *Journal of Consulting and Clinical Psychology, 43,* 683–688.

Barton, C., Alexander, J. F., Waldron, H., Turner, C. W., & Warburton, J. (1985). Generalizing treatment effects of functional family therapy: Three replications. *American Journal of Family Therapy, 13,* 16–26.

Bates, J. (1990). Conceptual and empirical linkages between temperament and behavior problems: A commentary on the Sanson, Prior, and Kyrios study. *Merrill–Palmer Quarterly, 36*(2), 193–199.

Baum, C. B., & Forehand, R. L. (1981). Long-term follow-up assessment of parent training by use of multiple-outcome measures. *Behavior Therapy, 12,* 643–652.

Blechman, E. A. (1984). Competent parents, competent children: Behavioral objectives of parent training. In R. F. Dangel & R. A. Polster (Eds.), *Parent training: Foundations of research and practice* (pp. 34–66). New York: Guilford Press.

Blechman, E. A. (1987). *Solving child behavior problems at home and at school.* Champaign, IL: Research Press.

Braswell, L., & Bloomquist, M. L. (1991). *Cognitive-behavioral therapy with ADHD children: Child, family, and school interventions.* New York: Guilford Press.

Bronfenbrenner, U. (1979). *The ecology of human development.* Cambridge, MA: Harvard University Press.

Brunk, M., Henggeler, S. W., & Whelan, J. P. (1987). A comparison of multisystemic therapy and parent training in the brief treatment of child abuse and neglect. *Journal of Consulting and Clinical Psychology, 55,* 171–178.

Campbell, S. B., & Ewing, L. J. (1990). Follow-up of hard-to-manage preschoolers: Adjustment at age 9 and predictors of continuing symptoms. *Journal of Child Psychology and Psychiatry, 31,* 871–889.

Campbell, S. B., Ewing, L. J., Breaux, A. M., & Szumowski, E. K. (1986). Parent-referred problem three-year-olds: Follow-up at school entry. *Journal of Child Psychology and Psychiatry, 27*(4), 473–488.

Carlson, C. I., Hickman, J., & Horton, C. B. (1992). From blame to solutions: Solution-oriented family–school consultation. In S. L. Christenson & J. C. Conoley (Eds.), *Home–school collaboration: Enhancing children's academic and social competence* (pp. 193–213). Silver Spring, MD: National Association of School Psychologists.

Centers for Disease Control and Prevention. (1990). *Youth Risk Behavior Surveillance System (YRBSS).* Atlanta, GA: Author.

Christenson, S. L. (1995). Supporting home–school collaboration. In A. Thomas & J. Grimes (Eds.), *Best practices in school psychology III* (pp. 253–267). Silver Spring, MD: National Association of School Psychologists.

Christenson, S. L., & Buerkle, K. (1999). Families as educational partners for children's school success: Suggestions for school psychologists. In C. R. Reynolds & T. B. Gutkin (Eds.), *Handbook of school psychology* (3rd ed., pp. 709–744). New York: Wiley.

Christenson, S. L., & Hirsch, J. (1998). Facilitating partnerships and conflict resolution between families and schools. In K. C. Stoiber & T. Kratochwill (Eds.), *Group interventions in the school and community* (pp. 307–344). Newton, MA: Allyn & Bacon.

Coie, J. D. (1990). Adapting intervention to the problems of aggressive and disruptive rejected children. In S. R. Asher & J. D. Coie (Eds.), *Peer rejection in childhood* (pp. 309–377). New York: Cambridge University Press.

Coie, J. D., Dodge, K. A., & Coppotelli, H. (1982). Dimensions and types of social status: A cross-age perspective. *Developmental Psychology, 18,* 557–570.

Comer, J. P., & Haynes, N. M. (1992). Parent involvement in schools: An ecological approach. *Elementary School Journal, 91*(3), 271–278.

Conduct Problems Prevention Research Group (CPPRG). (1992). A developmental and clinical model for the prevention of conduct disorder: The FAST Track program. *Development and Psychopathology, 4,* 509–527.

Conoley, J. C. (1989). The school psychologist as a community–family service provider. In R. C. D'Amato & R. S. Dean (Eds.), *The school psychologist in nontraditional settings: Integrating clients, services, and settings* (pp. 33–65). Hillsdale, NJ: Erlbaum.

Cox, R., & Gunn, W. (1980). Interpersonal skills in the schools: Assessment and curriculum development. In D. Rathjen & J. Foreyt (Eds.), *Social competence: Interventions for children and adults* (pp. 113–132). Elmsford, NY: Pergamon Press.

Dadds, M. R., Schwartz, S., & Sanders, M. R. (1987). Marital discord and treatment outcome in behavioral treatment of child conduct disorders. *Journal of Consulting and Clinical Psychology, 55,* 396–403.

Dodge, K. A. (1980). Social cognition and children's aggressive behavior. *Child Development, 53,* 620–635.

Dodge, K. A., & Coie, J. D. (1987). Social information processing factors in reactive and proactive aggression in children's peer groups. *Journal of Personality and Social Psychology, 53,* 1146–1158.

Dodge, K. A., & Frame, C. L. (1982). Social cognitive biases and deficits in aggressive boys. *Child Development, 53,* 620–635.

Dodge, K. A., Murphy, R. R., & Buchsbaum, K. (1984). The assessment of intention-cue detection skills in children: Implications for developmental psychopathology. *Child Development, 55,* 163–173.

Dodge, K. A., & Somberg, D. R. (1987). Hostile attribution biases are exacerbated under conditions of threat to self. *Child Development, 58,* 213–244.

Dubow, E. F., & Cappas, C. L. (1990). Reducing aggression in children through social interventions. In J. Edwards, R. S. Tindale, L. Heath, & E. J. Posavac (Eds.), *Social influence processes and prevention* (pp. 197–219). New York: Plenum Press.

Dumas, J. E., & Wahler, R. G. (1983). Predictors of treatment outcome in parent training: Mother insularity and socioeconomic disadvantage. *Behavioral Assessment, 5,* 301–313.

Eron, L. D., Huesmann, L. R., & Zelli, A. (1991). The role of parental variables in the learning of aggression. In D. J. Peplar & K. H. Rubin (Eds.), *The development and treatment of childhood aggression* (pp. 169–188). Hillsdale, NJ: Erlbaum.

Evelo, D. L., Sinclair, M. F., Hurley, C. M., Christenson, S. L., & Thurlow, M. L. (1996, December). *Keeping kids in school: Using Check and Connect for dropout prevention.* Minneapolis: Institute on Community Integration, University of Minnesota.

Family Services Research Center. (1995). *Multisystemic therapy using home-based services: A clinically effective and cost effective strategy for treating serious clinical problems in youth.*

Charleston: Department of Psychiatry and Behavioral Sciences, Medical University of South Carolina.

Farrington, D. P. (1991). Childhood aggression and adult violence: Early precursors and later-life outcomes. In D. J. Pepler & K. H. Rubin (Eds.), *The development and treatment of childhood aggression* (pp. 5–29). Hillsdale, NJ: Erlbaum.

Feldman, R. A., Caplinger, T. E., & Wodarski, J. S. (1983). *The St. Louis conundrum: The effective treatment of antisocial youths.* Englewood Cliffs, NJ: Prentice-Hall.

Feshbach, N. (1989). The construct of empathy and the phenomenon of physical maltreatment of children. In D. Cicchetti & V. Carlson (Eds.), *Child maltreatment: Theory and research on the causes and consequences of child abuse and neglect* (pp. 349–373). New York: Cambridge University Press.

Forehand, R. L., & Long, N. (1986). *A long-term follow-up of parent training participants.* Paper presented at the meeting of the Association for Advancement of Behavior Therapy, Chicago.

Forehand, R. L., & McMahon, R. J. (1981). *Helping the noncompliant child: A clinician's guide to parent training.* New York: Guilford Press.

Forehand, R. L., Sturgis, E. T., McMahon, R. J., Aguar, D., Green, K., Wells, K., & Breiner, J. (1979). Parent behavioral training to modify child noncompliance: Treatment generalization across time and from home to school. *Behavior Modification, 3,* 3–25.

Frick, P. J. (1994). Family dysfunction and the disruptive behavior disorders: A review of recent empirical findings. In T. H. Ollendick & R. J. Prinz (Eds.), *Advances in clinical child psychology* (pp. 203–226). New York: Plenum Press.

Frick, P. J., Lahey, B. B., Loeber, R., Stouthamer-Loeber, M., Christ, M. A., & Hanson, K. (1992). Familial risk factors to oppositional defiant disorder and conduct disorder: Parental psychopathology and maternal parenting. *Journal of Consulting and Clinical Psychology, 60*(1), 49–55.

Furlong, M. J., & Morrison, G. M. (1994). Introduction to mini-series: School violence and safety in perspective. *School Psychology Review, 23*(2), 139–150.

Goodman, J. F., Sutton, V., & Harkavy, I. (1995). The effectiveness of family workshops in a middle school setting: Respect and caring make the difference. *Phi Delta Kappan, 76*(9), 694–700.

Gordon, D. A., & Arbuthnot, J. (1987). Individual, group, and family interventions. In H. C. Quay (Ed.), *Handbook of juvenile delinquency* (pp. 290–324). New York: Wiley.

Greist, D. L., Forehand, R., Rogers, T., Breiner, J. L., Furey, W., & Williams, C. A. (1982). Effects of parent enhancement therapy on the treatment outcome and generalization of a parent training program. *Behaviour Research and Therapy, 20,* 429–236.

Greist, D. L., & Wells, K. C. (1983). Behavioral family therapy with conduct disorders in children. *Behavior Therapy, 14,* 37–53.

Haddad, J. D., Barocas, R., & Hollenbeck, A. R. (1991). Family organization and parent attitudes of children with conduct disorder. *Journal of Clinical Child Psychology, 20*(2), 152–161.

Hawkins, J. D., & Fraser, M. W. (1983). Social support networks in delinquency prevention and treatment. In J. K. Whitaker, J. Garbarino, & Associates (Eds.), *Social support networks: Informal helping in human services* (pp. 333–352). New York: Aldine.

Hawkins, J. D., & Weis, J. G. (1985). The social development model: An integrated approach to delinquency prevention. *Journal of Primary Prevention, 6,* 73–95.

Henggeler, S. W., Rodick, J. D., Bordin, C. M., Hanson, C. L., Watson, S. M., & Urey, J. R. (1986). Multisystemic treatment of juvenile offenders: Effects on adolescent behavior and family interaction. *Developmental Psychology, 22,* 132–141.

Herbert, M. (1987). *Conduct disorders of childhood and adolescence: A social learning perspective* (2nd ed.). Chichester, UK: Wiley.

Holleran, P. A., Littman, D. C., Freund, R., & Schmaling, K. B. (1982). A signal detection approach to social perception: Identification of negative and positive behaviors by parents of normal and problem children. *Journal of Abnormal Child Psychology, 10,* 547–557.

Hooper-Briar, K., & Lawson, H. A. (1994). *Serving children, youth, and families through interprofessional collaboration and service integration: A framework for action.* Oxford, OH: Institute for Educational Renewal, Miami University.

Horne, A. M. (1993). Family-based interventions. In A. P. Goldstein & C. R. Huff (Eds.), *The gang intervention handbook* (pp. 189–218). Champaign, IL: Research Press.

Hudley, C. A. (1994). Perceptions of intentionality, feelings of anger, and reactive aggression. In M. J. Furlong & D. G. Smith (Eds.), *Anger, hostility, and aggression: Assessment, prevention, and intervention strategies for youth* (pp. 39–56). Brandon, VT: Clinical Psychology.

Improving America's Schools Act of 1994, Public Law 103-382, Title IV, Safe and Drug Free Schools and Communities, § 4000, 20 U.S.C. § 7113.

Kauffman, J. M. (1985). *Characteristics of children's behavior disorders* (3rd ed.). Columbus, OH: Merrill.

Kazdin, A. E. (1985). *Treatment of antisocial behavior in children and adolescents.* Pacific Grove, CA: Brooks/Cole.

Kazdin, A. E. (1987a). *Conduct disorders in childhood and adolescence.* Newbury Park, CA: Sage.

Kazdin, A. E. (1987b). Treatment of antisocial behavior in children: Current status and future directions. *Psychological Bulletin, 102*(2), 187–203.

Kazdin, A. E., Mazurick, J. L., & Bass, D. (1993). Risk for attrition in treatment of antisocial children and families. *Journal of Clinical Child Psychology, 22*(1), 2–16.

Klein, N. C., Alexander, J. F., & Parsons, B. V. (1977). Impact of family systems intervention on recidivism and sibling delinquency: A model of primary prevention and program evaluation. *Journal of Consulting and Clinical Psychology, 45,* 469–474.

Kolko, D. J. (1994). Conduct disorder. In M. Hersen, R. T. Ammerman, & L. A. Sisson (Eds.), *Handbook of aggressive and destructive behavior in psychiatric patients* (pp. 363–394). New York: Plenum Press.

Kuperschmidt, J., & Coie, J. (1990). Preadolescent peer status, aggression, and school adjustment as predictors of externalizing behaviors in adolescence. *Child Development, 61,* 1350–1362.

Ladd, G. W. (1990). Having friends, keeping friends, making friends, and being liked by peers in the classroom: Predictors of children's early school adjustment? *Child Development, 61,* 1081–1100.

Lochman, J. E. (1987). Self and peer perceptions and attributional biases of aggressive and nonaggressive boys in dyadic interactions. *Journal of Consulting and Clinical Psychology, 55,* 404–410.

Loeber, R. (1990). Development and risk factors of juvenile antisocial behavior and delinquency. *Clinical Psychology Review, 10,* 1–41.

Loeber, R., & Dishion, T. J. (1983). Early predictors of male adolescent delinquency: A review. *Psychological Bulletin, 94,* 68–99.

Loeber, R., & Stouthamer-Loeber, M. (1986). Family factors as correlates and predictors of juvenile conduct problems and delinquency. In M. Tonry & N. Morris (Eds.), *Crime and justice* (pp. 129–149). Chicago: University of Chicago Press.

Loeber, R., & Stouthamer-Loeber, M. (1987). Prediction. In H. Quay (Ed.), *Handbook of juvenile delinquency* (pp. 325–382). New York: Wiley.

Mansfield, W., Alexander, D., & Farris, E. (1991, November). *Teacher survey on safe, disciplined, and drug-free schools* (Report No. NCES 91-091). Washington, DC: National Center for Educational Statistics, U.S. Department of Education.

McLoyd, V. C. (1990). The impact of economic hardship on black families and children: Psychological distress, parenting, and socioemotional development. *Child Development, 61,* 311–346.

McMahon, R. J., & Forehand, R. (1984). Parent training for the noncompliant child: Treatment outcome, generalization, and adjunctive therapy procedures. In R. F. Dangel & R. A. Polster (Eds.), *Parent training: Foundations of research and practice* (pp. 298–328). New York: Guilford Press.

McMahon, R. J., Forehand, R., & Greist, D. L. (1981). Effects of knowledge of social learning principles on enhancing treatment outcome and generalization in a parent training program. *Journal of Consulting and Clinical Psychology, 49,* 526–532.

McMahon, R. J., Forehand, R., Greist, D. L., & Wells, K. (1981). Who drops out of treatment during parent behavioral training? *Behavioral Consulting Quarterly, 1,* 79–85.

McMahon, R. J., Slough, N. M., & the Conduct Problems Prevention Research Group (CPPRG). (1996). Family-based intervention in the FAST Track Program. In R. D. Peters & R. J. McMahon (Eds.), *Preventing childhood disorders, substance abuse, and delinquency* (pp. 90–110). Thousand Oaks, CA: Sage.

Middlebrook, J. L., & Forehand, R. (1985). Maternal perceptions of deviance in child behavior as a function of stress and clinic versus nonclinic status of the child: An analogue study. *Behavior Therapy, 16,* 494–502.

Milich, R., & Dodge, K. (1984). Social information processing in child psychiatric populations. *Journal of Abnormal Child Psychology, 9,* 127–140.

Miller, G. E. (1994). Enhancing family-based interventions for managing childhood aggression and anger. In M. Furlong & D. Smith (Eds.), *Anger, hostility, and aggression: Assessment, prevention, and intervention strategies for youth* (pp. 83–116). Brandon, VT: Clinical Psychology.

Miller, G. E., & Prinz, R. J. (1990). Enhancement of social learning family interventions for childhood conduct disorder. *Psychological Bulletin, 108*(2), 291–307.

Miller, N. B., Cowan, P. A., Cowan, C. P., Hetherington, E. M., & Clingempeel, W. G. (1993). Externalizing in preschoolers and early adolescents: A cross-study replication of a family model. *Developmental Psychology, 29*(1), 3–18.

National Education Goals Panel. (1995). *The national education goals report* (Vol. 1). Washington, DC: U.S. Government Printing Office.

National Institute of Education. (1978). *Violent schools–safe schools: The safe school study report to the Congress* (Executive Summary). Washington, DC: Author.

Offord, D. R., & Bennett, K. J. (1994). Conduct disorder: Long-term outcomes and intervention effectiveness. *Journal of the American Academy of Child and Adolescent Psychiatry, 33*(8), 1069–1078.

O'Leary, K. D., & Emery, R. E. (1982). Marital discord and child behavior problems. In M. D. Levine & P. Satz (Eds.), *Middle childhood: Developmental variation and dysfunction* (pp. 345–364). New York: Academic Press.

Paavola, J. (1994). *Comprehensive and coordinated psychological services for children: A call for service integration.* Washington, DC: American Psychological Association.

Patterson, G. R. (1974). Interventions for boys with conduct problems: Multiple settings, treatments, and criteria. *Journal of Consulting and Clinical Psychology, 42,* 471–481.

Patterson, G. R. (1982). *Coercive family process.* Eugene, OR: Castalia.

Patterson, G. R. (1983). Stress: A change agent for family process. In N. Garmezy & M. Rutter (Eds.), *Stress, coping, and development in children* (pp. 235–264). New York: McGraw-Hill.

Patterson, G. R. (1986). Performance models for antisocial boys. *American Psychologist, 41*, 432–444.

Patterson, G. R., Capaldi, D., & Bank, L. (1991). An early starter model for predicting delinquency. In D. Pepler & K. H. Rubin (Eds.), *The development and treatment of childhood aggression* (pp. 139–168). Hillsdale, NJ: Erlbaum.

Patterson, G. R., & Chamberlain, P. (1988). Treatment process: A problem at three levels. In L. C. Wynne (Ed.), *The state of the art in family therapy research: Controversies and recommendations* (pp. 189–223). New York: Family Process Press.

Patterson, G. R., Chamberlain, P., & Reid, J. B. (1982). A comparative evaluation of a parent training program. *Behavior Therapy, 13*, 638–650.

Patterson, G. R., DeBaryshe, B. D., & Ramsey, E. (1989). A developmental perspective on antisocial behavior. *American Psychologist, 44*, 329–335.

Patterson, G. R., & Fleischman, M. S. (1979). Maintenance of treatment effects: Some considerations concerning family systems and follow-up data. *Behavior Therapy, 10*, 168–185.

Patterson, G. R., & Fleischman, M. S. (1985). Maintenance of treatment effects: Some considerations concerning family systems and follow-up data. *Behavior Therapy, 10*, 168–185.

Patterson, G. R., & Forgatch, M. S. (1985). Therapist behavior as a determinant for client noncompliance: A paradox for the behavior modifier. *Journal of Consulting and Clinical Psychology, 53*, 846–851.

Patterson, G. R., Reid, J. B., Jones, R. R., & Conger, R. W. (1975). *A social learning approach to family intervention* (Vol. 1). Eugene, OR: Castalia.

Pettit, G. S., Bates, J. E., & Dodge, K. A. (1993). Family interaction patterns and children's conduct problems at home and school: A longitudinal perspective. *School Psychology Review, 22*(3), 403–420.

Reid, J., Taplin, P., & Loeber, R. (1981). A social interactional approach to the treatment of abusive families. In R. Stewart (Ed.), *Violent behavior: Social learning approaches to prediction, management, and treatment* (pp. 83–101). New York: Brunner/Mazel.

Reid, J. B., & Patterson, G. R. (1976). Follow-up analyses of a behavioral treatment program for boys with conduct problems: A reply to Kent. *Journal of Consulting and Clinical Psychology, 44*, 299–302.

Reid, J. B., & Patterson, G. R. (1991). Early prevention and intervention with conduct problems: A social interactional model for the integration of research and practice. In G. Stoner, M. Shinn, & H. Walker (Eds.), *Interventions for achievement and behavior problems* (pp. 715–739). Silver Spring, MD: National Association of School Psychologists.

Richman, N., Stevenson, L., & Graham, P. J. (1982). *Pre-school to school: A behavioral study.* London: Academic Press.

Robins, L. N. (1978). Sturdy childhood predictors of adult antisocial behavior: Replications from longitudinal studies. *Psychological Medicine, 8*, 611–622.

Robins, L. N. (1981). Epidemiological approaches to natural history research: Antisocial disorders in children. *Journal of the American Academy of Child Psychiatry, 20*, 566–580.

Robins, L. N., & Ratcliff, K. S. (1980). Risk factors in the continuation of childhood antisocial behavior into adulthood. *International Journal of Mental Health, 7*(3–4), 6–16.

Rutter, M., & Giller, H. (1983). *Juvenile delinquency: Trends and perspectives.* Harmondsworth, UK: Penguin.

Rutter, M., Tizard, J., Yule, W., Graham, P., & Whitmore, K. (1976). Research report: Isle of Wight studies. *Psychological Medicine, 6*, 313–332.

Sheley, J. F., McGee, Z. T., & White, J. D. (1992). Gun-related violence in and around inner-city schools. *American Journal of Diseases of Children, 146*, 677–682.

Sheridan, S. M., & Kratochwill, T. R. (1992). Behavioral parent–teacher consultation: Conceptual and research considerations. *Journal of School Psychology, 30,* 117–139.

Short, R. J., & Shapiro, S. K. (1993). Conduct disorder: A framework for understanding and intervention in schools and communities. *School Psychology Review, 22*(3), 362–375.

Sturge, C. (1982). Reading retardation and antisocial behavior. *Journal of Child Psychology and Psychiatry, 23,* 21–31.

Thomas, A., & Chess, S. (1977). *Temperament and development.* New York: Brunner/Mazel.

U.S. Department of Education, Office of Special Education Programs. (1994). *Sixteenth annual report to Congress on the implementation of the Individuals with Disabilities Education Act.* Washington, DC: Author.

U.S. Department of Justice. (1993, May 19). *Bureau of Justice news release.* Washington, DC: Author.

Vaughn, B., Egeland, B., Sroufe, L. A., & Waters, E. (1979). Individual differences in infant–mother attachment at twelve and eighteen months: Stability and change in families under stress. *Child Development, 50,* 971–975.

Vostanis, P., Nicholls, J., & Harrington, R. (1994). Maternal expressed emotion in conduct and emotional disorders of childhood. *Journal of Child Psychology and Psychiatry, 35*(2), 365–376.

Wahler, R. G., & Afton, A. D. (1980). Attentional processes in insular and noninsular mothers. *Child Behavior Therapy, 2,* 25–41.

Wahler, R. G., & Dumas, J. E. (1984). Changing the observational coding styles of insular and noninsular mothers: A step toward maintenance of parent training effects. In R. E. Dangel & R. A. Polster (Eds.), *Parent training: Foundations of research and practice* (pp. 379–416). New York: Guilford Press.

Webster-Stratton, C. (1982). The long-term effect of a videotape modeling parent education program: Comparison of immediate and one year follow-up results. *Behavior Therapy, 13,* 702–714.

Webster-Stratton, C. (1984). A randomized trial of two parent training programs for families with conduct disordered children. *Journal of Consulting and Clinical Psychology, 52,* 59–69.

Webster-Stratton, C. (1985). Comparison of abusive and nonabusive families with conduct disordered children and their mothers in the clinic and at home. *American Journal of Orthopsychiatry, 55,* 59–69.

Webster-Stratton, C. (1990a). Long-term follow-up of families with young conduct problem children: From preschool to grade school. *Journal of Clinical Psychology, 19,* 144–149.

Webster-Stratton, C. (1990b). Stress: A potential disruptor of parent perceptions and family interactions, *Journal of Clinical Child Psychology, 19*(4), 302–312.

Webster-Stratton, C. (1993). Strategies for helping early school-aged children with ODD and CD: The importance of home–school partnerships. *School Psychology Review, 22*(3), 437–457.

Webster-Stratton, C. (1994). Advancing videotape parent training: A comparison study. *Journal of Consulting and Clinical Psychology, 62*(3), 583–593.

Webster-Stratton, C., & Herbert, M. (1993). What really happens in parent training? *Behavior Modification, 17*(4), 407–456.

Webster-Stratton, C., & Herbert, M. (1994a). Strategies for helping parents of children with conduct disorders. In M. Hersen, R. M. Eisler, & P. M. Miller (Eds.), *Progress in behavior modification* (Vol. 29, pp. 121–142). Pacific Grove, CA: Brooks/Cole.

Webster-Stratton, C., & Herbert, M. (Eds.). (1994b). *Troubled families–problem children.* New York: Wiley.

Weiss, H. M., & Edwards, M. E. (1992). The family–school collaboration project: Systemic interventions for school improvement. In S. L. Christenson & J. C. Conoley (Eds.), *Home–school collaboration: Enhancing children's academic and social competence* (pp. 215–243). Silver Spring, MD: National Association of School Psychologists.

Wells, K. C., & Egan, J. (1988). Social learning and systems family therapy for childhood oppositional disorder: Comparative treatment outcome. *Comprehensive Psychiatry, 29,* 138–146.

Wells, K. C., Forehand, R., & Greist, D. L. (1980). Generality of treatment effects from treated to untreated behaviors resulting from a parent training program. *Journal of Clinical Psychology, 9,* 271–219.

Williams, J. R., & Gold, M. (1972). From delinquent behavior to official delinquency. *Social Problems, 20,* 209–229.

Zins, J. E. (1981). Referral out: Increasing the number of kept appointments. *School Psychology Review, 10*(1), 107–111.

CHAPTER 15

Coping with the Consequences of School Violence

JAMES GARBARINO
ELLEN deLARA

SOCIAL SUPPORT AND SCHOOL SAFETY

Schools are many things—physical facilities, sets of people in interlocking roles, centers of academic resources. But one important aspect of the school, particularly as it relates to school safety and violence in the school, is its function as a "support system" for children and youth. The role of social support systems in preventing, controlling, and coping with violence lies in the linking of social nurturance and social control (Garbarino, 1987). Such support systems provide feedback to children and youth and validate their expectations about others. When this kind of feedback and affirmation is lacking in other social systems, such as the family, support systems in the school can help offset the deficiencies (Caplan, 1976; Naylor & Cowie, 1999).

These themes of social support in the school and its relation to safety and violence are illustrated by an intensive case study conducted in a relatively small and safe school (deLara, 2000; Garbarino and deLara, 2002). Some of the major conclusions of this study were these:

- Care from teachers and other school personnel is critical for students to feel safe at (and on the way to and from) school.
- Peer predictability is crucial for a sense of safety among students.
- Adults often underestimate students' feelings of danger and insecurity.
- Schools, as systems, can be either caring and supportive, or inadvertently maintain and enable hostile and unsafe environments.

This chapter builds on these conclusions to explore the role of social support in school safety.

SCHOOL-BASED SOCIAL SUPPORT INTERVENTIONS

Two corollary premises are embedded in a school-based strategy for increasing safety and decreasing violence. The first is that the support provided can be internalized by an individual in some manner and thus can have an effect beyond the period during which it is provided. The second is that the support can strengthen the individual's functioning in the school enough to have a significant positive effect on overall child health and development (Weiss & Halpern, 1991).

These concerns reverberate through all analyses of school-based programming in the form of two recurrent questions: Can support be "treatment," or must it be a condition of life? And can school-based programming succeed amid conditions of accumulated high risk? Both call our attention to the limiting factors on school support: whether it is possible to synthesize a positive school climate, and whether school-based support is feasible in the neediest communities. Beyond these fundamental issues of efficacy are a number of issues concerning process. For example, to what extent can and should school-based social support programs for violence prevention be staffed at least in part by volunteers and/or paraprofessionals? To what extent can and should efforts be aimed at assisting peers in helping one another? In short, to what extent is school-based programming to prevent violence inextricably tied to issues of empowerment?

To what degree is it necessary and feasible to train peers as natural helpers to function as violence prevention and control systems? This is one of the hot issues in the field of school-based support programs, and it has special relevance to programs addressing violence. Certainly one focal point of national efforts to reduce school violence is enlisting peers as sources of information for adults. Some programs parallel efforts aimed at drunk driving, such as the program using the adage "Friends don't let friends drive drunk."

One school of thought on this issue emphasizes the need for professionals to serve as consultants to natural helpers or central figures in peer groups. However, work with adults suggests that the use of paraprofessionals (in this case adolescent peer helpers) has limitations. Working with adults, Halpern (1990) found that paraprofessionals encountered problems in helping clients in emotionally charged areas—for adults, these areas were adolescent sexuality and the use of corporal punishment.

Extrapolating to adolescents, problems may arise from overidentification with a peer, projecting one's own situation onto a peer, or low expectations (Austin, 1978; Gibbs, Granville, & Goldstein, 1995). Students are at times reluctant to reveal personal matters to peers because they fear a loss of privacy. In addition, they fear possible ridicule as a result of making themselves vulnerable through disclosures to their classmates (deLara, 2000).

These issues give rise to domains of silence. Two of the issues in families most likely to invoke personal or cultural domains of silence are sexuality and aggression (Halpern, 1990; Musick & Stott, 1990). Consequently, peer helpers, without specific training, are not prepared to deal with issues of sexuality, harassment, aggression, and violence. Any effort to prevent or address the aftermath of school violence through social support systems relying on natural peer helpers must contend with this fact. Matters of sex and violence are potentially going to be approached in ways that adults may find less than satisfactory. The natural helpers' own experiences of victimization, teenage sexual activity, and corporal punishment can be powerful impediments in dealing with these issues openly (Hyman & Snook, 1999). This can limit the power of curricula aimed at employing peer helpers to identify and refer high-risk peers.

SELF-SELECTION OR SCHOOL EFFECTS?

One of the nagging problems facing school-based support interventions is the disentangling of selection and program effects. To what extent are schools safer and more supportive because of who goes there versus how the school is structured and managed? This issue at school parallels issues at the neighborhood and community levels. For example, research shows that as the proportion of a community's residents who know each other decreases, criminal activity increases. Evidence from schools suggests a parallel process: As kids experience school as an anonymous place, they are more likely to experience reduced predictability of fellow students, and this increases their sense of danger and general insecurity (deLara, 2000). We return to this issue when we discuss school size and its relevance to school safety.

Beyond even these obvious selection factors, schools differ on the basis of climate. Some schools are more vital and coherent than others, just as is the case among neighborhoods (Warren, 1978). And there are common problems. A survey in South Carolina (Melton, 1992) revealed that on a scale of 1–7 (with 7 indicating high involvement), the average score for neighborhood residents was 2+ in response to the question "How involved are you with other people's children?" The same survey revealed that most people could not name one agency that had been particularly helpful on behalf of children. Students in high school often exhibit this same sense of isolation when asked about adults in the school who are reliably caring (deLara, 2000).

UNDERSTANDING SOCIAL IMPOVERISHMENT IN THE SCHOOL

In research conducted in both small and large schools, deLara (2000, 2001) found that a critical aspect of students' sense of safety at school is what she has termed *peer predictability*. Being able to predict the behavior of one's peers was at the crux of a sense of security for the adolescents in her studies.

Students reported that in order for them to view someone as predictable, regardless of good or bad behavior, it was necessary to know that person. In knowing, or being familiar with other students' behaviors and ways of thinking, adolescents make continuous calculations or evaluations of their peers. These evaluations are the basis for what they believe to be more or less accurate predictions of the meaning of current behavior or the speculation of future behavior. The implied significance behind a remark can be calibrated as a harmless tease or as an explicit ridicule, harassment, or attempt to engage in physical fighting. Peer predictability is accomplished by having an extensive knowledge base of the other people in the social environment. If an adolescent feels he or she knows another student, then a comment or shove can be gauged as hostile, or merely off-hand, even playful. In knowing the other students, it is possible to measure whether someone is "taking it" wrong or harboring ill feelings. "Taking it wrong" can then be seen as a potential threat to the balance of interactions at the school. Various behaviors result from either being the subject of hostility or noticing someone else reacting poorly to being the victim. These responses include retaliation, speaking to an adult or friends, or trying to absorb the discomfort engendered by the circumstances—just "taking it." Students in smaller schools feel that they have an advantage over students from large schools. Those who had attended schools of both sizes reported feeling safer in the smaller schools because they had an opportunity to really know the other students; therefore, they could more readily predict their behavior. The lesson for adults is that secondary school students monitor their colleagues' behaviors on a more or less continuous basis and that this engages a large portion of their time and energy while at school. Consequently, although this strategy is effective for feeling safer at school, it takes away from the energy or attention students might be utilizing for academic reasons.

Identifying schools at high and low risk for violence takes place in a social as well as a psychological and cultural context. Prevention, treatment, and research should incorporate this contextual orientation (Garbarino & Crouter, 1978; Garbarino, 1987). For many purposes, this means examining high-risk schools, as well as individuals, as the contexts for violence (Garbarino, 1999). Research has sought to explore and validate the concept of "social impoverishment" as a characteristic of high-risk family environments and as a factor in evaluating support and prevention programs aimed at violence (most notably child maltreatment). The same approach can be applied to schools.

The starting point is identifying the environmental correlates of school and community violence (Garbarino, 1999; Garbarino & Crouter, 1978). This provides an empirical basis for "screening" to identify high- and low-risk schools. One aspect of the foundation for this approach is the link between accumulated risk and lack of developmental assets and most forms of violence (Garbarino, 1987; Pelton, 1978, 1981, 1992). By "developmental assets" is meant relationships and attributes that indicate positive, prosocial experiences with adults, peers, and institutions. For example, the Search Institute research reveals that the rate of serious violence among children with 31–40 developmental assets is 6%, whereas the rate for a child with 0–10 assets is 61%. From this association stem two conceptions of "high risk" as it applies to schools. The first is in regard to those children with a high absolute rate of violence (based on cases per 100 students). In this sense, concentrations of socioeconomically distressed children are most likely to be at high risk for violence. Data over 4 decades documents this association (despite the recent upsurge in school shootings among middle-class communities).

It is a second meaning of "high risk" that is of greater relevance here, however. "High risk" can also be taken to mean that a school has a higher rate of violence *than would be predicted* from a knowledge of its socioeconomic character. Thus, two schools with similar socioeconomic profiles may have very different rates of violence. In this sense, one is a "high-risk" school and the other is a "low-risk" school, although both may have higher rates of violence than schools in other, more affluent areas.

We recognize that adults and youth may differ in their perception of the importance and emotional significance of diverse acts of aggression. A complete analysis must take into account what the students themselves are experiencing as violence or "incidents" in their schools. Moreover, adults and adolescents may not similarly define "safe" or "violent." An example of a typical research effort on this subject is the Principal/ School Disciplinarian Survey on School Violence conducted by the U.S. Department of Education in 1997. In this document, the following statement is made: " . . . about 1,000 crimes per 100,000 students *were reported* in our nations' public schools. This included about 950 crimes per 100,000 that were not serious or violent crimes (theft, vandalism, fights or assaults without a weapon) . . . " *(http://nces.ed.gov/pubs98/ violence/98030005.html*; emphasis added*)*.

This statement poses the following questions: For whom is assault without a weapon, fighting, vandalism, and theft not serious or violent? And from whose perspective? Do students concur with this conclusion? Further, it is clear that many incidents of serious concern to students and parents occur in schools on a daily basis, which are never recorded at all and are not reported to the police. Thus, any use of conventional, adult-biased data may well present a somewhat distorted picture of what kids actually experience with regard to safety and danger at school.

Figure 15.1 illustrates our context concept of relative high and low risk. In the figure, schools A and B have high actual observed rates of violence (36 per 1,000 and 34 per 1,000, respectively). Schools C and D have lower actual rates (16 per 1,000 and 14 per 1,000). However, for schools A and C, the actual observed rates are higher than predicted rates (10 per 1,000 predicted for A and 7 per 1,000 for C), whereas for schools B and D, actual rates are

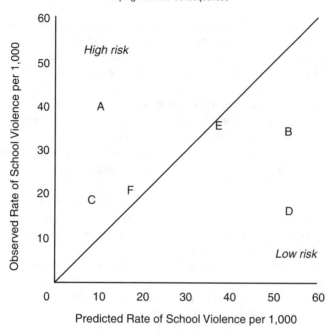

FIGURE 15.1. Two meanings of risk in assessing community areas.

lower than predicted rates (55 per 1,000 predicted for B and 54 per 1,000 D). In this sense, A and C are both high-risk, and B and D are both low-risk schools. Schools E and F evidence a close approximation between predicted and actual rates. This classification system can provide the basis for identifying contrasting social environments in schools. Unfortunately, this sort of relative, contextual risk analysis is lacking in most programmatic efforts aimed at preventing or dealing with the consequences of violence.

THE HUMAN SIGNIFICANCE OF SCHOOL RISK LEVELS

What do low- and high-risk social environments in schools look like? And do they look different to adults than they do to children? Answering these questions is important if we are to understand the essential elements and likely outcomes of social support programs seeking to prevent violence. One means of answering these questions involves examining pairs of real schools with the same predicted but different observed violence rates (i.e., one area at high risk and the other at low risk for violence). This permits a hypothesis that two such schools present contrasting environments and thus may impose contrasting differences in prevention and rehabilitation efforts.

In looking at schools as contrasting social environments, we must remember the role of individual variations in the children who "inhabit" them. There are a series of temperamental characteristics that favor active coping attempts and positive relationships with others, such as activity, goal orientation, and sociability rather than passive withdrawal. Beyond temperament, a stable emotional relationship with at least one parent or other reference person enhances coping. Similarly, an open, supportive educational climate and parental model of behavior that encourages constructive coping with problems increases the odds that a child will cope with environmental challenges. Social support from persons outside the family helps too. These factors have been identified as important when the stresses involved are in the "normal" range found in the mainstream of modern industrial societies (e.g., poverty, family conflict, childhood physical disability, and parental involvement in substance abuse). We presume that the same factors are relevant to dealing with the acute and chronic stresses of school attendance.

Of the seven factors identified in the research on resilience and coping, several are particularly relevant to our concerns (and some of the others are indirectly relevant). We are particularly interested in the factors of social support from persons outside the family; an open, supportive educational climate and parental model of behavior that encourages constructive coping with problems; and a stable emotional relationship with at least one parent or other reference person. These three factors constitute the beginning of an agenda for neighborhood support programs to prevent child maltreatment, and indeed for more macrolevel interventions as well (see Thompson, 1992).

The first factor is, of course, at the heart of our concern: "social support from persons outside the family." We see this as a generic affirmation of the validity of a social support approach. The importance of social support increases inversely with the inner resources of the family: The poorer need more help. Of course, here as elsewhere, we expect to find a kind of Catch-22 in operation: The more troubled and impoverished a family system is inside its boundaries, the less effective it will be in identifying, soliciting, and making effective use of resources outside its boundaries. This is the message of the research on neglecting families conducted by Polansky, Gaudin, and their colleagues (see Gaudin & Polansky, 1985). Neglecting parents are less ready, willing, or able to see and make use of social support in their neighborhoods, and more in need of such support, than other parents are. This vicious cycle has been demonstrated repeatedly in studies of child maltreatment (Garbarino, 1977; Vorrasi, deLara, & Bradshaw, in press). The second resilience factor explicitly targets the community's institutions. Schools, religious institutions, civic organizations, and other social entities are optimally what operationalize the concept of "an open, supportive educational climate." Programs and role models that teach and reward the reflective processing of experience are an essential feature of social support in the school.

The third resilience factor is "a stable emotional relationship with at least one parent or other reference person." How does this translate into our model of generic social support? It does so through repeated findings that depth—as opposed to simply breadth—is an important feature of social support (and one often neglected in programmatic approaches). In addition to having social support effectively available through friends, neighbors, co-workers, and professionals, parents (and children) need social support in its most intensive form: "someone who is absolutely crazy about you" (Bronfen-brenner, 1979). This is clear from research on parenting (children must have someone in this role), but it is also important in the functioning and development of youths and adults, including those in parenting roles.

It is important to remember that social support has at least two distinct dimensions. The first is its role in simply making the individual feel connected to others, which is important in its own right. The second is its role in promoting prosocial behavior (e.g., encouraging appropriate and respectful behavior among students). This offers an explanation for the finding that under conditions of social stress, families whose only social network is the kin network are more likely to abuse children than families whose network includes nonrelatives (Straus & Gelles, 1990). Kin networks are more likely than more diverse networks to offer consensus support for an interpretation of child behavior and a corresponding rationale for parent behavior. Considering the structure of social support without regard to its value and cultural content is insufficient. We can see further evidence of this by explicitly focusing on socially maladaptive methods of coping. Families forced to cope with highly stressful situations (such as the chronic danger and social impoverishment of many low-income neighborhoods, or the unstable and alienated neighborhoods that reflect community disruption even in the absence of poverty) may adapt in ways that are dysfunctional. The psychopathological dimensions of such adaptations are now widely recognized—most notably, posttraumatic stress disorder in the case of traumatic environments.

The social dimensions are equally worthy of attention, however. Families and individual family members may cope with highly stressful conditions by adopting a worldview or persona that is dysfunctional in many everyday situations in which they are expected to participate (e.g., school and other institutions of the larger community). Applying this concept to schools, we find that children who are forced to contend with highly stressful situations (such as chronic bullying, harassment, or fear of school shooting) may make adaptations that are dysfunctional and unhealthy to themselves and the school as a whole (Garbarino, 1999; Hawkins et al. 2000). For example, aggressive behavior may seem necessary and justified for the chronic crisis situations they encounter (Astor & Behre, 1997). However, such aggressive behavior may be maladaptive to school success, as it sometimes stimulates rejection by other students.

What is more, some adaptations to chronic threat and social impoverishment (such as emotional withdrawal) may be socially adaptive in the short run, but become a danger to the next generation when the individuals become parents. This phenomenon has been observed in studies of families of Holocaust survivors (Danieli, 1988). Physical withdrawal at school in the form of absenteeism is an adaptive response by some children to fears of school violence. Certainly this reaction cannot be judged maladaptive until schools can ensure safety—emotional and physical—for students. In the meantime, 160,000 children are absent each day and 9% of all students drop out each year in direct response to the danger they experience in regard to school (National Crime Prevention Council, 2001).

One of the most important contemporary efforts to place social support in the framework of youth development comes from the Search Institute (Benson, 1997). The Search Institute has put forth a way of looking at the entire social and psychological environment of children in terms of the presence or absence of a series of assets. Their research identifies 40 such assets. The more assets children or teenagers have, the less likely they are to be plagued with problems of violence (such as assaulting other children three or more times in the past 12 months), substance abuse (using illicit drugs such as cocaine, heroin, or amphetamines three or more times in the past year), and problem alcohol use (using alcohol three or more times in the past 30 days or become intoxicated one or more times in the past 2 weeks).

With 0–10 assets, 61% of the children were in the violent category; with 31–40 only 6%. The pattern is much the same for substance abuse (42% with 0–10 assets vs. 1% with 31–40) and for problem alcohol use (53% with 0–10 assets vs. 3% for 31–40). Although we cannot necessarily conclude that if we simply provide these assets kids will automatically become less violent, less drug involved, and less involved in problem alcohol use, we can conclude that the more assets children have in their lives the more likely it is that they will be acting as we hope they will act.

This view is consistent with the findings of the Search Institute when it comes to positive behaviors. For academic success (judged as getting mostly A's on a report card), valuing diversity (placing high importance on getting to know people of other races and ethnic groups), maintaining good health (paying attention to nutrition and exercise), and delaying gratification (saving money for something special rather than spending it all right now), the picture is a mirror image of the problem behaviors: The more assets kids have, the more positive they are. Whereas only 7% of children with 0–10 assets succeed in school, 53% of those with 31–40 assets do. Whereas only 27% of those with 0–10 assets delay gratification, 72% of those within the 31–40 range do.

The assets are grouped into eight categories. Some of these assets are under the direct control of parents in their role as parents—for example, "Parent(s) are actively involved in helping young person succeed in school." But many others are characteristics of the school or community—for example, "School provides a caring, encouraging environment" and "Neighbors take responsibility for monitoring young people's behavior." There is much to be done in support of children outside the actions of parents as parents, but even the parent-oriented assets can benefit from social support.

For example, it is easier to promote "reading for pleasure at least three hours per week" in a community that demonstrates its commitment to literacy via the public library. Actually getting kids to "spend three or more hours per week in lessons or practice in music, theater, or other arts" is more likely in a community that supports music and art in school and perhaps even has a community school of music and the arts. A 1995 Gallop poll conducted for *Parenting* magazine revealed that 90% of parents said they had talked to their children about God. That is a good start, but it is most likely to translate into the asset "Young person spends one or more hours per week in activities in a religious institution" in a community that is rich with religious institutions and other supports for spiritual practice. These are institutional supports for the assets children need to develop in a positive way. Schools play a decisive role, both as the site for assets and as a source of community leadership in promoting assets in other contexts (e.g. family, neighborhood, and community institutions).

SCHOOL SIZE AS A CASE STUDY

Second to what happens in their homes, perhaps the biggest immediate influences on youth are their peer groups and the schools they attend. An often overlooked feature of schools that contributes to the difficulties students face is the size of their schools—most notably the high schools. Put most simply, big high schools encourage spectatorship and the "herd feeling," (Barker & Gump, 1964) rather than participation, and exclude all but a small proportion of their students from leadership roles and other developmentally enhancing activities. As a result, they leave the majority of students at loose ends and the most vulnerable ripe for the destructive pressures of the socially toxic environment (Garbarino, 1980).

In contrast, small schools enhance affirmation and identity because they draw students into participation and leadership. They offer challenges that stimulate the development of competence. They can potentially monitor behavior more effectively. All these effects are strongest for the students most at risk for alienation and dropping out, the academically marginal students.

A visit to the smallest public high school in Nassau County, outside New York City, after a 30-year absence found that even academically and socially marginal kids had a sense of belonging there. They said things like, "It's like a family here. You know you can count on everyone. You know everyone." They said, "You can't get away with anything here. Someone always notices what you are doing." That is a good recipe for positive development in teenagers, to act so the kids will think: "People care about me, and they prove it by paying attention to what I do—both the good and the bad." This orientation lies at the core of "character."

The initial research on high school size, performed in the 1950s and 1960s, documented the superiority of small schools in providing a positive environment for teenagers. However, just as this evidence was becoming available, social forces and deliberate policy were closing and consolidating small schools in favor of big ones. This research—much of it conducted by psychologists Roger Barker and Paul Gump and their colleagues in Kansas—found that large schools tend to discourage students from meaningful participation in the social and extracurricular activities of the school.

As a result, their sense of personal ownership for what happens in the school and their sense of responsibility are diminished. Currently, research on the impact and effects of school size, both academically and socially, is again under way. The resurgence has happened in the wake of serious outbreaks of violence and is also due to the impact of school consolidation on communities as a whole. Similar results are being found as were reported in the early research (Gates, Boyter, Walker, & Hill, 1998; Raywid, 1998; Schroth & Fishbaugh, 2000).

The research demonstrated that although the large school provides more settings in which students can act, there are proportionately more adolescents to fill those spots (thus the large school has proportionately more people than positions). Small high schools, in contrast, have proportionately more positions than students to fill them. For example, although a large school may have both a chorus and a glee club, together these two settings can accommodate only a very small proportion of the student body, so it is still hard for any given student (particularly a student with little talent) to get into either activity. A small high school may have only one vocal group, but is apt to be so eager for voices that any student willing to make the effort to participate will be welcomed.

The kinds of satisfactions reported by students differ in the small schools versus large schools. Researchers find that students from small schools report satisfaction associated with the development of responsibility, competence, challenge, inclusion, and a sense of identity (Barker, 1986; Barker & Gump, 1964; deLara, 2000; Fanning, 1995; Garbarino, 1980; Garbarino & Bedard, 2001). They were being drawn into positions of responsibility and activity on behalf of prosocial goals—putting on concerts, organizing meetings, practicing and working in teams in preparation for competing in athletic events. This is the stuff of which healthy environments are made, particularly for children who do not bring to the situation all the internal resources and motivation needed to succeed *despite the social environment*.

In contrast, most students in large high schools emphasized vicarious, passive enjoyment, being part of a large crowd, watching the elite perform, and generally feeling part of a nameless, faceless crowd—what Barker and Gump (1964) called the "herd feeling." This may have been tolerable 50 years ago, when there were fewer children coming to school loaded with the family risk factors of separation and divorce, when there were not the same temptations of drugs that confront children today, when the mass media were tame by today's standards, when the larger structures of adult authority were largely intact, and when teenagers who dropped out of high school could still get on track occupationally. Today the costs are much greater, and the need to go to a school that compensates for the larger toxic society is dramatically greater.

In large high schools at-risk kids are superfluous; in small high schools they are needed. Although behavior that is inclusive or exclusive, that is respectful or disrespectful, by teachers, staff, or students is currently under assessment for its impact on all students (deLara, 2001; Garbarino & Bedard, 2001), what is central is the human ecology of the school. Psychologist Rudolph Moos (1974) uses the term "the principle of progressive conformity" to describe the fact that people tend to become what their environment elicits and rewards. Large schools elicit and reward passivity and marginal involvement among most students, and leadership and activity only among the elite. Small schools elicit and reward participation and responsibility among the whole student body as a matter of necessity.

What constitutes a big or small school? In the 1950s and early 1960s research concluded that after a school exceeds 500 students in grades 9–12 it quickly takes on the dynamics of bigness. From 1955 to 1975 the average size of U.S. high schools grew from approximately 500 to 1,500 students. Currently, many large high schools have the appearance and the atmosphere of factories—or even worse, of prisons. Elaborate security systems are in place in an attempt to keep track of students. But even so, the schools leak students all day long.

In contrast, small schools like the one in Nassau County, New York or those in rural areas do not typically suffer from a sense of anomie. Students are accounted for and feel that they are known by the staff and teachers.

But even small schools today are not immune to the forces at work in the society to undermine the successful development of our kids. One of us (E. deL.) undertook an in-depth study of how safe kids felt in a small high school located in a rural part of New York State. As it happened, she conducted the first part of her study in the fall of the 1998–1999 school year and then completed her study at the end of the spring term. This permitted her to observe the impact of the Columbine High School shooting on the perceived safety of the school.

What she found is disturbing. Prior to Columbine, 82% of the students said, "I can count on it that the teachers or other adults would stop someone from hurting me or anyone else in the classroom." After Columbine, only 60% of the same students agreed. Even the small high school is vulnerable to the corrosive effects of social toxicity in our society, but it does have many advantages for the students who attend and the parents who send them there. The small school is an asset for the community and for the families, and a setting easier to make safe.

CONCLUSION

The dynamic interaction of people, practices, and policies in the school itself is another factor that is relevant in the foundation for screening to identify high- and low-risk schools. Any given school may be functional or dysfunctional, healthy or unhealthy for the children and adults in its environment, just as in family functioning. The functioning of a school as a system must be taken into account in any appraisal of risk. The school, like any other organization, will work to maintain homeostasis (deLara, 2000; Dowling & Osborne, 1994; Gaynor, 1998). Typically, that means maintaining procedures and practices that are "tried and true" despite their questionable contemporary usefulness. An example of this is the idea of student empowerment through active involvement in policy decision making. In most schools students have little real power to influence educational decisions or school climate issues. It is exactly this sense of helplessness, however, that has a profound impact on adolescents' sense of safety at school (deLara, 2000). Young people need to be involved in a meaningful way in formulating and implementing decisions that directly affect their work environment—the school.

It is extremely difficult for parents and guardians to tolerate the idea that their children may attend a school that is anything but safe. That school may be a daily battlefield is anathema for any parent. If school is unsafe, how can a caring adult go about his or her day with any equanimity? Turning a blind eye, or only half knowing what is happening in the neighborhood elementary or secondary school, is what allows caregivers to continue to function in their already busy and stressful lives. Not knowing is what also permits the schools to continue to function in their current manner—whether that is adaptive or maladaptive, whether it is supportive, safe, and caring for children or only purporting to be so.

Violence is a symptom not only of troubled individual children at school, but also of the schools, families, and communities from which they come. Anxiety about the possibility of violence or fear of the threat of violence is an everyday experience for children in American schools today.

We know that many children can absorb and surmount the obstacles that one or two risk factors present to them; however, at this juncture, we cannot be certain about the impact of the accumulation of anxieties experienced by many youth on a daily basis in our schools. Research has yet to determine the correlation of fear of violence (as in taunting, harassment, and physical harm) with fear of, or isolation from, the school community. Research has yet to firmly establish the correlation between harassment and eventual violent acting out of students in a school system. What does seem clear is that adults are coping with violence at school by misplacing responsibility for prevention and intervention, shifting it from themselves, for the most part, to children and youth. This displacement of responsibility for prevention and intervention is, in itself, a symptom of an unhealthy school and community system and, if allowed to continue, will facilitate and enable violence in our schools.

All adult stakeholders in the school community must be willing to take responsibility for school safety by providing leadership and supervision. Students must be empowered through meaningful avenues of contribution to school policy and to their school climate.

REFERENCES

Astor, R. A., & Behre, W. (1997). Violent and nonviolent children's and parents' reasoning about family and peer violence. *Behavioral Disorders, 22,* 4, 231–245.

Austin, M. (1978). *Professionals and paraprofessionals.* New York: Human Sciences Press.

Barker, B. (1986). *The advantages of small schools* (Report No. ED 265 988). East Lansing, MI: National Center for Research on Teacher Learning. (ERIC Document Reproduction Service.)

Barker, R. G., & Gump, P. V. (1964). *Big school, small school: High school size and student behavior.* Stanford, CA: Stanford University Press.

Benson, P. (1997). *All our kids are our kids: What communities must do to raise caring and responsible children and adolescents.* San Francisco: Jossey-Bass.

Bronfenbrenner, U. (1979). *The ecology of human development: Experiments by nature and design.* Cambridge, MA: Harvard University Press.

Caplan, G. (1976). *Support systems and community mental health.* New York: Behavioral Publications.

Danieli, Y. (1988). The treatment and prevention of long-term effects and intergenerational transmission of victimization: A lesson from Holocaust survivors and their children. In C. Figley (Ed.), *Trauma and its wake.* New York: Brunner/Mazel.

deLara, E. W. (2000). *Adolescents' perceptions of safety at school and their solutions for enhancing safety and decreasing school violence: A rural case study.* Unpublished doctoral dissertation, Cornell University.

deLara, E. W. (2001). *Pre and post Columbine effect: Students' perceptions of safety at school.* Manuscript submitted for publication.

Dowling, E., & Osborne, E. (Eds.). (1994). *The family and the school: A joint systems approach to problems with children.* New York: Routledge.

Fanning, J. (1995). *Rural school consolidation and student learning* (Report No. ED 384 484). East Lansing, MI: National Center for Research on Teacher Learning. ERIC Document Reproduction Service.

Garbarino, J. (1977). The human ecology of child maltreatment: A conceptual model for research. *Journal of Marriage and the Family, 39,* 721–736.

Garbarino, J. (1980). Some thoughts on school size and its effects on adolescent development. *Journal of Youth and Adolescence, 9*(1), 19–31.

Garbarino, J. (1987). Family support and the prevention of child maltreatment. In S. Kagan, R. Powell, B. Weissbourd, & E. Zigler (Eds.), *America's family support programs*. New Haven, CT: Yale University Press.

Garbarino, J. (1999*) Lost boys: Why our sons turn violent and how we can save them*. New York: Free Press.

Garbarino, J., & Bedard, C. (2001*) Parents under siege: Why you are the solution, not the problem in your child's life*. New York: Free Press.

Garbarino, J., & Crouter, A. (1978). Defining the community context of parent–child relations. *Child Development, 49,* 604–616.

Garbarino, J., & deLara, E. (2002). *And words can hurt forever: Protecting adolescents from bullying, harassment, and emotional violence*. New York: Free Press.

Gates, G. S., Boyter, G. A., Walker, J. T., & Hill, H. (1998). School community: A better way for addressing school violence. *Rural Special Education Quarterly, 17*(3–4), 39–47.

Gaudin, J., & Polansky, N. (1985). Social distancing of the neglectful family: Sex, race, and social class influences. *Social Service Review, 58,* 245–253.

Gaynor, A. K. (1998). *Analyzing problems in schools and school systems: A theoretical approach*. Mahwah, NJ: Erlbaum.

Gibbs, J. C., Granville, B. P., & Goldstein, A. P. (1995). *The equip program: Teaching youth to think and act responsibly through a peer-helping approach*. Champaign, IL: Research Press.

Halpern, R. (1990). Community-based early intervention. In S. J. Meisels &J. A. Shonkoff (Eds.), *Handbook of early childhood intervention*. Cambridge, UK: Cambridge University Press.

Hawkins, J. D., Herrenkohl, T. I., Farrington, D. P., Brewer, D., Catalano, R. F., Harachi, T. W., & Cothern, L. (2000). *Predictors of youth violence*. Washington, DC: U.S. Department of Justice.

Hyman, I., & Snook, P. (1999). *Dangerous schools: What we can do about the physical and emotional abuse of our children*. San Francisco: Jossey-Bass.

Melton, G. (1992). It's time for neighborhood research and action. *Child Abuse and Neglect, 16,* 4.

Moos, R. (1974). Systems for the assessment and classification of human environments: An overview. In R. H. Moos & P. M. Insel (Eds.), *Issues in social ecology*. Palo Alto, CA: National Press Books.

Musick, J., & Stott, F. (1990). Paraprofessionals, parenting and child development: Understanding the problems and seeking solutions. In S. J. Meisels & J. P. Shonkoff (Eds.), *Handbook of early childhood intervention*. Cambridge, UK: Cambridge University Press.

National Crime Prevention Council. (2001). [On-line]. Available: *http://www.ncpc.org*

Naylor, P., & Cowie, H. (1999). The effectiveness of peer support systems in challenging school bullying: The perspectives and experiences of teachers and pupils. *Journal of Adolescence, 22,* 467–479.

Pelton, L. (1978). Child abuse and neglect: The myth of classlessness. *American Journal of Orthopsychiatry, 48,* 608–617.

Pelton, L. (1981). *The social context of child abuse and neglect*. New York: Human Sciences Press.

Pelton, L. (1992). *The role of material factors in child abuse and neglect*. Washington, DC: U.S. Advisory Board on Child Abuse and Neglect.

Raywid, M. A. (1998). Small schools: A reform that works. *Educational Leadership, 55*(4), 34–39.

Schroth, G., & Fishbaugh, M. S. (2000, March 16–18). Increasing caring and reducing violence in rural schools. In *Capitalizing on leadership in rural special education: Making a difference for children and families.* Conference Proceedings, Alexandria, VA. ERIC Document Reproduction Service No. ED 439 869.

Straus, M., & Gelles, R. (1990). *Physical violence in American families.* New Brunswick, NJ: Transaction Publications.

Thompson, R. (1992). *Social support and the prevention of child maltreatment.* Washington, DC: U.S. Advisory Board on Child Abuse and Neglect.

Vorrasi, J. A., deLara, E. W., & Bradshaw, C. P. (in press). Psychological maltreatment. In A. Giadino (Ed.). *Child maltreatment: A clinical guide and reference.* St. Louis, MO: G.W. Medical Publishing.

Warren, R. (1978). *The community in America.* Boston: Houghton Mifflin.

Weiss, H., & Halpern, R. (1991). *Community-based family support and education programs: Something old or something new?* New York: National Center for Children in Poverty, Columbia University.

CHAPTER 16

The Real World
Good Ideas Are Never Enough

JANE CLOSE CONOLEY
JEREMY R. SULLIVAN

This book contains the latest and best evidence-based programs to increase school safety. A chasm exists, however, between effective programs and successful school-based implementation. This chasm is caused not only by ignorance of new programs, but also by the lack of attention to program implementation challenges.

The distance between the best answer and the disturbing problem must be traversed by principals, consultants, and staff members armed with state-of-the-art information about school safety, school culture, and innovation dissemination. This chapter is about getting schools ready to use evidence-based school safety programs. In particular, the purpose of the chapter is to provide practical guidance to anyone whose responsibility includes assisting others in solving problems and implementing programs related to preventing school violence. Knowing about school safety programs is necessary, but insufficient, to guarantee success. If merely knowing about something were sufficient to cause change, the only challenge at hand would be information dissemination. Clearly, this is not the case.

This chapter is meant to facilitate the adoption of school safety programs by focusing on creating systemic contexts that are open to change and have the resilience to maintain innovation. This work may be termed *intervention priming* because the target is to assist the system's readiness for and use of programs. Anyone who has worked in a school (or almost any other organization) realizes the wisdom of the ancient parable that suggests seeds spread on hard ground will not germinate. Preparing the system for change is as important as introducing the correct change.

There is an annotated list of related research at the end of the chapter. Those who wish to develop skills in preparing systems for change may benefit from studying some of these references in depth.

WHOSE JOB IS IT?

School personnel are vitally concerned with school safety, but school safety is not a school's primary mission. Teaching and learning are the missions of school. Thus, no one in a school is called a safety system primer or system change agent, although such a role is badly needed and can be assumed by a number of individuals. School principals, superintendents, counselors, psychologists, and special education teachers are likely candidates for the work described here. All of these people may have broad access across a school building or organization and may have training backgrounds that include consultation and system change theory and practice.

The exact job title of the person is of less importance than his or her having a repertoire of skills and attitudes necessary for success. Position does hold some power, however, in predicting influence. Clearly, a principal or superintendent who cultivates a system to be open to new ideas and programs does so with greater structural power than does a school psychologist or counselor. Yet, the principal's position may interfere with his or her receiving authentic feedback from teachers, resulting in the adoption of programs that are maintained only to satisfy a boss rather than as a true change in the way schooling is accomplished. The appearance of new programming as a sham may be more damaging than no programming at all. Myriad half-hearted attempts at change fuel the perception among many teachers either that nothing is really effective in improving a troublesome situation or that a passive, resistant approach will outlast any change effort.

WHAT IS YOUR ROLE?

Leaders

If you are a system administrator/leader, your role is to hire the right people, to create human systems that support and reinforce people who are willing to adopt effective innovations, and to fire people who do not perform. Sounds simple? In fact, many school leaders inherit most of their staff from previous regimes, and even the people they select will likely have difficulty staying abreast of every promising program aimed at increasing school safety.

Administrators have the advantage, however, of being able to complete needs assessments in their organizations. This is a powerful technique to create a felt need for change and provide some signposts for possible program development. Collecting and using data that bring an issue into sharp focus is a first and vital step in getting a system ready to change. People must come to believe that change is unavoidable and desirable. They often come to such realizations when the magnitude of a problem becomes known or the costs of inaction are outlined in ways that create motivation for change. For example, when the costs of cleaning up graffiti or replacing vandalized equipment are shown to impact the day-to-day well-being of individuals, they can find the energy to support a new prevention program.

In addition, leaders can sponsor big events and ongoing booster sessions to educate entire schools in particular approaches to classroom management, family relationships, or teamwork. The principal can reward teachers and other professionals who experiment with the new techniques by offering them time to plan and time to receive advanced training. When successes are showcased, interventions can spread across school buildings and districts.

Of course, persistence is the key to change. Superintendents, principals, and other supervisors must have realistic time lines and recognize the need to continue to offer support to veteran staff, as well as training to novices. Organizational change, unless occurring amid a crisis situation, is often a 3–5 year adventure. A pattern of adopting and then dropping programs, on an annual basis, interferes with teachers', parents', and students' embracing new programs as part of their everyday expectations.

In addition to persistence, most leadership people must cultivate a leadership team to ensure that systems are ready for change. The leadership team must be cohesive and have great clarity of purpose. If there is disagreement among members of the leadership team, staff members will be left to choose whether to take part in innovative programming.

A system is primed for flexibility when the goals are clear and the leadership team gives consistent messages about purpose and strategies. Clear and frequent communication provides security for staff members about how they can succeed. Of course, such communication need not be unidirectional. The best plans are often the products of systemwide discussion and contribution.

Consultants

Anyone can be a consultant in getting a system ready for change. Consultation is a change strategy that is embedded in the relationship between a consultant and his or her consultees (e.g., educators, parents, and other professionals) working to improve a client situation (e.g., insubordinate speech from students). The consultant strives to offer another point of view for consultees to consider. This alternative perspective may deal with an individual client (e.g., a student) or an entire system. A consultant is preeminently a support for problem solving within a system. Common wisdom suggests that many problems cannot be solved at the same level of their creation. That is, for example, we cannot improve a child's behavior only by working with the child. We strive therefore to "think outside the box." Consultants assist consultees in overcoming lacks in skills, knowledge, or attitudes that interfere with discovering and applying solutions.

Consultants can play a key role in priming systems for interventions to reduce school violence. They can assess systems in terms of the skills of the staff and the need for and motivation for change. To ensure success, consultants must identify the real power brokers in a system and how decisions are actually made. In some schools, a few powerful senior teachers with political connections to the school board can make or break any program. If these individuals are not targeted for investment in a program, little progress is likely.

Consultants can identify and deliver resources needed for adoption—for example, training in particular programs. In the best of cases, conversations with a consultant leave a consultee with an increased number of available choices and clear road maps toward more resources for problem solving. In contrast to supervision, this approach permits consultees to decide whether to accept alternatives offered by consultants. Ideally, the relationship is confidential and built on peer respect.

Consultation can be focused on facilitating change in an individual student or group (e.g., classroom of children or parents). For example, a consulting psychologist may assess a child's social skills and offer information about social skills training programs that can teach the child to negotiate differences rather than to punch adversaries. This approach is called client-centered consultation because the target for change is primarily the client.

In contrast, consultee-centered consultation focuses on developing new skills in the client's caregiver (e.g., teacher, parent, principal). A consultant uses this approach when consultees are missing some important skills, knowledge, or attitudes. Consultees who have inaccurate or missing knowledge bases can be unsuccessful in large numbers of cases, even those that are not particularly challenging. An example of this approach is a consulting special education teacher assisting a regular education teacher to revise curriculum tasks to make them more appropriate for children with reading disabilities. Such revisions can allow the child with a disability to be successful and engaged in academic tasks, rather than disruptive and angry at failure.

Finally, program-centered consultation is oriented toward helping systems identify and adopt new programs to solve problems. The consultant's role is not to market a particular approach but to help consultees choose among available alternatives, adapt programs to local situations, evaluate effectiveness, and ensure institutionalization of positive changes. Program-centered consultation may be particularly important in system priming.

A consultant who is well versed in the research that supports various school safety programs can be invaluable to a system looking for an intervention. Such expertise allows for informed choice and full knowledge of the inevitable caveats associated with any program (e.g., not well researched with children from the inner city; takes significant amount of a teacher's time and attention; available only with English-language supporting materials). Further, a well-prepared consultant can assist the school system in establishing and conducting formative and summative evaluations. Continuous data streams are vital in adjusting programs and in keeping participants' motivation high.

In practice, of course, the expert consultant uses all approaches blended to meet a system's needs. The important aspect of considering these models separately, however, is that their use keeps the consultant facilitating change at multiple levels. For a complete discussion of models of consultation, see Caplan (1970) and Conoley and Conoley (1992).

The following section discusses some personal skills necessary for getting systems ready for change. We call the system-priming change agent a *consultant* to indicate that anyone in a school can occupy this role.

PERSONAL SKILLS NECESSARY FOR SYSTEM CHANGE

What does a consultant need to know in order to be successful? The key consultation skills are as follows:

- System assessment skills
- Communication skills
- Problem-solving skills

System Assessment

Most school-based practitioners engage in child-centered assessment. Such assessments may relate to cognitive, social, emotional, or behavior skills. Because most assessment is individually focused, most of the difficulties schools have with challenging children are conceptualized as residing within the children. In consultation language, this conceptualization describes problems as residing inside the client and suggests the use of client-centered consultation. Although a common approach, complete reliance on strategies for effecting change in a child is likely to be unsuccessful. Most people have difficulty with change, and almost all troubling children do not believe that the problem is their fault. Their lack of insight and motivation to change make them particularly challenging change targets.

Throughout this book, successful direct interventions have been described. All, however, depend on the willingness of many of the adult caregivers in a system to change in order to support improvement in the troubling child. The vital importance of caregiver change is very often overlooked. In fact, one of the major obstacles to a system's embracing a needed change is the belief or attitude that "others must change—not I!"

The consultant must be able to assess the conditions within an individual and the individual's life space (e.g., classroom, interactions with peers or parents, success with academic tasks) and be skilled at assessing the more macro-level environments that surround the troubling child (including, for example, schoolwide discipline practices, poverty, racism, chaotic neighborhoods). In fact, the skill of shifting among and between levels of assessment may be one of the most valuable perspectives a consultant can offer a school.

For example, a consultant who can determine that the trip to school through a sinister neighborhood is a factor in school absenteeism opens up a new world of intervention possibilities for a community concerned with its children's academic success. Rather than punitive visits from an attendance officer, a school might sponsor "walk your children to school days" or work with community police to position extra officers during morning and afternoon entries and exits from school.

Teachers, who are involved in the day-to-day hassles of responding to challenging children, may have tremendous difficulty in considering anything but child-focused coercive interactions (e.g., yelling, punishments, and time out). In fact, however, alternative approaches to analyze the behavior must be discovered. These may include the following:

- Another understanding of the child (e.g., a child with street smartness may be channeled to academic success by a focus on leadership)
- Additional training for teachers to enable them to have multiple approaches to problem solving (e.g., social skills, cooperative learning, social-emotional approaches, parent involvement)
- More classroom personnel (e.g., aides or student teachers who can give one-on-one attention to troubling individuals)
- A schoolwide commitment to a particular way of responding to insubordinate children (e.g., zero tolerance for minor verbal disrespect, resulting in small-group training for children)

Any or all of these approaches may be absolutely necessary to increase the safety of a school building, and all require the adults to shift targets for change in order to create the desired result of pleasant teacher–student interactions. Facilitating change among the adult caregivers in a school is quite a task, but one that must be successful if school buildings are to become contexts that elicit peaceful, task-oriented behavior among the entire community.

Communication

Readers may be tempted to skip a section on communication skills. Is there anything really new? Perhaps there is little new information about successful communication, but there is a huge gap between knowledge and action. Our experience suggests that the greatest single cause of program failure in schools is not the poor worth of the program but the poor communication surrounding it.

Priming a system to accept change requires that a program be clearly understood and that program implementers have created investment in the program's success among a large number of, or a key faction of, the adult caregivers. The absolute value or research base of a program may have very little to do with its adoption and maintenance.

Listening

The basic skills learned by many educators in beginning counseling classes are still valuable. Listen to what the consultee says about situations that interfere with program implementation. Verbally repeat, reflect, or paraphrase what is heard to ensure that true understanding has been achieved. Elaborate on what consultees say, rather than immediately introducing new information, so that consultees see their influence on program development. Ask clarifying questions about situations faced by consultees so they know that the consultant really appreciates the dilemmas and challenges they face. Offer tentative alternatives, rather than dogmatic truths, so that consultees always have the experience of being in control of program development and implementation.

Positive Reinforcement

Other very basic skills include a willingness and ability to express affection or positive statements regarding the consultee. The best consultants sound, and *are*, quite accepting of others. Their words and actions are congruent. They are empathic, perceptive individuals who hear the words said by consultees as well as the emotional music that plays in the background. Although consultants do not necessarily follow up on every emotional expression from a consultee, they do assess whether particular emotions or stresses are likely to interfere with problem solving and adjust their behavior accordingly. For example, teachers who have just had a very upsetting interaction with a child or a parent may need support, not more advice about how to do better in the future.

Summarizing

Consultants must be flexible. Because their role is to help systems solve problems, they do not assume rigid control of interactions or topics. This flexibility is balanced, however, with the skill of pursuing important issues. Although consultees may wander a bit in their reports of program difficulties, the consultant picks out the important issues and pursues these so that both can have a sense of direction and momentum toward problem solving. A companion skill to pursuing issues is the ability to sum up well. A surprising amount of information can be saved and used if consultants take time to periodically sum up the main points of a conversation with an emphasis on decisions made and action steps planned. Follow-up notes and visits are vital to keeping verbal promises in the forefront for busy consultees.

Reframing

Somewhat more advanced communication skills are also necessary. Consultants know the power of positive reframing and connotation. Successful use of this technique challenges the consultant to find the kernel of truth or good intention in any statement. For example, the consultee who expresses doubt about the worth of a change or a program can be complimented for being a healthy skeptic and for considering change thoughtfully.

This skill is surprisingly effective at disarming the resistance many people feel at the mere suggestion of change. Practice makes using positive connotation or reframing an almost automatic skill.

For example, during a recent conversation a consultant encountered a rather racist attitude in a young white teacher who was struggling to fit into a school dominated by black teachers. She felt that she was being misunderstood and stereotyped by the older black teachers and not allowed to show her true skills and attitudes. She bemoaned the effect "those people" were having on her. The consultant listened with care and wondered aloud whether her experiences might be paralleling those of young black teachers in schools dominated by older white teachers. The consultant congratulated the consultee on having the courage to examine these feelings and expressed confidence that she would use the experience to better understand the plight of others who are in minority groups. With some surprise, the consultee began to consider that the anger, disengagement, and futility she felt as a consequence of her minority status might be the same that black teachers and students feel in majority-dominated contexts.

Attributional Language

Another more slightly advanced communication skill for consultants to perfect is the use of attributional language. In both their self-talk and public conversations with consultees, consultants are well advised to use internal and unstable explanations for behavior. Thus, consultants should emphasize that personal effort and dedication can cause change. We are not the victims of our environments. At the same time, consultants should focus on the truth that behavior, once understood, can be changed. Consultees must believe (as consultants must) that problems are amenable to change through effort. Such beliefs run counter to the common wisdom prevalent in many schools that much of what is wrong with children is out of the control of teachers and that some people/families/ethnic groups/social classes are "just that way" (e.g., lazy, uncaring, unmotivated) and cannot be changed.

For example, a consultant can talk about success stories related to families and children who are similar to the population served by a particular school. By providing examples of success associated with personal effort, a consultee's hopeless attitudes may be ameliorated. Further, the consultant should always seize upon opportunities to compliment the consultee for making changes through personal effort—no matter how trivial these may seem.

Self-Disclosure

Another advanced communication skill necessary for consultation success is understanding how much self-disclosure by a consultant is helpful for system improvement. A certain degree of personal openness is valuable. Consultees can learn from consultants about how to cope with stress or how to conceptualize and problem solve if consultants are overt in sharing personal processes. Yet too much self-disclosure about personal and private matters is very likely to reduce consultation effectiveness. Not only does it detract from engaged problem-solving time, but too much self-disclosure is likely to create gratuitous issues between a consultee and a consultant. These may include political, religious, or personality conflicts with one or more individuals or cliques in a school. Sharing too much information can undermine perceptions of a consultant's expertise, objectivity, and commitment to confidentiality.

Consultants can, however, share positive self-views and reinforcing information about others. They can tell how they have dealt with conflict in open and relationship-enhancing ways. They can describe how they have learned from others who have been willing to be direct. Consultants who describe their own initial uneasiness about taking risks can provide coping models to consultees. Consultees may need support to expect success or to trust that recovery from mistakes is possible.

Giving Feedback

Change agents must be skilled at giving and getting feedback. Feedback is information we offer to another person about how that person's behavior affects us or the implementation of a program. Most people would rather eat worms than offer candid appraisals to others! This reluctance prevents valid data from getting into the hands of people who need it. There are some simple steps to follow in giving feedback, however, that are likely to reduce defensiveness and give others a chance to improve their performance.

1. *Timing.* Give feedback closely after the behavior being noted, but do not overload people with information. If a teacher is drained after a tough day with disruptive children, focus on positives and aspects of the program that were well executed. Save constructive criticism until the teacher's energy and outlook may enable him or her to learn.

2. *Specifics.* Give feedback that is specific about a behavior and about a behavior that is observable. Telling people they are "negative" or "positive" does not give them much to go on. Mentioning that you are impressed with their use of reinforcement when children raised their hands can be the basis of behavior enhancement. Mentioning that you were concerned when you overheard them using profanity in front of children gives them a clue about what is not acceptable.

3. *Needs of the receiver.* Feedback is meant to assist the receiver, not to make the giver appear insightful or to allow the giver to express hostility. Whether or not the receiver can use this feedback must be a primary consideration. Letting me, the receiver, know that my Muslim heritage is an obstacle for some parents in a school does not give me anything to change, just something to worry about.

4. *Tentative delivery.* The best feedback is delivered often in a rather gentle manner. Dogmatic feedback may lead to dogmatic resistance. A style like this, "From my perspective, your handling of the fight among the fifth graders today didn't get you the result you probably intended. Am I right?" keeps the door open for additional conversation. In contrast, saying, "You did not follow program guidelines in dealing with that fight" is likely to invite a defensive reaction.

5. *I-statements.* A beginning rule in communication is to weight your messages with "I-statements" rather than "you-statements." Labeling yourself as concerned or excited or wary is safe. Labeling others is always dangerous. This rule suggests that people are less defensive and resistant to hearing about how others experience events and more defensive about hearing themselves being rated or interpreted. For example, a consultant can say, "When DeNeetra began to talk in the group, I felt elated. It seemed your strategies were really paying off." This is better than saying, "You must have been happy to finally see some results from your work with the social skills group." The first approach communicates the consultant's admiration. The second approach invites the teacher to dispute how well the group performed or whether or he or she is satisfied with progress.

Getting Feedback

If consultants are working effectively in moving a system toward change, they will attract attention. It is very likely that other members of the system will have feedback for them. Following some simple rules about receiving feedback can keep communication lines open. Such openness is critical for system priming. People must experience their influence on any program if it is to be adopted in a meaningful way.

Think about receiving feedback in seven steps. First, take a deep breath and, second, really listen. Third, ask clarifying questions about the feedback—that is, *when, where,* and *how often* questions that let the speaker know that you are taking the information seriously. Fourth, reflect on what you have heard and attempt to link it to other input you have received. For example, the fifth person who mentions that your tendency to interrupt makes you a difficult team member may be giving you some valid information. Fifth, do not give excuses. Thank the person for sharing the information and let him or her know that you will think about it (especially if it is negative information) or that you are most thankful for it (especially if it is positive information). No one needs to hear that your rudeness (e.g., interrupting) is due to poor parental models or that your success is just accidental. Sixth, if the feedback indicates that your behavior is having a troubling effect on others, get over it. Effective change agents do not get mired in personal reactions to emotional content. It is easy to like and to approach those who are always supportive and complimentary. It is much more difficult to keep approaching those who have been critical. A willingness to keep relationships with both supporters and critics, however, separates change agents from mere members of an organization. Finally, step seven is to move on to action. If consultees are delighted with what you are doing, then do more. If your behavior is unsettling to the group, get some supervision about how to be more facilitating.

Sometimes the feedback a consultant receives is about the program being implemented. It is common for program consultants to develop a sense of ownership of particular program parts or goals and therefore to be defensive about hearing others' distaste for a program. Getting a system ready for change and resilient enough to maintain the change, however, demands that the consultant keep the focus on relationships among the adults in the system. Defending a program may give some momentary satisfaction, but losing the investment of others in program implementation may be the long-term outcome. People implement programs and so must receive support, interest, and guidance.

Summary of Communication Skills

People who are consultants must rely on their personal skills to help others consider change. Even leadership individuals learn that skills in motivating and supporting change are more important than the power to command a change. To be successful in the work of supporting change, consultants must be able to:

- Confront situations in helpful and nondefensive ways.
- Anticipate situations and individuals' reactions to stress
- Take risks in introducing new information into systems and be persistent in championing new approaches to old problems.
- Believe in the competence of the consultees so that the internal resources and problem-solving skills of a system are supported and reinforced.

- Be an expert in giving and receiving feedback so all the intended and unintended consequences of a particular program can be explored and accommodated.

Problem Solving

Another set of much described, but rarely practiced, skills are involved in problem solving. Our experience is that many of the disturbances faced by school systems are ignored or reacted to with very general strategies. Getting a system ready to adopt a change demands that a problem or a goal become shared by a number of key individuals. Once a critical number of people agree that something must be done, for example, to increase students' skills in using polite conversation, the problem solving can begin. Obstacles to this first step are pessimism, apathy, helplessness, and hopelessness. All that has been described earlier in this chapter is meant to help the members of the system avoid the trap of feeling powerless to change a troubling situation. A can-do attitude with a belief in each member's ability to make a difference is absolutely essential to problem solving. Without that, no amount of problem analysis will lead to changed behaviors.

Once the participants in an organization agree to put their energies into solving a problem, the effective next steps are simple to teach.

1. *Analyze problem antecedents and consequences.* The most direct way to eliminate a problem is to eliminate the conditions that cause it to happen or the conditions that reinforce its appearance. If fights among students are most common during class transitions, a reasonable approach is to reduce or eliminate the number of times students are all in the hall together. Removing the setting that is used to display a certain behavior is often the most effective in stopping the behavior. Alternately, if graffiti is ruining the appearance of a school, implicated students can be invited to paint murals on certain surfaces after taking part in a graffiti cleanup program. Many schools in inner cities have all but eliminated graffiti vandalism by using student talents in new and even more reinforcing ways.

2. *Identify responsible parties.* Many problem-solving efforts fall apart because people responsible for implementing agreed-upon strategies are not clearly named and held accountable. How many times have you left a meeting during which many ideas were shared, but no assignment of responsibility was given? This pattern plagues system readiness for change because it creates a sense that action is futile. People mistake the act of talking about interventions for the responsibility to actually do something different.

3. *Plan the evaluation before implementing the strategy.* If forced to name the markers or variables that will indicate program success and to create a system for collecting data on those markers, problem solvers will develop a better plan and a way to monitor delivery and outcomes. Too often we rush to implement a new strategy without a clear understanding of what problem

is being attacked and how we will know whether we are successful. For example, if the problem is impolite verbalizations from students that escalate into verbal combat between students and teachers, the markers for success may be a reduction in student- generated profanity or interruptions of teacher talk. Markers could also be teachers' use of ignoring of provocative statements followed by respectful probes for academic information. In other words, the problem may be a pattern of interaction in which both teachers and students are pulled into hostile and coercive statements. Both student and teacher change may be necessary to measure whether an authentic evaluation is to be accomplished.

4. *Establish a timeline.* Always plan a follow-up meeting to check on program implementation and unexpected consequences. Tell everyone that there will be unintended consequences to every good idea. This inoculates the group to the pains involved in change. Agree that everyone will try a new effort for a specified time but will meet at intervals during the implementation. This creates a stronger sense of accountability and allows those who are having trouble with program implementation a low-threat way of receiving booster information to facilitate success.

5. *Throughout the implementation of the program, the consultant must continue to work on relationship building.* There are no "silver bullets" for increasing school safety. The first choice of a program may not be the best choice. The consultant must stay in touch with individuals, acting as a coach, cheerleader, mentor, and confidante. The people in a system will keep trying new approaches if they feel appreciated and valued. They will attempt some change just to please a much loved principal or superintendent. Again, the actual scientific foundation of the program may have little to do with its implementation. People do things for other people.

6. *Finally, debrief and celebrate.* If change is occurring based on the efforts of individuals in the system, ascertain this and make it known. Success leads to more success. If formative evaluation shows little change, be ready to reanalyze the problem and bring in other supports. Many systems are notorious for more-of-the-same approaches to problem solving. For example, if yelling at students does not stop their fights, some teachers yell louder or actually join in the fray. Although we can think of situations that do benefit from more of the same (e.g., consistent praise, unflappable respect toward students; persistent approaches to family involvement), we can think of many more in which being stuck in a particular approach is counterproductive. A relevant example may be the pattern still existing in many schools that allow corporal punishment as a consequence for negative behavior. Some children will, after no or just one experience with corporal punishment, never misbehave in order to avoid the paddle. Although it is an odious technique that models aggression as problem solving, corporal punishment is effective in suppressing behavior with that group of young people. However, a much larger proportion of children not only do not change following physical punishment, but derive certain secondary gains from infuriating adults and/or

withstanding ever increasing numbers of slaps. More of the same actually promotes the very behaviors it is meant to eliminate, because the young people discover the joys of beating the system through subterfuge or by assuming a tough kid persona that is enhanced by increasing punishments.

ACCEPTABILITY OF INTERVENTIONS

An important consideration is the acceptability of various programs. *Acceptability* means how likely is it that consultees will say and believe that the program is relevant to the problem, possible to implement, and likely to cause the desired change. Various programs and interventions probably do vary in acceptability just by the nature of what is required for comprehensive implementation. For example, programs that demand a lot of teacher attention to individual students are often seen by educators as unacceptable. Some educators simply cannot shift focus away from their whole groups to individual students for significant periods of time without experiencing a loss of control of the larger group.

Other programs may be attractive, or not, because of their theoretical underpinnings. If teachers like behavioral approaches, they may find the social cognition themes in some interpersonal problem-solving programs too theoretical or too indirect to be attractive.

The educational jargon that characterizes a lot of material can make it unacceptable, as teachers or other professionals resist having to learn a new language in order to become proficient. Programs that come with ready-made supporting material (e.g., handouts, evaluation plans, and videos) may be very attractive to others because they imply turnkey implementation.

What affects acceptability, however, are not simply the variables in the particular program under discussion. Other, perhaps more subtle, forces make participants in a system more or less likely to embrace a new program.

Acceptability, Implementation, Maintenance

Acceptability should be seen as a three-part problem. First, will professionals in a system agree to try an approach? Second, having given a verbal commitment, will individuals actually implement a strategy? Finally, once it is implemented successfully, will people continue with the program? This final point is interesting because most school consultants can list many examples of successful interventions that are never used after an initial application. Success is not a guarantee to institutionalization. This fact punctuates the reality that people in systems do not act from simple motivations. They make complex and subtle decisions about the costs and benefits of any program and may choose to continue or not for reasons far removed from the precipitating problem.

The first predictor of acceptability is the perceived seriousness of the problem. Trivial annoyances are unlikely to mobilize action, and overwhelming threats can paralyze a system unsure of its capacity to meet a huge test. Making or keeping a system ready for change means describing problems in ways that illustrate the dangers of inaction for small disturbances while promoting a sense of competence in meeting serious confrontations. This is delicate work, because without a felt need to change, nothing will happen. Yet too much focus on the crisis aspect of an issue can convince people that they are incompetent to be part of the solution.

For example, children are likely to be better behaved when supervised by adults. Getting teachers to stand outside their classroom doors or walk the halls during classroom transitions will reduce rough horseplay, bullying, and teasing. Of course, busy teachers can find other things to do during these brief breaks between classes. How can they be motivated to make their presence known during changes of classes?

A principal who mentions that noise levels are unacceptably high during class changes may generate little enthusiasm in teachers who may not experience transitional noise as very annoying. However, a principal who worries about fights with knives and guns during class transitions may scare teachers back into their classrooms. Some balance is necessary that communicates that the current situation, although not a crisis, is likely to escalate into one without timely intervention. Problems have to be serious enough to warrant a change in preferred patterns of behavior, but not so serious as to allow people to opt out of being part of the solution.

Another aspect of acceptability is the perceived cause of a problem or the purpose of a problem behavior. If educators believe that nothing they do can overcome a negative home life or chaotic neighborhood situation, they will not engage in activities to increase school safety. In addition, if they see a child's behavior as purposefully aimed at making them miserable or as indicative of serious emotional disturbance, they will be reluctant to intervene with any positive strategies. A system-priming consultant must help members of the organization understand that they do have power to make positive changes even for children from very challenging and risky environments. Further, the consultant must complicate everyone's thinking about the causes and purpose of behaviors. Behavior rarely has a single cause or purpose. A child who carries a weapon to school is often doing so to increase his or her own sense of security, not with a motive to hurt others. Although no child can be permitted to bring a weapon to a school, understanding that the child is seeking safety can give rise to creative problem solving, not just long-term expulsion. Vulnerable children can be assigned buddies. Community policing can provide a comforting presence within a building for children who are fearful. Metal detectors, open lockers, dress codes, and constant adult monitoring can communicate that the adults are in charge and the children are safe.

Sophisticated educators are also attentive to whether the program under consideration seems like a good match to the agreed-upon problem description. If the problem is tardiness to classes that results in classroom disruption by an identified group of youngsters, most educators will resist a program that targets improvement in young people's self-esteem. A link may exist, but tenuous and distal connections increase resistance to change. A better approach would be a schoolwide program that rewards promptness and punishes tardiness while providing backup to teachers who are dealing with frequent and organized classroom disruptions by a particular subset of young people.

Most educators will deny allowing their feelings toward particular children or parents to influence their actions. If they were not affected, however, they would be unique in humankind. All of us do more for those who admire and like us. All of us are tempted to offer less to those who demean or exhibit hostility toward us. These feelings are normal and can be handled only through open discussion about the limits we all face in dealing with difficult clients.

For example, it is clear that young people are better off and safer in schools than in many other contexts. Further, it is undeniable that most youngsters who fail to finish high school are at a tremendous life-long economic disadvantage. Despite these two well-documented truths, schools all over the United States (and probably the world) stop encouraging certain students to come to school by the end of ninth grade. The students they let slip through the drop-out cracks are difficult and insubordinate. Some of these students are not behavior problems, but have such limited English skills that teachers feel hopeless about helping them "catch up" with the others. When these students are in school, teachers and administrators are tense and poised for confrontations. Educators experience relief at their absence.

Surmounting the very real tendency to do less for those who need most requires a well-functioning team that provides support and respite for all involved. Some young people need alternative settings to typical high schools, and these should be established to offer a chance for the widest array of learning styles. In every school district in which we have worked, there is a small cadre of tough-talking, tough-love-acting teachers. These professionals are especially gifted at connecting with the most challenging students. Such educators must be identified and nurtured, because every school system needs them. They must not, however, be overused to the point of exhaustion. These are the educators who can teach us how to find the child looking for acceptance under the gang member's surly expression, or the mother in search of support behind the angry parent's complaint.

Once people agree to try a new set of strategies and take some beginning steps at implementation, what predicts whether they will maintain the program? Already alluded to are the time and effort required for implementation. A principal may see that regular meetings with a school–community safety council are very important, but may simply become overwhelmed with responding to critical incidents and begin to ignore the preventive planning time offered by the council. Better strategies, of course, would be to have a backup person who can attend the meeting or to give the council the task of analyzing the conditions in the school that maintain a fire-fighting mentality among the leadership staff. A common contributor to this constant crisis-fighting problem is that teachers have not received the appropriate training to deal with minor difficulties or are not organized to be supports for one another when a challenge occurs. Both of these deficits can pull the school administrator into every disturbance.

If a program seems to be working, it is more likely that people will continue with it. Program effectiveness is not, however, a guarantee of long-term adoption. One reason for this apparent paradox was mentioned earlier. Implementing the program may be punishing to the educator because of the time and effort involved or because the program demands that the teacher stay in relationship with children who used to be sent to the office or excluded from school. Consultants working on the challenge of institutionalizing best practices must be aware of this very real threat and help system participants to find ways of supporting each other or accessing additional external resources.

Another threat to adoption of effective programs is our tendency to think of childhood disturbances as existing within the child. If, for example, consultees implement a schoolwide program that catches both children and teachers doing something good, they will very likely notice an increase in prosocial behavior by everyone. If they imagine that they have now taught others to be prosocial and them stop the program, it is very likely that prosocial behavior levels will return to low preintervention levels. Why? The maintenance of prosocial behavior demands a reinforcing environment. If we want positive behavior from others, we must offer positive behavior to them. Positive behavior is not established once and then available in any environment. It is, most often (at least among troubled children), quite dependent on particular contexts that are designed to elicit it.

We have all heard that dieting is not an effective way to lose weight. Rather, what is necessary is a permanent change in the food choices we make and in our activity levels. No one likes the message that to get what we want, we must change forever. Resisting this truth interferes with program adoption in schools. Everyone can be enthusiastic for brief periods of time, but accepting that we create the climates in our buildings by our everyday actions is an onerous realization. It is also, however, a realization of the great power held by the system participants. This part of the message must be highlighted to keep everyone's energy sustained over the long haul of program institutionalization.

A final aspect of acceptability that bears mentioning is that you, as system change agent, are likely the latest in a rather long line of people suggesting that others adopt some innovation. Your success will be affected, at least initially, by consultees' experiences with past consultants. If the experiences have been positive and supportive, you will benefit. If the past has taught your consultees to distrust those who come bearing new ideas, you will have to win their confidence. In most cases, system change is a journey that requires a long relationship, persistence, and high levels of trust among the participants. If you know of a history of failed attempts at improvement or negative dealings with previous consultants, you will be forewarned to focus first on relationship building and on contributing to the welfare of the system by your own activities. Only after you have proved yourself are others likely to commit to adopting new programs or policies.

CONCLUDING THOUGHTS

This chapter has focused on the challenging problem of helping people adopt good ideas. The thesis that good ideas are never enough has been offered, with many supporting examples. The answer to system priming or helping a system be open to innovation is based in strategic actions—for example, needs assessments, educational events, booster sessions—and a focus on relationships. Whoever aspires to make lasting change in order to help schools to be safer places for children must know the literature and research on what works with children and young people. In addition, such aspirants must:

- Understand the constraints of each system (e.g., the current skills of the teachers in dealing with troubling children).
- Figure out the hierarchy of actual power so the right people can be targeted for change.
- Give ideas away so that people in the system can be the owners of the innovation.
- Understand the vision that guides the school and build the program around that goal.
- Give credit to others so that everyone feels good about involvement in the program.
- Build trust as the foundation for any lasting change.
- Search for early success and disseminate it aggressively.
- Check back frequently with those program pioneers willing to take a chance on new approaches, so the consultant can offer support and help and keep them accountable for program integrity.
- Provide resources as often as possible to reduce the time and effort involved in personal and organizational change.
- Stay positive and never critical of others' efforts. Systems need valid feedback, but they also need cheerleaders who will look for evidence of success.
- Understand the readiness of consultees and clients to change and suggest alternatives that allow successive approximations to improvement.

- Respect the consultee's construction of the problem and build interventions that reflect those understandings. Consultees who feel listened to and understood are likely to take risks with the consultant in trying new approaches..
- Whatever the outcome of a conversation, maintain contact with all members of the organization. Change agents cannot afford to belong to factions.

Throughout this chapter we have alluded to caveats to our suggestions for incremental change. It can happen that a crisis occurs (e.g., a school shooting that results in student and/or teacher deaths) that mobilizes an organization to adopt dramatic changes. Systems that have adequate coping skills can be propelled into very high functioning by dramatic events. In addition, some educational leaders are endowed with such powerful charisma that their personal influence is sufficient to create momentum for system change.

Obviously, we cannot hope for or plan on such exceptional circumstances. More often, systems are made ready for change through persistent efforts to build the capacity of its members to accept new challenges and to build a level of trust and confidence that allows people to take risks and operate outside previous comfort zones. Believing in people and their abilities to transcend the past is a necessary ingredient.

REFERENCES

Caplan, G. (1970). *The theory and practice of mental health consultation.* New York: Basic Books.
Conoley, J. C., & Conoley, C. W. (1992). *School consultation: Practice and training* (2nd ed.). Boston: Allyn & Bacon.

ANNOTATED BIBLIOGRAPHY: INTERVENTION PRIMING

Chamley, J., Caprio, E., & Young, R. (1994). The principal as catalyst and facilitator of planned change. *NAASP Bulletin, 78*(560), 1–7.—Good principals are sensitive to the risks teachers take when they make changes. They encourage change in teachers. Principals should facilitate and not dictate change. Implementing change involves three phases: (1) the creation of new roles and expectations; this phase includes making suggestions to the staff and reviewing past efforts; ambivalence is often prominent; (2) the mobilization of those in favor of change; principals use those in favor of change to move forward; (3) the implementation process and staff resistance; changes cause conflict, which can be helpful for change; principals can manage resistance by instilling ownership in the staff, engaging in site-based management, and delegating leadership. The principal as catalyst creates a "change-sensitive environment" (p. 5).

Ehrhardt, K. E., Barnett, D. W., Lentz, F. E., Stollar, S. A., & Reifin, L. H. (1996). Innovative methodology in ecological consultation: Use of scripts to promote treatment acceptability and integrity. *School Psychology Quarterly, 11*(2), 149–168.—There is concern that consultees do not always follow the intervention plans that have been constructed for them. Four single-case studies were presented demonstrating a new approach for studying treatment acceptability. Researchers developed naturalistic scripts that described the intervention steps. Children were identified through Head Start centers and preschools. Consultees were classroom teachers or parents. Researchers used structured consultation techniques that included problem-solving interviews, observations, development of intervention scripts, and collaborative evaluation of the treatment. Scripts were basically step-by-step outlines of what the teacher had to do once an unacceptable behavior occurred. Consultees found the scripts acceptable, and thus intervention increased. In addition, the integrity of the interventions improved as well.

Elliott, S. N. (1988). Acceptability of behavioral treatments: Review of variables that influence treatment selection. Professional Psychology: *Research and Practice, 19,* 68–80.–Elliott analyzes factors involved with treatment acceptability. Psychological jargon, teacher's philosophies about behavior changes, teacher's resources, and the severity of the child's problem are important variables to consider. Twenty studies are reviewed regarding treatment acceptability. Four general conclusions can be reached: (1) It is important to quantify consultee's evaluation of treatments; (2) treatment acceptability is influenced by many factors (child, teacher, and psychologist); (3) consultees accept positive interventions more often than negative interventions; (4) there is a strong relationship between pretreatment acceptability and the perceived effectiveness of the intervention. Overall, acceptability research is still in its infancy.

Evans, D. A. (1973). Problems and challenges for the mental health professional consulting to a community action organization. *Community Mental Health Journal, 9*(1), 46–52.–This article looks at consultation in community agencies. Specifically, two models of consultation, Schein's process consultation model and Caplan's consultee-centered administrative consultation model were utilized within an antipoverty agency (the United Communities against Poverty). Evans used the techniques for 5 months, with an extended follow-up report. This author discovered that the positive changes that came from the consultation did not last (cohesiveness, flexibility of leadership, group decision making). Evans also found that the models were inappropriate for antipoverty agencies. The models overpredicted the personal resourcefulness of the staff. Consultants misunderstood the system constraints and the length of time necessary to engage in the consultation process.

Gainey, D. (1994). The American high school and change: An unsettling process. *NAASP Bulletin, 78*(560), 26–34.–The most common reaction to change is resistance. Change in U.S. high schools needs to take place between principals, students, and staff, not at the school board level. Principals are important as change agents. They can identify the collective needs of those they serve. Unfortunately, high schools are fragmented into many departments. Principals in this environment should become "problem seekers" (p.30). They should also understand the belief systems that need to be reinforced and those that need to be changed. Principals have to meet with groups and come up with cooperative solutions. They should always seek the input of the relevant groups before taking action. Principals also need to determine if the vision for change can become a reality. A plan of action must be developed, considering all opinions. A principal should make the plan clear to all and then gather support. Regular evaluation of the plan should occur. Finally, principals should realize that change is a "never-ending cycle" (p. 33). They must also instill in others the importance of a common vision for the school.

Glidewell, J. C. (1959). The entry problem in consultation. *Journal of Social Issues, 15*(2), 50–59.–To become an effective consultant, one must understand the problems that can occur in the entry process. Entry can be defined as the attachment of a new person to an existing system. Overall, consultation is a process of goodness of fit. For example, the consultant and consultee must share the same perceptions of need, role equity, availability of resources, and the like. Consultant and consultee must have congruence in their value systems and must have complementary roles.

Kazdin, A. E. (1981). Acceptability of child treatment techniques: The influence of treatment efficacy and adverse side effect. *Behavior Therapy, 12,* 493–506.—Two experiments were conducted to evaluate treatment acceptability. In the first study, 112 undergraduates participated. The first experiment examined whether acceptability of treatment was influenced by its therapeutic effects. Participants rated audiotaped interventions applied to children who had aggressive behavior or mental retardation. Each participant heard two tapes, the first presenting a case description of a child and the second describing treatments administered. Results of the first study indicate that reinforcement was rated more acceptable than positive practice, time out, and medication. In the second experiment, the same participants reviewed side effects (i.e., emotional reactions, aggressiveness after treatment was applied) that occurred after the supposed intervention took place. The purpose was to determine whether side effects detracted from the acceptability of some or all of the interventions. Side effects were found to influence acceptability ratings. As a side effect increased in intensity the intervention associated with the side effect was subsequently rated lower in acceptability.

Martens, B. K., Witt, J. C., Elliott, S. N., & Darveaux, D. X. (1985). Teacher judgments concerning the acceptability of school-based interventions. *Professional Psychology: Research and Practice, 16,* 191–198.—In this article, researchers investigated several factors that might influence treatment acceptability (severity of behavior problem, interventionist, and modality of case presentation). Fifty-four teachers participated in the study. Teachers viewed a videotape or read a written account of interventions applied to two behavior problems (daydreaming and destruction of property). Teachers completed an intervention rating profile to assess their views about the interventions. Interventionist variables were also evaluated. Two interventions were used in the study, which varied in the length of time, effort, and skill the teacher needed to implement. Results indicate that severity of behavior and interventionist affected teacher's acceptability of interventions. Specifically, results contradicted previous research in the area. Typically, teachers prefer interventions that are less time-consuming; however, not so in this study. The authors suggest that having control over the implementation of the intervention may make a time-consuming intervention acceptable. In addition, the more severe a child's behavior, the more likely a teacher is to accept an intervention.

Noell, G. H., & Witt, J. C. (1999). When does consultation lead to intervention implementation? Critical issues for research and practice. *Journal of Special Education, 33*(1), 29–35.— This article is a theoretical discussion about the issues surrounding consultation research. Most research until now has been flawed or has not asked the right questions. For example, many studies look at teacher satisfaction after consultation, but this does not tell the consultant whether the teacher actually implemented the intervention. The authors argue that first the field must operationally define terms like consultation and collaboration. Fortunately, much progress has been made in operationally defining consultation procedures (since the late 1970s). Variables must also be measured accurately during consultation to determine the effect of the intervention and its implementation. There is an inherent problem in defining what the independent and dependent variable(s) are, because of the triadic nature of consultation. The implementation of an intervention can be both an independent and a dependent variable. The authors looked at some consultation research and discovered that very few existing studies accurately assess intervention implementation. They state that examining the variables related to intervention implementation is an emerging area of research.

Soo-Hoo, T. (1998). Applying frame of reference and reframing techniques to improve school consultation in multicultural settings. *Journal of Educational and Psychological Consultation, 9*(4), 325–345.—This article is a theoretical discussion of the unique circumstance of multicultural consultation. Consultation with multicultural groups requires extra sensitivity. Soo-Hoo suggests using two techniques in these settings—namely, frame of reference and reframing. Frame of reference means understanding the problem the consultee is facing within the sociopolitical context. The consultant must get inside the client's world. Culture greatly enhances the consultees' worldview. It influences the way they think; however, each individual within the cultural group will interpret the culture in a slightly different way. Understanding the history of a cultural group is also important (i.e., racism, oppression, discrimination). School psychologists must be sensitive to the cultural worldview of the child, too. Reframing means changing the way a person views an event. It can help consultees view situations differently. Reframing should consider cultural factors as well. A case example is presented to demonstrate how the techniques can be used.

PART VI
Special Topics

CHAPTER 17

School Violence
and Cultural Sensitivity

GWENDOLYN CARTLEDGE
CAROLYN TALBERT JOHNSON

A person's culture provides for a set of common experiences that influences the way in which the individual interprets the environment and behaves. The social behaviors of youths from racial and ethnic minorities need to be studied and addressed within a cultural context. As U.S. society becomes more diverse and certain groups of long-term residents remain entrenched in subcultures, the image of a melting pot is increasingly changing to one of a mosaic. Although cultural diversity provides for a social richness that should be celebrated, cultural differences appreciably determine the social patterns observed in the classroom and may present certain challenges in terms of cognitive and social development. These cultural differences may cause children and adolescents from diverse backgrounds to respond to environmental events in different or nonproductive ways and may cause their actions to be misperceived by peers and adults who do not share the same cultural orientation. School personnel are challenged to interpret accurately the behaviors of culturally different learners, to distinguish social skill differences from deficits, and to employ instructional strategies that will be effective in helping these learners acquire the most productive interpersonal and cognitive skills.

Our focus in this chapter is on the unique patterns that are instructive for these purposes; however, it is imperative to remain cognizant of the universality of children's behavior. No group is a monolith, and the variability within each culture must be respected. Nevertheless, certain patterns do prevail, and these distinctions are highlighted here for each of the four largest minority cultural groups in the United States (Hispanic/Latino American, African American, Native American, and Asian American). As important as their distinguishing characteristics are the school factors that uniquely affect these young people and the ways in which educators may program the learning environment to the developmental advantage of culturally different students.

VIOLENCE AND CULTURAL DIVERSITY

Aggressive, violent behaviors of children and youths have become a major concern of our schools. Numerous studies show that teachers in the United States are distressed about the increasing levels of violence in and around public schools (Metropolitan Life Insurance Company, 1995). Hughes and Cavell (1995), for example, report a dramatic increase of aggressive behaviors among school-age youths, including destruction of property and verbal or nonverbal behaviors that harm others. A graphic illustration of the increased concern can be seen in two surveys conducted with public school teachers over a 50-year period (Volokh & Snell, 1998). In 1940 teachers listed their seven top disciplinary concerns as talking out of turn, chewing gum, making noise, running in the hall, cutting in line, dress code violations, and littering, as compared with the seven top concerns in 1990: drug abuse, alcohol abuse, pregnancy, suicide, rape, robbery, and assault.

Aggressive or violence-prone youth often evidence poor school performance, poor interpersonal relationships, and a tendency to violate existing rules or norms (e.g., being truant from school). These and other characteristics are predictive of dropping out of school (Parker & Asher, 1987), as well as of later-life criminality (Eron, Huesmann, & Zelli, 1991). The rise in school violence is accompanied by a corresponding increase in the incidence of weapons in schools, particularly guns. Felgar (1992) suggests that this increase is partly driven by drug trafficking and gangs, but most youths contend that their weapons are intended primarily for protection. Gun possession also appears to bolster the self-esteem and assurance of many students, in that the size of the gun is equated with toughness: The larger the gun, the "badder" or more esteemed the owner (Felgar, 1992).

Violence in the schools is not restricted to racial or cultural minorities, but for these groups cultural and racial factors need to be addressed in order for effective interventions to be designed. One such issue is ethnic identity and its relationship to psychosocial development and adaptive behavior. Ethnic identity is considered to provide a sense of belonging and to be particularly important for disparaged or disenfranchised minority groups (Phinney, 1990; Smith, 1991). Adaptive behavior is believed to be at least partly based on the way the individual views his or her own ethnic group and that of others. Ethnic identity formation, according to one model presented by Phinney (1990), is a three-stage evolutionary process. At the first stage, "unexamined identity," the individual has not been exposed to ethnic identity issues and shows a preference for the dominant culture. The second stage, "exploration," occurs when the individual begins to study and become involved in his or her own culture. "Ethnic identity," the third stage, is achieved when the individual acquires a deep appreciation of his or her own culture, often manifested in a positive attitude toward the culture and participation in cultural activities. The third stage is associated with a positive attitude toward the dominant group or culture as well, and represents the best psychological adjustment. Another identity model, described by Vargas (1994), involves four parts: (1) "ideal self" (what a person would like to be), (2) "feared self" (what the person would not like to be), (3) "claimed self" (what the person would like others to think he or she is), and (4) "real self" (what the person believes he or she is).

Although most of the research on ethnic identity has been conducted with college populations, there is some evidence of a connection between identity issues and adaptive behaviors for school-age populations. To illustrate, Vargas (1994) proposes that young people struggling with self-identity issues may gravitate toward desired selves (e.g., macho selves) to cover for the insecurity of their real selves. Others theorize that youths, most alienated from the dominant culture tend to engage in "cultural inversion" or oppositional social identity, in which they consider behaviors typical of the dominant group as inappropriate for their own group members (Bemal, Saenz, & Knight, 1991). For example, the most alienated Hispanic and African American youths have been observed to disparage and label as "acting white" the achieving and socially compliant behaviors of their same-group peers (Fordham, 1988; Matute-Bianchi, 1986). Alienated young people from low-status groups may redefine the values of the dominant culture in oppositional, self-destructive ways. For example, some African American elementary school males of low socioeconomic status (SES) described their role as that of "being bad" (a role at which their teacher felt many of them excelled) and felt that "the badder they were, the greater their social status" (Elrich, 1994, p. 14).

Undoubtedly, the effects of this emphasis on being tough or bad can be seen in the data on the violent death rate among U.S. youths. Between 1980 and 1986 the rate of white and black juvenile offenders were approximately the same, but following that period there was an explosion of juvenile violence largely attributed to black youth (Hawkins, Laub, Lauritsen, & Cothern, 2000). Vargas (1994) reported that within the period from 1985 to 1990, there was a 13% increase (from 62.8 to 70.9 per 100,000) in the violent death rate for teens between 15 and 19 years of age, and these increases were most pronounced for ethnic or racial minorities. For example, in the state of New Mexico for the period between 1988 and 1990, the male homicide rate per 100,000 for 15–24-year-olds was 56.7 for African Americans, 53.6 for Native Americans, 34.1 for Hispanic Americans, and 7.9 for Anglo Americans (Vargas, 1994). Since the mid 1990s the picture has changed, in that there have been substantial declines in juvenile violence, with black youth accounting for the major portion of these reductions (U. S. Department of Justice, 1999).

Albeit encouraging, these lowered rates of juvenile violence remain un-acceptably high, especially for minorities. These youth are far more likely to be arrested and to be treated harshly by the juvenile justice system (Feld, 1997). African American adolescents, for instance, are seven times more likely to be arrested than white adolescents for minor offenses and twice as likely to be arrested for serious crimes. Minority youth in general are more likely to be sent to correctional facilities than are white youth who commit similar offenses. The differences of social class in serious criminal activity are not unusual, resulting in an overrepresentation among the poor. In light of the fact that many young adolescents grow up in inner cities, gang vio-lence and victimization are chronic problems. Most researchers agree that vi-olence and aggression among youth are strongly linked to poverty, for a num-ber of reasons. First, when families live in impoverished neighborhoods, parents are less effective in nurturing and monitoring their children, and this diminished effectiveness leads to increased aggression and crime (Sampson & Laub, 1994). Second, concentrated poverty upsets the social fabric of a neighborhood, making it more difficult for adults and social institutions to provide the guidance and supervision that adolescents need (Sampson, 1992). Third, in many inner-city communities devastated by unemployment, aggression is used by males to demonstrate their standing and power—characteristics that are typically demonstrated in middle-class communities through occupational success (Wilson & Daly, 1985). Finally, repeated expo-sure to violence—whether in the home or in the neighborhood—breeds violence itself (DuRant, Cadenhead, Pendergrast, Slavens, & Linder, 1994). Beyond the culture of poverty, other factors that may provide some explana-tions for youth violence include the drug culture, which encourages students to arm themselves; population mobility, which contributes to anonymity; discrimination, promoting anger within minority students; and violence in the media, which desensitizes youth to the effects of violence (Volokh & Snell, 1998).

Other data show that youth from diverse backgrounds (i.e., African American, Hispanic American, and American Indian) living in the inner city are disproportionately likely to be the victims of violent crime (Hutson, Anglin, & Pratts, 1994; U.S. Department of Justice, 1999). Despite the data evidencing the disproportionate impact of violence for minority popula-tions, relatively little effort has been made to study the social behaviors of children and youths in each group.

African Americans

Currently, African Americans constitute 16% of the U.S. public school popu-lation (King, 1993). Many of the studies of African American male delin-quency have also focused on the disparate schooling experience and degree of school identification among these students (Voelkl, 1997). For example, on the average, levels of academic achievement are higher among white than African American students, and African Americans are disproportionately tracked into lower-ability class (Oakes, 1990), suspended from school more frequently and for longer duration (Cartledge, Tillman, & Talbert-Johnson, 2001), and punished more severely in school (Office for Civil Rights, 1992). In light of these findings, Noguera (1995) posits that the disproportionate involvement of African Americans, particularly young males, in the criminal justice system may constitute a national crisis. Some criminologists blame the disparities on racial discrimination (Baer & Chambliss, 1997), whereas others assert that social class biases account for the differences (Blau & Blau, 1982).

Schools have not tended to address students' behavior problems according to cultural/racial background. The few existing studies on social skill assessments by teachers show race to be an influential factor, with teachers giving African American students lower behavioral ratings than their other-race peers (Feng & Cartledge, 1996; Keller, 1988; Lethermon et al., 1984; Lethermon, Williamson, Moody, & Wozniak, 1986). Feng and Cartledge (1996) studied the social skills of African American, Asian American, and European American fifth-grade low-SES students. As compared with their other-race peers, the African American students received from their teachers lower mean social skill ratings and higher problem behavior ratings, resulting in a relatively distinct behavioral profile. The teachers did rate African American students highly in people-oriented behaviors, noting that they were inclined to be friendly and to interact readily with others. Yet, the teachers also perceived these students to have poor self-control (i.e., distractible, excessive movement) and poor conflict management skills. Some of the highly rated problem behaviors pertained to being argumentative and likely to interrupt the conversations of others.

In her discussion of their culture, Irvine (1990) points out that African Americans' arguing style tends to be direct, entering a heated argument without following the turn-taking rule. The energetic, fast-paced, confrontational manner in which many of these youngsters are socialized may be misunderstood as aggression and may be in conflict with the culture of the classroom. An example of cultural differences is given in a description of girls of two cultures playing volleyball in the school gymnasium. The team in one gym consisted of African American girls, and in another, Hmong girls. The noise level was very high in the gym with the African American girls—laughing, screams of encouragement, hollering—whereas in the other gym the only noise that could be heard was the contact of hands with the volleyball. The elevated movement and peer interaction may be seen by some school personnel as undesirable and an occasion for reprimands (Delpit, 1995).

The tendency for some minority youth to subscribe to aggressive options (e.g., Feng & Cartledge, 1996) is a point of valid concern. Aggression is extremely problematic for African American youths, especially males, who are disproportionately singled out for disciplinary actions in schools (Irvine, 1990) and punishment for delinquent activities in the community (Prothrow-Stith, 1991). The tendency to believe in aggressive alternatives is typical of low-income individuals—particularly those from urban, violence-prone areas, where children are often socialized to counteraggress, ostensibly as a means for survival (Hudley & Graham, 1993). Accordingly, children are taught not to seek assistance from adults or to negotiate these problems, but to respond in kind with verbal or physical aggression. This orientation probably explains the lowest mean self-ratings by African American students on items pertaining to asking for help or ignoring peer conflict in the Feng and Cartledge (1996) study. These conditions are exacerbated by drug trafficking and the easy accessibility of guns. Excessive verbal and physical aggression are some of the most serious behavior problems encountered among schoolchildren; they are predictive of academic failure, delinquency, and various types of adult psychopathology (Patterson, Capaldi, & Bank, 1991). Constructive interventions are needed to reduce distractible, combative behaviors while reinforcing the positive qualities of generous, people-oriented patterns.

Hispanic Americans

Hispanic Americans now constitute the largest group of people of color in the United States (U.S. Census Bureau, 2001). There is considerable diversity in areas of ethnic origin (i.e., Cuban, Mexican, Puerto Rican, etc.), socioeconomic status, and degree of assimilation. Language, which also varies somewhat, is the most common unifying factor.

The literature on the school-based social behaviors of Hispanic Americans is sparse. Mexican American elementary students have been described as cooperative, quiet, and obedient (Carlson & Stephens, 1986; Casas, Furlong, Solberg, & Carranza, 1990), and Moore (1988) reports that teachers viewed Hispanic American females as passive and docile. The interpersonal difficulties noted for these students tend to be linguistically based: They evidence problems with being verbally assertive, initiating statements, discussing feelings, and offering opinions (Carlson & Stephens, 1986; Moore, 1988).

An area of considerable concern for Hispanic American students is school failure, in terms of both graduation rates and school achievement (Bernal et al., 1991; Casas et al., 1990; Matute-Bianchi, 1986). In 1997, only 55% of Hispanics 25 years and older had graduated from high school and 7.4% had graduated from college (Valverde, 2000). Valencia (2000) asserts that these students have inferior educational opportunities and are exposed to teachers and school administrators who have low academic expectations for them. Despite evidence of a strong desire to get an education, Casas et al. (1990) found that Mexican American students felt that falling behind in school or helping out at home was a viable reason for dropping out of school.

Family, community, and ethnic group are all central to the life of many Hispanic/Latino students. Therefore, these students often develop a sense of community. They are generally taught to be cooperative and to have a strong sense of group membership (Carrasquillo, 1991). This means that Hispanic/Latino children tend to be warmer, more concerned about others, and more physically affectionate than children in mainstream society (e.g., touching is an important part of interpersonal communication in the culture). Language and cultural differences often make schools alien environments for Hispanic American students. Communication and perception problems can lead to home–school tensions; students may resent being singled out for remedial instruction; teachers may be unaccepting of students' unorthodox productions; and students' behavior may be in conflict with the strict behavioral standards of the school (Mulhern, 1995; Seda & Bixler-Márquez, 1994).

Hispanic American students report more daily stressors and depression than do their nonminority peers (Aguilar-Gaxiola & Gray, 1994; Casas et al., 1990; Hoernicke, Kallam, & Tablada, 1994). The stressors include being in new classes, peer pressures, fear for physical safety, inadequate English, worries about maintaining their primary language, poverty, and racial and ethnic intolerance. These stressors undoubtedly contribute to interpersonal problems and substance abuse. According to Ramirez (1989), Mexican Americans are 14 times as likely as their Anglo American counterparts to abuse inhalants, and the use of other substances (e.g., alcohol, stimulants, tranquilizers, and heroin) is significantly higher in small Mexican American communities than the national average. As Hispanic American children move into the teen years, issues such as aggression and violence gain in importance. Hispanic youths make up approximately 33% of the current gang membership in the United States (Soriano, 1993), and their homicide rates are estimated to be three or four times greater than those of their nonminority age mates (Hammond & Yung, 1993).

Native Americans

Native Americans, who constitute slightly less than 1% of the U.S. population, are the smallest of the four major racial and ethnically diverse groups (U.S. Census Bureau, 2001). As with other groups, there is considerable within-group diversity. About 10% of school-age Native American children are born and reared in cities (Grant & Gomez, 2001). The research on these students' social skills is even more limited than that for the other groups, but there is evidence showing that the social behavior profiles of elementary-age Native American children resemble those noted previously for Hispanic children. That is, comparisons with nonminority children have shown differences in language-based behaviors of verbal assertion (Powless & Elliott, 1993). Native American children were perceived to make fewer verbal initiations, but there were no differences between the two groups in problem behaviors. Other behavioral characteristics commonly attributed to some Native American groups include tendencies to (1) avoid eye contact, as a sign of respect to adults, (2) avoid initiating conversations within mixed-age groups, and (3) emphasize self-management (i.e., the locus of control is internal rather than external or adult oriented).

Emphasis is often placed on the group and the importance of maintaining harmony within the group; the needs of the group are often considered over the needs of the individual. Because of strong feelings of group solidarity, cooperation, rather than competition, is the desirable mode of operation. Native American children are often hesitant to show themselves as superior, especially if this would present someone else in a poor light (Cleary & Peacock, 1998). Furthermore, Native American children often feel more comfortable participating in class after they have had time to consider their responses or practice their skills. They also are apt to delay answering questions.

The impoverished and stressful living conditions of many Native Americans account for the major risk factors that mark the lives of at least 50% of their youths: poor education, substance abuse, and suicide. The estimates for high school dropouts are as high as 85–90%, and at least one-third of the population is considered illiterate (LaFromboise & Low, 1989). As compared with the non-Native rate of 5%, nearly 33% of Native Americans between 7th and 12th grades are reported to use marijuana and alcohol regularly (Oetting et al., 1983). From 1950 to 1986, suicide rates for Native American adolescents have tripled and are the highest for any group in the United States (Grossman, Milligan, & Deyo, 1991).

These conditions are interrelated and predictive of one another. Although Native Americans are family- and relationship-oriented people, their children are disproportionately removed from their close family networks to attend schools in non-Native cultures, intensifying feelings of alienation and isolation. LaFromboise and Low (1989) point out their sense of anonymity upon entering school: "Many of them speak an entirely different first language, practice an entirely different religion, and hold different cultural values than the dominant culture, and yet they are expected to perform successfully according to conventional Anglo educational criteria" (p. 119).

Asian Americans

Asian Americans currently represent 3.6% of the U.S. population and are the fastest-growing minority group in the country (U.S. Census Bureau, 2001). Between 1980 and 1990, their numbers increased from 3,500,000 to 7,274,000, representing a 107.8% increase. Most Asian Americans in this country originate from East Asia (China, Japan, and Korea), but other members of this group include those from Southeast Asia, India, and the South Pacific islands.

Teacher evaluations consistently profile Asian American students as co-operative, self-controlled, and task oriented (Cartledge & Feng, 1996). Although teachers tend to value such school-oriented behaviors, others question whether these behaviors are emphasized at the expense of peer-based behaviors and the opportunities to develop interpersonal social skills (Schneider & Lee, 1990). A multimethod study conducted by Feng and Cartledge (1996) showed that although Asian American students received the highest sociometric peer ratings from their other-race peers, were the objects of fewer negative statements, and made proportionately more outer-group statements than students from the other two groups, they also had lower peer interaction rates than their European and African American classmates. Howes and Wu (1990) also found that Asian American students had lower communication rates but were more likely to enter cross-ethnic interactions than their African American, European American, and Latino American elementary peers.

Asian Americans are a unique minority group in the United States, in that greater percentages of their population have more education and higher incomes than the national average (U.S. Census Bureau, 1999). As compared with 8.8% of whites, however, 13% of Asian-Americans fall below the poverty line and thus are subjected to many of the same stressors as other impoverished U.S. minority groups. A distinctive at-risk subgroup consists of recent arrivals from East and Southeast Asia. Since 1975 almost 1 million refugees have entered this country from Southeast Asia (i.e., Laos, Vietnam, and Cambodia) (Cowart & Cowart, 1993); there have also been tremendous increases from China, Hong Kong, and Taiwan (Chin, 1990). Many of the newly arrived young people are unaccompanied by parents or guardians. Their school adjustment is particularly difficult: In addition to experiencing language problems, many are placed in classes with much younger cohorts, where they are frustrated with their own efforts to learn the subject matter. Learning, disciplinary, and other problems lead to leaving school early, so that, for example, Asian Americans represent more than 25% of all dropouts in the New York City schools (Los Angeles Unified School District, 1991).

Increasingly, the emerging profile for a subset of Asian American youths is one of school failure and growing criminality (Chin, 1990; Cowart & Cowart, 1993; Los Angeles Unified School District, 1991). These youngsters frequently victimize members of their own ethnic community, who often do not report incidents to officials outside the community. Cowart and Cowart (1993) propose that gang membership is attractive to these youths because it offers a sense of belonging, support, and respect, as well as a common language. This sense of community helps to counter the "detachment experienced by the disruption of their families caused by war and/or immigrant status. For those with intact families, gang membership may offer freedom from the restraints of family and school, yet provide support and identity.

The cultural features that apparently contribute to more positive teacher and peer reviews of Asian Americans may also cause significant problems to go undetected. The stereotypical view of them as hard-working, high-achieving students may cause teachers to see them as self-sufficient and thus to overlook many of their problems. Teachers and other professionals need to be aware of and attend to the special problems presented by Asian American youths, especially those who are recent arrivals in the United States.

SCHOOLS: THEIR FAILINGS AND POTENTIAL FOR MINORITY STUDENTS

Socially conscious authorities increasingly assert that U.S. schools are failing their students and disproportionately failing poor students of color (Bettmann & Moore, 1994; Gomez, 1994; Grossman. 1995; Kozol, 1991). Bettmann and Moore (1994) point out that schools appear to ignore the multicultural nature of the United States and are preparing students for a monocultural existence. They suggest that the schools' worldview represents the dominant male culture and devalues the contributions of members from other groups. Bettmann and Moore (1994) label the school inequities of tracking, biased testing, monocultural curricula and teaching staff, inhospitable school climate, and instructional methods that fail to capitalize on the learners' abilities and background as unjust; they contend that "social injustice is a catalyst for violence" (p. 15).

These authors go on to argue that if we hope to help students develop nonviolent skills to manage conflict there is a need to change classroom environments that promote conflict through an emphasis on competition, distrust, inappropriate expression of feelings (e.g., aggressive expressions of anger), inflexible rules, bigotry, and discrimination. According to Bettmann and Moore (1994), other policies and practices that lead to student unrest include (1) failure to validate the voices of students or their parents, (2) unequal allocation of financial resources, and (3) stereotypical programming in terms of educational placement and discipline.

Similar themes of injustice are registered by other authors. Kozol (1991), for example, notes the extreme inequities in school funding, which unquestionably have an impact on students' cognitive, social, and psychological development. Kozol describes schools within the same district that range from attractive, well-equipped settings for affluent majority students to dilapidated, overcrowded facilities with inadequate supplies and materials for poor minority pupils. Ladson-Billings (1995) suggests that as students observe these differences, they will begin to associate these conditions with the respective groups and to regard these inequities as normal. These unhealthy thought patterns are most destructive for poor and minority students, for they color the students' self-perceptions and the expectations they have for themselves. Such associations undoubtedly gave rise to the self-deprecating statements made by Elrich's (1994) Hispanic and African American students, referred to earlier in this chapter. This distorted thinking led these young males to take pride in their disruptive, antisocial behaviors.

Teachers as a Factor

The continuing trends of an increasingly greater proportion of minority students in the public school population and a teaching corps of largely white females set the conditions for "cultural discontinuities" that potentially undermine the learning of students and serve to frustrate teachers. Many African American and Mexican American students continue to attend highly segregated schools where, as compared with their white peers, they are more likely to experience noncredentialed teachers, ill-prepared to assume teaching responsibilities with culturally diverse students in urban settings (Darling-Hammond, 1995; Valencia, 2000). Gomez (1994) addresses teacher attitudes and actions as follows:

> These new teachers working in inner cities, small towns, and rural areas were more likely to cite influences outside of school as challenging students' ability to learn than were their counterparts teaching in suburbia. Teachers working with students of color and students from low-income families were also more likely to point to outside-of-school influences as detrimental to students' learning and achievement. Taken together, these responses from novice teachers indicate that early in their careers, many teachers locate problems of learning and achievement not as outcomes of teachers' beliefs about and behaviors towards children in school, but as consequences of children's outside-of-school lives—beyond the purview of teachers, schools and schooling. (p. 321)

Teachers' beliefs are extremely important; they influence teachers' expectations and judgments about students' abilities, effort, and progress in school. These beliefs dictate whether teachers recognize a student's need, assume responsibility for addressing this need, or shift the responsibility to others. Winfield and Manning (1992) observed that in many urban schools, the wide array of supplementary programs permits some teachers to become "general contractors" who relegate the responsibility for the development of their students to others in the school.

The actions of a black child are likely to be viewed negatively by a white middle-class teacher who fails to distinguish a cultural style from a behavior disorder (Irvine, 1990). The language, style of walking, glances, and dress of black males have engendered fear, apprehension, and overreaction in many teachers and school administrators. Both the nonverbal and verbal communication styles of black students baffle school personnel, especially white teachers, who fail to understand black students' expressive language (Cartledge & Loe, 2001; Irvine, 1992). According to Irvine, verbal ability is valued as highly as physical ability among black males; whenever black males, young and old, assemble, a boasting or teasing encounter usually ensues. This contest of words (known among blacks as "playing the dozens") is an important male ritual in the black community. Cartledge and Milburn (1996) give one young white teacher's real-life account of her misinterpretation of one such ritual and the resulting interpersonal conflicts.

A prescription proposed by Miller-Lachmann and Taylor (1995) is that teachers first need to recognize and directly confront their biases. Second, they need to understand the influence of culture in order to diagnose children's learning and behavior problems correctly and, finally, acquire knowledge of other cultures in order to see things from other perspectives.

Educational Programming

Typical educational programming and placements speak volumes to culturally and racially diverse students; unfortunately, many of the messages conveyed are negative. A particularly pernicious practice is academic tracking, labeled by Kuykendall (1992) as a "caste system" and by Irvine (1990) as the creation of "educational ghettos." These inequitable learning opportunities accompany poor academic achievement, less challenging classes, greater rates of grade retention, higher dropout rates, and lower rates of college matriculation (Valencia, 2000), leading to lowered self-images for academic achievement.

The power of this "self-stereotyping" can be seen in the research conducted by Claude Steele and Joshua Aronson, as reported by Elaine Woo (1995). According to Woo, Steele and Aronson believe that "pervasive negative stereotypes about blacks' intellectual ability create a 'situational pressure' that distracts them and depresses their academic performance" (p. 6B). In a study with university students, Steele and Aronson found that blacks who were told that a test was intended to measure verbal reasoning ability scored significantly lower than those who were given no information that intellectual prowess was being assessed. Findings from this and other confirming studies led the researchers to theorize that suggestions of intellectual abilities trigger blockers among blacks, causing them to "labor harder, but with ill effect . . . they reread questions . . . work less efficiently and make more mistakes" (Woo, 1995, p. 6B).

The effects of these negative stereotypes are equally damaging to more able African-American students, if not more so. Woo (1995), for example, reports evidence from Steele indicating that black university students with higher Scholastic Aptitude Test scores failed and dropped out more often than black students with lower scores. At the elementary and secondary levels, these perceptions are aggravated by poor learning conditions, causing students to devalue school as well as themselves and their same-race peers. Poor achievement and social adjustment are obvious outcomes.

Disciplinary Measures

The way in which school personnel view discipline for racially or culturally different populations is critical for curbing violence in our schools. Containment or punishment policies tend to be overemphasized. Demographic studies repeatedly show that minority youths, especially African American and Hispanic American males, are disproportionately referred for behavior and learning problems as compared with their majority counterparts (Executive Committee, Council for Children with Behavioral Disorders [CCBD], 1989; Hilliard, 1980; Maheady, Algozzine, & Ysseldyke, 1985). Other research shows that black students are two to five times more likely to be suspended at a younger age and to receive lengthier suspensions (Irvine, 1990).

Leal (1994) observes that within poor districts, attitudes toward school safety and discipline tend to be more authoritarian, stressing "get tough" policies that increase imprisonment, the length of prison sentences, and the involvement of the police and courts. Leal contends that the public's perception is distorted, leading to the pursuit of actions that have little impact on violent crime, particularly among young people. He attributes major culpability to the mass media, noting that murders account for less than 1% of all the crime in U.S. society but receive 87% of all crime coverage on TV. Along the same lines, the print media tend to overemphasize crime through regular columns with titles such as "Crime Watch" and "Most Wanted Fugitives," which suggest the ubiquitous and ominous presence of criminal activity. The reality tends to be far less than all this coverage would suggest, and little if any attention is given to mediation programs designed to help all students develop nonviolent problem-solving skills. Instead, Leal argues, the public is focused on these costly and unredemptive "get tough" practices.

Not only do educators and other authorities resort excessively to punitive models, but punishments also appear to be administered with racial and cultural bias. Perhaps this is seen most vividly in the "zero tolerance" popularized in the mid-1990s with the advent of a rash of school shootings. By 1997, at least 90% of United States public schools had zero-tolerance policies that mandated predetermined consequences or punishments for specific offenses (U.S. Department of Education, 1998). These policies have led to dramatic increases in student expulsions and suspensions, and, accordingly, not only deny a free and public education but also are likely to contribute to problems such as grade retentions, dropping out of school, academic failure, and recidivism (Costenbader & Markson, 1998; Morgan-D'Atrio, Northup, Ladler, LaFleur, & Spera, 1996). Other researchers contend that excessive expulsions/suspensions invariably lead to marginalization, as exhibited in poverty, poor living conditions, mental health disorders, and criminality (Blyth & Milner, 1993).

Students of color, particularly African American, are most vulnerable for school policies that emphasize expulsions/suspensions (Blyth & Milner,

1993; Larson, 1998), in addition to referrals for disciplinary actions (Gregory, 1995; Irvine, 1990), and for more restricted educational placements (U.S. Department of Education, 1999). For example, in a study of 620 middle and high school students, Costenbader and Markson (1998) found that black students made up 25% of the school population but 40% of the students suspended from school. Another finding in this study was that 45% of the black students reported that they had been externally suspended from school as compared with rates of 12% for whites and 18% for Hispanics. Similarly, other studies have found that black students are suspended/expelled two to five times more often than white students, with evidence of more severe punishments for the same infractions (Claiborne, 1999; Pauken & Daniel, 1999).

Beyond race or ethnicity is the issue of gender. From infancy, males are socialized to be aggressive, dominant, competitive, and assertive, but in the classroom, where the teacher is likely to be a white female, these behaviors may be viewed as threatening if not pathological. Boys are punished more often than females (Kehrberg, 1994), and when racial diversity is combined with male status, poor school outcomes are even more predictable. Black males, as compared with white males regardless of socioeconomic level, are much more likely to be suspended at a younger age, to receive lengthier suspensions, to be placed in special education classes, to be programmed into punishment facilities such as juvenile court rather than referred for treatment, and to be given more pathological labels than warranted (Carmen, 1990; Council for Children with Behavioral Disorders, 1989; Ewing, 1995; Forness, 1988; Irvine, 1990 McFadden, Marsh, Price, & Hwang, 1992).

To illustrate the effects of race and gender, in a study of the office referral disciplinary data for an urban elementary school (87% African American), Lo and Cartledge (2001) found that 50% of the student body had at least one office referral and that 32% of the students had been suspended over the school year. Disciplinary referral guidelines developed by Sprague, Sugai, Homer, and Walker (1999) advise that schoolwide interventions are warranted when office referrals exceed 20% of the student population. For the school in the Lo and Cartledge study, suspensions alone substantially exceeded this 20% criterion, not to mention the 50% office referrals. The African American males in this school were suspended at a level 10% higher than their representation in the school, whereas African American females were suspended at a level 10% lower than their school enrollment. These data for this school may be somewhat extreme, but they do provide an example of the excessive punitive measures in low socioeconomic black schools as compared with the data compiled by Sprague et al. (1999) of mainstreamed U.S. elementary schools. Another observation in the Lo and Cartledge (2001) study is that as the school year progressed, disciplinary measures systematically increased, suggesting that these punishing consequences were more likely worsening rather than relieving behavior problems in the school.

More important than punishment is the need to help students develop skills that will enable them to deal with conflict without violence (Leal,

1994). Rather than being viewed as simply a means to control students' behaviors, conflict resolution skills should be practiced by both students and staff for the social development of all students (Bettmann & Moore, 1994; Leal, 1994).

INTERVENTIONS

The schooling of students from culturally diverse backgrounds must stress positive approaches, designed to promote intellectual and social growth. Schools should be inviting places where students feel welcomed and valued. Schools should also be proactive, equipping students with strategies and ways of thinking about conflict in order to prevent or minimize problem situations. In recent years researchers and other authorities have increasingly recognized the greater beneficial effects of preventive positive interventions rather than simply reacting to students' behaviors with punitive consequences (e.g., Lewis & Sugai, 1999). These procedures call for employing school- and classwide incentives to motivate students to want to follow rules and explicitly teaching students the desired behaviors. Social skill instruction is a positive, direct method for helping schoolchildren acquire critical prosocial behaviors. Social skill instruction incorporates behavioral and social learning principles into an instructional sequence of social modeling, guided practice, feedback, and behavior transfer. There are several curriculum programs and texts that provide teaching guidelines, instructional materials, and varying versions of this basic learning sequence (e.g., Cartledge & Kleefeld, 1991, 1994; Cartledge & Milburn, 1995; Goldstein & McGinnis, 1997; Guerra, Moore, & Slaby, 1995; McGinnis & Goldstein, 1997; Richardson & Evans, 1997; Stephens, 1992).

Direct Instruction

Direct instructional approaches tend to be preferred and most beneficial to each of the minority groups discussed in this chapter (Cartledge & Milburn, 1996). Each of these groups is rooted in a culture that emphasizes direct teachings or instruction as a means to mold social behavior; simple stories or folktales are often used to illustrate the desired ways of living. To make skills training procedures most relevant, social skills trainers need to attend especially to the skills targeted for instruction, the communication styles of the learners, the manner in which the scripts are developed and presented, and the developmental level of the learners.

Social Skill Instruction

Although we do not wish to present these groups stereotypically, we believe it is important to note that certain groups of children are often socialized in ways that are inconsistent with the larger society. The dominant Western culture, for example, values verbal assertiveness and expects children to articulate their needs easily and readily in order to achieve their goals. For the four targeted groups, less heavily language-based social skills tend to distinguish them from their Anglo peers and may place them in danger of misperceptions by others or may impede the development of verbal communication skills (Carlson & Stephens, 1986; Feng & Cartledge, 1996; Powless & Elliott, 1993).

A teacher's constant misinterpretations of a student's behavior can cause tensions that may contribute to conflict or fear and thus interfere with desired social development. For instance, Feng and Cartledge (1996) found that in their study of low-SES fifth-grade students, the Asian Americans were significantly more likely than their African American or European American peers to state that they would say or do nothing when encountering unfair treatment. Another finding was that whereas European American students made more negative statements than either of the other two groups, African Americans emitted more verbally aggressive statements. Although the level of verbal aggression found in this study was almost negligible, teachers are likely to judge and deal with the minimal verbal aggression much more severely than the verbal negativity occurring at much higher rates. Along the same lines, the passivity expressed by the Asian Americans is likely to be overlooked.

These data indicate that substantial numbers of children in all three groups evidenced social communication difficulties that may appear to warrant intervention, with a slightly different focus for each group. The Asian American students in this study, for example, may benefit from teachings emphasizing the importance of relating unfair treatment and ways to communicate these events appropriately. The African American students, however, may be helped most in assessing ambiguous events and in responding to provocation in nonaggressive ways. Finally, instruction for the European American students may stress reducing authoritarian or caustic peer communication.

Although members within each group would benefit from instruction in each of these areas, certain behavior patterns found in each group as a whole could be the basis for guiding interventions. Extensive instruction designed to establish the importance of communicating wrongdoing, for instance, may be poor use of valuable time for the African American and European American students in the Feng and Cartledge (1996) study. Within each group there were students who evidenced very passive, assertive, and aggressive social communication behaviors. But because the students tended to interact largely along racial lines and were likely to return to rather segregated conditions in their neighborhoods, the likelihood that the identified distinctive behaviors would be reinforced was great.

When educators are targeting social skills from a cultural perspective, it is just as important to recognize a group's strengths as its deficits, if not more so. In the Feng and Cartledge (1996) study, several of the differences among groups indicated, desirable interpersonal qualities. African American students were observed to be more people oriented and significantly more generous in their indications of liking their peers, regardless of race. Asian American students engaged in more cross-race interactions than either of the other two groups, and European Americans had the highest rate of positive statements made to their peers. If differences among individuals or groups are viewed only in terms of deficits, distortions can occur. For example, an educator who assumes that every African American male will respond with verbal aggression, and that such acts are signs of serious disorders or pathology, is likely to miss such a youngster's humanity and to react to him in counterproductive ways.

Social skill interventions are not to be viewed as a means for controlling students for the comfort of teachers, or for homogenizing students so that they conform to some middle-class prototype designated by the majority group in U.S. society. Inherent in the concept of culturally relevant social skill instruction is a reciprocal process in which the educator (1) learns to respect each learner's cultural background, (2) encourages the learner to appreciate the richness of this culture, (3) when needed, helps the learner to acquire additional or alternative behaviors as demanded by the social situation, and (4) similarly employs and practices the taught behaviors. The African American male who engages in good-natured verbal sparring with his peers need not be rebuked for this behavior, but may have to learn alternative ways to assert himself under conditions where the sport of "playing the dozens" would be misunderstood. Likewise, the teacher may become more knowledgeable about this cultural exchange and explore variations in African American literature that can serve as the basis for academic as well as social learnings (see Cartledge & Milburn, 1996; Foster, 1974; Irvine, 1990; Wynn, 1992a).

Along the same lines, for language-different children, the initial point of intervention may be for the teacher to understand the learners through the learners' form of communication. Mulhern (1995) presents a case study of a young Mexican American female who started to thrive in school when her teachers began to celebrate her writing and learn about her world through the child's stories. Mulhern attributed this progress to an "environment in which children can understand and be understood" (p. 22). Viewing the child's life from a broader perspective, Mulhern saw ways in which the child and her family were unfairly blamed, leading her to conclude "that educators need to pay closer attention to the sociocultural worlds of children and to move past initial perceptions or "assumptions about children from low-income and/or minority families" (p. 24).

Culturally sensitive instruction permits the teachers to affirm the students and the students' background. This step is critical to increasing the learners' receptivity to the needed social learning. At the same time, the teachers increase their own cultural understanding; this enables them to respond to the students in accepting, nonstereotypical ways. The legitimacy of these teachings is enhanced greatly when they are demonstrated and practiced by the school staff. For example, if teachers want students to respond to provocation in nonaggressive ways, then confrontations regarding students' misbehavior should be handled accordingly—that is, in an assertive, decisive manner without verbal or physical acts intended to inflict harm.

In addition to an understanding of and respect for the culture of the learner, culturally sensitive direct social skill instruction requires relevance in terms of a variety of factors, including stimulus materials, models, and group composition (Cartledge & Milburn, 1996). The model for direct instruction often begins with the provision of some rationale for the skill (Cartledge & Milburn, 1995). This rationale can be presented in various forms, including stories, films, videos, or real-life events. It is important that these scenarios be culturally relevant and pertinent to the students' everyday experiences. Hammond (1991), for example, presents a series of videotapes relevant to the lives of many African American males by using scenes of common experiences (e.g., confronting a peer about a pair of missing athletic shoes).

Social skill trainers are likely to use commercial or teacher-prepared scripts. Even if these scripts contain a culturally relevant context, the language style may still be unfamiliar to the students and thus reduce the lesson's effect. In one study, urban adolescent males increased their attention to and participation in social skill instruction after being permitted to design scenarios and develop scripts with their own wording and language styles (Moore, Cartledge, & Heckaman, 1995). Prior to this "co-scripting" between teachers and students, the students displayed minimal interest and tended to change the scenes and words of the teacher-developed scripts. A statement such as "You aren't that good. Your jump shot is no good," for example, would be changed to "You ain't all that now. Your 'J' is broke." As the students assumed more responsibility in developing the instruction, there was evidence of a corresponding increase in the importance they attached to these social skills. The researchers also observed the students using statements from their scripts to prompt peer behavior under regular school conditions. Improvements were found in game-related social behaviors in the targeted students.

Effective Instruction

To be most effective, interventions must be based on the behavioral profiles presented by the specific population. In the Lo and Cartledge (2001) study, for example, disciplinary referrals revealed that the teachers' concerns centered mainly on (1) classroom disruptions, (2) peer-on-peer aggression, and (3) insubordination. Furthermore, the main reason for school suspension was aggression followed by insubordination. These findings have direct implications for the most critical teachings needed by these students. Classroom disruptions, which involved more male than female students, suggested that the students were not effectively engaged in the classroom instruction. Elementary-age boys often have high energy levels and require attractive, well-structured instructional activities for sustained attention.

Heward (1994, 2000) offers strategies, classified as active student responding (ASR), useful for increasing students' academic responding and adaptive classroom behavior. ASR is designed so that all students are able to respond simultaneously to questions; this is in contrast to typical classroom instruction where only one child at a time responds to teacher questioning, giving other students the opportunity to drift cognitively or physically. During these periods highly active students, especially males, will become disengaged from the lesson and begin to distract other students and disrupt the class. One technique proposed by Heward is the use of response cards, whereby students have either preprinted or wipe-off cards to respond to each question posed by the teacher. Students have an opportunity to respond continuously throughout the lesson, which accordingly guides them to be more attentive and less disruptive. Lambert (2001) trained teachers to use response cards during math class with their urban general education students. Using a single-subject reversal design, a functional relationship was observed between the use of response cards and a reduction in disruptive behavior. Corresponding improvements were found in correct student responding—that is, during the response card condition, students were less likely to be disruptive and more likely to respond correctly to the academic material.

Behavior Management

In addition to using instructional strategies that keep students continually and meaningfully engaged, teachers need to become skilled in management techniques that are proactive, effective, and culturally responsive. No child likes to be corrected in front of his or her peers, but children of some cultures find it more demeaning than others (Grant & Gomez, 2001). Children who are part of cultural groups that value group (or familial) membership over the individual find public retribution particularly humiliating and may respond in a manner that is not socially acceptable to a teacher. Teachers must be aware of the individual needs of these children as they solve problems with dignity by addressing them in private. Failing to do so leads to power struggles, which is a lose-lose situation for both school personnel and the student

A basic principle for avoiding frequent power struggles is to review the rules and the consequences for not following the rules, and point out to the learner that it is his or her choice to either follow the rules or suffer the consequences. The teacher must be prepared to follow through with the consequences; note also that the consequences must be structured so that students find it more rewarding to follow the rules than to experience the consequences. There are classroom strategies for dealing with noncompliance, which are requisite for schools/classrooms with high levels of insubordination (e.g., McEwan, 2000; Rhode, Jenson, & Reavis, 1992; Watson, 1998).

Intervening with children before they develop ingrained antisocial behaviors can be an important dimension of reducing violence in youth (Straub, 1996). It is imperative that any behavioral intervention program for culturally diverse learners include strategies for teaching these learners effective ways of managing conflict. Such instruction equips the students with tools to regulate their own behavior, monitor the behavior of others, and to respond appropriately. Slogans, campaigns, and scare tactics will not work. Hammond (1991; Hammond & Yung, 1993) present a series of culturally sensitive videotapes in which peer role models demonstrate ways to negotiate and deal with problem situations. Reports indicate that participating students had fewer violence-related offenses than nonparticipants.

Dealing with Stress

The living conditions of many low-income and minority students force them to deal with many more stressors than their nonminority peers must confront. Hispanic Americans, for example, report more daily stressors and depression than their Anglo counterparts (Casas et al., 1990; Hoemicke et al., 1994; Ramirez, 1989). Some of the more universal stressors for culturally different youths include (1) being new or feeling different in classes, (2) fearing for physical safety, (3) fearing premature death, (4) maintaining their primary language and conversing effectively in English as well, (5) racial and ethnic intolerance by others, and (6) peer pressure (Casas et al., 1990).

Walker, Colvin, and Ramsey (1995) report data indicating that high school students of all backgrounds believe that race relations in the United States are getting worse, and that most minority youths (i.e., 71% of African Americans, 79% of Asian Americans, and 60% of Latino Americans, as compared with 33% of whites) feel that they have experienced racial or ethnic discrimination. Within-group stressors are noted by several researchers for African American (Fordham, 1988), Hispanic American (Matute-Bianchi, 1986), Native American (Deyhle, 1986), and Asian American (Chin, 1990) youths, who are ridiculed by their same-race peers either for engaging in achievement-oriented behaviors (labeled "acting white') or for failing to measure up to the mainstreamed standards for speech, dress, and so forth.

These conditions, which undoubtedly contribute to maladaptive behaviors such as persistent peer conflict, substance abuse, and violence, suggest the need to emphasize skills and strategies designed to cope with and reduce stress. Young people need to be helped to think positively and constructively about themselves and to learn ways to react to the misguided or unkind actions of others. Curriculum programs such as that provided by Goldstein & McGinnis (1997) often present a set of skills that include dealing with stress-related situations, such as group pressure and being left out. These skills and related instruction can be refined to address directly the racial or ethnic issues confronting students. For example, peer taunts centering on either rejecting one's ethnicity or acting too ethnic may be rooted in unresolved identity issues, both for the taunter and for the taunted. Instruction on helping students to cope with peer pressures in this area might explore healthy and unhealthy attitudes toward one's racial or ethnic background and incorporate related facilitating thoughts into coping self-statements. Meichenbaum (1977) provides a stress inoculation training model designed to help the learner recognize the source of the stress, prepare for it, employ self-statements to handle the stressful event, recognize the accompanying emotions, evaluate the outcome, and reinforce accomplishments.

Students who disparage their same-group peers often have identity issues suggesting negative feelings about their minority group and themselves. For instance, African American or Hispanic American males who attribute antisocial characteristics to themselves and view such behaviors positively (e.g., Elrich, 1994) may be expressing "sour grapes" as a means of avoiding the stress of trying to achieve under formidable odds. These students would benefit from empowering experiences such as those discussed later in this chapter. Similar interventions are recommended for students at the other extreme, who experience mainstream success but devalue their same-group peers who persist in typical ethnic ways and speech.

Early Intervention

If educators and other professionals hope to have a positive effect on children's social behavior, especially on antisocial patterns such as aggression and delinquency, they have to begin their interventions with very young children. Ideally, such teaching would begin in the home, but in too many cases parents are either unaware of or unable to equip their children with the critical skills needed for positive social interaction and school success. This is particularly true in low-income situations, where both children and parents are often overwhelmed by the stressors that typically accompany poverty, and find that the unwholesome lessons from the immediate environment and the mass media are more powerful than the relatively healthier ones that may be provided in the home. In addition to poverty other stressors (e.g., marital conflict, parental psychiatric disorders, or parental drug abuse), combined with a biological dysfunction within a child (e.g., an attention disorder), frequently lead to poor family management practices, resulting in antisocial behavior in the child (Patterson, 1986; Whalen, 1989).

Preschool and Head Start programs are excellent sites for early direct instruction in social skills. Young children can begin to learn to use nonaggressive words to express their needs and feelings. They can learn appropriate ways to negotiate and compromise with their peers in order to manage disputes and conflict. They can also be prompted in ways to be more empathic and helpful to fellow students and others. Middleton used a primary-level curriculum (Cartledge & Kleefeld, 1991) to reduce the aggression (Middleton & Cartledge, 1995) and increase the prosocial behaviors (Middleton, 1994) of inner-city African American kindergarten, first-grade, and second-grade students. The requisite and typically greater involvement of parents in the school programs of younger children makes social skill instruction for this age group even more attractive. In both of her studies, Middleton was successful in getting parents to prompt, reinforce, and report the behaviors at home that their children had been taught at school.

Parental Involvement

Cultural sensitivity is extremely relevant to the assumptions made about the home. Parents of low-income and minority children are often characterized as underinvolved in the schooling of their children (Chavkin, 1989; Shea & Bauer, 1985), but there is also evidence that teachers are less inclined to contact minority parents than middle-class parents, because they assume indifference on the part of minority parents (Turnbull & Turnbull, 1986). In addition, teachers disproportionately contact minority parents for disciplinary actions (Marion, 1980), and miscommunications between the school and minority homes are likely to occur (Mulhern, 1995). When home–school relations are tense and revolve largely around negative events, parents tend to withdraw and resist overtures from the school.

School personnel need to cultivate more productive family approaches, such as learning about a child's culture before making an initial contact. In many traditional Hispanic families, for example, the father is addressed first. Other suggestions include making first contacts positive ones, conducting individual conferences with parents (in their homes, if necessary), establishing a system for regular home–school communication, and involving the parents in some ongoing way in the children's social skill instructional program. An example of the last of these is given by Middleton (Middleton & Cartledge, 1995; Cartledge & Middleton, 1996): African American parents received a weekly form (a Gaining Appropriate Behaviors, or GAB, sheet) detailing the "skill being taught in school that week, questions or activities that were to be conducted with the students as homework, and a way to evaluate their children's performance. Prior to intervention for the Middleton studies, parents received a hour in-service" session on ways to teach social skills and the potential benefit of such teaching to their children. Parents responded favorably to the project, and corresponding improvements were noted in their children's social skills.

Cultural Learning

Central to any discussion of cultural sensitivity and social behaviors are issues of ethnic or racial identity and self-esteem. According to Nieto (1995), an important step in becoming socially competent is developing a good sense of one's dignity and self-worth, resulting from a strong identity. Nieto demonstrates through case studies of "subjugated and economically depressed" adolescents the transformative power of culturally specific curriculum and pedagogy to bring about more adaptive academic and social behaviors. Accordingly, it is felt that social skill instruction put in a culturally relevant context can be more effective for minority populations than traditional approaches can be.

Among the principal means for transmitting cultural information are literature and other media, such as films and tapes. Since the 1970s the number of authentic books written by and about minority populations has increased substantially. Many of these works—both fiction and nonfiction—contain valuable information relative to ethnic or racial background, along with important content relative to social learning and character development. Cartledge and Milburn (1996) have identified many of these books according to the ethnicity and age of the learner. The reader is also referred to annotations that list books for children and adolescents by race, country of origin, and/or issue (e.g., Cartledge & Kiarie, 2001; Miller-Lachmann, 1992; Rudman, 1995).

Despite the recent increase in culturally diverse literature, it is important to note that many of the works are published by small publishing houses and may not be easily accessible, and that materials for adolescents are particularly limited (de Cortes, 1992). Equally important, if not more so, is the realization that the students at greatest risk for disruptive or violent behavior in our schools are those least likely to have the skills or motivation to pursue a wide range of reading. And if they do read, there is little assurance that they will attend to the most salient points to promote self-identity and social development. These observations indicate the need to take several steps in order to foster social adjustment through cultural knowledge. First, to increase the quantity of reading material, teachers and other professionals might draw upon various community resources—community leaders, churches, civic organizations, local libraries, and so forth. Books by and about minorities have a relatively short shelf life and often are not widely publicized. Therefore, more effort may have to be expended to compile an adequate set of high-quality books.

While collecting these books, teachers might conduct informal surveys of youngsters and adults to determine which books are favorites among youths and potentially have the greatest impact. Because males are less likely than females to engage in independent reading (Rudman, 1995), and males are more closely associated with physical aggression or violence than females, teachers will have to do much more than simply make reading assignments. To help reading become an integral part of young people's daily lives, from preschool throughout the senior grades, daily school periods have to be set aside for extended reading, both oral and silent. Even at the high school level, teachers may find it beneficial to read to their students. This is especially true for social skill instruction, inasmuch as students prone to violent behavior are likely to overlook the desired lessons. Oral readings also circumvent the problems of students with reading deficits who cannot master the reading selections independently. Along with oral readings, another powerful motivator, particularly for adequate readers, is to allocate in-school time for independent reading. Gloeckner (1995), for example, found this strategy resulted in dramatic increases in the independent reading of her high school students, who then were more inclined to continue their reading outside of class. Cartledge and Kiarie (2001) give guidelines for selecting and using books for social learning.

Many of the recent books written for young children deal with the pain and stresses of being different. These are contemporary stories that are intended to be informative and affirming. For example, in *The Adventures of Connie and Diego/Las Aventuras de Connie y Diego* (Garcia, 1987), a Hispanic American sister-and-brother pair, born in a fictitious land, tire of being taunted because of their skin color and run away. During their adventures they learn to appreciate differences and to accept themselves. Another example for a black child is *Amazing Grace* (Hoffman & Binch, 1991). Grace, who has a penchant for drama, wants the lead role of Peter Pan in the school play but is discouraged by her classmates, who tell her it is not a role for a black female. Comforted by members of her family, who make her aware of a black ballerina with the lead role in *Romeo and Juliet* in a local theater, Grace wins the part of Peter Pan and is convinced of her potential to be whatever she wants to be. These and similar stories, such as *Angel Child, Dragon Child* (Surat, 1983) for Asian Americans and *Sequoia* (Cwiklik, 1989) for Native Americans, can help young readers learn valuable lessons about themselves (positive self-statements, personal goals, personal interests, perseverance, and so forth.).

For older youths, there are noteworthy books that deal realistically with the pressures and challenges experienced by specific populations. An award-winning author of such a book is Walter Dean Myers. In his book *Hoops* (1981), for example, a talented 17-year-old basketball player must decide between immediate gratification with possible punishing consequences or persevering toward a delayed but more worthwhile goal. This easy-to-read book is authentic in its portrayal of urban teenage life and provides provocative, useful content for social learnings. Other such books by Myers include *Scorpions* (1988), focusing on youth gang life and its outcomes, *Motown and Didi: A Love Story* (1984), which addresses values, racial identity, and relationships, and *Monster* (2001), an award-winning book that vividly depicts the thoughts and circumstances of a youth inadvertently caught up in the criminal justice system. Stories about typical social experiences for Hispanic teens can be found in *Baseball in April: And Other Stories* (Soto, 1990).

Perhaps most useful for social awareness are autobiographies or biographies that depict individuals overcoming obstacles similar to those encountered in the daily lives of violence-prone youths. An especially compelling biography is *Makes Me Wanna Holler* by Nathan McCall (1994). McCall, currently a journalist with the *Washington Post*, describes his growing up as a young black male in the 1970s. He takes the reader through his thought processes and life events as he decided to ignore academics and pursue a life of drugs and criminal activity. The scenes of prison life are vivid, and McCall details his thoughts about his various actions, his misgivings about his behavior, and the specific steps he took to put his life on a more productive course. Teachers and other professionals should be cautioned about the explicit nature of such material, since some youngsters may glamorize the unsavory. This work should be read with the students, discussing the essential points and helping them to make personal applications where appropriate. Other books with themes for urban culturally diverse youth include *Our America* (Jones & Newman, 1997), *Living to Tell about It* (Dawsey, 1995), and *Freedom Writers Diary* (Gruwell, 1999).

Contemporary literature for many minority children and youths, particularly recent immigrants, focuses on biculturalism and the expected conflicts that occur in language, between parents and peers, and in adapting to different customs. These young people are often troubled and embarrassed by their differences. The stress of trying to cope under these conditions causes some to retreat from mainstreamed classes, to drop out of school, and to pursue criminal activity within their communities as one means of survival (Chin, 1990; Matute-Bianchi, 1986). a book entitled *I Speak English for My Mom* (Stanek, 1989) details the difficulties encountered by an immigrant female-headed Hispanic family in which the young daughter is required to translate everything for her mother. The strong mother–daughter relationship is further strengthened when the young girl helps her mother to learn English and become more self-sufficient.

The literature for immigrant youths with Asian and South Pacific origins is limited (Chu & Schuler, 1992), but there are some books available that provide narratives about the difficulties, adjustments, and successes such teens experience in the United States—for example, *Into a Strange Land: Unaccompanied Refugee Youth in America* (Ashabranner & Ashabranner, 1987), *New Kids on the Block: Oral Histories of Immigrant Teens* (Bode, 1989), and *Dark Sky, Dark Land: Stories of the Hmong Boy Scouts of Troop 100* (Moore, 1989). These books give information about the young people's countries of origin and provide firsthand accounts of ordeals encountered in both their native and new lands; the youths offer advice on ways to meet the challenges of adjusting to a new land. Personal narratives are also provided for contemporary Native American youths in *To Live in Two Worlds: American Indian Youth Today* (Ashabranner, 1984), which depicts Native teens' efforts to overcome the difficulties of traversing two cultures. The same theme, along with issues of alcoholism and related self-destructive behavior, is effectively presented in the fictional work *Ceremony of the Panther* (Wallin, 1987).

The use of literature by and about minority groups is beneficial to all students, not only those who are members of the specific group targeted in a particular story or book (Walker et al., 1995). All young people need to be validated and affirmed in their own minds, as well as in the eyes of others. The respectful presentation of the traditions and lives of all groups for all group members is one means of helping to achieve this goal. Maladaptive behaviors often grow out of misguided attempts at self-validation by youths from subjugated groups. Current books with contemporary issues and solutions can be a valuable resource for social learning. With these materials. it is possible for readers to identify with the principal characters, analyze the characters' thought processes and management styles, and consider various approaches for dealing with their own personal situations. At the very least, it can be reassuring for young people to realize that their external and internal conflicts are experienced in similar ways by others. Educators should read and discuss these works with students, making sure that the important messages are understood.

Valuing Students

Schools should be important, empowering environments for all students, including those from racially and ethnically diverse backgrounds. Within schools, students need to feel welcomed and valued, and they should be given the opportunity to develop a sense of competence, usefulness, and belonging (Vargas, 1994; Walker et al., 1995). Passive educational climates tend to dominate our schools; students are expected to keep quiet; be attentive, and follow the teacher's directions. This atmosphere may be conducive to certain types of school performance, particularly rote learning, but does little to help a learner become an active participant in the schooling process and develop a sense of value and purpose.

For many minority youths, the message they perceive from authority figures toward them is one of indifference, invisibility, or second-class citizenship. These young people may be attending schools where they have no expectation of full participation in school activities (e.g., student groups focused on drama, journalism, science, etc.). Assuming that such endeavors are reserved for members of the dominant group or for only the highest achievers in the school, these youngsters are likely to avoid and belittle most wholesome school activities. To complicate matters further, the policies of many schools prohibit students with poor academic or discipline records from engaging in extracurricular activities, even if they display a special talent or interest in such an activity. Although the rationale for these rules is understandable, they tend to discriminate disproportionately against students with cultural differences and mild disabilities, placing vulnerable students at even greater risk. A major challenge for the schools is to identify ways to engage marginal students actively, so that school becomes a meaningful, productive experience. Possible strategies for this purpose include providing special-interest and extracurricular activities, peer mediation, peer tutoring, and cooperative environments.

Special-Interest and Extracurricular Activities

Some schools offer or allow for small-group mentoring activities designed specifically for minority students. An adult leader who is of the same racial or ethnic background as the students meets with a small group of students two or three times weekly to carry out various activities. Students selected for these programs tend to be those most at risk for negative outcomes. Through an emphasis on self-awareness and character development, these programs intend to counter destructive social influences and to prevent violence, substance abuse, school failure, premature parenting, and so forth. Wynn (1992a) has developed a 10-step approach that includes activities typically used in these groups. The program, entitled Empowering African-American Males to Succeed, is focused on helping these youths "think and . . . do for themselves in ways that are morally sound and socially acceptable" (Wynn, 1992a, p. xix). Following is a summary of this 10-step program, which Wynn presents in the form of a pyramid. Each step is viewed as a building block laid upon the previous one to complete the pyramid with step 10.

1. *Cultural understanding.* Understanding the youngster's culture in terms of role models, family environment, specific characteristics (e.g., clothes, hair, etc.), personality (e.g., leadership skills, self-esteem), and personal goals is basic to teaching and motivating the learner to succeed. Teachers often know little about the background, interests, or aspirations of specific students. Exercises are provided to highlight this point and to help teachers increase their knowledge about their students. At least two critical understandings must be acquired and employed. First, the culturally specific behavior of minority youths should be viewed as differences, not as deficits. Their backgrounds are not inherently inferior, and our goal is not that they should discard their ways of being in order to emulate totally the styles of European Americans. Second, African American males are humanistic and strongly desire to be valued and respected. When affection and respect are not evident, anger and rebelliousness are likely to result. Specific suggestions are given for dealing with two pervasive culturally based behaviors: "playing the dozens" and the "showdown."

2. *Mutual respect/character development.* A desired outcome of successful schooling is that young people exhibit disciplined and ordered lives. Teachers are not to strive to "make" students behave, but to motivate students to *want* to behave. Young African American males display extraordinary discipline for desired goals in sports, music, and other areas of personal interest School-based discipline is at least partly predicated on mutual respect between teachers and students. Instead of superimposing rules and engaging in power struggles, teachers and students should jointly carve out a code of acceptable behaviors. Students understand the importance of these regulations, and when they take some ownership in developing them, they are

more likely to follow and enforce them with their peers. The resulting rules are often comparable to, or even more stringent than, those the teacher initially had in mind, but this collaborative process is a valuing and motivating experience for students. A sample code of conduct is given that includes behaviors such as affirming each other, showing respect for self and others, and avoiding verbal and physical aggression.

3. *Personal responsibility.* Learning to take responsibility for one's behavior is a critical aspect of personal development. Parents, teachers, and others must refrain from making excuses for a youngster's poor conduct, but insist that the young person acknowledge his or her actions and fully accept them. It is not enough for young people simply to *attend school*; teachers and students must assume responsibility for the students' full participation and productivity. Teaching procedures that facilitate responsible behavior include helping students to develop a sense of mastery through successfully meeting desired goals, providing students an active voice in classroom decision making, and assigning daily classroom responsibilities. Such responsibilities may include taking attendance, providing a daily quote, collecting homework, and giving oral quizzes.

4. *Teacher/parent expectations.* Adults often have low expectations of the eventual achievements of minority students, which are either directly or indirectly communicated to these young people. There is good evidence, however, of excellence among minority youths when they are expected to excel. Teachers are advised to raise their expectations for African American males. Exercises such as helping students set and achieve *extraordinary* goals are given as a means for helping teachers and students raise their expectations for academic and social behavior.

5. *Focusing on/identifying goals.* Closely aligned to step 4, this step deals with helping students to set specific goals confidently. Discouraging students from setting goals perceived to be unrealistic may weaken their spirit and cause them to lose interest in many valuable activities. Students who are encouraged to pursue their goals are more likely to remain engaged in the schooling process and become successful in some worthwhile endeavor. Exercises are given for this purpose. Despite the odds, for example, a student who strives to be another Michael Jordan, is encouraged to keep this dream and to prepare for it by researching the life of Michael Jordan, exploring colleges and scholarship opportunities, learning about contracts with the National Basketball Association, engaging in mock media interviews, and so forth.

6. *Visualization.* It is important that low-income minority youths see themselves as successful, rather than succumbing to despair and a sense of hopelessness about ever being able to emerge from their present condition. Teachers are encouraged to set aside "quiet time" each day for students to visualize great expectations, such as getting all A's, writing great books, giving great speeches, or being a doctor. Through various means (e.g., field trips or guest speaker), real-life examples of these dreams should be produced. Such

efforts can help to maintain motivation and to extend these youths' dreams beyond the typical ones (e.g., professional sports).

7. *Affirmation.* African American males are confronted daily with negative, demeaning messages suggesting failure and inferiority. These youngsters are in critical need of affirmations. Teachers can be affirming, helping them to believe that they can be successful and achieve their worthwhile goals.

8. *Integrating curriculum and home.* Teachers can incorporate what is known about the lifestyles and culture of African American males to motivate classroom learning. For example, these males participate more in team sports (e.g., basketball, football) than in individualistic ones (e.g., gymnastics, swimming). Classroom academics might be structured according to interactive groups along the principles of cooperative or "family-style" learning. Other suggestions include drawing upon oral history traditions. so that students get an opportunity to discuss the subject matter vigorously, and respecting students' efforts and being careful not to embarrass them in front of peers.

9. *A passion for excellence.* Failure is not expected or accepted in these young men. They are urged to aim constantly for excellence, and teachers are charged to help them develop the confidence, pride, and dignity needed for this quest One suggested activity is a poetry recitation designed to help students respond in ways that involve gradually increasing displays of confidence, pride, and dignity.

10. *Empowerment.* At this level, young people evidence self-confidence, respect for self and others, and a conviction that they can achieve their dreams. Through diligent study and culturally relevant readings, the spirit of empowerment can be maintained. These youngsters need to read, write, and speak about their heritage and to develop socially appropriate visions for the future.

Wynn (1992b) also provides a workbook with exercises for each of the pyramid blocks. Although not extensive, these exercises can be useful to the educator or professional initiating an "empowering" program for students from culturally diverse backgrounds. Even though the book specifies African American males and incorporates an Africentric focus, Wynn (1992a) points out that this model can be adapted to any group. Interventions of this nature, however, are of critical importance for African American males because they are at the greatest risk for violent outcomes (Prothrow-Stith, 1994).

Participation in other regular school activities is equally important for at-risk students from culturally diverse backgrounds. To the extent possible, these students need to be included in mainstream school activities where they are helped to feel like full citizens, to assume ownership for school functions, and to take pride in their successes (no matter how small). Students who are left to languish on the margins of the school community tend to feel devalued and are likely to develop antischool attitudes and behaviors. Special efforts must be made to tap the talents and interests of each student in order to engage the student in one or more of the full range of school activities (e.g., music, journalism, drama, sports, and visual arts). Each student has some unique, noteworthy abilities. Involvement in the school community is a goal for each student and should not be based on superior skills; however, students should be assessed individually to determine where the best match might occur. For example, a student who has limited written communication skills but enjoys interacting with others might be given "roving reporter" assignments for the school newspaper. The semi scripted interviews can be tape-recorded and transcribed by this student or by a fellow student with adequate word-processing or computer skills. Another example is to engage these youngsters as cross-age tutors or playground monitors for their youngster and less-skilled peers.

To be effective in this "full-inclusion" effort, school involvement must begin during a child's early years, before antischool attitudes are entrenched. At-risk students can be identified in the primary grades. Schools have to look for students evidencing poor academic performance, high rates of aggressive behaviors, and social skill deficits. Minority males who exhibit this profile are at the greatest risk and should receive priority attention for participation in esteem-building school-based and culturally specific activities.

Peer Mediation

All students need to learn to regulate their own behavior and manage conflict. Skills in conflict mediation and management should be explicitly included in the school's curriculum. Mediation is important for both young people and adults, because mediation focuses on understanding a conflict and arriving at a mutually acceptable resolution, rather than simply on exercising control over other persons' behavior. Schools often emphasize controlling students and maintaining order, at the expense of helping students develop the problem-solving and cognitive skills required to effectively manage everyday problems in living.

The use of peer mediation in the schools is increasing, with documented evidence of its beneficial effects (Johnson & Johnson, 1994; Koch, 1988; Lane & McWhirter, 1992; McCormick, 1988). Students are trained to be mediators to assist their peers to minimize conflict and resolve problems peacefully. As mediators, students are expected to follow the following sequence: (1) They determine whether the disputants want mediation and then specify the rules (e.g., no name calling, being honest, no interrupting), (2) they listen to the events detailed individually by each disputant, (3) they determine what each person wants to happen, (4) they engage the disputants in deciding what they can do to agree on a problem solution, avoid future problems, and dispel rumors, and (5) they congratulate the disputants for their hard work (Lane & McWhirter, 1992).

Lane and McWhirter (1992) recommend selecting a specific group of students to be trained to serve as peer mediators. However, Johnson and

Johnson (1991,1994) believe that because students are involved in conflict daily, a "total student body approach," in which all students are trained to use these procedures, will produce the most effective and widespread results. Furthermore, Johnson and Johnson suggest that conflict mediation procedures be taught and employed throughout the 12 years of schooling. Prothrow-Stith (1991) also provides guidelines for conflict management, with an emphasis on urban, minority settings. Accordingly, issues pertaining to violence and homicide are stressed, and students are guided to examine possible contributing factors in order to identify ways to avoid these outcomes.

Students from racial and cultural minorities may be particularly well served by peer mediation procedures. First, these youths are often less trusting of members of the dominant group and may be more receptive to messages from their peers, especially same-race peers. Second, mediation with peers takes place within a climate of mutual respect and minimal stress. Students choose to air the problem within a nonauthoritarian atmosphere without the imminent threat of possible punishing consequences. In addition, each disputant has an equal opportunity to be heard, and students can take pride in achieving their own solutions. This can be an empowering experience, which is sorely needed by students who are constantly confronting their subjugated status in the larger society. Finally, the success of a mediated event can cause some conflict-prone youths to want to serve as mediators. Acting as mediators can have a substantial effect on young people's behavior. School personnel should take steps to include as many students as possible as mediators, particularly students from culturally or racially diverse backgrounds who are at risk for violent outcomes. Curricula are available for training young (e.g., Johnson & Johnson, 1991) and older (e.g., Guerra et al., 1995) students to manage conflict.

Peer Tutoring and Teaching

Peer tutoring can be an extremely effective tool for improving academic achievement (Berliner & Casanova, 1988), but under certain conditions it can also have beneficial effects on self-esteem (Giesecke, Cartledge, & Gardner, 1993) and social skills (Cochran, Feng, Cartledge, & Hamilton, 1993). Model students are typically singled out to be tutors for their lower-achieving same-age peers. This high-status assignment can enhance the tutors' self-regard, but the students being tutored may experience greater embarrassment and lowered self-esteem (e.g., Seda & Bixler-Márquez, 1994).

Although some form of remedial intervention is necessary and strongly encouraged for low-achieving students, the negative effects of remedial instruction may be softened somewhat by making similar empowering opportunities available to the remedial recipients. For example, in both the Giesecke et al. (1993) and Cochran et al. (1993) studies, low-achieving students served as cross-age tutors for their younger peers. Gains were observed for tutors and tutees in both studies. In the Cochran et al. study, low-achieving fifth-grade inner-city African American males with behavior disorders tutored low-achieving second-grade males in reading. Results showed academic gains for both tutors and tutees, as compared with their nontutoring peers, as well as sustained high levels of positive interactions during tutoring for the experimental students.

More recently, Blake, Wang, Cartledge, and Gardner (2000) conducted a set of studies in which students with behavior disorders were trained to teach small groups of their peers socially appropriate behaviors. Instead of employing the one-on-one interactions as described earlier, these studies utilized students to teach their peers in small groups of three. In one study that focused on verbally aggressive behavior, the trainer used the students with the poorest skills as trainers and found that the trainers showed the greatest growth in verbally supportive behaviors.

Cooperative Groups

Children from the four groups discussed in this chapter have their cultural backgrounds in collectivistic rather than individualistic societies (Cartledge & Milburn, 1996; Schneider, 1993). Extended family units and a historical emphasis on working for the betterment of the group, rather than competing for personal gain, are characteristic of each group. This philosophy reflects the underlying principles of cooperative learning, which is thought to have special advantages for members reared within a collectivistic orientation. Specific strategies for devising cooperative groups are described by various authors (e.g., Johnson & Johnson, 1987; Slavin, 1978). In the simplest form, children are organized into small groups and assigned to work together to accomplish a task. For example, as a group they may be required to complete one worksheet, to write a report on some topic, or to make certain that all group members are able to read or spell a set of designated words. To increase the likelihood that they will work as a group, all students in the group receive the same evaluation, based on the productivity of the group. This specification motivates students to work to assist the less skilled members of their group, and it aids in bringing about full participation of all the students. Alternative versions of cooperative learning include groups working as competitive teams (Slavin, 1978) or each student's assuming responsibility to teach specific subject matter to the other group members (Aronson, 1978).

Cooperative learning can be a vehicle to help students improve their social interaction skills, tolerance of peers, and academic achievement (Slavin, 1990). To participate effectively in these groups, children and youths must develop an array of subskills that may need to be taught directly. Cartledge and Cochran (1993) found that young students with emotional and behavior disorders required specific instructions in a set of rudimentary cooperative skills, such as (1) getting started, (2) asking for help, (3) responding to requests, (4) giving help, and (5) making support- ive statements. These skills have to be identified, demonstrated, practiced, and programmed for generality. A direct instruction paradigm was used to teach these behaviors, so that each skill was modeled by the trainer and re- hearsed several times by the students before they were to apply them in co- operative groups.

Cooperative techniques must be modeled and reinforced in the school. Initial efforts should be brief and simple, focusing more on performing the desired behaviors appropriately than on achieving some academic or social goal. As students become more skilled in participating in cooperative groups, the academic and social demands can be increased systematically. Eventually, it is hoped, students will recognize and become convinced of the beneficial effects of working together. That is, positive, constructive interac- tions may result in more gains—academically, socially, and personally—than environments that are intensively competitive with overtones of acrimony. Several authorities note the special predisposition of African American (Haynes & Gebreyesus, 1992), Asian American (Cook & Chi, 1984), Native American (Slavin & Oickle, 1981), and Hispanic American (Ravetta & Brunn, 1995) students toward cooperative environments and the beneficial returns of cooperative groups for these students.

CONCLUSIONS

All children and youths, regardless of race or ethnic background, have more commonalities than differences, but culture does influence the way they be- have and are perceived. Within pluralistic U.S. society, subcultural groups are affected differentially by various mitigating conditions (e.g., segregated communities. poverty, and recent immigrant status) that further alter life- styles and resulting social behaviors. The behaviors children bring to school must be interpreted and treated within a cultural context.

Schools for culturally diverse populations often reflect the harsh condi- tions children experience in the larger society. For some youngsters, schools fail to be valuing and empowering environments; rather, they are agents of control and containment, typically reacting to students' misbehavior with pu- nitive measures while giving little attention to positive interventions that fos- ter social development. Under these conditions, tensions and feelings of alienation are increased, and these can lead to more disruptive, violent behavior.

This is not meant to suggest that students should be allowed to misbe- have without consequences. But if schools hope to stem the tide of violence among their students, they must become proactive, intervening early in chil- dren's lives to provide social learning and affirming experiences that will be effective in countering antisocial, disruptive behaviors. Social skill instruc- tion has to be an explicit component of the curriculum throughout the 12 years of formal schooling; students must be helped to learn prosocial ways of being, ways to manage conflict, and ways to cooperate with others and contribute to the common good. Schools have to become places where children, regardless of their abilities and backgrounds, grow in the regard they have for themselves and others. Schools that teach from a monocultural perspective disenfranchise and further subjugate a significant minority of their constituencies. Students need to develop and maintain cultural competence, and their culture should serve as a vehicle for social skill teachings.

REFERENCES

Aguilar-Gaxiola. S. A., & Gray, T. (1994, August). *Diagnostic concordance between computerized and paper-and-pencil Spanish versions of the mood disorders section of the SCID-P in Hispanics*. Paper presented at the 102nd Annual Convention of the American Psychological Association, Los Angeles.

Aronson, E. (1978). *The jigsaw classroom*. Beverly Hills, CA: Sage.

Ashabranner, B. (1984). *To live in two worlds: American Indian youth today*. New York: Dodd, Mead.

Ashabranner, B., & Ashabranner, M. (1987). *Into a strange land: Unaccompanied refugee youth in America*. New York: Putnam.

Baer, J., & Chambliss, W. (1997). Generating fear: The politics of crime reporting. *Crime, Law, and Social Change, 27*, 87–107.

Berliner, D., & Casanova, U. (1988). Peer tutoring: a new look at a popular practice. *Instructor, 97*, 14–15.

Bernal, M. E., Saenz, D. S., & Knight, G. P. (1991). Ethnic identity and adaptation of Mexican American youths in school settings. *Hispanic Journal of Behavioral Sciences, 13*, 135–154.

Bettmann, E. H., & Moore, P. (1994). Conflict resolution programs and social justice. *Education and Urban Society, 27*, 11–21.

Blake, C., Wang, W., Cartledge, G., & Gardner, R. (2000). Middle-school students with serious emotional disturbances (SED) serve as social skill trainers/reinforcers for peers with SED. *Behavioral Disorders, 25*, 280–298.

Blau, J., & Blau, P. (1982). The cost of inequality: Metropolitan structure and violent crime. *American Sociological Review, 47*, 114–129.

Blyth, E., & Milner, J. (1993). Exclusion from school: A first step in exclusion from society. *Children and Society, 7*, 255–268.

Bode, J. (1989). *New kids on the block: Oral histories of immigrant teens*. New York: Franklin Watts.

Carlson, P. E., & Stephens, T. M. (1986). Cultural bias and identification of behaviorally disordered and learning disabled students. *Behavioral Disorders, 3*, 191–199.

Carmen, B. (1990, April 14). More blacks are disciplined. *Columbia Dispatch*, p. 1D.

Carrasquillo, A. L. (1991). *Hispanic children and youth in the United States: A resource guide* [Reference Books on Family Issues, Vol. 20]. New York: Garland.

Cartledge, G., & Cochran, L. L. (1993). Developing cooperative learning behaviors in students with behavior disorders. *Preventing School Failure, 37*, 5–10.

Cartledge, G., & Feng, H. (1996). Asian Americans: Culture and social skills. In G. Cartledge & J. F. Milburn (Eds.), *Cultural diversity and social skills instruction: Understanding ethnic and gender differences* (pp. 87–131). Champaign, IL: Research Press.

Cartledge, G., & Kiarie, M. (2001). Children and adolescent literature as a vehicle for social learning. *Teaching Exceptional Children, 7*, 255–268.

Cartledge, G., & Kleefeld, J. (1991). *Taking part: Introducing social skills to children.* Circle Pines, MN: American Guidance Service.

Cartledge, G., & Kleefeld, J. (1994). *Working together: Building children's social skills through folk literature.* Circle Pines, MN: American Guidance Service.

Cartledge, G., & Loe, S. (2001). Cultural diversity and social skill instruction. *Exceptionality, 9*, 33–46.

Cartledge, G., & Middleton, M. (1996). African Americans: Culture and social skills. In G. Cartledge & J. F. Milburn (Eds.), *Cultural diversity and social skills instruction: Understanding ethnic and gender differences* (pp. 133–203). Champaign, IL: Research Press.

Cartledge, G., & Milburn, J. F. (1995). *Teaching social skills to children and youth: Innovative approaches* (3rd ed.). Needham Heights, MA: Allyn & Bacon.

Cartledge, G., & Milburn, J. F. (Eds.). (1996). *Cultural diversity and social skills instruction: Understanding ethnic and gender differences.* Champaign, IL: Research Press.

Cartledge, G., Tillman, L. C., & Talbert-Johnson, C. (2001). Professional ethics within the context of student discipline and diversity. *Teacher Education Special Education, 24*, 25–27.

Casas, J. M., Furlong, M. J., Solberg, V. S., & Carranza, O. (1990). An examination of individual factors associated with the academic success and failure of Mexican-American and Anglo students. In A. Barona & E. E. Garcia (Eds.), *Children at risk: Poverty, minority status, and other issues in educational equity* (pp. 103–118). Washington, DC: National Association of School Psychologists.

Chavkin, N. F. (1989). Debunking the myth about minority parents. *Educational Horizons, 67*, 119–123.

Chin, K. (1990). *Chinese subculture and criminality.* New York: Greenwood Press.

Chu, E., & Schuler, C. V. (1992). United States: Asian Americans. In L. Miller-Lachmann (Ed.), *Our family, our friends, our world* (pp. 92–120). New Providence, NJ: Bowker.

Claiborne, W. (1999, December 17). Disparity in school discipline round: Blacks disproportionately penalized under get-tough policies, study says. *The Washington Post*, p. A03.

Cleary, L. M., & Peacock, T. D. (1998). *Collected wisdom.* Boston: Allyn & Bacon.

Cochran, L., Feng, H., Cartledge, G., & Hamilton, S. (1993). The effects of cross-age tutoring on the academic achievement, social behaviors, and self-perceptions of low-achieving African-American males with behavior disorders. *Behavioral Disorders, 18*, 292–302.

Cook. H., & Chi, C. (1984). Cooperative behavior and locus of control among American and Chinese-American boys. *Journal of Psychology, 118*, 169–177.

Costenbader, V., & Markson, S. (1998). School suspension: a study with secondary school students. *Journal of School Psychology, 36*, 59–82.

Council for Children with Behavioral Disorders (1989). Best assessment practices for students with behavioral disorders: Accommodation to cultural diversity and individual differences. *Behavioral Disorders, 14*, 263–278.

Cowart, M. T., & Cowart, R. E. (1993, December). Southeast Asian refugee youth and the cycle of violence. *NASSP Bulletin*, pp. 40–45.

Cwiklik, R. (1989). *Sequoia.* Englewood Cliffs, NJ: Silver Burdett.

Darling-Hammond, L. (1995). Inequality and access to knowledge. In J. A. Banks & C. A. M. Banks (Eds.), *Handbook of research on multicultural education* (pp. 465–483). New York: Macmillan.

Dawsey, D. (1995). *Living to tell about it: Young Black men in America speak their piece.* New York: Anchor Books.

de Cortes, O. G. (1992). United States: Hispanic Americans. In L. Miller-Lachmann (Ed.), *Our family, our friends, our world* (pp. 121–154). New Providence, NJ: Bowker.

Delpit, L. (1995). *Other people's children': Cultural conflict in the classroom*. New York: New Press.

Deyhle, D. (1986). Break dancing and breaking out Anglos, Utes, and Navajos in a border reservation high school. *Anthropology and Education Quarterly, 17*, 111–127.

DuRant, R., Cadenhead, C., Pendergrast, R., Slavens, G., & Linder, C. (1994). Factors associated with the use of violence among urban black adolescents. *American Journal of Public Health, 84*, 612–617.

Elrich, M. (1994). The stereotype within. *Educational Leadership, 51*, 12–15.

Eron, L. D., Huesmann, L. R., & Zelli, A. (1991). The role of parental variables in the learning of aggression. In D. J. Pepler & K. H. Rubin (Eds.), *The development and treatment of childhood aggression* (pp. 169–188). Hillsdale, NJ: Erlbaum.

Ewing, N. J. (1995). Restructured teacher education for inclusiveness: A dream deferred for African, American children. In B. A. Ford, F. E. Obiakor, & J. M. Patton (Eds.), *Effective education of African American exceptional learners: New perspectives* (pp. 189–207). Austin, TX: Pro-Ed.

Executive Committee, Council for Children with Behavioral Disorders. (1989). Best assessment practices for students with behavioral disorders: Accommodation to cultural diversity and individual differences. *Behavioral Disorders, 14*, 263–278.

Feld, B. (1997). Juvenile and criminal justice systems' responses to youth violence. In M. Tonry & M. Moore (Eds.), *Crime and justice* (Vol. 17, pp. 197–280). Chicago, IL: University of Chicago Press.

Felgar, M. (1992). Children on the edge. *Journal of Emotional and Behavioral Problems, 1*, 9–12.

Feng, H., & Cartledge, G. (1996). Social skills assessment of innercity Asian, African, and European American students. *School Psychology Review, 25*, 227–238.

Fordham, S. (1988). Racelessness as a factor in black students' school success: Pragmatic strategy or pyrrhic victory? *Harvard Educational Review, 58*, 54–84.

Forness, S. R. (1988). Planning for the needs of children with serious emotional disturbance: The National Special Education and Mental Health Coalition. *Behavioral Disorders, 13*, 127–139.

Foster, H. L. (1974). *Ribbin', jivin', and playin' the dozens: The unrecognized dilemma of inner city schools*. Cambridge, MA: Ballinger.

Garcia, M. (1987). *The adventures of Connie and Diego/Las aventuras de Connie y Diego*. San Francisco: Children's Book Press.

Giesecke, D., Cartledge, G., & Gardner, R. (1993). Low-achieving students as cross-age tutors: The effects on sight-word acquisition and self-concept. *Preventing School Failure, 37*, 34–43.

Gloeckner, J. (1995). *Effects of allotted class time and public posting on independent reading behavior of ninth grade students with learning disabilities*. Unpublished master's thesis, Ohio State University.

Goldstein, A. P., & McGinnis, E. (1997). *Skillstreaming the adolescent*. Champaign, IL: Research Press.

Gomez, M. L. (1994). Teacher education reform and prospective teachers' perspective on teaching "other people's" children. *Teaching and Teacher Education, 10*, 319–334.

Grant, C. A., & Gomez, M. L. (2001). *Campus and classroom: Making schooling multicultural*. Upper Saddle River, NJ: Merrill/Prentice-Hall.

Gregory, J. F. (1995). The crime of punishment: Racial and gender disparities in the use of corporal punishment in U.S. public schools. *Journal of Negro Education, 64*, 454–462.

Grossman, D. C., Milligan, C., & Deyo, R. A. (1991). Risk factors for suicide attempts among Navajo adolescents. *American Journal of Public Health, 81,* 874.

Grossman, H. (1995). *Special education in a diverse society.* Needham Heights, MA: Allyn & Bacon.

Gruwell, E., & The Freedom Writers (1999). *The freedom writers diary: How a teacher and 150 teens used writing to challenge themselves and the world around them.* New York: Main Street Books, Doubleday.

Guerra, N. G., Moore, A., & Slaby, R. G. (1995). *Viewpoints: A guide to conflict resolution and decision making for adolescents.* Champaign, IL: Research Press.

Hammond, W. R. (1991). *Dealing with anger: Givin' it, takin' it, workin' it out.* Champaign. IL: Research Press.

Hammond, W. R., & Yung, B. R. (1993). Psychology's role in the public health response to assaultive violence among young African-American men. *American Psychologist, 48,* 142–154.

Hawkins, D. F., Laub, J. H., Lauritsen, J. L., & Cothern, L. (2000). *Race, ethnicity, and serious and violent juvenile offending.* Washington, DC: U.S. Department of Justice, Office of Justice Programs, Office of Juvenile Justice and Delinquency Prevention.

Haynes, N. M., & Gebreyesus, S. (1992). Cooperative learning: A case for African-American students. *School Psychology Review, 21,* 577–585.

Heaviside, S., Rowand, C., Williams, C., & Farris, E. (1998). *Violence and discipline problems in U.S. public schools: 1996–97* (NCES 98–130). Washington, DC: U.S. Department of Education, National Center for Education Statistics.

Heward, W. L. (1994). Three "low-tech" strategies for increasing the frequency of active student response during group instruction. In R. Gardner III, D. M. Sainato, J. O. Cooper, T. E. Heron, W. L. Heward, J. Eshleman, & T. A. Grossi (Eds.), *Behavior analysis in education: Measurably superior instruction* (pp. 283–320). Monterey, CA: Brooks/ Cole.

Heward, W. L. (2000). *Exceptional children: An introduction to special education* (6th ed.). Upper Saddle River: Merrill/Prentice-Hall.

Hilliard, A. G. (1980). Cultural diversity and special education. *Exceptional Children, 46,* 584–588.

Hoernicke, P., Kallam, M., & Tablada, T. (1994). Behavioral disorders in Hispanic-American cultures. In R. L. Peterson & S. Ishii-Jordan (Eds.), *Multicultural issues in the education of students with behavioral disorders* (pp. 115–125). Cambridge, MA: Brookline Books.

Hoffman, M., & Binch, C. (1991). *Amazing Grace.* New York: Dial Books for Young Readers.

Howes, C., & Wu, F. (1990). Peer interactions and friendships in an ethnically diverse school setting. *Child Development, 61,* 537–541.

Hudley, C., & Graham, S. (1993). An attributional intervention to reduce peer-directed aggression among African-American boys. *Child Development, 64,* 124–138.

Hughes, J. N., & Cavell, T. A. (1995). Enhancing competence in aggressive children. In G. Cartledge & J. F. Milburn (Eds.), *Teaching social skills to children and youth: Innovative approaches* (3rd ed., pp. 199–236). Needham Heights, MA: Allyn & Bacon.

Hutson, H., Anglin, D., & Pratts, M. (1994). Adolescents and children injured or killed in drive-by shootings in Los Angeles. *New England Journal of Medicine, 330,* 324–327.

Irvine, J. J. (1990). *Black students and school failure.* New York: Greenwood Press.

Irvine, J. J. (1992). Making teacher education culturally responsive. In M. E. Dilworth (Ed.), *Diversity in teacher education: New expectations* (pp. 79–92). San Francisco: Jossey-Bass.

Johnson, D. W., & Johnson, R. T. (1987). *Learning together and alone: Cooperative. competitive, and individualistic learning.* Englewood Cliffs, NJ: Prentice-Hall.

Johnson, D. W., & Johnson, R. T. (1991). *Teaching students to be peacemakers*. Edina, MN: Interaction.

Johnson, D. W., & Johnson, R. T. (1994, April). *Teaching students to be peacemakers: Results of five years of research*. Paper presented at the annual meeting of the American Educational Research Association, San Francisco.

Jones, D. L., & Sandidge, R. F. (1997). Recruiting and retaining teachers in urban schools: Implications for policy and the law. *Education and Urban Society, 29*, 192–203.

Jones, L., & Newman, L. (1997). *Our America*. New York: Scribner.

Kehrberg, R. S. (1994). Behavioral disorders and gender/sexual issues. In R. L. Peterson & S. Ishii-Jordan (Eds.), *Multicultural issues in the education of students with behavioral disorders* (pp. 184–195). Cambridge, MA: Brookline Books.

Keller, H. R. (1988). Children's adaptive behaviors: Measure and source generalizability. *Journal of Psychoeducational Assessment, 6*, 371–389.

King, S. H. (1993). The limited presence of African-American teachers. *Review of Educational Research, 63*, 115–149.

Koch, M. (1988, January). Resolving disputes: Students can do it better. *NASSP Bulletin*, pp. 16–18.

Kozol, J. (1991). *Savage inequalities*. New York: Crown.

Kuykendall, C. (1992). *From rage to hope: Strategies for reclaiming black and Hispanic students*. Bloomington, IN: National Educational Service.

Ladson-Billings, G. (1995). But that's just good teaching! The case for culturally relevant pedagogy. *Theory into Practice, 34*, 159–165.

LaFromboise, T. D., & Low, K. G. (1989). American Indian children and adolescents. In J. T. Gibbs, L. N. Huang, & Associates, *Children of color* (pp. 114–147). San Francisco: Jossey-Bass.

Lambert, M. C. (2001). *The effects of increasing active student responding with response cards during mathematics instruction on the disruptive behavior of fourth-grade urban learners*. Unpublished doctoral dissertation, Ohio State University, Columbus, OH.

Lane, P. S., & McWhirter, J. J. (1992). a peer mediation model: Conflict resolution for elementary and middle schoolchildren. *Elementary School Guidance and Counseling, 27*, 15–23.

Larson, J. (1998). Managing student aggression in high schools: Implications for practice. *Psychology in the Schools, 35*, 283–295.

Leal, R. (1994). Conflicting views of discipline in San Antonio schools. *Education and Urban Society, 27*, 35–44.

Lethermon, V. R., Williamson, D. A., Moody, S. C., Granberry, S. W., Lemanek, K. L., & Bodiford, C. (1984). Factors affecting the social validity of a role-play test of children's social skills. *Journal of Behavioral Assessment, 6*, 231–245.

Lethermon, V. R., Williamson, D. A., Moody, S. C., & Wozniak, P. (1986). Racial bias in behavioral assessment of children's social skills. *Journal of Psychopathology and Behavioral Assessment, 8*, 329–337.

Lewis, T. J., & Sugai, G. (1999). Effective behavior support: a systems approach to proactive school-wide management. *Focus on Exceptional Children, 31*, 1–24.

Lo, Y.-Y., & Cartledge, G. (2001). *Disciplinary office referrals: Implications for behavioral interventions*. Unpublished manuscript, Ohio State University, Columbus, Ohio.

Los Angeles Unified School District. (1991). *Issues facing the Asian immigrant learner* (Report No. L000100). Los Angeles: Author.

Maheady, L., Algozzine, B., & Ysseldyke, J. E. (1985). Minorities in special education. *Education Digest, 51*, 50–53.

Marion, R. L. (1980). Communicating with parents of culturally diverse exceptional children. *Exceptional Children, 46*, 616–623.

Matute-Bianchi, M. E. (1986). Ethnic identities and patterns of school success and failure among Mexican-descent and Japanese-American students in a California high school: An ethnographic analysis. *American Journal of Education, 95*, 233-255.

McCall, N. (1994). *Makes me wanna holler: A young black man in America.* New York: Random House.

McCormick, M. (1988). *Mediation in the schools: An evaluation of the Wakefield Pilot Peer Mediation Program in Tucson, Arizona.* Washington, DC: American Bar Association.

McEwan, B. (2000). *The art of classroom management: Effective practices for building equitable learning communities.* Columbus, OH: Merrill.

McFadden, A. C., Marsh, G. B., Price, B. J., & Hwang, Y. (1992). A study of race and gender bias in the punishment of school children. *Education and Treatment of Children, 15*, 140-146.

McGinnis, E., & Goldstein, A. P. (1997). *Skillstreaming the elementary school child.* Champaign, IL: Research Press.

Meichenbaum, D. (1977). *Cognitive-behavior modification: An integrative approach.* New York: Plenum Press.

Metropolitan Life Insurance Company. (1995). *The American teacher, 1984-1995: Old problems, new challenges.* New York: Author.

Middleton, M. B. (1994). *The effects of social skills instruction and parent participation on aggressive behaviors, antisocial behaviors, and prosocial skills exhibited by primary-age students.* Unpublished doctoral dissertation, Ohio State University.

Middleton, M. B., & Cartledge, G. (1995). The effects of social skills instruction and parental involvement on the aggressive behaviors of African American males. *Behavior Modification, 19*, 192-210.

Miller-Lachmann, L. (Ed.). (1992). *Our family. our friends, our world.* New Providence, NJ: Bowker.

Miller-Lachmann, L., & Taylor, L. S. (1995). *Schools for all: Educating children in a diverse society.* Needham Heights, MA: Allyn & Bacon.

Moore, D. L. (1989). *Dark sky, dark land: Stories of the Hmong Boy Scouts of Troop 100.* Eden Prairie, MN: Tessera.

Moore, H. (1988). Effects of gender, ethnicity, and school equity on students' leadership behaviors in a group game. *Elementary School Journal, 5*, 514-526.

Moore, R. J., Cartledge, G., & Heckaman, K. (1995). The effects of social skill instruction and self-monitoring on game-related behaviors of adolescents with emotional or behavioral disorders. *Behavioral Disorders, 20*, 253-266.

Morgan-D'Atrio, C., Northup, J., LaFleur, L., & Spera, S. (1996). Toward prescriptive alternatives to suspensions: A preliminary evaluation. *Behavioral Disorders, 21*, 190-200.

Mulhern, M. M. (1995, April). *Mexican-American child's home life and literacy learning from kindergarten through second grade.* Paper presented at the annual meeting of the American Educational Research Association, San Francisco.

Myers, W. D. (1981). *Hoops.* New York: Dell.

Myers, W. D. (1984). *Motown and Didi: A love story.* New York: Viking.

Myers, W. D. (1988). *Scorpions.* New York: Harper & Row.

Myers, W. D. (2001). *Monster.* New York: HarperCollins.

Nieto, S. (1995, April). *On the brink between triumph and disaster: Exploring tensions between traditional secondary school and academically unsuccessful students through two case studies.* Paper presented at the annual meting of the American Educational Research Association, San Francisco.

Noguera, P. A. (1995). Preventing and producing violence: A critical analysis of responses to school violence. *Harvard Educational Review, 65*, 189-212.

Oakes, J. (1990). *Multiplying inequities: The effects of race, social class, and tracking on opportunities to learn mathematics and science.* Santa Monica, CA: Rand.

Oetting, E. R., Beauvais, F., Edwards, R., Waters, M. R., Velarde, J., & Goldstein, G. (1983). *Drug use among Native American youth: Summary of findings (1975–1981).* Fort Collins: Colorado State University.

Office for Civil Rights. (1992). *Elementary and secondary civil rights survey, 1990: National summaries.* Arlington, VA: Direct Broadcast Satellite.

Parker, J. G., & Asher, S. R. (1987). Peer relationships and later personal adjustment Are low-accepted children at risk? *Psychological Bulletin, 102,* 357–389.

Patterson, G. R. (1986). Performance models for antisocial boys. *American Psychologist, 41,* 432–444.

Patterson, G. R., Capaldi, D., & Bank, L. (1991). An early starter model for predicting delinquency. In D. J. Pepler & K. H. Rubin (Eds.), *The development and treatment of childhood aggression* (pp. 139–168). Hillsdale, NJ; Erlbaum.

Pauken, P. D., & Daniel, P. T. K. (1999, December). Race and disability discrimination in school discipline; a legal and statistical analysis. *Education Law Reporter, 139,* 759–790.

Phinney, J. S. (1990). Ethnic identity in adolescents and adults; Review of research. *Psychological Bulletin, 108,* 499–514.

Powless, D. L., & Elliott, S. N. (1993). Assessment of social skills of Native American preschoolers: Teachers' and parents' ratings. *Journal of Psychology, 31,* 293–307.

Prothrow-Stith, D. (1991). *Deadly consequences.* New York; HarperCollins.

Prothrow-Stith, D. (1994, April). Building violence prevention into the curriculum. *The School Administrator,* pp. 8–12.

Ramirez, O. (1989). Mexican American children and adolescents. In J. T. Gibbs, L. N. Huang, & Associates, *Children of color* (pp. 224–250). San Francisco; Jossey-Bass.

Ravetta, M. K., & Brunn, M. (1995, April). *Language learning, literacy and cultural background: Second language acquisition in a mainstreamed classroom.* Paper presented at the annual meeting of the American Educational Research Association, San Francisco.

Rhode, G., Jenson, W. R., & Reavis, H. K. (1992). *The tough kid book: Practical classroom management strategies.* Longmont, CO: Sopris West.

Richardson, R. C., & Evans, E. T. (1997). *Connecting with others: Lessons for teaching social and emotional competence.* Champaign, IL: Research Press.

Rudman, M. K. (1995). *Children's literature: An issues approach* (3rd ed.). White Plains, NY: Longman.

Sampson, R. (1992). Family management and child development: Insights from social disorganization theory. In J. McCord (Ed.), *Advances in criminological theory* (Vol. 3, pp. 63–93). New Brunswick, NJ: Transaction.

Sampson, R., & Laub, J. (1994). Urban poverty and the family context of delinquency: A new look at structure and process in a classic study. *Child Development, 65,* 523–540.

Schneider, B. H. (1993). *Children's social competence in context: The contributions of family, school, and culture.* Tarrytown, NY: Pergamon Press.

Schneider, B. H., & Lee, Y. (1990). A model for academic success: The school and home environment of East Asian students. *Anthropology and Education Quarterly, 21,* 358–377.

Seda, M., & Bixler-Márquez, D. J. (1994). The ecology of a Chicano student at risk. *Journal of Educational Issues of Language Minority Students, 13,* 195–208.

Shea, T. M., & Bauer, A. M. (1985). *Parents and teachers of exceptional students.* Boston: Allyn & Bacon.

Slavin, R. E. (1978). Student teams and achievement divisions. *Journal of Research and Development in Education, 12,* 39–49.

Slavin, R. E. (1990). Research on cooperative learning: Consensus and controversy. *Educational Leadership, 47,* 52–54.

Slavin, R. E., & Oickle, E. (1981). Effects of cooperative learning teams on student achievement and race relations: Treatment by race interactions. *Sociology of Education, 5,* 174–180.

Smith, E. J. (1991). Ethnic identity development: Toward the development of a theory within the context of majority/minority status. *Journal of Counseling and Development, 70,* 181–188.

Soriano, F. (1993). Cultural sensitivity and gang intervention. In A. P. Goldstein & C. R. Huff (Eds.), *The gang intervention handbook* (pp. 141–161). Champaign, IL: Research Press.

Soto, G. (1990). *Baseball in April: And other stories.* Orlando, FL: Harcourt Brace Jovanovich.

Sprague, J. R., Sugai, G., Homer, R., & Waker, H. M. (1999). Using office discipline referral data to evaluate school-wide discipline and violence prevention interventions. *OSSC Bulletin, 42,* 1–18.

Stanek, M. (1989). *I speak English for my mom.* Niles, IL: Albert Whitman.

Stephens, T. M. (1992). *Social skills in the classroom.* Odessa. FL: Psychological Assessment Resources.

Straub, E. (1996). Cultural-societal roots of violence. *American Psychologist, 51,* 117–132.

Surat, M. M. (1983). *Angel child, dragon child.* Milwaukee: Raintree.

Turnbull, A. P., & Tumbull, H. R. (1986). *Families, professionals, and exceptionality: A special partnership.* Columbus, OH: Merrill.

U.S. Census Bureau. (1999). *Our diverse population: Race and Hispanic origin, 1999.* http://www.census.gov/dmd/www/2kresult.htm.

U.S. Census Bureau. (2001). *Demographic profiles: Census 2000.* Public Information Office. http://www.census.gov/Press-Release/www/2001/demoprofile.html.

U.S. Department of Education. (1999). *20th annual report to Congress on the implementation of the Individuals with Disabilities Education Act.* Washington, DC: Author.

U.S. Department of Justice, Office of Justice Programs (1999). American Indians and crime. http://www.ojp.usdoj.gov/bjs/abstract/aic.

Valencia, R. R. (2000, Summer). Inequalities and the schooling of minority students in Texas: Historical and contemporary conditions. *Hispanic Journal of Behavioral Sciences, 22,* 445–459.

Valverde, L. A. (2000). Executive director's corner. *The Hispanic Border Leadership Institute Adelante Newsletter, 2*(3), p. 2.

Vargas, A. M. (19947 August). *Culture focused group therapy: Identity issues ill gang involved youth.* Paper presented at the 102nd Annual Convention of the American Psychological Association. Los Angeles.

Voelkl, K. E. (1997). Identification with school. *American Journal of Education, 105,* 29–18.

Volokh, A., & Snell, L. (1998). *School violence prevention: Strategies to keep schools safe.* Policy Study No.234. Reason Public Policy Institute, Reason Foundation, Los Angeles. Available at: http://lwww.rppi.org/ps234.html.

Walker, H. M., Colvin. G., & Ramsey. E. (1995). *Antisocial behavior in school: Strategies and best practices.* Pacific Grove, CA: Brooks/Cole.

Wallin, L. (1987). *Ceremony of the panther.* New York: Bradbury.

Watson, G. (1998). *Classroom discipline problem solver: Ready-to-use techniques and materials for managing all kinds of behavior problems.* West Nyak, NY: Center for Applied Research in Education.

Whalen, C. K. (1989). Attention deficit and hyperactivity disorders. In T. H. Ollendick & M. Hersen (Eds.), *Handbook of child psychopathology* (2nd ed., pp. 131–169). New York: Plenum Press.

Wilson, M., & Daly, M. (1985). Competitiveness, risk taking, and violence: The young male syndrome. *Ethology and Sociobiology, 6,* 59–73.

Winfield, L. F., & Manning, J. B. (1992). Changing school culture to accommodate student diversity. In M. E. Oilworth (Ed.), *Diversity in teacher education: New expectations* (pp. 181–214). San Francisco: Jossey-Bass.

Woo, E. (1995, December 17). Stereotypes "psych out" students. *The Columbus Dispatch,* p. 68.

Wynn, M. (1992a). *Empowering African-American males to succeed: A ten-step approach for parents and teachers.* Marietta, GA: Rising Sun.

Wynn, M. (1992b). *Empowering African-American males to succeed: A ten-step approach for parents and teachers. Teacher/parent workbook.* Marietta, GA: Rising Sun.

CHAPTER 18

Student Alienation Syndrome

The Other Side of School Violence

IRWIN HYMAN
MATTHEW MAHON
IAN COHEN
PAMELA SNOOK
GRETCHEN BRITTON
LOUISA LURKIS

School violence, as reported in the media over the past decade, has generated unrealistic public fears about the nature and extent of victimization of schoolchildren (Hyman & Snook, 1999a). In the first edition of this text (Hyman, Weiler, et al., 1997) and previous presentations and publications, we documented the reality that school violence is not epidemic and has remained relatively steady since 1978 (Hyman & D'Alessandro, 1984; Hyman & Snook, 1999a; Hyman & Snook, 2000; Hyman, Snook, Lurkis, Aldrete-Phan, & Britton, 2001; National Institute of Education, 1978a, 1978b; Office of Juvenile Justice, 2001; U.S. Department of Education/U.S. Department of Justice, 2000).

Unfortunately, alarmist rhetoric has largely contributed to the public's misperceptions. Conservative politicians' fear-inducing polemics have resulted in counterproductive, overpunitive school-safety-oriented policies. These have led to increasing introduction of ineffective punitive policies and measures, such as zero tolerance, drug screening, the use of metal detectors, unnecessary police presence in many schools, and others, which undermine students' faith in democracy and the Constitution. Paralleling these school policies have been punishment alternatives such as boot camps, wilderness camps, mandatory sentencing for drug offenses, and case adjudications of delinquents as if they were adults (Hyman & Snook, 1999a, 2000).

Shootings, such as those that have occurred in Pearl, Mississippi, in 1997 and later events at Columbine High School in Colorado and Santee High School in California, have perpetuated the public's fear of this extremely low-incidence, traumatic type of event. In fact, figures from the National Center for School Safety from 1998 to 1999, when homicides in schools were at the highest recorded level in recent years, indicate that there were about 30 deaths. At that time, with more than 52 million students in U.S. schools, the chance of any individual being killed was about 0.0576 for every 100,000 students. Research by Vossekuil, Fein, Reddy, Borum, and Modzeleski (2002) indicates that less than 1% of homicides of school-age children occur in and around schools. This age group (5–19 years) is much more likely to be killed by lightning (Hyman & Snook, 1999a) or in their homes, than in school (Hyman, Dahbany, et al., 1997).

The problem of school violence is actually exacerbated when the same people calling for more punitive "law and order" practices mask the routine victimization of students by teachers and other school personnel (Hyman, 1997). Acquiescence, trivialization, and cover-ups of student maltreatment can create a climate that increases student anger, aggression, violence, and criminal behaviors. These issues are rarely discussed in the media, in research on school violence, or in the most frequently used survey textbooks on school discipline (Blum, 1994). Although isolation of students and police tactics may be necessary in some extreme situations, they do not address the underlying issues that involve student and staff attitudes, school climate, formal and implied contracts, and school discipline policies. Most punitive approaches lack empirical support and do not reduce recidivism (e.g., boot camps), yet they continue to be funded (American Psychological Association, 1993; U.S. Department of Health and Human Services, 2001).

There is ample evidence, as demonstrated in this text, that preventive, mental-health-oriented approaches to violence are successful (Cunningham & Henggeler, 2001; Durlak, 1995, 1997, 1998). The prevention of school violence includes recognition of a complex interaction of personal, social, and ecological factors in the lives of schoolchildren. For instance, risk factors such as students' knowing at least one victim of violence, having witnessed violent acts, and having been victimized in the past are major predictors of violent behavior (Weist, Acosta, & Youngstrum, 2001). Life stress, both chronic and acute, is a predictor of maladjustment and violence among youth. When the school becomes a place of stress and when victimization predominates a student's experience, it is likely that the victim will develop a range of negative emotional reactions, including anger, hostility, and aggression. One study indicated that three-quarters of school shooters felt bullied, threatened, or persecuted prior to carrying out violent acts at school (Vossekuil et al., 2002).

Many people fail to recognize the complex relationship between all of the factors just mentioned and the modeling of violence by teachers and peers. For instance, the United States is one of the few remaining democracies that allow teachers to paddle students, an act in which a teacher models the infliction of pain as a method of changing behavior. Further, studies (Hyman & Snook, 1999b) suggest that more than half of U.S. students suffer from some form of maltreatment by teachers or peers, which causes various stress symptoms. One to two percent of the victims of maltreatment by teachers or peers suffer sufficient symptoms to warrant a diagnosis of posttraumatic stress disorder (PTSD) (Lambert, 1990; Savage, 1999; Snook, 2000; Vargas, 1991; Zelikoff, 1986).

This chapter describes our research on the traumatic events students experience in the school setting and, specifically, how these events may be precursors to violence. We propose a hypothetical construct, student alienation syndrome (SAS). We begin with a brief overview of two issues of school violence that are rarely discussed—corporal punishment and psychological maltreatment by educators. We then turn to the importance of "belongingness" within a school community. Next, we examine research on the development of SAS, an outgrowth of the construction of a scale to measure PTSD. We describe the Student Alienation and Trauma Scale (SATS) and its revised version (SATS-R) and the three-pronged approach for prevention, intervention, and treatment in schools. The chapter concludes with a case study that illustrates the use of SATS/SATS-R in the prevention of school violence.

SMACKING AND WHACKING: IS CORPORAL PUNISHMENT A FORM OF VIOLENCE?

"Corporal punishment" is generally defined as the purposeful infliction of pain or confinement as a penalty for an offense (Hyman & Wise, 1979). Among the 22 states that allow it, corporal punishment often involves the use of a wooden paddle in the schools. However, corporal punishment has many forms, including the reported use of straps, fists, bats, hoses, forced exercise drills, and forced eating of noxious substances (Hyman, Clarke, & Erdlen, 1987; Hyman & Wise, 1979). Because disciplinary procedures that directly inflict pain are varied, "corporal punishment" should be broadly defined to include unreasonable confinement in a restricted space (Hyman, 1988), inappropriate uses of time out, forcing children to assume fixed postures for unreasonable periods of time, exposure to painful environments, and/or certain types of psychological maltreatment that cause emotional pain. The data clearly demonstrate that the potential duration, intensity, and frequency of psychological symptoms resulting from traumatic physical and psychological assaults are the same (Hyman, 1990).

Since 1974 the research, advocacy, and policy efforts to abolish the use of corporal punishment in U.S. education have revealed pervasive and troubling attitudes of approval for the infliction of pain on children (Greven, 1980, 1990; Hyman, 1990; Hyman & Pokalo, 1992; Straus, 1991). In 1974, only New Jersey and Massachusetts forbade paddling schoolchildren; in the rest of the country, estimates suggested at least 3 million paddling incidents per school year (Glackman et al., 1978; Hyman, 1990). By 2001, 28 states had outright prohibitions of corporal punishment, and another 11 states, by local rules, banned such punishment of more than half of the children in their public schools. By 1997 there were approximately 450,000 yearly paddlings of U.S. students.

There is a great deal of evidence connecting early physical abuse by caregivers with the development of conduct disorder and violent behavior. Therefore, using corporal punishment on emotionally disturbed students whose pathology was shaped by the use of physical violence is further damaging and may cause or increase symptoms of PTSD (Berna, 1993, Curcio-Chilton, 1994; Hyman, 1990; Hyman & Gasiewski, 1992; Kohr, 1995; Rea, 1995; Vargas-Moll, 1991; Vargas-Moll & Hyman, 1992). Practitioners and researchers recognize that the physical pain caused by bruises, welts, and lacerations rarely lasts more than a month. However, it is the psychological effects of the physical pain that often have lasting effects. Further, there is strong evidence that psychological maltreatment by caregivers, even when physical pain is not inflicted, can have the same traumatic effect on victims (Hyman & Snook, 1999a). Therefore, we turn to a brief overview of the concept of psychological maltreatment as it occurs in schools.

PSYCHOLOGICAL MALTREATMENT IN SCHOOLS

Psychological maltreatment by educators may consist of (1) discipline and control techniques that are based on fear and intimidation, (2) a low quantity of human interaction, whose quality communicates a lack of interest, caring, and affection for students, (3) limited opportunities for students to develop adequate skills and feelings of self-worth, (4) encouragement to be dependent and subservient, especially in areas where students are capable of making independent judgments, (5) denial of opportunities for healthy risk taking, such as exploring ideas that are not conventional and approved by the teacher, (6) verbal assault, (7) ridicule, (8) isolation and rejection, (9) punitive sanctions, (10) allowing or ignoring peer humiliation, and (11) sexual harassment or corruption (Brassard, Hart, & Germain, 1987; Hyman, 1987; Hyman, 1990; Hyman, Zelikoff, & Clarke, 1988). Educators may also maltreat students by being overdemanding or perfectionistic with children who already have these traits as a result of parental pressure or self-demands. Other types of emotional maltreatment include overrestrictive bathroom policies, unrealistic expectations for students to go from one class to another in large buildings, beginning school times that run counter to adolescent developmental sleeping needs, and extraordinary demands on students' time outside of school due to excessive homework requirements.

Victimization of students consists of (1) isolation, (2) ridicule, involving name-calling, scapegoating, and mocking children who are different, (3) intimidation by threats, and (4) spreading rumors to others in the school community. Obviously, the various practices that constitute psychological maltreatment conflict with the legal, moral, and historical obligations of schools (Brassard et al., 1987).

THEORETICAL UNDERPINNINGS OF STUDENT ALIENATION SYNDROME

Physical and psychological student victimization causes a large and unknown number of students to become alienated from schools. Although for many the alienation may be mild and temporary, some develop deep feelings of resentment, anger, and hostility. Some of these alienated students act out their feelings by vandalizing property, threatening school staff with anonymous phone calls, and physically attacking teachers, peers, and other school staff. On the average, fewer than 30 students actually commit homicides each year (U.S. Department of Health and Human Services, 2001; Vossekuil et al., 2002). We believe that many of these students suffer from "student alienation syndrome" (SAS), which directly results from experiences occurring within the school community.

Ecological theorists and environmental psychologists have long posited that behavior and misconduct are a function of the interaction between individuals and their environments (Barker, 1968; Lewin, 1951; Proschansky, Ittelson, & Rivlion, 1970). This orientation focuses on how individuals behave within a particular context and the degree to which communities and contexts support individual functioning. This systems theory approach can be applied to understanding the way students function within the school setting (Baker, 1998; Fine, 1986; Gottfredson & Gottfredson, 1985; Hyman & Perone, 1998; Plas, 1994). When students feel a sense of belonging within a school community, there is great potential to reduce feelings of isolation and anger (Osterman, 2001). Conversely, when students feel ridiculed, mistrusted, verbally or physically attacked, or ignored by the school staff or their peers, they can develop feelings of victimization and alienation potentially resulting in various psychological manifestations. Therefore, examining the school context is critical in determining students' levels of comfort within the system (Howard, Howell, & Brainard, 1987; Hyman, Dahbany, et al., 1997).

BELONGINGNESS AND THE SCHOOL COMMUNITY

A sense of belonging to the school community has long been recognized as vital to students' educational and psychological growth (Osterman, 2001). In the early 1900s John Dewey (1985) articulated an educational philosophy of community, which is at the core of the American educational system. It focuses on the role of the community in the learning process. More recent theorists emphasize the relational bonds between individuals that allow them to forge shared values and ideals in pursuit of a meaningful common goal

(Sergiovanni, 1994). Community-oriented schools engender a spirit of commitment and shared purpose in students and, in so doing, work against the feelings of alienation that can lead to acts against the community (Noddings, 1988). Students' connections to the school environment affects acceptance of educational values, motivation, and commitment to school and has also been found to be essential to school completion and satisfaction (Fine, 1986; Kagan, 1990). However, climate alone cannot be blamed entirely for acts of school violence. Students may come to school with preexisting pathologies, which can be exacerbated by the school environment.

For instance, Dodge's (1986) hypothesis of information processing and anger arousal in aggressive children suggests that cognitive errors and distortions among aggressive children contribute to heightened anger, which they may bring to school. They typically misinterpret and overreact to the perceived aggression of others. In addition to perceiving their environment to be more threatening than their peers perceive it, these children also lack the behavioral skills to mediate conflict. A self-fulfilling prophecy is played out as the angry child reacts to perceived slights, thereby precipitating anger, rejection, and aggressive counterresponses from peers (Lochman, White & Wayland, 1991). Alienated youth view school as a battleground where they must constantly defend themselves from attacks on their self-esteem and physical safety. These students are often both victims and victimizers (Metropolitan Life Survey of the American Teacher, 1999; Olafsen & Viemero, 2000; Smith & Brain, 2000).

It is clear that a variety of factors may lead to SAS (Bai, 1999; Begley, 1999; Belluck & Wilgoren, 1999; Johnson, 1999). A comprehensive discussion of theoretical underpinnings and research findings is beyond the scope of this chapter. However, most practitioners and researchers would agree that the measurement of alienating climates and of individual students' responses to those climates will go a long way in identifying both institutional and individual pathology.

RISK ASSESSMENT FOR SCHOOL VIOLENCE

Despite the relatively recent and horrendous murders in schools, the fact is that school violence is not epidemic; yet government authorities have been quick to attempt to develop politically salient solutions. A beginning analysis suggests three categories of resolutions. These include punishment, profiling, and prevention. In the first category, adherence to zero tolerance policies embraces erring on the side of caution. This means mandatory suspension and expulsion of any student deemed a threat as a result of verbal, written, or physical expressions of aggression. The problem with this approach, which appears to be based on the unconstitutional assumption that one is guilty until proven innocent, is that many students who commit minor, relatively innocent, and sometimes stupid offenses are punished. A glaring example is the 4-week suspension of a first grader who brought a 2-inch paper clip–knife–bottle opener to school (Gostomski, 2000). The youngster had received this as a gift from the United States Marines' Toys for Tots program.

Concomitant with increasing police tactics in the schools, the FBI has suggested that profiling of potentially violent students might be effective in identifying them (Band & Harpold, 1999). Although this approach suggests preventive potential, it casts too wide a net. Some of the indicators, such as fire setting, cruelty to animals, and bed-wetting beyond a developmentally appropriate age, are research based. However, the list of 20 violence indicators also includes low self-esteem, rejection of romantic pursuits, and watching 40 hours or more a week of violent video entertainment. These are manifestations of relatively common events in the lives of many students. The vast majority do not commit violent acts. Furthermore, a recent report of 40 school shooters interviewed following violent acts on school grounds indicated that potentially violent students have varied characteristics in terms of such factors as family support, academic achievement, and socioeconomic status (Vossekuil et al., 2002). We believe that in comparison to the aforementioned approaches, the SATS/SATS-R offers a solution for violence prevention that is based on sound ecological, psychometric, and mental health principles.

STUDENT ALIENATION TRAUMA SURVEY
AND STUDENT ALIENATION TRAUMA SURVEY—REVISED

Brief Overview of the SATS/SATS-R

We believe that the Student Alienation and Trauma Survey-Revised (SATS/SATS-R), which is briefly described here, provides an ideal vehicle for researchers and practitioners interested in identifying and ameliorating the problem of student victimization. As a result of early experience with previous versions of the scale, the concept of educator-induced posttraumatic stress disorder (EIPTSD) emerged (Hyman, 1990; Hyman & Snook, 1999a).

The SATS-R is the latest version of our attempts to measure SAS. A complete history of the development of the SATS-R (Hyman & Snook, 1999b) is beyond the scope of this chapter. We began with the notion that common and acceptable traumatic events, such as paddling, spanking, excessive time outs, and verbal maltreatment by caregivers, can cause many children to develop stress symptoms and some children to develop PTSD (Hyman, 1990). Our research led to the development of the My Worst Experience Scale (MWES) and a parallel form for schools called the My Worst School Experience Scale (MWSES). The scales have different beginning formats in Part I, which address the settings and type of trauma that occurred. Part I of the MWES was developed to identify a wide range of stressors, including war, rape, natural disasters, and loss of a loved one. Part I of the SATS and SATS-

R was specifically developed to indicate school-related stressors, including maltreatment by educators and peers.

The SATS-R contains 58 school stressors, including both common and low-incidence events. The most current study using the SATS and SATS-R allowed students to indicate if a peer, educator, or both caused the traumatic experience (Halkias et al., 2002, 2003). An earlier version of the SATS-R provided the first factor analytic information for Part I. Fifty-three of the current 58 items generated a factorial structure that includes: (1) physical assaults, (2) sexual acts, (3) denigration acts, (4) unfair disciplinary procedures, and (5) yelling, ignoring, or isolating (Aldrete-Phan, 2001). These factors, in terms of peer bullying, are consistent with previous research (Mynard & Joseph, 2000). A recent cross-national study of a total of 450 Israeli, Greek, and U.S. college students' remembered traumas yielded a slightly different factor structure: (1) being excluded, (2) physical abuse, (3) criminal acts, (4) physical coercion, (5) school problems, (6) group harassment, (7) embarrassment, and (8) sexual abuse. Since this study aggregated the traumas and did not separate out when they were done, a current large study utilizing thousands of subjects' responses is now being conducted.

Part II of the MWES and the SATS/SATS-R are identical. Most of the statistical properties of the scale are based on an analysis of the 105 symptoms of Part II of both scales. The scales have good psychometric properties, which have been established over a 15-year period (Hyman, Snook, Berna, DuCette, & Kohr, 2002). The major purpose of the scale is to aid in the assessment of PTSD for children and adolescents who have experienced a variety of stressors, including excessive disciplinary procedures, sexual and physical abuse, natural disasters, and interpersonal assaults (Hyman, Snook, et al., 2002; Hyman et al., 1988).

The 105 symptom items in Part II are written at a third- to sixth-grade level according to the Fry (1968) Readability Formula. Estimation of readability, using a more conservative approach (Thomas, Hartley, & Kinkaid, 1975), yields a sixth-grade level and a Flesch Reading Ease score of 70, in the "Fairly Easy" category.

A study using an earlier version of the scale in an urban school sample of 63 regular students and 43 students diagnosed with learning disabilities (LD) offers an example of the types of worst school events experienced by this sample (Aldrete-Phan, 2001). In this study, students could choose whether their worst experience was caused by a school staff member or by a peer. The worst school experience was being made fun of (18.6% for regular education students and 12.7% for students with LD). Other frequent responses by the LD group included (1) being suspended for no reason (9.3%), (2) being yelled at (7%), (3) being hit with a ruler, paddle, or something else (7%), and (4) someone lying about them so they got in trouble (7%). In addition, 7% of the respondents chose "other" as their worst school experience. Other frequent responses by the regular education group included (1) seeing a person do something bad to someone else (11.1%), (2) being made to feel not as good as everyone else (7.9%), (3) being ignored when asking for help (7.9%), (4) being told that something bad would happen (6.3%), and (5) being punched (6.3%). In addition, 11.1% of the respondents chose "other" as their worst school experience.

A study by Savage (1999) of 179 community college students, also using an earlier version of the SATS-R and asking only about educator maltreatment, offers further insight into the nature and extent of stressors. In this case, rather than identifying the worst experience of each respondent, the researcher analyzed all of the traumatic experiences indicated. The following percentages do not total 100%, because they represent multiple bad experiences by each respondent. The most common stressors were teachers yelling (75%), making fun of students (56%), put-downs that made a student feel not as good as everyone else (50%) and put-downs for not doing well (50%), ridicule in front of other students (45%), threats (39%), ignoring (29%), name calling related to the student's physical appearance, and (20%) encouraging peers to tease the student.

Subscales of the SATS/SATS-R

Four subscales meet the DSM-IV-TR (American Psychiatric Association, 2000) criteria for diagnosis of PTSD: Impact of Event (IMPACT), Reexperiencing the Trauma (REEX), Avoidance and Numbing (AVOID), and Increased Arousal (AROUS). Impact of Event (IMPACT) has 4 items that describe disorganized and agitated behavior that is often observed among youngsters who have experienced trauma. Reexperiencing the Trauma (REEX) has 10 items and is a hallmark of PTSD. Research and clinical practice indicate that children, however, are unlikely to experience the dramatic flashbacks often reported by adults with PTSD. Children are more apt to reexperience the trauma in different ways according to their age (i.e., distressing dreams in younger children and difficulty concentrating in school-age children). Avoidance and Numbing (AVOID) consists of 24 items and is associated with avoiding thoughts about the trauma, avoiding the victimizer, and repressing certain aspects of the trauma. Children are more apt to experience avoidance than numbing. Finally, Increased Arousal (AROUS) consists of 21 items and is often seen as sleep disturbances, hypervigilance, irritability, and anger.

The MWES/SATS/SATS-R symptom subscales emerged from normative studies of large samples of children and adolescents: the subscales measure distress in seven distinct symptom areas: Depression (DEP), Hopelessness (HOPELS), Somatic Symptoms (SOM), Oppositional Conduct (OPP), Hypervigilance (HYPER), Dissociation/Dreams (DISSOC), and General Maladjustment (MAL). In addition to a total score (TOT), the instrument yields an inconsistency-of-responding scale to determine the validity of responses. The symptom subscales are particularly useful in identifying symptom patterns that may not qualify for a diagnosis of PTSD, but may be indicative of pressing problems. As with the DSM-IV-TR criteria scales, clinically significant scores of 60T or higher on any of these subscales should be considered to indicate the presence of a disturbance and suggest the need for clinical follow-up.

The Student Alienation Index

Thus far, we have provided a framework for positing the concept of SAS and have presented a brief overview of the SATS/SATS-R, which can be used to assess a student's level of alienation. This paradigm will, of course, require further conceptualization, research, and refinement. However, we believe that the SATS/SATS-R provides subscales that clearly describe the type of ideation that differentiates traumatized students with hostile and aggressive feelings from those individuals who tend to internalize their emotions and may be less likely to act out. Interestingly, and consistent with previous literature (Garbarino, 1999), externalizing behaviors such as fighting, truancy, and delinquency are often associated with internalizing, depressive symptomatology. This intermixing of depression and anger is illustrated in the factor scores that form the subscales for the Oppositionality, Hopelessness, and Hypervigilance symptoms on the SATS/SATS-R, which constitute the Student Alienation Index (SAI). These three symptom subscales form a Student Alienation Index (SAI). Students with high T scores on the SAI are at risk for aggressively acting out their feelings and are candidates for further evaluation. They are often victims who transform their feelings of helplessness, hopelessness, and fearfulness into a rage, which when acted upon, can result in horrendous acts of violence. They are at risk because of their potential for hurting themselves and others. Studying students with similar characteristics, for instance, Vossekuil et al. (2002) found three-quarters of school shooters felt bullied, threatened, or persecuted prior to carrying out violent acts in school.

Responses of "a lot" or "all the time" to certain items included in the SAI should be of concern. Clinicians wishing to make risk assessments for the potential to act out will have to use their own judgment, based in part on probing about the meaning of specific responses to items in the SAI. Examples of such items on the Oppositional Conduct (OPP) scale include "I got very angry for no reason" (#1), "I got angry very fast" (#19), "I did whatever I wanted even if people didn't like it" (#88), and "I felt like fighting all the time" (#50). Examples on the Hypervigilance (HYPER) scale include "I thought about things to get back at the person who hurt me" (#10), "I didn't trust people as much as before" (#94), and "I was always waiting for something to happen to me" (#105). Examples from the Hopelessness (HOPELS) scale include "I didn't care about the future" (#14), "I didn't seem to care what happened to me"(#25), and "I felt like a failure" (#62).

Clinicians should be alerted to T scores of 60 or above on these three subscales of the SAI. High scores suggest the need for further evaluation of students who are at risk for the combination of self-destruction and interpersonal aggression, which is characteristic of school shooters and other violent offenders. These are the students who have characteristics of both victims and victimizers and who may express their sense of helpless rage in acts of violence.

The scales that constitute the SAI must be conceptualized within the framework of PTSD. This is important to note, inasmuch as diagnosis, prevention, and treatment of the hypothetical construct of SAI fall within the rubric of PTSD, for which there is a well-developed body of clinical literature and research. As noted previously, the 105 symptoms presented on the SATS/SATS-R are identical to those on the MWES and offer a sound psychometric basis for screening for PTSD in general and the kind associated with school-related traumas. The latter is an additional and important feature of the SATS/SATS-R as compared with the MWES. The SATS/SATS-R, Part I, provides a list of possible traumatic incidents caused in the educational setting. These offer the potential for institutional assessment of the nature and extent of student victimization, which can lead to primary and secondary prevention.

Mental Health Audits to Identify Student Alienation Syndrome

In terms of *primary prevention*, the SATS/SATS-R can be used to conduct mental health audits of schools in order to determine the number and proportion of students who have been traumatized by educators or peers. For purposes of determining the level of SAS as a function of traumatization fostered by school climate, anonymity will probably result in a larger percentage of accurate responses. Although this measure will provide levels of traumatization, it will not allow for identification of those individuals who may require ecological intervention or individual treatment. The scales may be easily administered to large groups of students, and scoring is readily accomplished with the use of scanning techniques.

The concept of mental health audits has been developed since the most recent school shootings, and therefore we cannot present any normative data, although data available provide normative information regarding students' aggressive feelings to school traumatization. It seems reasonable to assume that schools with high rates of traumatized students are more likely to harbor the possibility for student acting out. Whether this scale will predict school homicides is not yet known; however, normative data will certainly provide useful information about school climates, student victimization, and the levels of traumatic symptomatology. To provide further validation for the concept of SAS, it will be necessary to correlate numbers and proportions of aggressive acts within the school with the proportion of alienated students as indicated on the SATS/SATS-R.

Secondary prevention, using large-scale screening, requires that students record their names on the scoring sheet. This provides a format for screening individual students for potential and significant traumatic symptomatology related to maltreatment by peers and educators. Items that tap aggressive and vengeful ideation can be identified by use of the three subscales Oppositionality, Hopelessness, and Hypervigilance, which constitute the SAI. Although the original intent of the SATS/SATS-R and MWES was to identify PTSD, the SATS/SATS-R can also be used to ascertain the group of victims of PTSD who are more likely to act out aggressively. These identified students will require both ecological and psychological interventions, as discussed in regard to the TREAT model in a later section.

The SATS/SATS-R can be used for *tertiary prevention* to check symptomatology of students at least 1 month following traumatic school or community events that impact large numbers of students. These events may include acts of interpersonal violence and terrorism, such as shootings, school kidnappings, or rapes. The SATS/SATS-R may also be used following events such as hurricanes, tornadoes, and other natural disasters that can impact an entire school population. Victims of trauma may develop internalizing and externalizing symptoms, and some may not be easily recognizable if the major manifestation is internalization. Identification of students with potential PTSD requires a moral and financial commitment to provide further diagnosis and treatment.

Clinical experience has demonstrated that not all victims of educator maltreatment develop sufficient symptomatology to necessitate treatment. Students studied have been the victims of excessive corporal punishment, psychological maltreatment, and the overzealous use of police tactics, such as strip searches (Hyman & Snook, 1999a). Case records spanning more than 15 years clearly indicate that educator maltreatment can cause aggressive ideation toward educators and schools. In some cases, teachers have directly encouraged peers to abuse a targeted student. In other cases, educators' maltreatment of students has indirectly caused bullying by peers (Hyman & Snook, 1999b; Snook, 2000).

A comprehensive discussion of schoolwide intervention strategies based on mental health audits is beyond the scope of this chapter and is discussed elsewhere throughout this book. Further, because audits of this type have not been conducted, it would be unwise to promote a particular approach. However, it is clear that schools that are seriously concerned about traumatization of students, which may lead to SAS, will not have great difficulty in developing intervention plans. For instance, if large numbers of students indicate that their worst school experience consists of repeated types of verbal abuse by either teachers or peers, such as "I was yelled at," "I was put down for not doing well," and "I was made fun of," then the intervention must address these issues. Teachers need to be educated about, or, if necessary, forbidden from, verbally assaulting children. If students are the perpetrators, intervention programs must focus on training in empathy, conflict resolution, and moral responsibility. If large numbers of students indicate bullying activities by peers with high scores on such items as "I was pushed," "I was slapped," and "Other children were allowed to hit, push, or slap me," it is clear that a bully intervention program must be initiated (Elliot, 1999; Olweus, 1996; Batsche & Knoff, 1994).

We offer a note of caution regarding implementation of schoolwide screening. "Political" considerations by school authorities may well prevent most officials from using the SATS/SATS-R for mass screening. The reluctance of schools to gather problematic data, which may be embarrassing, is an unfortunate example of the "no news is good news" paradigm. Despite this potential problem, the SATS/SATS-R is a valid and reliable instrument to aid in the diagnosis of PTSD related to school traumas and to determine whether SAS is evident. It is well known that prevention, although well accepted in the area of public health, is not as fully embraced when it crosses into the field of education and mental health. In the short term, prevention is more costly than crisis management, which follows events that mobilize and coalesce entire communities. Nonetheless, in the long run, prevention is less costly and more effective because it targets problems before they occur (Durlak, 1995, 1997, 1998). Despite the difficulties associated with schoolwide screenings, the SATS/SATS-R can be extremely effective as a component of diagnosis and preventative treatment with individuals.

THE TREAT MODEL OF DIAGNOSIS AND TREATMENT OF STUDENT ALIENATION SYNDROME

As noted earlier, the various scales, which have evolved into the MWES and the SATS/SATS-R, have been grounded in research and clinical experience with PTSD. Parallel to development of the scales, one of us (I. H.) has developed a treatment approach to dealing with PTSD in children and adults. It is a multimodal approach derived from the literature, research, and clinical successes. It is important to recognize the unique aspects of this type of PTSD inasmuch as it occurs within an institutional setting. In many cases, school authorities ignore, trivialize, or inappropriately deal with the institutional sources of the more common stressors such as peer bullying and teacher denigration of students. A comprehensive discussion of these issues and the TREAT model is beyond the scope of this chapter and is presented in detail elsewhere (Hyman, 1990; Hyman & Snook, 1999a, 2000).

Effective treatment of PTSD is especially dependent on comprehensive diagnosis. After the initial interview and administration of the SATS/SATS-R, it is important to do a complete family history, with clinical probes for anxiety and depression. Educational history should include anecdotal records of the student, in addition to grades and clues to identification of possible learning, attention, and/or emotional problems that may make the child more vulnerable to intense stress symptoms.

In addition to formal scoring of the SATS/SATS-R, the clinician should discuss qualitative factors related to the student's responses. For instance, what are the meanings of symptoms to the victim? How have they changed the student's life? Experienced clinicians will know how to conduct this part of the evaluation. In addition to the SATS/SATS-R, the clinician may wish to base the diagnosis on an extensive clinical interview, other paper-and-pencil tests, and projective techniques. Because of the nature of PTSD, diagnostic information must include an analysis of overt behavior, feelings, thoughts, ecological factors, family support, and the meaning of the event to the student and his or her family. Also an important part of the diagnostic picture and the treatment plan is information from school staff, and sometimes even peers who witnessed the event. This is especially crucial, because most of the cases we have treated required actual school interventions. Once the diagnosis is made, the treatment plan, based on TREAT, can be implemented. The TREAT model includes five steps, which may not necessarily occur in any particular order: Treat symptoms that respond to behavioral techniques such as relaxation and systematic desensitization; Reframe dysfunctional cognitions and feelings by use of cognitive restructuring techniques promoted by cognitive-behavioral therapy, rational-emotive therapy, and the like; Explore the need for medication if other techniques do not yield a significant reduction in symptoms; Address existential/spiritual issues, which examine the meanings the individual ascribes to his or her experiences; Tackle ecological impediments related to school, family, and peers. This involves identifying traumatic events, eliminating those events when possible, developing alternative strategies to change the traumatic environmental antecedents, and ensuring places of safety and nurturance. The following case example illustrates how this model has been used in practice.

CASE EXAMPLE–THE WARY WRESTLER: HAZING WITHOUT END

Bob, a 15-year-old, was referred by the school counselor in October of his sophomore year to the senior author of this chapter (I. H.) for what appeared to be a complete lack of academic motivation and a string of disciplinary infractions. Bob was chronically tardy, skipped classes, frequently failed to hand in homework, and failed almost all of his exams. He claimed he hated school and all the students in it. He felt wary toward most of the school community and constantly felt in danger. He begged his parents to send him to a different school.

During the referral, the guidance counselor indicated that Bob had been severely hazed as a new member of the wrestling team in January of the previous year. After one of the beginning practice sessions, Bob was initiated into the team. He was pushed around in the shower, shoved to the floor, and urinated on by several senior wrestlers. He felt humiliated, ashamed to tell anyone, and fearful that the hazing would continue. He reluctantly reported the hazing to his parents, who insisted that the school investigate. It was discovered that this was a common practice, although the coaches claimed to be totally unaware of it. The offending students were suspended, and the witnesses were put on probation. They all blamed Bob for ending the tradition.

Bob was censured by his teammates for the duration of the school year. Further, when other classmates found out about the incident, he was victimized by intense bullying—both verbal and physical. Much of the bullying focused on allegations that Bob was not a "real man" because he could not take a little hazing. Classmates started calling him a "fag" and other derogatory names. In the hall, students "accidentally" knocked his books out of his hand or bumped into him. However, he did not report these events for fear of further retaliation. The bullying resumed in the fall, especially on the school bus. By the end of September it was obvious that Bob was having problems. Teachers referred him to the guidance counselor, as he appeared preoccupied, disorganized, depressed, and sometimes explosive.

A review of records, family interview, and consultation with teachers revealed that Bob had been diagnosed at the age of 4 as having a possible learning disability and attention-deficit/hyperactivity disorder. He had an average IQ, but had trouble following directions and getting along with peers in a group. He tended to be shy, to misinterpret social cues, and was quite disorganized. After an initial interview and developmental/educational history, Bob was given the SATS. He included his account of the worst school experience: "After the guys peed on me, I was sexually harassed by both guys and girls. They said I was gay and would touch me and pretend they were gay and come on to me. They tripped me, and several guys threw me into the girls' bathroom and lockers."

Assessment revealed that Bob was a vulnerable student with low self-esteem. Although the hazing was a precipitating event, it is clear that the ensuing bullying contributed significantly to Bob's emotional distress. His total T score on the SATS was 66 (94th percentile). On the DSM-IV-TR criteria scores, Bob clearly met the criteria for PTSD. The symptom subscale scores revealed the extent of the PTSD associated symptoms. Clinically significant scores included Depression (T score 64), Hopelessness (T score 62), Oppositional Conduct (T score 70), Increased Arousal (T score 67), and Hypervigilance (T score 67). Bob scored particularly high on the Oppositional Conduct subscale, indicating that he felt angry and hostile and had vengeful ideation almost all of the time.

Note that Bob's scores on the Student Alienation Index are all in the clinically significant range ($T \geq 60$), including Hopelessness and Hypervigilance. It is especially significant that the Oppositional Conduct score, the highest of the three, is in the extreme range ($T \geq 70$). Bob was angry, vengeful, and depressed. He obsessed about thoughts of revenge. He responded that "all of the time" he kept thinking about revenge, fear of being hurt, and hatred of school. Interestingly, Bob indicated that only "a few times" did he feel badly about things he had done to break school rules, which he had been doing quite frequently.

Bob's family was concerned about his hurting himself or others. Fortunately, the family did not have any weapons in the house and tended to be nonviolent. Further, Bob did not have a history of aggression. He did have suicidal ideation, but said that he was too scared to actually follow through. However, the interview and scores on the SATS suggested the potential for a major hostile action against selected peers or the school in general. The scores on the SATS indicated the need for further evaluation, which included the MMPI-A, the Social Skills Rating System—Teacher form, the Symptom Checklist-90-R, and intensive clinical interview.

It was clear that Bob needed intensive treatment, possible medication, and immediate ecological interventions. His parents were told that because of comorbidity, he would probably need long-term psychotherapy, to begin with intensive treatment over the short term. In this case, the parents were both high-level executives who traveled frequently. They assured cooperation but were rarely available for family therapy or to work with the school. They put much of that responsibility on the psychologist. The following is a brief overview of the TREAT approach in this very difficult case.

Treat Symptoms That Respond to Behavioral Techniques

Bob's major symptoms that might respond to behavioral techniques, at the time he was referred, were his obsessive thoughts of revenge. He also obsessed about what a failure he was, how the school had transformed him into a victim, and his hatred of the school, most of the students, and the school staff. He was chronically breaking school rules. He smoked on school grounds, illegally used the computers, cut classes, and often refused to pay attention in class. Underlying much of this was his intense anger and desire to be transferred to another school, which was theoretically possible but not probable, given the wishes of his parents and the school authorities.

Two early therapeutic goals were anger management and dealing with his constant state of vigilance against verbal assaults. He admitted that he had trouble controlling his angry thoughts. He often had fantasies of revenge, especially in regard to specific peers whom he considered ring leaders. The usual approach of meditation and relaxation was tried, although he did not practice the procedure as was suggested. However, after several sessions he began to cooperate and was able to obtain a reasonable state of relaxation. Bob was taught, that when he started to get angry, to take three deep breaths and say the words "calm and relaxed," which were part of the posthypnotic suggestion he taught himself as the cue to achieving a relaxed state.

Reframe Dysfunctional Cognitions and Feelings

Bob's self-concept in school was quite negative. He saw himself as a victim who was basically an outsider. Except for the students in his therapy group, he had few friends. In his mind, and to some extent by many of his class-mates, he was perceived as a loser. He felt he was stupid, even though IQ tests showed him to have average intelligence. He felt unattractive to girls, even though he had several girlfriends outside of school. He expressed fears that he was crazy, even though he was able to function appropriately and show good judgment when he tried. He felt unlikable and unsupported by school staff, even though one particular teacher became a strong advocate for him and the assistant principal was always lenient with him for infrac-tions and moved aggressively against bullies. On the positive side, he devel-oped an interest in several outside-school activities such as skiing and scuba diving and made friends around those activities. Cognitive-behavioral tech-niques were used to challenge his inaccurate and distorted core beliefs and automatic thoughts.

After Bob's trust was secured through individual therapy and demon-strated effectiveness in convincing school authorities to take appropriate ac-tions, he joined group therapy with a mixed group of students who had diffi-culties with anxiety, depression, underachieving, low self-esteem, alienation, and poor social skills. The group commiserated with Bob and spent much time supporting the belief that there were too many bullies and ineffectual countermeasures by school staff. They bonded around this theme and began to develop both individual and group strategies to identify interventions and thinking that would help solve their problems in a nonviolent manner. As a result of encouragement and support from the therapist, they readily sought out staff they felt would help them.

It was soon apparent to the group that Bob was eager to dominate them when describing his own problems. However, he had a real problem in at-tending to others in the group while they were speaking. It took more than a year to teach Bob the skills needed to attend to others, to try to observe their behaviors, and to interpret the meanings of their behaviors. The therapist and the group focused on the concept of empathy and what is needed to feel it. Bob had a problem moving from victim to survivor and empathizer.

Through social skills training, the group helped Bob to determine how to counter bullying behavior. He began to realize that his overreactions and catastrophic thinking were self-destructive. He needed to rethink and then role-play how to deal with verbal taunts, especially the accusations that he was gay. Because he was clearly interested in girls and had girlfriends from other schools, this issue became secondary.

Explore Need for Medication

Bob's parents were quite eager to explore medication to help him calm down. He had been taking Ritalin for many years, though very sporadically. Unlike many of the students with ADHD that claim that psychostimulants re-ally help, Bob claimed the Ritalin did not help. As the therapist, I (I. H.), dis-cussed the problem of comorbidity and the possibility that medication might work, but I pointed out that much of his difficulty was related to ecological factors. Despite this advice, Bob was periodically medicated by a psychiatrist who never consulted with the school or the psychologist. He was tried on several selective seratonin reuptake inhibitors, but none seemed to work, because he claimed they caused too many side effects.

Address Existential/Spiritual Issues

When the bullying began, Bob's sense of safety was undermined and, as a result, life seemed meaningless. Bob could never feel completely safe in school, even though he reported no significant bullying during his senior year. The failure of the school and his parents to effectively protect him during the ongoing bullying changed his perception of his world. Furthermore, he had no spiritual or existential compass to guide him. Bob and his family had no interest in religion, so this was not a source of support. Existentially, the meaning of life for Bob was bifurcated. There were, in essence, two Bobs. Out of school he had a car, enough money to do things he wanted, hobbies that he liked, and the ability to have girlfriends. He realized that his parents were affluent and that he would probably never have real financial problems. He had successfully worked at jobs and found that when he wanted to, he could concentrate and learn, despite the ADHD. In school, he was angry, alienated, and rejected.

The group was extremely helpful to Bob in helping him to change his perceptions of his school experiences. For instance, during one group session he described his experience with a girl who kept putting him down. The group assured him that she did that to everyone because she herself was such a poor student and had a lousy home life. With support from the group, he was able to deal with the other minor, periodic put-downs and sarcasm that are part of high school life. As a result, Bob was able to take on a different perception of past events, though he never felt a sense of belonging to the school community.

Tackle Ecological Impediments Related to School, Family, and Peers

Unfortunately, in this case, the parents were rarely available to deal with the school on a regular basis unless there was a crisis. In relation to the ecological domain, one goal was for Bob to view his therapist as an advocate who would represent him to school staff who initially trivialized and ignored many of his complaints. This was done for two reasons. First, Bob's parents were resistant to participating in family therapy and were often not available to intervene in school matters when needed. Second, it is important in cases of this type that the therapist take an active role in helping the school understand the nature of student alienation and the possible consequences of inappropriate actions by school authorities.

During the first year of therapy, the psychologist (I. H.) worked regularly with school staff in the area of ecological consultation. The school cooperated in order to help Bob feel protected. In addition, one of the school counselors sponsored an antibullying program presented by a local Quaker group. The assistant principal became an advocate for Bob and took swift disciplinary actions when he was bullied. Considering Bob's comorbid problem, one of the major goals was to get him through high school and that was accomplished. So, despite his problems, he could view himself as a survivor, who made it in the face of all the odds against him. Also on the positive side, as a result of psychotherapy in the group, he felt optimistic that in college, where he was not yet known, he had a good chance for an upbeat experience.

Even if the parents are willing and to intervene in schools, they need the support of an experienced psychotherapist who understands schools. In cases of peer bullying and ineffectual interventions or direct maltreatment by faculty, schools frequently are defensive and fearful to admit their own mistakes. Sometimes it requires a concerted effort to force school authorities to actively intervene in order to completely stop all maltreatment that could trigger vengeful action by the victim. It is also necessary, as was done in this case, for adjustment in teachers and classes so that the student feels safe and protected.

In summary, we have presented a case in which the SATS played an important role in early screening and diagnosis. The scale helped to identify the intensity and frequency of Bob's feelings of hostility, alienation, and obsession with revenge. He had the potential to act out his angry feelings. Administration of the scale at periodical intervals during treatment helped to determine the frequency and intensity of his symptoms when he was first assessed. He had strong enough feelings of hopelessness and helplessness not to care whether his aggressive behavior hurt him or others. The use of the SATS also helped to determine treatment strategies. It is particularly useful in large high schools where victimized students go virtually unnoticed by school staff. However, as with any well-designed instrument of this type, clinicians must depend on good training, adequate experience with schools, creativity, and common sense.

Although the MWES and SATS/SATS-R have met the usual psychometric standards of reliability and validity, we caution that the SAS is still a hypothetical construct. Despite this limitation, it offers fertile ground for further exploration. Like all paper-and-pencil instruments, the MWES and SATS/SATS-R should not be the sole basis for a definitive diagnosis, but they can contribute to a comprehensive assessment. Further, resistant respondents may not report all symptoms. The instruments may not be completely valid in individual cases without verification by an adult familiar with the respondent. For instance, adolescents may not wish to report symptoms such as crying. To account for this limitation, it is useful to probe about possible symptoms that often occur in clusters but are not all reported. Any adult can easily administer the scales as a screening instrument, but because of these factors, skilled clinicians, such as school psychologists, should interpret them.

SUMMARY AND CONCLUSIONS

In this chapter, we have proposed a paradigm termed "student alienation syndrome," which has grown out of our research on Educator-Induced PTSD. We have discussed problems of defining, investigating, preventing, and treating student alienation, which appears to be one factor related to a recent spate of school homicides and attempted homicides by students. We have framed this issue within the general context of the public's misperceptions about the nature and extent of school violence and policy makers' overreaction in implementing unnecessarily punitive and counter-productive methods in violence prevention approaches.

In conclusion, we hope that this chapter provides a useful guideline for clinicians interested in diagnosing and treating trauma related to school events, and in further conceptualizing the SAS. Further research agendas should include the development of a national database to assess the climates of various schools. This could lead to an examination of the relationship between climate, SAS, and school disruption. It could also lead to the development of prevention and intervention programs to ameliorate alienation. We recognize that the agenda proposed here is expensive and time-consuming, as are all efforts related to prevention. However, we believe that these efforts are necessary in reducing student alienation and victimization, and that the concepts presented offer tremendous potential to reduce aggression in schools.

REFERENCES

Aldrete-Phan, C. (2001). *A comparison of stress responses of children with learning disabilities and others.* Unpublished doctoral dissertation, Temple University, Philadelphia.

American Psychiatric Association. (2000). *Diagnostic and statistical manual of mental disorders* (4th ed., text rev.). Washington, DC: Author.

American Psychological Association. (1993). *Violence in youth: Psychology's response. Vol I: Summary report of the American Psychological Association commission for violence and youth.* Washington, DC: Author.

Bai, M. (1999, May 3). Anatomy of a massacre. *Newsweek,* pp. 24–31.

Baker, J. A. (1998). Are we missing the forest for the trees? Considering the social context of school violence. *Journal of School Psychology, 36*(1), 29–44.

Band, S. R., & Harpold, J. A. (1999, September). School violence: Lessons learned. *FBI Law Enforcement Bulletin, 68*(9), 9–16.

Barker, R. G. (1968). *Ecological psychology.* Stanford, CA: Stanford University Press.

Batsche, G. M., & Knoff, H. M. (1994). Bullies and their victims: Understanding a pervasive problem in school. *School Psychology Review, 23*(2), 166–174.

Begley, S. (1999, May 3). The roots of violence. *Newsweek,* pp. 32–35.

Belluck, P., & Wilgoren, J. (1999, June 29). Caring parents, no answers in Columbine killers' past. *The New York Times,* pp. A1, A14.

Berna, J. (1993). *The worst experiences of adolescents from divorced and separated parents and the stress responses to those experiences.* Unpublished doctoral dissertation, Temple University, Philadelphia.

Blum, M. (1994). *The pre-service teacher's educational training in classroom discipline: A national survey of teacher educational programs.* Unpublished doctoral dissertation, Temple University, Philadelphia.

Brassard, M., Hart, S., & Germain, B. (Eds.). (1987). *Psychological maltreatment of children and youth.* Elmsford, NY: Pergamon Press.

Cunningham, P. B., & Henggeler, S. W. (2001). Implementation of an empirically based drug and violence prevention and intervention program in public school settings. *Journal of Clinical Child Psychology, 30*(1), 221–232.

Curcio-Chilton, K. (1994). *Stress symptoms of special education students diagnosed with conduct disorder.* Unpublished doctoral dissertation, Temple University, Philadelphia.

Dewey, J. (1985). *John Dewey: The middle works, 1899–1925: Vol. 9. Democracy and education–1916.* Carbondale, IL: Southern Illinois Press.

Dodge, K. A. (1986). A social information processing model of social competence in children. In M. Perlmutter (Ed.), *Minnesota symposium on child psychology* (pp. 77–125). Hillsdale, NJ: Erlbaum.

Durlak, J. A. (1995). *School-based prevention programs for children and adolescents.* Thousand Oaks, CA: Sage.

Durlak, J. A. (1997). *Successful prevention programs for children and adolescents.* New York: Plenum Press.

Durlak, J. A. (1998). Why program implementation is important. *Journal of Prevention and Intervention in the Community, 17,* 5–12.

Elliot, D. (Ed.). (1999). *Blueprints for violence prevention: Bullying prevention program.* Boulder: Center for the Study and Prevention of Violence, University of Colorado at Boulder.

Fine, M. (1986). A systems-ecological perspective on home–school intervention. In M. Fine & C. Carlson (Eds.). *The handbook of family school intervention: A systems perspective.* Boston: Allyn & Bacon.

Fry, E. (1968). A readability formula that saves time. *Journal of Reading, 11*(4), 513–516.

Garbarino, J. (1999). *Lost boys.* New York: Free Press.

Glackman, T., Berv, V., Martin, R., McDowell, E., Spino, R., & Hyman, I. (1978). The relation between corporal punishment, suspensions, and discrimination. *Inequality in Education, 23,* 61–65.

Gostomski, C. (2000, January 14). Toy not intended for tot. *York Dispatch/York Sunday News,* p. A-1.

Gottfredson, G., & Gottfredson, D. (1985). *Victimization in schools.* New York: Plenum Press.

Greven, P. (1980). *The Protestant temperament.* New York: Knopf.

Greven, P. (1990). *Spare the child: The religious roots of punishment and the psychological impact of physical abuse.* New York: Knopf.

Halkias, D., Fakinos, M., Hyman, I., Cohen, I., Akrivos, D., & Mahon, M. (2003, May). *Victimization of children in Greek schools: Stress and trauma symptoms related to school bullying.* Paper presented at the 9th Panhellenic Conference on Psychological Research, Rhodes, Greece.

Halkias, D., Fakinos, M., Hyman, I., Cohen, I., Akviros, D., Mahon, M., Snook, P., & DuCette, J. (2002, July). *Victimization of children in schools: Traumatic symptoms and stressors in Greek and American students.* Paper presented at the XVI Congress of the International Association for Cross-Cultural Psychology, Yogyakarta, Indonesia.

Howard, E., Howell, B., & Brainard, E. (1987). *Handbook for conducting school climate improvement projects.* Bloomington, IN: Phi Delta Kappa Educational Foundation.

Hyman, I. (1987). Psychological correlates of corporal punishment and physical abuse. In M. Brassard, S. Hart, & B. Germain (Eds.), *Psychological maltreatment of children and youth.* Elmsford, NY: Pergamon Press.

Hyman, I. (1988, August13). *Eliminating corporal punishment in schools: Moving from advocacy research to policy implementation.* Paper presented at the 86th Annual Convention of the American Psychological Association, Atlanta, GA.

Hyman, I. (1990). *Reading, writing, and the hickory stick: The appalling story of physical and psychological abuse in American schools.* Lexington: Lexington Books.

Hyman, I. (1997). *The case against spanking: How to discipline your child without hitting.* San Francisco: Jossey-Bass.

Hyman, I., Clarke, J., & Erdlen, R. (1987). An analysis of physical abuse in American schools. *Aggressive Behavior, 13,* 1–7.

Hyman, I., Cohen, I., Glass, J., Kay, B., Mahon, M., Siegel, N., Tabori, A., & Weber, M. (2003, June). *School bullying: Theory, research, assessment, and interventions.* Workshop presented at the Annual Convention of the Pennsylvania Psychological Association, Harrisburg, PA.

Hyman, I., Dahbany, A., Blum, M., Brooks-Klein, V., Weiler, E., & Pokalo, M. (1997). *School discipline and school violence: The teacher variance approach.* Needham Heights, MA: Allyn & Bacon.

Hyman, I., & D'Allesandro, J. (1984). Good old-fashioned discipline: The politics of punitiveness. *Phi Delta Kappan, 66,* 39–45.

Hyman, I., & Gasiewski, E. (1992, March). *Corporal punishment, psychological maltreatment and conduct disorders: A continuing American dilemma.* Paper presented at the 24th Annual Convention of the National Association of School Psychologists, Nashville, TN.

Hyman, I., & Perone, D. (1998). The ecology of school violence: Introduction to the special theme section on school violence. *Journal of School Psychology, 36*(1), 36.

Hyman, I., & Pokalo, M. (1992, May). *Spanking, paddling, and child abuse: The problem of punitiveness in America.* Paper presented at the Eighth Biennial National Symposium on Child Victimization, coordinated by the Children's National Medical Center, Washington, DC.

Hyman, I., & Snook, P. (1999a). *Dangerous schools: What we can do about the physical and emotional abuse of our children.* San Francisco: Jossey-Bass.

Hyman, I., & Snook, P. (1999b, April). *Use of the My Worst Experience Scales for diagnosis and treatment of posttraumatic stress disorder in children.* Paper presented at the National Association of School Psychologists Annual Convention, Las Vegas, NV.

Hyman, I., & Snook, P. (2000, August). *Student alienation syndrome: Theory, assessment and application.* Paper presented at the 108th National Convention of the American Psychological Association, Washington, DC.

Hyman, I., Snook, P., Berna, J., DuCette, J., & Kohr, M. (2002). *Manual for the My Worst Experience Scale.* Los Angeles: Western Psychological Services.

Hyman, I., Snook, P., Lurkis, L., Aldrete-Phan, C., & Britton, G. (2001, August 27). *Student Alienation and Trauma Scale: Assessment, research and practice.* Paper presented at the 109th National Convention of the American Psychological Association, San Francisco.

Hyman, I., Weiler, E., Perone, D., Romano. L., Britton, G., & Shanock, A. (1997). Victims and victimizers: The two faces of school violence. In A. P. Goldstein & J. C. Conoley (Eds.), *School violence intervention: A practical handbook* (pp. 426–459). New York: Guilford Press.

Hyman, I., & Wise, J. (Eds.). (1979). *Corporal punishment in American education.* Philadelphia: Temple University Press.

Hyman, I., Zelikoff, W., & Clarke, J. (1988). Psychological and physical abuse in the schools: A paradigm for understanding post-traumatic stress disorder in children and youth. *Journal of Traumatic Stress, 1,* 243–267.

Johnson, S. (1999, May 3). One father's unique perspective. *Newsweek,* p. 38.

Kagan, D. M. (1990). How schools alienate students at risk: A model for examining proximal classroom variables. *Educational Psychologist, 25,* 105–125.

Kohr, M. (1995). *Validation of My Worst Experience Survey.* Unpublished doctoral dissertation, Temple University, Philadelphia.

Lambert, C. (1990). *Factorial structure and reliability of a scale measuring stress responses as a result of maltreatment in the schools.* Unpublished doctoral dissertation, Temple University, Philadelphia.

Lewin, K. (1951). Psychological ecology. In D. Cartwright (Ed.), *Field theory in social science: Selected theoretical papers by Kurt Lewin.* New York: Harper & Row.

Lochman, J. E., White, K. J., & Wayland, K. K. (1991). Cognitive-behavioral assessment and treatment with aggressive children. In P. C. Kendall (Ed.), *Child and adolescent therapy: Cognitive-behavioral procedures.* New York: Guilford Press.

Metropolitan Life Survey of the American Teacher, 1999: Violence in America's public schools–5 years later. (1999, May). New York: Louis Harris and Associates.

Mynard, H., & Joseph, S. (2000). Development of the multidimensional peer-victimization scale. *Aggressive Behavior, 26*(2), 169–178.

National Institute of Education. (1978a). *School crime and disruption: Prevention models.* (NIE contract NIE-P-77–0193). Washington, DC: U.S. Government Printing Office.

National Institute of Education. (1978b). *Violent schools–safe schools: The safe school study report to the Congress* (Vols. 1–3). Washington, DC: U.S. Government Printing Office.

Noddings, N. (1988). An ethic of caring and its implications for instructional arrangements. *American Journal of Education, 96,* 215–230.

Office of Juvenile Justice and Delinquency Program. (2001). *www.ojjdp.ncjrs.org*

Olafsen, R. N., & Viemero, V. (2000). Bully/victim problems and coping with stress in school among 10–12-year-old pupils in Aland, Finland. *Aggressive Behavior, 26*(1), 57–65.

Olweus, D. (1996). *Bullying at school.* Cambridge, MA: Blackwell.

Osterman, K. (2001). Students' need for belonging in the school community. *Review of Educational Research, 70*(3), 323–367.

Plas, J. M. (1994). The development of systems thinking: A historical perspective. In M. Fine & C. Carlson (Eds.), *The handbook of family–school intervention: A systems perspective.* Boston: Allyn & Bacon.

Proschansky, H. M., Ittelson, W. H., & Rivlion, L. G. (1970). *Environmental psychology: Man and his physical setting.* New York: Holt, Rinehart & Winston.

Rea, C. (1995). *Comparisons of patterns of traumatic stress symptoms in adolescents with and without overt behavior difficulties.* Unpublished doctoral dissertation. Temple University, Philadelphia.

Savage, S. (1999). *Academic stress and student alienation: A descriptive study of worst school experiences.* Unpublished doctoral dissertation, Temple University, Philadelphia.

Sergiovanni, T. J. (1994). *Building community in schools.* San Francisco: Jossey-Bass/Pfeiffer.

Smith, P., & Brain, P. (2000). Bullying in schools: Lessons from two decades of research. *Aggressive behavior, 26*(1), 1–9.

Snook, P. (2000). *A comparison of traumatic symptomatology of the My Worst Experience and the My Worst School Experience Scales.* Unpublished doctoral dissertation, Temple University, Philadelphia.

Straus, M. A. (1991). Discipline and deviance: Physical punishment of children and violence and other crime in adulthood. *Social Problems, 38*(2), 133–154.

Thomas, G., Hartley, R. D., & Kincaid, J. P. (1975). Test–retest and inter-analyst reliability of the Automated Readability Index, Flesch Reading Ease Score, and the Fog Count. *Journal of Reading Behavior, 7,* 149–154.

U.S. Department of Education/U.S. Department of Justice. (2000). *Indicators of school crime and safety, 1998.* Washington, DC: U.S. Government Printing Office.

U.S. Department of Health and Human Services. (2001). *Youth violence: A report of the surgeon general.* Rockville, MD: Author.

Vargas, I. (1991). *A descriptive study of school induced stressors among inner city Hispanic students.* Unpublished doctoral dissertation, Temple University, Philadelphia.

Vargas-Moll, I., & Hyman, I. (1992, March 6). *Psychological and physical maltreatment of inner city Hispanic school children.* Paper presented at the 11th Annual Conference on the Future of Psychology in the Schools, School Psychology Program, Temple University, Philadelphia.

Vossekuil, B., Fein, R., Reddy, M., Borum R., & Modzeleski, W. (2002). *The final report and findings of the safe school initiative: Implications for the preventions of school attacks in the United States.* Washington, DC: U.S. Secret Service National Threat Assessment Center and the United States Department of Education.

Weist, M. D., Acosta, O. M., & Youngstrom, E. A. (2001). Predictors of violence exposure among inner-city youth. *Journal of Clinical Child Psychology, 30*(2), 187–198.

Zelikoff, W. (1986). *Evidence for a new diagnostic construct: Educator-induced posttraumatic stress disorder.* Unpublished manuscript, National Center for the Study of Corporal Punishment and Alternatives, Temple University, Philadelphia.

CHAPTER 19

Law and School Safety

MICHAEL E. ROZALSKI
MITCHELL L. YELL

Efforts to create safer schools have intensified in the last decade. Concern about the seriousness of violence in schools has compelled federal, state, and local legislatures and policy makers to act. These actions have ranged from "get tough" legislation that has created harsher penalties for violent offenders to the adoption of school curriculums that attempt to prevent violence through education.

This chapter examines the legal forces that have affected schools' efforts to prevent and control school violence, and discusses the legal implications for administrators and teachers. It begins by presenting an overview of federal legislation intended to create safer schools. Next, it briefly examines several U.S. Supreme Court decisions that have shaped the school–student relationship in regard to discipline. Finally, it offers recommendations to schools, intended to provide a foundation from which school districts may develop legally correct policies regarding the creation of safer schools.

FEDERAL LEGISLATIVE ATTEMPTS TO CREATE SAFER SCHOOLS

Compelled by their constituents' concerns, federal and state legislative bodies have passed laws designed to create safer schools. This section briefly reviews some of the federal legislative efforts.

The U.S. Constitution limits the power of the federal government by specifying in the Tenth Amendment that "the powers not delegated to the United States by the Constitution, nor prohibited by it to the states, are reserved to the states." Because the Constitution does not explicitly reserve the right of the federal government to provide public education, the Tenth Amendment prevents the U.S. Congress from legislating how public schools are operated. Congress, however, can influence a state's effort to govern public schools either by offering federal grants to state or local education agencies or by withholding federal money from those states that do not pass laws similar to national statutes. Over the last decade, the U.S. Congress has addressed the issue of school safety by passing a wide variety of legislation. See details in the following discussion and the summary in Table 19.1.

Improving America's Schools Act of 1994

The Improving America's Schools Act of 1994 (IASA; formerly the Elementary and Secondary Education Act of 1965) included several subsections that helped foster the creation of safer schools. Both the Safe and Drug-Free Schools and Communities Act of 1994 (SDFSCA) and the Gun-Free Schools Act of 1994 (GFSA) were included in the IASA's efforts to prevent school violence. In passing the IASA, Congress relied on both its ability to both provide additional funding through grant programs and to withhold funding if states did not pass laws similar to national statutes.

TABLE 19.1. Federal Legislative Attempts to Create Safe Schools

Law	Relation to school safety
Safe and Drug-Free Schools and Communities Act of 1994	Provided federal grant money to educational institutions for comprehensive violence and drug abuse prevention programs.
Gun-Free Schools Act of 1994	Compelled states, in order to receive federal IASA funds, to pass legislation requiring public schools to expel, for 1 year, any student who brings a weapon to school or to a school function.
Violent Crime Control and Law Enforcement Act of 1994	Provided federal grant money to community–school cooperatives for youth crime prevention in high-poverty and high-crime communities.
Safe Schools Act of 1994	Provided federal grant money to schools for assessment of problems of violence and for coordination of prevention efforts with community agencies.
Individuals with Disabilities Education Act of 1997	Compelled states, in order to receive federal IDEA funds, to pass legislation requiring schools to follow specific discipline procedures for students in special education who exhibit violent behavior problems.

Thus, Congress was able to legislate how states improved the safety of the nation's public schools.

Safe and Drug-Free Schools and Communities Act of 1994

The Safe and Drug-Free Schools and Communities Act of 1994 (SDFSCA) was designed to address the seventh National Education Goal, which stated that "by the year 2000, every school in the United States will be free of drugs, violence and the unauthorized presence of firearms" (Goals 2000: Educate America Act, 20 U.S.C. §5812(7)(A), 1994). One of the main purposes of the SDFSCA was to reduce the threat and reverse the trend of increasing violence in schools and communities by funding violence prevention programs.

To accomplish this goal, the SDFSCA made federal grant monies available to state educational agencies, local educational agencies, institutions of higher education, and nonprofit organizations. Through the grant programs, schools could (1) disseminate information about violence prevention and the promotion of school safety, (2) develop and implement character education programs, (3) provide training and technical assistance for teachers, (4) purchase and install metal detectors, and (5) hire additional security personnel. Recognizing that the impact of students' violent behavior and drug use was felt beyond the schoolhouse walls and that the "tragic consequences of violence . . . are not only felt by students . . . but by such students' communities and the Nation" (SDFSCA- §7102(5), 1994), SDFSCA also provided federal assistance to coordinate community-based services, like programs that established "safe zones of passage" (SDFSCA- § 7116(b)(5), 1994) for students traveling to and from school.

Gun-Free Schools Act of 1994

The Gun-Free Schools Act of 1994 (GFSA) was Congress's attempt to revise a law, the Gun-Free School Zones Act of 1990 (GFSZA), that the U.S. Supreme Court found unconstitutional (see *U.S. v. Lopez*, 1995). The main purpose of the GFSA was to compel states to adopt "zero tolerance" disciplinary policies for weapon-toting students.

The GFSA required that to receive funding under the IASA, a state must pass a law that required the local educational agency to expel, for not less than 1 year, any student who brought a weapon (e.g., gun, bomb, grenade, rocket, or missiles; by federal definition, the Gun Control Act of 1968- § 921(g)(2), a knife is not a weapon) to school. To allow for fair treatment under the law, school district administrators were allowed to modify the expulsion requirement on a case-by-case basis. States that did not have a similar law in place by 1995 faced the cutoff of all federal IASA funds. Congress thus avoided the constitutional problems associated with the GFSZA by creating a law that was tied to federal funding, rather than directly imposing federal school and firearms requirements on the states.

Violent Crime Control and Law Enforcement Act of 1994

In recognition that violent behavior had become a severe threat to our communities, Congress passed the Violent Crime Control and Law Enforcement Act of 1994 (VCCLEA). The VCCLEA was designed to broadly address violence by providing additional resources to the crime-fighting effort (e.g., expanding "juvenile correctional facilities or pretrial detention facilities for juvenile offenders"; VCCLEA- § 13705(c)), while also funding community-based crime prevention initiatives. Toward the latter aim, VCCLEA provided grants to improve opportunities for youth in poverty and high-crime areas by fostering the development of projects that encouraged community participation and school cooperation.

The Ounce of Prevention Council was authorized to fund a variety of mentoring or tutoring programs that encouraged the active involvement of strong adult role models, such as DARE America and the Boys and Girls Clubs of America. To encourage general community support, monies were also available to develop and run after-school programs, like midnight sports leagues, job placement training, and economic development activities (VCCLEA- § 13841, 1994). The key requirement for obtaining these grants was to create a comprehensive planning and implementation team, including educators, community residents, business and civic leaders, and representatives from religious organizations, law enforcement, public housing and other public agencies, that extended the prevention efforts beyond the school.

Safe Schools Act of 1994

Like the SDFSCA, the Safe Schools Act of 1994 (SSA) was designed to address the seventh National Education Goal to create safe, disciplined, and drug-free schools. The SSA, however, focused more explicitly on "identifying and assessing school violence and discipline problems" (§ 5965(a)(1)) prior to making funds available for the development and implementation of violence prevention activities and materials.

Under the SSA, schools were required to carefully coordinate their research and intervention efforts. For example, the local educational agency was to conduct needs assessment activities in consultation with representatives from law enforcement, judicial, health, social services, and juvenile justice agencies. Data from schools were to be collected in order to (1) evaluate research and programs for youth violence prevention in conjunction with the Coordinating Council on Juvenile Justice and Delinquency Prevention of the Department of Justice (SSA- §5968, 1994) and (2) "develop a written safe schools model ... that enable[d] all students to participate" (SSA- §5966, 1994).

Individuals with Disabilities Education Act Amendments of 1997

The predecessor to the Individuals with Disabilities Education Act Amendments of 1997 (hereafter IDEA '97), the Education for All Handicapped Children Act (EAHCA, 1975), guaranteed a free appropriate public education (FAPE) for students with disabilities. Every few years, the EAHCA was reauthorized and amended. In 1990, the EAHCA was renamed the Individuals with Disabilities Education Act (IDEA), and in 1997, Congress amended the IDEA to specifically address the issue of school discipline. The 1997 changes were made, in part, to alleviate the concerns of school administrators and teachers about their inability to effectively discipline students with disabilities who engaged in violent behavior in school.

The IDEA '97 attempted to safeguard the educational right of students with disabilities to an FAPE, while providing school administrators the means to discipline students with disabilities. To achieve this aim, the IDEA '97 outlined specific procedures that school officials must follow to remove students with disabilities from school. For example, school officials can place a student with disabilities in an interim alternative educational setting (IAES) for up to 45 days if the student brings a weapon to school or to a school function, or if the administrators can convince an impartial hearing officer that a student with disabilities presents a danger to him- or herself, or to others.

The specific discipline provisions of IDEA '97 are beyond the scope of this chapter; for additional information concerning the discipline of students with disabilities, see the more extensive discussions (e.g., Conroy, Clark, Gable, & Fox, 1999; Katsiyannis & Maag, 1998; Yell, Katsiyannis, Bradley, & Rozalski, 2000; Yell, Rozalski, & Drasgow, 2001).

Attempting to address concerns for the safety of students in U.S. schools, Congress has passed legislation designed to reduce violence in schools. This legislation has influenced how states have created safer schools by providing additional funding through grant programs and withholding funding to states that did not pass laws similar to the federal statutes. The U.S. Supreme Court has also influenced the creation of safer public schools by interpreting these laws and other statutes. The next section reviews some of the more important Supreme Court rulings as they relate to the prevention of school violence.

THE U.S. SUPREME COURT AND THE CREATION OF SAFE SCHOOLS

As we have conceptualized the creation of safe schools, the U.S. Supreme Court has issued a single ruling, in *U.S. v. Lopez* (1995), that directly ad-

dresses school violence. The high court, however, has addressed broader issues of students' rights to free speech, due process, and reasonable searches,
which have shaped the way school administrators must attend to school discipline and violence prevention. This section reviews these court cases; Table
19.2 provides a summary.

U.S. v. Lopez (1995)

Earlier we referred to Congress's first attempt at legislating school violence
prevention, the Gun-Free School Zones Act of 1990, which made it a federal
crime to possess a firearm within 1,000 feet of a public, parochial, or private
school building. This statute was first tested in 1992 when a 12th-grade stu-

TABLE 19.2. The U.S. Supreme Court and School Safety

Supreme Court case	Ruling as it relates to school safety
U.S. v. Lopez (1995)	The Gun-Free School Zones Act of 1990 was unconstitutional because it illegally extended Congress' power to legislate public schools.
Tinker v. Des Moines (1969)	Students are entitled to basic constitutional protections, and schools must be able to clearly justify that restrictions to those protections are based on legitimate educational concerns.
Bethel v. Fraser (1986)	Schools should provide advanced verbal and written notification to students regarding behavior that may interfere with the educational process and the consequences for those violations.
Goss v. Lopez (1975)	Students have due process protections and must be able to hear the charges leveled against them and the rationalization for their suspension, and be given an opportunity to present their side of the story.
Honig v. Doe (1988)	Limited schools' authority to remove dangerous and disruptive students with disabilities from school by mandating that, pending administrative review, a student must remain in the current placement unless school officials and parents agree otherwise.
New Jersey v T.L.O. (1985)	When conducting searches, schools must meet a standard of reasonableness, which holds that a search must be justified at inception, motivated by violations of school rules, related to the rule violation that led to the initial search, and conducted in the least intrusive manner possible.
Vernonia v. Acton (1995)	To protect against unreasonable searches, a school should have a clearly stated and publicly developed policy that announces a decreased expectation for privacy.

dent brought a concealed and loaded .38 caliber handgun to school. School authorities confronted the student after receiving an anonymous tip. When the student admitted that he was carrying the weapon, he was promptly arrested for violating Texas law. A day later, state prosecutors dropped their complaint when federal charges were brought under GFSZA.

The United States District Court for the Western District of Texas convicted the student. The student appealed, claiming that the law unconstitutionally extended the power of the federal government to legislate control over public schools by violating the Constitution's commerce clause (for a detailed explanation, see Safra, 2000). Agreeing with the student, the U.S. Court of Appeals for the Fifth Circuit reversed the district court's conviction. In 1995, the U.S. Supreme Court affirmed the appeals court's ruling and ruled that the GFSZA was unconstitutional. By then, the Gun-Free Schools Act, which established the same moratorium on gun possession on school grounds, had been passed.

Tinker v. Des Moines Independent Community School District (1969)

Tinker v. Des Moines Independent Community School District (hereafter *Tinker*) did not explicitly address the issue of school violence, but helped define students' constitutional right to freedom of speech. To protest the hostilities in Vietnam, three students wore black armbands to school. Because the school had a policy that required a student wearing an armband to remove it upon request or be suspended, the three students were sent home. The U.S. District Court for the Southern District of Iowa found, and the U.S. Court of Appeals for the Eighth Circuit affirmed, that the school authorities' action did not violate the students' right to free speech because the suspension reasonably attempted to prevent the disruption of school discipline.

In 1969, the U.S. Supreme Court reversed the earlier rulings, stating that students do not "shed their Constitutional rights . . . at the schoolhouse gate" (*Tinker*, p. 506). The high court reasoned that (1) students are also entitled to basic protections under the Constitution and (2) schools must be able to justify that restrictions to those protections are based on legitimate educational concerns. In this case, wearing armbands to publicize a political view was not disruptive to the school environment and therefore should not concern school officials.

Bethel School District No. 403 v. Fraser (1986)

Bethel School District No. 403 v. Fraser also addressed students' right to free speech. In this case a high school student gave a sexually suggestive nomination speech for a friend running for a student government office to an assembly of about 600 students. School officials suspended him for 2 days and removed his name from a list of potential graduation speakers for violating the disciplinary rule that prohibited the use of obscene language when it interfered with the educational process. The student filed suit against the district. The U.S. District Court for the Western District of Washington found, and the U.S. Court of Appeals for the Ninth Circuit affirmed, that the school had violated the student's rights under the First and Fourteenth Amendments.

In 1986, the U.S. Supreme Court reversed the decision. The high court reasoned that the student's obscene speech could have a disruptive effect on the education process and was not protected by the First Amendment. Further, the Court found that the school did not violate the Fourteenth Amendment's due process protections because (1) the student had been warned in advance by two teachers that the speech could lead to severe consequences and (2) a 2-day suspension was not severe enough to trigger extensive due process protections.

Goss v. Lopez (1975)

Like *Tinker, Goss v. Lopez* did not explicitly address the issue of school violence, but instead more clearly defined the due process procedures that schools must follow when suspending or expelling students. In this case, nine students at two high schools and one junior high school were suspended from school for misconduct without a hearing. The students filed a complaint, claiming that they had been denied due process of law under the Fourteenth Amendment.

In 1975 the case went to the Supreme Court. Although the high court acknowledged that school officials have the authority to set expectations for appropriate behavior, they ruled against the school. The court reasoned that students' overriding right to a public education entitled them to some due process protections under the Fourteenth Amendment when faced with suspension or expulsion. The Supreme Court further clarified its position by emphasizing that schools could rely on suspension when necessary to maintain order, but that students would have the right to (1) hear the charges leveled against them and the rationalization for their suspension and (2) be given an opportunity to present their side of the story.

Honig v. Doe (1988)

Honig v. Doe (hereafter *Honig*) was a case that addressed how students with disabilities are disciplined. In this case two students with emotional disabilities had been suspended and recommended for expulsion from the San Francisco public school system following separate incidents of serious misbehavior. In accordance with California law, the suspensions were continued indefinitely while the expulsion proceedings were being held. When attorneys for the students filed a joint lawsuit (*Doe v. Maher*, 1986), the federal district court issued an injunction that prevented the school district from suspending any student with disabilities for misbehavior causally related to the student's disability. The school district appealed to the U.S. Court of Appeals for the Ninth Circuit. The circuit court ruled that expelling a student protected under the IDEA amounted to a change in placement and that no student with a disability, regardless of the danger presented by the student, could be excluded from school pending administrative review (the "stay-put" provision). In response, the California superintendent of public instruction, Bill Honig, filed a petition of *certiorari* with the U.S. Supreme Court, contending that the circuit court's interpretation of the stay-put provision was untenable. He argued that a literal reading of this provision would require schools to return potentially violent and dangerous students to the classroom, a situation Congress could not have intended.

On January 20, 1988, the U.S. Supreme Court ruled that expulsion constituted a change in placement. The high court rejected Honig's argument that Congress did not intend to deny schools the authority to remove dangerous and disruptive students from the school environment. Stating that Congress had intended to strip schools of their unilateral authority to exclude students with disabilities from school, the high court declined to read a dangerousness exception into the law. The Court found that pending administrative review, the student must remain in the then current placement unless school officials and parents agree otherwise.

The high court, however, noted that its decision regarding the stay-put provision did not leave educators helpless to discipline students with disabilities. Schools could rely on time out or suspension for up to 10 days when the prompt removal of a dangerous student was necessary. If a serious danger existed and formal efforts "to persuade the child's parents to agree to an interim placement" (*Honig*, p. 605) failed, then school officials could immediately seek the aid of the courts. According to the Supreme Court, the stay-put provision did not preempt the court's authority to grant an injunction to temporarily remove the student from the school.

New Jersey v. T.L.O. (1985)

New Jersey v. T.L.O. (hereafter *TLO*) addressed the issue of student searches as conducted by school officials. In this case, a teacher found a high school freshman smoking in the bathroom. When brought to and then confronted by the assistant vice principal, the student denied that she had been smoking. The assistant vice principal searched her purse and found a pack of cigarettes, cigarette rolling papers, marijuana, and two letters implicating the student in dealing marijuana. The student was referred to a New Jersey juvenile court, where she was found delinquent and sentenced to a year of probation. Eventually the Supreme Court of New Jersey heard the case and ruled that because the search of the purse was not reasonable, the evidence could not be used against the student.

In 1985, the U.S. Supreme Court reversed the decision and ruled that the marijuana was admissible as evidence. The high court reasoned that, although students are protected by the Fourth Amendment from unreasonable searches and seizures, school officials are not required to meet as stringent standards as police officers. In the interest of maintaining discipline and security in school, administrators are neither required to (1) obtain a warrant in order to conduct a search nor to (2) strictly adhere to the requirement that searches be based on probable cause. According to the Supreme Court, school officials must meet a reasonableness standard, which holds a search justified if a reasonable person would have cause to suspect that evidence of illegal activities might be present. Specifically, a search must be (1) justified at inception, (2) motivated by violations of school rules or policies, (3) related to the rule violation that led to the initial search, and (4) conducted in the least intrusive manner possible (Susswein, 2000).

Vernonia School District v. Acton (1995)

Like *TLO, Vernonia School District v. Acton* was a case that addressed students' protections against unreasonable search and seizure. In this case, rising concern over drug use and discipline problems prompted school officials, with parent approval, to adopt a urinalysis drug testing policy for student athletes. The policy required any student participating in school-sponsored athletics to consent to a preseason drug test and in-season random testing; parents of the athletes were also required to provide written consent. A seventh grade student and his parents refused to sign the forms and filed a complaint. The U.S. District Court for the District of Oregon dismissed the suit, but the United States Court of Appeals for the Ninth Circuit reversed the ruling, arguing that drug testing policy violated the Fourth Amendment.

In 1995, the U.S. Supreme Court vacated the district court's opinion. The high court reasoned that because the district's drug problems, especially involving student-athletes, were severe enough to warrant intervention, the schools could act. Further, because the drug testing policy was reasonable, given that (1) the clearly stated and publicly developed policy announced a decreased expectation for privacy and (2) the search was relatively unobtrusive, the policy did not violate the student's right to be free from unreasonable searches under the Fourth Amendment.

The federal government has been involved in a variety of efforts to prevent and contain school violence. Having reviewed how the U.S. Congress has passed federal legislation and the U.S. Supreme Court has interpreted some of these laws, we now offer seven recommendations to schools attempting to develop legally correct policies regarding the creation of safer schools.

RECOMMENDATIONS FOR CREATING LEGALLY CORRECT POLICIES

By themselves, schools are not going to prevent school violence (Paige, 2000). An effective effort to create safer schools will require intense collaboration with a number of key players, including community agencies, researchers, and the students who commit these acts (e.g., Brooks, 2000). School districts, however, can greatly impact the successfulness of violence prevention efforts by being proactive. The following discussion explains how administrators and teachers can proactively create legally correct programs and procedures to help prevent the occurrence and limit the impact of school violence. The recommendations are summarized in Table 19.3.

Know the Law

Without knowledge of the federal and state laws that address school safety, and the court cases that have shaped the understanding of those laws, schools cannot develop legally correct policies and procedures. Although all schools must follow the federal laws (e.g., the Individuals with Disabilities Education Act Amendments of 1997, the Gun-Free Schools Act of 1994), some states have

TABLE 19.3. Recommendations for Creating Legally Correct Policies

Broad recommendation	Considerations
Know the law.	Require a representative from the school district's legal department, who understands both federal and state laws, to work with your district policy-making team
Follow the law.	Ensure that administrators better understand the need to adhere to legal guidelines, and that they have the tools they need to properly follow the dictates of the law.
Train all school staff.	Train staff to understand the characteristics of safe and unsafe schools and students, and how to respond to violence as it is occurring or after it has occurred.
Involve the community.	Publicly announce existing policies and procedures and encourage community members to participate in planning committees for violence prevention initiatives.
Evaluate the issue.	Review district and school policies, design measures of school violence that can be tracked, conduct audits of resources, and prioritize recommendations for intervention.
Intervene.	Fix deficiencies identified in the evaluation stage, consider adopting prevention programs or schoolwide discipline policies, and create a crisis-response team and procedures.
Monitor your progress.	Measure progress, document efficacy, modify programs as needed, and provide ongoing staff training.

added additional requirements that extend the federal statutes. In these cases the school districts are required to meet the more stringent state requirements. The creation of legally correct policies and procedures therefore requires intimate knowledge of the law. Because this knowledge is ever changing (e.g., new court cases are decided, laws are amended), some authors have suggested that district policy-making teams include persons, such as representatives from the school district's legal department, who understand both federal and state legislation (Kyle & Hahn, 1995).

Follow the Law

When states and school districts are required to adopt policies or risk losing the appropriation of funds (e.g., IDEA '97, GFSA), there is increased pressure to follow the procedural requirements of a law (Yell et al., 2001). For example, IDEA '97 requires that certain procedures be followed when disciplining a student with disabilities who exhibits violent problem behavior (e.g., bringing a weapon to school). Districts, however, are struggling to properly follow these discipline procedures. (For extensive discussion regarding the legal guidelines for disciplining students with disabilities, see Yell et al., 2001). Smith (2000) noted that schools often lose due process hearings and court cases when they are challenged. This does not imply that schools are negligent in following the law, but rather that extensive training is needed to ensure that school administrators (1) understand the need to adhere to legal guidelines and (2) have the tools they need to properly follow the dictates of the law.

Train All School Staff

Because the need for violence prevention extends beyond the classroom, all staff members, including administrators, teachers, administrative assistants, paraprofessionals, librarians, bus drivers, and cafeteria and custodial staff, should be trained to help prevent violence (Goldstein, 1999). Failure to train staff adequately to prevent violence may leave districts open to lawsuits in the event of a violent incident (Hermann & Remley, 2000; Kyle & Hahn, 1995). We have previously suggested that training include "(1) understanding the characteristics of safe and unsafe schools, (2) managing and disciplining students in the classroom, (3) identifying and responding to warning signs of possible violent behavior, (4) using safe and effective intervention procedures, and (5) responding to violence after it has occurred" (Yell & Rozalski, 2000, p. 195). In addition to training school staff, community participants must be informed about school safety procedures and policies.

Involve the Community

As emphasized by federal legislation, (e.g., the Safe and Drug-Free Schools and Communities Act of 1994), community involvement in preventing school violence is essential (Schwartz, Weiner, White, & Joe, 2000). School policy makers should involve community members when attempting to create safer schools by (1) publicly announcing existing policies and procedures, (2) hosting forums to discuss possible school violence prevention initiatives, and (3) encouraging community members to participate in school-sponsored training and as team members on planning and implementation committees. For example, a school can first mail pamphlets or newsletters that outline current policies and procedures, then invite parents, child and family service agencies, local law enforcement organizations, and business representatives to a town meeting to discuss the revision of school safety plans and crisis response procedures. Fostering public discussion of violence prevention initiatives can increase community cooperation and support and, in the event of violent situation in a school, help to minimize negative publicity and legal liability.

Create Safe School Teams

Creating a single point of contact for coordination of violence prevention efforts is essential. Districts and schools should develop a Safe School Team that has the time and financial resources needed to identify and implement violence prevention plans. The primary responsibility of the team should be to (1) evaluate the seriousness of school violence and the resources currently available for violence prevention, (2) coordinate intervention efforts, and (3) monitor the effectiveness of the programs. Additional details are given in the following sections.

Evaluate the Issue

The creation of safer schools will not happen after a single community meeting. Efforts to prevent violence will require that school and community participants make comprehensive plans to evaluate how students' violent behavior does and may affect their schools. Schools will be required to assess their current problems before developing plans to prevent future violent incidents. This evaluation will require schools to (1) review district- and school-level policies, (2) revise or design measures of school violence that can be tracked for long-term evaluation, (3) conduct physical audits of schools, and (4) prioritize recommendations for intervention. Because community involvement is crucial in the assessment stage, it is important to recruit knowledgeable members. For example, in conducting physical audits of schools, law enforcement officials can be asked to help assess how secure the physical plant is and identify areas that need improvement (Dwyer, Osher, & Warger, 1998; Walker & Gresham, 1997).

Intervene

After a school-based team has evaluated a school for its ability to prevent and respond to violent problem behavior, a thoughtful plan must be developed. Common approaches to creating safe schools are to (1) address deficiencies based on the evaluation of the procedures and physical plant, (2) adopt prevention programs, (3) implement schoolwide discipline policies, and (4) develop a crisis response team and procedures.

Fix What's Broken

If the Safe School Team identifies shortcomings in the policies, procedures, or physical plant when evaluating a school for its ability to prevent or address violence, the school should fix them. For example, if a school's policy does not clearly specify prohibited weapons (e.g., is a pellet gun a weapon?) or suspension procedures are inflexible (e.g., mandatory 1-year suspension with no review of mitigating circumstances), revise policy statements. A reasonable discipline policy should allow flexibility while creating clear and nondiscriminatory standards (Uhler & Fish, 2001).

Adopt Prevention Programs

The importance of preventing violence through educational programs (Meyer & Farrell, 1998) and positive behavioral interventions that do not rely on coercion or punishment for behavior change (Dunlap & Koegel, 1999) has been well established. When adopting various violence prevention programs, schools must be careful to rely on empirically based strategies and match the target audience to the program. For example, students at risk for developing behavioral problems may be exposed to a conflict resolution curriculum such as Second Step (Frey, Hirschstein, & Guzzo, 2000; Grossman et al., 1997), whereas students with more severe behavior problems may require a multiple-component behavior change program to replace their inappropriate behaviors (Drasgow, Yell, Bradley, & Shriner, 1999).

Implement Schoolwide Discipline Policies

Schools use rules and consequences to establish expectations for students' behavior. Comprehensive efforts to prevent violence should include schoolwide discipline plans that have understandable rationales, clearly communicated behavioral expectations, and fairly administered consequences that are reasonable, given the transgression (Hartwig & Reusch, 2000; Yell et al., 2000). To be successful, schoolwide discipline plans must also include specific procedures for correcting problem behavior and a means of establishing and monitoring staff commitment to the schoolwide implementation of the discipline plan (Colvin, Kameenui, & Sugai, 1993; Lewis, Sugai, & Colvin, 1998; Sugai, 1999).

Develop a Crisis Response Team and Procedures

Violence is not always predictable. Schools must therefore be prepared to respond to violent incidents within their premises by establishing both a crisis response team and procedures in advance of an actual emergency. A crisis response team must have clear leadership and an established chain of command, but should not be composed only of members of the Safe School Team. Crisis procedures must include (1) a communication system that allows for both efficient notification of internal staff (e.g., "code blue in the library" over an intercom system) and external emergency support (e.g., law enforcement, medical personnel, trauma counselors) and (2) staff training in safe and effective interventions during and following crises. Additional procedures for investigating a violent incident after the school has been secured and for handling the media are also necessary (Dwyer et al., 1998).

Monitor Your Progress

To successfully create safer schools, officials must recognize that comprehensive planning and intervening is followed by further evaluation and training. For example, schools should monitor their progress by tracking changes in the number, location, and times of office referrals (Sugai, 1999) and violent or criminal behavior. Further, the Safe School Team, in coordination with administrators and outside agencies, can conduct exercises to assess the school's readiness to respond to a serious violent incident and can ensure that staff are promptly informed of procedural updates through in-service training (Stephens, 1994). Without conducting ongoing assessments to (1) document the efficacy of a school's prevention efforts, (2) make needed program adjustments, and (3) determine staff training needs, a school's labor to create a safer environment is likely to be ineffective.

SUMMARY

Federal, state, and local legislatures and policy makers have guided efforts to create safer schools. This chapter has provided an overview of the legal forces that have impacted schools' efforts to prevent school violence and made recommendations for schools attempting to develop legally correct policies and procedures. Schools must be proactive in how they create programs and procedures to prevent the occurrence and limit the impact of school violence.

REFERENCES

Bethel School District No. 403 v. Fraser, 478 U.S. 675 (1986).

Brooks, S. L. (2000). Therapeutic and preventive approaches to school safety: Applications of a family systems model. *New England Law Review, 34,* 615–622.

Colvin, G., Kameenui, E. J., & Sugai, G. (1993). Reconceptualizing behavior management and schoolwide discipline in general education. *Education and Treatment of Children, 16,* 361–381.

Conroy, M., Clark, D., Gable, R., & Fox, J. (1999). A look at IDEA 1997 discipline provisions: Implications for change in the roles and responsibilities of school personnel. *Preventing School Failure, 43,* 64–70.

Doe v. Maher, 793 F.2d 1470 (9th Cir. 1986).

Drasgow, E., Yell, M. L., Bradley, R., & Shriner, J. G. (1999). The IDEA amendments of 1997: A schoolwide model for conducting functional behavioral assessments and developing behavior intervention plans. *Education and Treatment of Children, 22,* 244–266.

Dunlap, G., & Koegel, R. L. (1999). Welcoming introduction. *Journal of Positive Behavior Interventions, 1,* 2–3.

Dwyer, K., Osher, D., & Warger, C. (1998). *Early warning, timely response: A guide to safe schools.* Washington, DC: United States Department of Education. Available: *http://www.air-dc.org/cecp/cecp.html*

Education for All Handicapped Children Act, 20 USC § 1400 (1975).

Frey, K. S., Hirschstein, M. K., & Guzzo, B. A. (2000). Second Step: Preventing aggression by promoting social competence. *Journal of Emotional and Behavioral Disorders, 8,* 102–112.

Goals 2000: Educate America Act, 20 U.S.C. § 5801 (1994).

Goldstein, A. P. (1999). *Low-level aggression: First steps on the ladder to violence.* Champaign, IL: Research Press.

Goss v. Lopez, 419 U.S. 565 (1975).

Grossman, D. C., Neckerman, H. J., Koepsell, T. D., Liu, P., Asher, K. N., Beland, K., Frey, K., & Rivara, F. P. (1997). Effectiveness of a violence prevention curriculum among children in elementary school: A randomized control trial. *Journal of the American Medical Association, 277,* 1605–1611.

Gun Control Act, 18 U.S.C. § 921 (1968).

Gun-Free Schools Act, 20 U.S.C. § 8921 (1994).

Gun-Free School Zones Act, 18 U.S.C. § 922(q) (1990).

Hartwig, E. P., & Ruesch, G. M. (2000). Disciplining students in special education. *Journal of Special Education, 33,* 243–250.

Hermann, M. A., & Remley. T. P., Jr. (2000). Guns, violence, and schools: The results of school violence—Litigation against educators and students shedding more constitutional rights at the school house gate. *Loyola Law Review, 46,* 389–439.

Honig v. Doe, 484 U.S. 305 (1988).

Improving America's Schools Act, 20 U.S.C. § 6301 et seq. (1994).

Individuals with Disabilities Education Act Amendments, 20 U.S.C. § 1400 (1997).

Individuals with Disabilities Education Act Amendments of 1997 Regulations, 34 C.F.R. § 300 et seq.

Katsiyannis, A., & Maag, J. (1998). Disciplining students with disabilities: Issues and considerations for implementing IDEA '97. *Behavioral Disorders, 24,* 276–289.

Kopka, D. L. (1997). *School violence.* Santa Barbara, CA: Contemporary School Issues.

Kyle, J. W., & Hahn, B. W. (1995). Violence and the school as a workplace. In *Violence in the schools: Causes, prevention, and crises management (Handbook of the Violence in the Schools Conference)*. Horsham, PA: LRP.

Lewis, T. J., Sugai, G., & Colvin, G. (1998). Reducing problem behavior through a schoolwide system of effective behavioral support: Investigation of a schoolwide social skills training program and contextual interventions. *School Psychology Review, 27*(3), 446–459.

Meyer, A. L., & Farrell, A. D. (1998). Social skills training to promote resilience in urban sixth grade students: One product of an action research strategy to prevent youth violence in high-risk environments. *Education and Treatment of Children, 21,* 461–488.

New Jersey v. T.L.O., 469 U.S. 325 (1985).

Paige, R. (2000). Safety above all else. *Houston Law Review, 37*(1), 111–116.

Safe and Drug-Free Schools and Communities Act, 20 U.S.C. § 7101 (1994).

Safe Schools Act, 20 USCS § 5961 (1994).

Safra, S. J. (2000). The amended Gun-Free School Zones Act: Doubt as to its constitutionality remains. *Duke Law Journal, 50*(2), 637–663.

Schwartz, I. M., Weiner, N. A., White, T., & Joe, S. (2000). School bells, death knells, and body counts: No apocalypse now. *Houston Law Review, 37*(1), 1–19.

Smith, C. R. (2000). Behavioral and discipline provisions of IDEA '97: Implicit competencies yet to be confirmed. *Exceptional Children, 66,* 403–412.

Stephens, R. D. (1994). Planning for safer and better schools: School violence prevention and intervention strategies. *School Psychology Review, 23*(2), 204–215.

Sugai, G. (1999, October). *Prevention focused schoolwide discipline programs: Key features in creating schoolwide systems of positive behavioral support.* Paper presented at the meeting of the Council for Children with Behavior Disorder, Dallas, TX.

Susswein, R. (2000). The New Jersey school search policy manual: Striking the balance of students' rights of privacy and security after the Columbine tragedy. *New England Law Review, 34,* 3, 527–564.

Tinker v. Des Moines Independent Community School District, 393 U.S. 503 (1969).

Uhler, S. F., & Fish, D. J. (2001). Zero-tolerance discipline in Illinois public schools. *Illinois Bar Journal, 89, 256–260.*

U.S. v. Lopez, 514 U.S. 549 (1995).

Vernonia School District v. Acton, 515 U.S. 646 (1995).

Violent Crime Control and Law Enforcement Act, 42 U.S.C. § 13701 (1994).

Walker, H. M., & Gresham, F. M. (1997). Make schools safer and violence-free. *Intervention in School and Clinic, 32*(4), 199–204.

Yell, M. L., Katsiyannis, A., Bradley, R., & Rozalski, M. (2000). Ensuring compliance with the disciplinary provisions of IDEA '97: Challenges and opportunities. *Journal of Special Education Leadership, 13,* 3–18.

Yell, M. L., & Rozalski, M. E. (2000). Searching for safe schools: Legal issues in the prevention of school violence. *Journal of Emotional and Behavioral Disorders, 8,* 187–196.

Yell, M. L., Rozalski, M. E., & Drasgow, E. (2001). Disciplining students with disabilities. *Focus on Exceptional Children, 33*(9), 1–20.

PART VII
Summary and Challenges for the Future

CHAPTER 20

The Known, Unknown, and Future of Violence Reduction

JANE CLOSE CONOLEY
ARNOLD P. GOLDSTEIN

The incidence of violence in our schools is growing rapidly and demands a response. It is vital, however, to keep the problem of school violence in some perspective. The overwhelming majority of schoolchildren are not involved in or even affected by violence. Although there is cause for concern, there is no cause for panic among educators, families, or other community members. Drastic overreactions that put a narrow focus on the schools are unlikely to be effective. Schools reflect an increasingly violent society; they are not the sources of such violence.

The previous chapters have outlined in useful detail the components of multilevel, multimodal, school-based programs to prevent and respond to violence. It is of critical importance that school personnel who are serious about developing such programs understand that simplistic attempts to reduce threats of vandalism, assaults, and gang violence are doomed to failure. The contributing authors of this book have illustrated that a culture of violence exists because of the following factors:

- Individual skills deficits
- Domestic abuse
- Poverty
- Racism
- Unemployment
- Inadequate classrooms
- Easy access to weapons, as well as to alcohol and other drugs
- Alienation from a cultural heritage
- Lack of supervision and of constructive outlets for young people

- Reduced influence of socializing institutions, such as churches and the family
- A popular media that models and glorifies aggressive solutions

Serious attempts to intervene require plans that target as many of these factors as possible, while avoiding aggressive responses to young people such as overuse of suspension from school, reliance on corporal punishment, and the building of so-called boot camps. These, like the many violence prevention programs that are currently available (our last count is 215 programs) have little or no research to support effectiveness; rather, their assessment relies on   anecdotes, impressions, or prevailing political philosophies.

WHAT WE DO KNOW

The authors who have contributed to this book have illustrated that violence in schools can be combated or prevented, at least in the short run, by making adjustments to the physical plant; improving the skills of students, teachers, and administrators; developing schoolwide discipline plans; improving relationships with parents; planning responses to crises; making changes in curriculum delivery systems; increasing community involvement; developing good relationships with the police; increasing extracurricular activities; having a good knowledge of the law; implementing parent training programs; and improving adult relationships within the schools. It is clear that early intervention maximizes a child's academic and social success and that positive academic and social involvement is a great buffer against violence.

The risk factors that threaten a child's ability to succeed in school and avoid aggressive behavior are known, and promising interventions are available. The escalation in violence is not occurring because we lack hopeful new responses to the ecology of aggression.

WHAT WE DO NOT KNOW

There is a dearth of research to support the long-range outcomes of even the most favorable programs, and much of what we do know is based on limited samples of children and young people, with a paucity of data on the developmental course of the interventions. The differential effectiveness of programs across cultural/ethnic groups is also largely unknown.

Continued research can respond to both of these concerns. Carefully controlled studies will eventually tell the professional community what treatments work best at what ages and with which ethnic/social groups. Gender differences are likely to be illuminated with appropriate research as well.

What are likely to elude researchers, however, are strategies to create a political and economic will to use the interventions that already exist and those that are likely to be developed. The best interventions must be implemented to have the desired effects, but the best interventions are expensive and require that many adults in schools, families, and communities change to create environments and treatment approaches that will reduce violence. Gathering the resources necessary to support the necessary changes will require the collaboration of individuals at many levels of the public and private sectors. The current political climate—which emphasizes a reduction of services to distressed families, and punishment and exclusion for troubled children—suggests that creating the needed will to intervene will be difficult.

The need for psychologists to advocate for their science is clear. There is a large gap between knowing what to do and having the resources to implement even the most wonderful program.

STEPS TOWARD THE FUTURE

Our optimistic prediction is that psychology is nearing the point at which effective ways of responding to violence in schools will be known. To maximize the benefits of these research triumphs, however, teams of psychologists, social workers, teachers, administrators, and parents must work together to select and implement violence prevention and treatment programs. It is vital that teams of concerned adults become invested in particular approaches and stay committed over long periods of time.

The efforts of families will be thwarted if children must pass through dangerous drug- and weapon-infested streets on their way to school. The success of school personnel will be limited if alliances with families are impossible. Neither schools nor families alone can combat violence. Even their powerful partnership requires the support of other systems, such as elected officials, the welfare system, the police, the judicial system, and mental health services.

Every coalition of importance is started and nurtured by a small group of committed individuals. We conclude this volume with a call for educational psychologists to take on the role of forming such coalitions. Psychologists are in a good position to initiate the needed collaborations that will make a community effort to facilitate safe schools possible. Psychologists understand aggression. They have contact with children, families, and school administrators. They know about the social psychology of organizations and can use this knowledge to plan strategic cooperation among agencies.

This role will be of the utmost importance to schools and communities. Individuals willing to take on the role will be indispensable to their agencies.

Some of the former roles available for mental health professionals in schools are disappearing because of new legislation and budgetary constraints. Constructing the role of coordinator of programs to create safe schools will be both a service to children and a way to expand the influence of empirically supported psychological science into education.

Index

531

S